THE HANDBOOK OF CHRONIC PAIN

959.78

THE HANDBOOK OF CHRONIC PAIN

SHULAMITH KREITLER
DIEGO BELTRUTTI
ALDO LAMBERTO
AND
DAVID NIV
EDITORS

Nova Biomedical Books
New York

For permission to use material from this book please contact us:
Telephone 631-231-7269; Fax 631-231-8175
Web Site: http://www.novapublishers.com

NOTICE TO THE READER

Library of Congress Cataloging-in-Publication Data
Handbook of chronic pain / Diego Beltrutti ...[et al.]. editors.
  p. ; cm.
Includes bibliographical references and index.
ISBN-13: 978-1-60021-044-0
ISBN-10: 1-60021-044-9
1. Chronic pain- -Handbooks, manuals, etc. 2. Chronic pain- - treatment- -Handbooks, manuals, etc.
[DNLM: 1. Pain- -therapy. 2. Chronic Disease. 3. Pain- -diagnosis. WL 704 H2356 2006] I. Beltrutti, Diego.
 RB127.H33 2006
 616'.0472--dc22
                            2006003985

Published by Nova Science Publishers, Inc.   New York

Contents

About the Editors

PROFESSOR SHULAMITH KREITLER, PH.D.

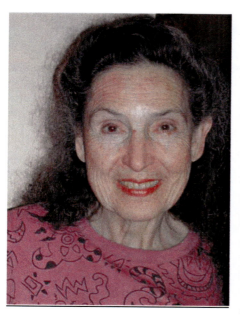

Got her Ph.D. in Psychology from Bern University, Switzerland, Summa cum Laude. She is Full Professor of Psychology at Tel-Aviv University from 1988 up to date and from 1996 up to date, head of Psychooncology Unit, at the Tel-Aviv Sourasky Medical Center (Ichilov Hospital). She has been a Visiting Professor of Psychology at Harvard University, Princeton University, and Yale University in the U.S. and several European universities; is a well-known researcher in psychology, mainly in the fields of cognitive psychology, personality, and health psychology, specializing in pain and psychooncology. Her major contributions are in the study of meaning, predicting and changing behavior and the psychological risk factors for health disorders. She has written 9 books and over 300 articles in scientific papers; has studied the psychosocial aspects of pain, its effects on quality of life and the pain-prone personality; and is a member of the editorial board of The Pain Clinic.

DR. DIEGO BELTRUTTI

Fellow at Emory University in Pain Management (1979). Founder of the Pain Center at Santa Croce Hospital in Cuneo (1980), he served as Director for thirteen years. Presently

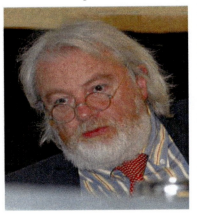 Head Department of Anesthesia, Resuscitation and Pain Medicine in Bra. Member of IASP (1975), AISD (1976). Presently Past President of the World Society of Pain Clinicians. Founder of the "Guido Moricca Prize": international award for scientists who gave an outstanding contribution to the Pain Medicine. Member of the WIP Alumni. Founder in 2000 of SIMED: Italian School of Pain Medicine. President of LICD, Italian League Against pain: an association of chronic pain patients. Author of more than 120 articles and several books in the pain field.

PROFESSOR DAVID NIV, M.D. FIPP

He was born in Bulgaria (1950), immigrated to Israel at the age of 3 months, and died under tragic circumstances in Tel Aviv (Feb. 6, 2007). He got his M.D. at the university of

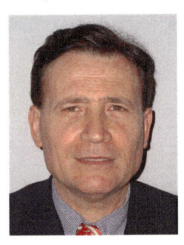 Bologna, Italy (1977), his specialization and certification in anesthesiology and critical care medicine at the Tel-Aviv Sourasky, Medical Center (1978-1983), was a researcher at Royal Medical School, London (1982), and a visiting professor at the University of L'Aquila, Italy (1992). At Tel-Aviv Sourasky Medical Center he was a member at the Multidisciplinary Center for Pain Medicine (1980 – 1988), director of the Multidisciplinary Center for Pain Medicine and Pain Research Lab. (1988-2007); at the medical school, Tel-Aviv University he was coordinator of postgraduate studies in anesthesia and intensive care (1987-1990), founder and chair of postgraduate studies on pain (1992-1995), and professor in anesthesia and critical care medicine (1996-2007). Further, he was Chief Advisor on Pain to the General Surgeon, Israel Defense Force (1989- 2007); secretary of the Israel Society of Anesthesiologists (1984-1987); founding member of the Israel Pain Association (Chapter of IASP), its secretary (1985 – 1988), and president (1988 – 1992); founder of the World Institute of Pain (WIP) (1995), its vice president (1999 – 2002), president (2002 – 2005) and founder of its Fellow Interventional Pain Practice (FIPP) Examination Board (2002); founder and coordinator of the initiative "Medical Specialties meet Pain Medicine" (2005-2007); chairman of EFIC Committee on Public Awareness (2000-2007); founder of Europe Against Pain Initiative (2000) and the first European Week Against Pain (2001);

drafter of EFIC's Declaration "Chronic Pain is a Disease in its own right" (2001); member of the editorial board of 10 international pain journals; organizer and chairman of Nine international meetings on pain; and recipient of 11 international awards for his achievements in pain. He authored over 120 scientific articles and co-edited five books on pain. His most prominent studies are on intrathecal and systemic analgesic properties of benzodiazepines and their antagonists, on systemic and spinal opioid analgesia, and on thermal sensory testing in various painful conditions.

ALDO LAMBERTO, PH.D.

Received his degree in Pedagogy in 1976 from the University of Torino and his degree in Psychology in 1986 from the University of Padua, and is Member of Register as Psychologist

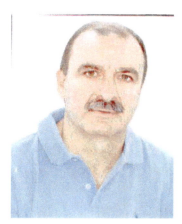

and as Psychotherapist. At present he is Senior Consultant in Psychology, Department of Anesthesia and Intensive Care, Pain Management Unit, Santa Croce e Carle General Hospital, Cuneo, Italy; Coordinator Master Palliative Care, University East Piedmont, Novara, Italy and Consultant at the University L'Aquila, Italy. Dr. Lamberto has conducted clinical research on the psychology of pain and especially on low back pain and headache patients. He has published over 40 scientific articles and book chapters, and has authored (with. D.P.C. Beltrutti) Psychological aspects of chronic pain: From evaluation to therapy (in Italian). He is a member of the editorial board of The Pain Clinic and Painomore.net.

Preface

S. Kreitler, D. Beltrutti, A. Lamberto and D. Niv

This book is the result and expression of several convictions shared by the editors, which have made it possible for us to create the conception of the book, implement the conception, persevere in carrying it out, and finally bring the project to completion despite all the difficulties and hardships encountered on the way. Probably the most important conviction has been that the starting point is the human being rather than the pain. Pain exists neither in a void nor is something that needs to be embedded in a context. It is something that defines its nature, role, and effects quite naturally if we start at the right place – which is evidently the human being as a whole. A second allied conviction was that freedom from pain is the right of the human being, a basic right that cannot be abrogated, and allows no compromises. This belief draws its strength from the focal statement in the American Declaration of Independence that the pusuit of happiness is an inalienable right of all human beings. Pain and suffering are undoubtedly one major obstacle that stands in the way of improving the well-being of human beings and enabling them to strive for the attainment of happiness.

These two convictions led us to the conclusion that as health professionals and as human beings we are called upon to join forces in order to do our best for controlling pain. Each of us four editors has had long experience of working in the domain of pain, studying pain and treating pain patients. On the basis of this long exposure to the issues and problems of pain we were convinced that chronic pain can best be treated by a multidisciplinary team, that includes representatives from the major health professions – medicine, nursing, psychology, physical therapy, occupational therapy and social workers. This conclusion conformed well also to our basic conviction that the starting point for managing pain should be the human being as a whole. Addressing pain in the context of the holistic approach to the individual requires as a *sine qua non* joining foces on the part of health professionals from the different disciplines. This is also the evident implication supported by the ubiquous bio-psycho-social model of pain.

Indeed, many pain researchers and clinicians have reached a similar conclusion and have tried to implement it in pain clinics and other setups for pain therapy all over the world. Actually, multidisciplinary treatment of pain seems to be the rule. Several studies, reviews and meta-analyses have been done to evaluate the results of this approach. Most of the findings showed that the effects of the comprehensive treatment programs on pain reduction and the patients' quality of life were positive and more often than not were maintained to some extent also for some time after termination of the treatment programs (e.g., Basler, Jäkle and Kröner-Herwig, 1997; Buchner, Zahlten-Hinguranage, Schiltenwolf et al., 2006; Dysvik, Natvig, Eikland et al., 2005; Flor, Fydrich and Turk, 1992; Greitemann, Dibbelt and Buschel, 2006). Further, it was shown that improvements in multidisciplinary pain treatment were associated with significant increases in the radiness of patients to undertake self-management of their pain (Jensen, Nielson, Turner, Romano et al., 2004). Most importantly, there is evidence that the beneficial effects on pain reduction were accompanied by and correlated with the expected changes in psychosocial variables, mainly beliefs about pain and coping mechanisms (Jensen, Turner & Romano, in press). Yet, not all results were positive (Joos, Uebelhart, Michel et al., 2004; Linssen and Spinhoven, 1992; Vollenbroek-Hutten, Hermens, Wever et al., 2004) and most of the findings were at best moderate, and in any case not as high as everyone would have expected and desired (Guzman, Esmail, Karjalainen et al., 2001; 2002; Huppe and Raspe, 2003, 2005; Karjalaine, Malmivaara, van Tulder et al., 2003; Lang, Liebig, Kastner et al., 2003).

This state of affairs may be considered as surprising, especially in view of the theoretical support and the seriousness of the endeavours applied for implementing the multidisciplinary approach in regard to pain management. However, on the basis of our experience with multidisciplinary teams, these findings did not appear to us wholly unexpected. The reason is that multidisciplinary cooperation requires more than theoretical conviction and motivation. A necessary condition for its success is sufficient cross-disciplinary sharing of information. As matters are at present, medical doctors and psychosocial professionals possibly hold each others' expertise in sufficiently high respect to try to cooperate but do not know enough of it to be able to cooperate successfully. Multidisciplinary treatment in not merely application of diverse methods in parallel but needs to be based on cooperation. A cooperation of this kind cannot take place in the present state of affairs when most psychosocial experts do not know enough about the medical aspects of pain and its treatment, and medical doctors do not know enough about the psychological and other aspects and treatment options of pain.This insight led us to the decision to try to improve the situation by providing the necessary tools. The present book is the result of this decision.

There are enough books about pain from the medical viewpoint and enough books about pain from the psychosocial viewpoint. But we think that there were none that deal with both aspects and certainly none that cover all the major aspects of pain and its treatment.

Accordingly, the objective of the book is to promote and enable closer cooperation between different health professionals in treating pain, by introducing psychosocially oriented team members to the medical aspects of pain, and medically oriented team members to the psychosocial aspects. The structure of the book clearly mirrors this objective. The book has nine parts, arranged according to a balanced plan. Parts I and II deal with theoretical (basic science) approaches to pain, whereby Part I focuses on the medical approaches and Part II on the psychosocial ones. Part III is devoted to pain evaluation and assessment, whereby chapter 9 deals with the medical aspects, chapter 10 with the psychophysiological and psychiatric aspects, and chapter 11 with the psychological psychometric approach, describing different commonly used questionnaires for assessing various aspects of pain.

Parts IV to Part VII are devoted to treatment of pain. Part IV focuses on medical treatments, Part V on psychological treatments, Part VI on palliative approaches, and Part VII on complementary approaches (mainly those supported by enough research and evidence). Part VIII focuses on particular pain syndromes, those that are most frequent in the practice of pain, emphasizing both medical and psychological aspects in each chapter. Finally, Part IX deals with the practice of treating pain – in chapter 29 with the facilities and pain centers, namely, the locations where the integration of the described approaches to pain is expected to take place, and in chapter 30 with the problems of the health professional that treats pain.

The objective of the book to promote and enable multidisciplinary cooperation is reflected also in the background and expertise of the authors. It will be noted that the book is the joint product of experts from both the medical and psychosocial domains. Of the four editors, two are M.Ds and two are Ph.Ds. The authors are a group of 43 international experts, doctors and other health professionals, representing diverse domains in the medical and psychosocial aspects of pain management, from various pain centers in different countries. It is to be hoped that if the goal of the book is attained then multidisciplinary management of pain will be promoted in the benefit of patients all over the world.

REFERENCES

Basler, H. D., Jäkle, C., and Kröner-Herwig, B. (1997). Incorporation of cognitive-behavioral treatment into the medical care of chronic low back patients: A controlled randomized study in German pain treatment centers. *Patient Education and Counselling*, 31, 113-124.

Becker, N., Sjørgen, P., Bech, P., Olsen, A. K., and Eriksen, J. (2000). Treatment outcome of chronic non-malignant pain patients managed in a Danish multidisciplinary pain centre compared to general practice: A randomized controlled trial. *Pain*, 84, 203-211

Buchner, M., Zahlten-Hinguranage, A., Schiltenwolf, M., and Neubauer, E. (2006). Therapy outcome after multidisciplinary treatment for chronic neck and chronic low back pain: a prospective clinical study in 365 patients. *Scandinavian Journal of Rheumatology*, 35, 363-367.

Dysvik, E., Natvig, G. K., Eikland, O-J., and Brattberg, G. (2005). Results of a multidisciplinary pain management program: A 6-. and 12-months follow-up study. *Rehabilitation Nursing*, 30, 198-206.

Flor, H., Fydrich, T., and Turk, D. C. (1992). Efficacy of multidisciplinary pain treatment centers: A meta-analytic review. *Pain*, 49, 221-230.

Greitemann, B., Dibbelt, S. and Buschel, C. Multidisciplinary orthopedic rehabilitation program in patients with chronic back pain and need for changing job situation – long-term effects of a multimodal, multidisciplinary program with activation and job development [German]. *Zeitschrift für Orthopedie und ihre Grenzgebiete*, 144, 255-266.

Guzman, J., Esmail, R., Karjalainedn, K., Malmivaara, A., Irvin, E. and Bombardier, C. (2001). Multidisciplinary bio-psycho-social rehabilitation for chronic low back pain. *British Medical Journal*, 322, 1511-1516.

Guzman, J., Esmail, R., Karjalainedn, K., Malmivaara, A., Irvin, E. and Bombardier, C. (2002). Multidisciplinary bio-psycho-social rehabilitation for chronic low back pain. *Cochrane Database Syst Rev.* (1):CD000963.

Huppe, A. and Raspe, H. (2003). Efficacy of inpatient rehabilitation for chronic back pain in Germany: a systematic review 1980-2001. *Rehabilitation (Stuttg.)*, 42,143-154.

Huppe, A. and Raspe, H. (2005). Efficacy of inpatient rehabilitation for chronic back pain in Germany: update of a systematic review. *Rehabilitation (Stuttg.)*, 44, 24-33.

Jensen, M. P., Nielson, W. R., Turner, J. A., Romano, J. M. and Hill, M. L. (2004). Changes in readiness to self-manage pain are associated with improvement in multidisciplinary pain treatment and pain coping. *Pain*, 111, 84-95.

Jensen, M. P., Turner, J. A., and Romano, J. M. (in press). Changes after multidisciplinary pain treatment in patient pain beliefs and coping are associated with concurrent changes in patient functioning. *Pain.*

Joos, B., Uebelhart, D., Michel, B. A., and Sprott, H. (2004). Influence of an outpatient multidisciplinary pain management program on the health-related quality of life and the physical fitness of chronic pain patients. *Journal of Negative Results in Biomedicine*, 3, 1-10.

Karjalainen, K., Malmivaara, A., van Tulder, M., Roine, R., Jauhiainen, M., Hurri, H. and Koes, B. (2003). Multidisciplinary biopsychosocial rehabilitation for subacute low back pain among working age adults. *Cochrane Database Systematic Review*, (2): CD002193.

Lang, E., Liebig, K., Kastner, S., Neundorfer, B. And Heuschmann, P. (2003). Multidisciplinary rehabilitation versus usual care for chronic low back pain in the community: effects on quality of life. *Spine Journal*, 3, 270-276.

Linssen, A. C., and Spinhoven, P. (1992). Multimodal treatment programmes for chronic pain: a quantitative analysis of existing research data. *Journal of Psychosomatic Research*, 36, 275-286.

Vollenbroek-Hutten, M. M. R., Hermens H. J., Wever, D., Gorter, M., Rinket, J., and Ijzerman, M. J. (2004). Differences in outcome of a multidisciplinary treatment between subgroups of chronic low back pain patients defined using two multiaxial assessment instruments: the multidimensional pain inventory and lumbar dynamometry. *Clinical Rehabilitation*, 18, 566-579.

List of Contributors

Adunsky, Abraham, M.D
Head of Geriatric Medicine
Senior Lecturer
Sheba Medical Center, Israel
Affiliated to the Tel Aviv University
Tel: work: +972.3.5303411
    home:+972.3.5409224
Home Address: Sinai Str.2, Ramat Ha Sharon. 47420, Israel
E-mail:adunger1@sheba.health.gov.il

Ashwini D. Sharan, M. D
Assistant Professor
Department of Neurosurgery
Thomas Jefferson University
909 Walnut Street
3rd Floor
Philadelphia, PA 19107
(215) 955-7000 Main
(215) 955-4589 Direct
(215) 308-0880 Pager
(215) 380-9520 Cell

11 Yearling Chase
Mt. Laurel, NJ 08054
(856) 638-0052 Home
<ashwini.sharan@jefferson.edu>

Barak, Frida, M.D.
Director, Oncology Unit, Barzilai Medical Center,
Hahistdrut Street, Ashkelon 78306, Israel
Counsellor Sick Fund Maccabi, and Sick Fund Leumit
Residence: P.O. Box 6754, Ashdod, 77440, Israel
Te. +972-8-8654111
E-mail: frida_bar@barzi.health.gov.il

Barolat, Giancarlo, M.D.
Director of Neurosurgical Services, of Neuro-Implant Program and
of the Division of Functional Neurosurgery Department of Neurosurgery
Thomas Jefferson University H1015 Chestnut Street Suite 1400
Philadelphia, PA 19107
Fax: (215) 923-8072
gbarolat@verizon.net

730 Genesee Mountain Rd.
Golden CO 80401-0000
USA
Tel. (215) 955-2364
Fax: (303) 526-1504
E-mail:gbr@bellatlantic.net

Beltrutti, Diego M. D., FIPP
Head, Professor, Department of Anaesthesia,
Intensive Care and Pain Medicine, ASL 18 Alba/Bra, Italy
Via V. Emanuele 3, 12042 Bra, Italy
Hospital 0039-0172-420806
E-mail : dbeltrutti@asl18.it

Benedetti, Fabrizio M.D.
Department of Neuroscience
Rita Levi-Montalcini Center for Brain Repair,
University of Turin Medical School,
Corso Raffaello 30, 10125.
Turin, Italy
Tel. +39-011-6707709; Fax +39-011-6707708
E-mail: fabrizio.benedetti@unito.it

Beneforti, Elisabetta, M. D.
Department of Critical Care Medicine
E-mail: elisabetta.beneforti@unifi.it
Tel: (055) 412063
Fax: (055) 4378638

Bercovitch, Michaela, M.D
Oncological Hospice "Friedman House"
Research and Information Coordinator
Lecturer
Sheba Medical Center,
Affiliated to the Tel Aviv University
Home Address: Ha Yasmin Str. 123,
                    Shoham, 73142 Israel
Tel: work +972.3.530.50.70:+972.3.5303290
    home:+972.3.977.28.26
E-mail: almi@sheba.health.gov il

Carasso, Rafael L, Prof. M.D. M.Sc.
Director, Department of Neurology, Pain Clinic and Clinic of Complementary Medicine
Medical Center Hillel-Yaffe
Hadera, Israel
Address of clinic: 173, Ibn Gvirol Street, Tel-Aviv, Israel
Tel. +972-3-6053869
E-mail: carasso@hillel-yaffe.health.gov.il

Chaves, John F. Ph.D.
Professor & Vice Dean for Dental Education
School of Dental Medicine
State University of New York at Stony Brook
Stony Brook, NY 11794-8704
Phone: 631-632-6986
FAX: 631-632-9105
E-mail: John.Chaves@sunysb.edu

Di Santo, Salvatore, M.D
Department of Anaesthesia,
Intensive Care and Pain Medicine,
ASL 18 Alba/Bra, Italy
Via V. Emanuele 3, 12042 Bra, Italy
Hospital 0039-0172-420806

Eisenberg, Elon M.D.
Pain Relief Unit
Rambam Medical Center
P.O.B. 9602. Haifa, 31096, Israel.
Tel: (+) 972-4-8542578
FAX: (+) 972-4-8542880
E-mail: e_eisenberg@rambam.health.gov.il

Fogliardi, Alfredo, M.D.
Palliative Care and Pain Therapy Unit,
Ospedale Santa Croce,
Fano, Italy
Address: Via V. Veneto, Fano 61032, Italy
afogliardi@yahoo.it
Residence: Via A. Diaz 19, Pesaro 61100, Italy
Tel Home 0039 0721-32665
Tel Hospital 0039 0721- 882339

Marion Good, Ph.D, RN, FAAN
Professor
Frances Payne Bolton School of Nursing
Case Western Reserve University
10900 Euclid Avenue
Cleveland OH 44106-4904
Phone 216-368-5975
Fax 216-368-3542
mpg@po.cwru.edu
http://fpb.case.edu/PainStudy/index.shtm
http://fpb.case.edu/PainStudy/about.shtm

Guerci, Antonio, M.D.
Professor of Anthropology
University of Genoa, Italy
E-mail: guerci@dibe.unige.it

Imbe, Hiroki, D.D.S., Ph.D.
Department of Oral Anatomy,
Osaka Dental University,
Hirakata City 573-1121, Japan
E-mail: imika@js9.so-net.jp

Kashiba, Hitoshi, Ph.D.
Department of Physiology,
Kansai College of Oriental Medicine,
Sennan, Osaka 590-0433, Japan
E-mail: kashiba@kansai.ac.jp

Kreitler, Michal M.

Psychooncology Unit,

Tel-Aviv Sourasky Medical Center,

6 Weizman St., Tel-Aviv 64239, Israel

Tel. +972-3-6973874, Fax +972-3-6973496

E-mail: psy_onc@tasmc.health.gov.il, mika@tasmc.health.gov.il

Kreitler, Shulamith, Prof. Ph.D.

Department of Psychology

Tel-Aviv University

Israel

Tel. +972-3-5227185 Cellular: +972-544-526434

Fax +972-3-5225371

e-mail: krit@netvision.net.il

Director, Psychooncology Unit

Tel-Aviv Sourasky Medical Center

6 Weizman st.,

Tel-Aviv 64239, Israel

Tel. +972-3-6973874

Fax +972-3-6973496

e-mail: psy_onc@tasmc.health.gov.il

Lamberto, Aldo, Ph.D.

Consultant Psychologist,

Pain Control Center and Palliative care,

Ospedale Santa Croce e Carle,

Cuneo, Italy

Via M. Coppino, 26 – Cuneo 12100, Italy

Tel:

lamberto@gem.it

Lang, Eric M.D.

Pharmaceutical Licensing Group

Johnson & Johnson

1125 Trenton-Harbourton Road

Titusville, N.J. 08560

U.S.A.

Tel. +609-730-3650

Fax +609-730-2941

E-mail: elang@janus.jnj.com

Lewandowski, Wendy Ph.D RN CS
Assistant Professor
Kent State University
College of Nursing
Kent, Ohio 44242
5431 Brainard Road,
Solon, Ohio 44139
440-248-9211
USA
wlewando@kent.edu

Livengood, **Janice M., Ph.D., HSP**
Director, Psychological Services
Vanderbilt Pain Control Center
Vanderbilt Pain Center at Cool Springs
2009 Mallory Lane/
Associate Professor of Anesthesiology
Vanderbilt School of Medicine
Vanderbilt University Hospital and Medical Center//
Department of Anesthesiology
Suite 324 Medical Arts Building
1211 21st Avenue South
Nashville, TN 37212
USA
E-mail: janice.livengood@Vanderbilt.Edu
Tel. +615-771-7580 EXT. 234
Fax: +615-771-7025

Loreto, Mariello, M.D.
Assistant fellow Anaesthesia and Intensive Care
Second University of Naples (S.U.N.)
Mariello Loreto Dirigente Medico I livello ASL SA1-Servizio di Anestesia e
Rianimazione Ospedale "Umberto I" Nocera Inferiore 84014 (prov. Salerno)
cellular 3496143893
Tel and Fax 081926669
marialor@libero.it

Maltsman-Tseikhin, Alexander, **M.D.**
Pharmaceutical Licensing Group
Johnson & Johnson
PO Box 300
Mail Stop 2628
Raritan, NJ 08869
USA

Marchetti, Giuseppe, M.D.
Head, Department of Radiotherapy.
"S. Croce e Carle" General Hospital, Cuneo, Italy
Via M. Coppino, 12100 Cuneo
Italy
tel/fax 00390171697316
E-mail: marchetti@et.unipv.it

Marino, Francesco, M.D.
Unità di Terapia del Dolore e Cure Palliative,
Casa di Cura Beato Matteo,
Vigevano, Italia

Merismsky, Ofer, Prof., M.D.
Professor of Oncology
Director, Unit of Lung and Tissues
Oncology Institute
Tel-Aviv Sourasky Medical Center
6 Weizman Street, Tel-Aviv 64239, Israel
E-mail: oferm@tasmc-health.gov.il
Address of clinic: 1, Cordova St., Tel-Aviv
E-mail: merimsky@zahav.net.il
Tel. +972-52-2336679

Mosek, Amnon M.D.
The Pain Control Unit, Sourasky Medical Center,
6 Weizman St., Tel-Aviv 64239, Israel
School of Medicine, Tel Aviv University,
Tel Aviv 69978, Israel.
Tel. 03-6973155
E-mail: mosekamnon@roshhelp.co.il

Nicoscia, Mauro, M.D.
Service of Anesthesia, Resuscitation and Pain Therapy
Garrison S. Hospital Worker, Carl – Voltri
A. S. L. 3 Genova, Italy
E-mail: mauro_nic@libero.it

Niv, David, M.D. Prof. FIPP
Director, Center for Pain Medicine
Tel - Aviv Sourasky Medical Center
6 Weizman st. 64239 Tel-Aviv, Israel
Tel: 972-3-6974477/4716 fax: 6974583
Email work: davidniv@tasmc.health.gov.il
Email home: tamir_niv@bezeqint.net

Ostrowsky, Lev, M. D.
Anesthesiologist, Home Care Unit for Chronic Patients,
Sick Funds Leumit & Maccabi, Israel

Pergolizzi, Stefano M.D.
Head, Radiotherapy Unit
"S. Vincenzo" Hospital, Taormina (ME),
Contrada Sirina. Taormina 98039
Italy
Tel. +339-942-579527
And
Department of Radiologic Sciences,
University of Messina,
Viale Gazzi,Policlinico. Messina 98100
Italy
Tel. +339-90-2212930
stefano.pergolizzi@unime.it

Pollo, Antonella, M.D.
Department of Neuroscience
Section of Physiology
University of Turin Medical School,
Corso Raffaello No. 30 – 10125,
Torino, Italy
Tel. +39 011670.7701
Fax +39 011670.7708
E-mail: antonella.pollo@unito.it

Rauck, Richard L., M.D.
Medical Director, Carolinas Pain Institute
Clinical Associate Professor of Anesthesiology
Wake Forest University Health Sciences
Winston Salem, North Carolina
E-mail: rrauck@ccrpain.com

P. Prithvi Raj, M.D.
Professor and Co-Director, Pain Services
Texas Tech University Health Sciences Center
Department of Anesthesiology
Lubbock, Texas 79430 USA
1097 Cameron Glen
Cincinnati, Ohio 45245
E-mail: prithviraj@fuse.net

Rappaport, Zvi Harry, Prof. M.D.
Department of Neurosurgery, Rabin Medical Center
Tel Aviv University School of Medicine
49100 Petah Tiqva, Israel
Fax:(972) 39219774
E-mail: zhr1@internet-zahav.net

Russi, Elvio Grazioso M.D.
Vice-Director, Department of Radiotherapy
"S. Croce e Carle" General Hospital, Cuneo,
Via M. Coppino, 12100 Cuneo, Italy
erussi@libero.it
tel/fax 00390171697316

Savoia, Gennaro, M. D.
Director, Paediatric Anaesthesia and Intensive Care IV Service
" A. Cardarelli" National Hospital-Naples
Direttore UOC Anestesia e Rianimazione Pediatrica AORN "A.Cardarelli"- Napoli Via
A.Cardarelli, 9
80134 Napoli cell. 3396344751 tel e fax 003981747256
gennarosavoia@libero.it

Scharf, Shimon, M.D.
Director General, Barzilai Medical Center,
Hahistdrut Street, Ashkelon 78306, Israel
Tel +972-8-6745600
E-mail: hanhala@barzi.health.gov.il

Senba, Emiko, MD, Ph.D.
Dept. of Anatomy & Neurobiology
Wakayama Medical University
811-1 Kimiidera,
Wakayama 641-8509, Japan
Tel & Fax: 73-441-0617
E-mail: esenba@wakayama-med.ac.jp

Shiri, Shimon, M.A.
Psychologist, Department of Physical Rehabilitation,
Hadassa Hospital, Mount Scopus, Jerusalem
E-mail: shimonshiri@hotmail.com
Tel. Cellular - +972-55-282733
Residence: Harlap 27/5, Jerusalem 92341, Israel

Zoppi, Massimo, Prof., M.D.
Department of Internal Medicine
University of Florence
Viale G. Pieraccini 18
50139 Florence
Italy
tel.: 0039055412063
fax: 00390554296536
E-mail: m.zoppi@dmi.unifi.it

LIST OF EMAIL ADDRESSES

adunger1@sheba.health.gov.il
frida_bar@barzi.health.gov.il
almi@sheba.health.gov.il
bercom@post.tau.ac.il
giancarlo.barolat@tju.academic.us
gbr@bellatlantic.net
gbarolat@verizon.net
stefano.pergolizzi@unime.it
fabrizio.benedetti@unito.it
John.Chaves@sunysb.edu
carasso@hillel-yaffe.health.gov.il
elisabetta.beneforti@unifi.it
l_eisenberg@rambam.health.gov.il
mpg@po.cwru.edu
afogliardi@yahoo.it
guerci@dibe.unige.it
kashiba@kansai.ac.jp
psy_onc@tasmc.health.gov.il
mika@tasmc.health.gov.il
wlewando@kent.edu
elang@janus.jnj.com
janice.livengood@Vanderbilt.edu

marialor@libero.it
marchetti@et.unipv.it
merimsky@zahav.net.il
mosek@tasmc.health.gov.il
mauro_nic@libero.it
antonella.pollo@unito.it
prithviraj@fuse.net
rrauck@ccrpain.com
zhr1@internet-zahav.net
gennarosavoia@libero.it
esenba@wakayama-med.ac.jp
hanhala@barzi.health.gov.il
ashwini.sharan@jefferson.edu
shimonshiri@hotmail.com
m.zoppi@dfc.unifi.it
davidniv@tsmc.health.gov.il
beltrutti@painclinicians.org
lamberto@gem.it
esenba@wakayama-med.ac.jp
imika@js9.so-net.jp
Krit@netvision.net.il
erussi@libero.it,m.zoppi@dmi.unifi.it

Part I: Medical and Physiological Considerations

In: The Handbook of Chronic Pain
Editors: S. Kreitler, D. Beltrutti, et al., pp. 3-23
ISBN 978-1-60021-044-0
© 2007 Nova Science Publishers, Inc.

Chapter 1

Anatomical and Physiological Bases of Nociception

Antonella Pollo and Fabrizio Benedetti

INTRODUCTION

Behind what we feel and describe as "pain" there is a bewildering array of phenomena, ranging from acute tissue injury, which prompts us to escape the noxious stimulus, to chronic states, which apparently do not subserve any useful function. Sometimes pain can be accurately localized and ascribed to a precise origin, sometimes it is so diffuse and difficult to define that in ancient times it was often attributed to supernatural causes (in today's common terminology, we still speak of "elf strike" to indicate the low back sudden pain due to nerve compression by a disk hernia). The most widely accepted general definition of pain is that approved by the International Association for the Study of Pain (IASP): "Pain is an unpleasant sensory and emotional experience associated with actual or potential tissue damage, or described in terms of such damage" (IASP, 1979).

From an anatomical and physiological point of view, the processes underlying the different painful experiences are numerous and distinct. A definition of a few terms is necessary in order to address specific categories of pain. *Nociception* refers to the process of transduction, encoding and transmission to the central nervous system (CNS) of stimuli provoking tissue damage. By *nociceptive pain* it is meant that evoked by the stimulation of the nociceptors and the consequent activation of the Aδ and C fibres. On the other hand, injury at different levels of the neuraxis forms the substrate of *neuropathic pain*, in which the original evolutionary role of pain, i.e. avoidance of harm, is lost, and a pathological nature is established. Pain sensation is not only the result of signals rigidly conveyed from the periphery to higher CNS centres along immutable pathways, but rather the product of the interplay of plastic processes, whereby the nociceptive neuron activity can be modified on a short- or long-time scale. In other words, following protracted noxious stimulation, the sensory system undergoes permanent changes which can maintain a chronic pain state independently of the original cause. Examples of these plastic processes are *peripheral* and *central sensitisation,* and phenomena such as *primary* and *secondary hyperalgesia.*

Another aspect of pain physiology is the elaboration in the CNS of nociceptive information giving rise to the different components of the pain experience. To what extent are the sensory-discriminative, emotional-affective-motivational and cognitive elements of pain perception processed in separate pathways? In which parts of the brain are they integrated? Does one component influence the others? Does a "pain center" exist? This approach has profited mainly from the neuroimaging techniques, such as functional magnetic resonance imaging (fMRI) and positron emission tomography (PET).

This chapter will present an overview of the anatomical organization of the nociceptive fibers from the periphery to the dorsal horn and hence to the thalamus and other relay stations in the neuraxis, followed by an outline of the brain areas involved in pain perception. Attention will be focused on the physiological mechanisms of pain transmission, with special emphasis on the changes of neuronal reactivity and connectivity, i.e. neuroplasticity. More extensive reviews are available elsewhere (Wall and Melzack, 1999, Willis, 1985, Willis and Coggeshall, 1991, Gebhart, 1995, Dubner and Bennett, 1983, Besson et al., 1995, Besson and Chaouch, 1987, Belemonte and Cervero, 1996, Millan, 1999).

NOCICEPTORS AND PRIMARY AFFERENT FIBRES

The receptors responsible for the initiation of pain signals in the periphery are termed *nociceptors* (Sherrington, 1906). They are free nerve endings located in most of the body structures and can be associated to two groups of primary afferent fibres (PAF): Aδ and C. The most thoroughly studied are the cutaneous nociceptors, sensitive to mechanical, thermal and chemical stimuli.

Unmyelinated, thin (0.4-1.2µm in diameter) and slowly conducting (0.5-2m/s) C fibres are activated mainly by a class of receptors termed polymodal, because they are responsive to all modalities. They are also named C-fibre mechano-heat nociceptors (CMHs), mechanical and heat stimuli being those systematically used to study them. Their response increases monotonically with stimulus intensity and their receptive field is very small, in the range of a few squared millimetres. These fibres can account for up to 70-90% of the primate nociceptive C fibre population. However, specific low-threshold mechanical, chemical or thermal nociceptors (these last two types also known as mechanically-insensitive afferents, MIAs) have also been described (Raja et al., 1999). Moreover, C fibres responsive to cold noxious stimuli seem to be localized not in the skin, but along the wall of cutaneous veins (Klement and Arndt, 1992).

Myelinated, medium-calibre (2-6µm) and medium-conducting (12-30m/s) Aδ fibres are classically linked to two main kinds of receptors: type I and type II mechano-heat nociceptors (AMHs). Type I AMHs are high-threshold mechanoreceptors showing long latency and slow adaptation; their receptive fields range between 1 and 8cm^2; by contrast, type II AMHs display smaller receptive fields and respond rapidly with a quick adaptation (Treede at al., 1991). Both types are also sensitive to heat, with type I displaying a somewhat higher threshold (52 vs. 43°C; Treede et al., 1995).

In addition to Aδ and C fibres, myelinated, large (>10μm in diameter), fast conducting (30-100m/s) Aβ fibres can also be involved in nociception. These fibres are excited by weak mechanical stimuli (hence the use of referring to them as "low-threshold", in opposition to "high-threshold" nociceptors). In normal conditions, their function deals only with touch and other non-noxious modalities, but in pathological situations (e.g. tissue injury and/or nerve lesion) they can become responsible for the phenomenon of mechanical allodynia, i.e. the perception of a normally innocuous stimulus as painful (see below).

By applying noxious heat stimuli to the hairy skin of human subjects, a double pain sensation can be evoked: a pricking acute and very brief impression ("first" pain) is followed after some delay by a dull burning feeling ("second" pain). Substantial evidence links the first to the activity of AMHs type II and the second to that of polymodal C receptors. Moreover, AMHs type I are likely to be engaged in the sustained discharge throughout long-duration stimuli, after CMHs adaptation. Consistently, no first pain is felt on the glabrous skin of the hand where, at least in primates, no type II AMHs have been found (Campbell and LaMotte, 1983).

Discharge in nociceptive PAFs does not automatically imply pain perception. By correlating microneurographic recordings with psychophysical curves in human subjects, it was observed that activation is possible at levels of mechanical stimulus intensity below pain threshold. Also, the pain level induced by the same electrical activity of a C fibre can differ by varying stimulus modality (heat or pressure). As with any sensory system, final perception and evaluation of the stimulus depends on signal processing and integration at subsequent stages, and phenomena like spatial summation or co-activation of other fibres may also play a role (Van Hees and Gybels, 1981).

The cell body of PAFs is located in the dorsal root ganglia (and in the gasserian ganglion of the trigeminal nerve). They contain neurones with large and small cell bodies: nociceptors belong to this second group. Glutamate, contained in small electron-translucent synaptic vesicles, is their main neurotransmitter, but often the same presynaptic terminals also release a variety of neuropeptides, e.g. substance P, from large, dense-core vesicles (Willis and Coggeshall, 1991).

In recent years, many attempts have been made to further characterize nociceptive neurons on the basis of their receptor expression, growth factor sensitivity, neurotransmitter and neuromodulator content, in the hope to distinguish with biochemical and neurobiological means specific neuronal populations performing separate functions along parallel pathways. Thus, at least in rodents, two major classes of C fibres have been identified. A first tentative division was based on alternative content of fluoride-resistant acid phosphatase (FRAP) or peptides (somatostatin and substance P) in dorsal root ganglion cells (Nagy and Hunt, 1982). Later, the FRAP-positive cells were shown in co-localization studies to selectively stain for the histochemical marker isolectin IB4 (a plant lectin from *Griffonia Simplicifolia*), the enzyme thiamine monophosphatase (TMP), a subtype of purine receptor (P2X3) and to display distinctive expression of the glial cell line-derived neurotrophic factor (GDNF) receptor complex, consisting of the tyrosine kinase c-Ret and a lipid-anchored alpha receptor, GFRα. The second class, somatostatin and substance P-positive, contains the calcitonin-gene-related peptide (CGRP) and expresses the tyrosine kinase trkA receptor with high affinity for the nerve growth factor, NGF (Vulchanova et al., 1998, 2001; Silverman and Kruger, 1990;

Bennett et al., 1998; Averill et al., 1995). Although this division is far from clear-cut, and the two populations present some degree of overlapping, further support comes from some anatomical findings. In fact, while sharing common peripheral distribution, CGRP- and substance P-containing neurones terminate with their central branch in lamina I and in the outer part of lamina II (substantia gelatinosa) of the dorsal horn, while FRAP-positive cells end preferentially in the deep part of lamina II. IB4-positive, non-peptidergic and IB4-negative, peptidergic cells also display distinct electrophysiological properties (Stuchy and Lewin, 1999). It has been suggested that the two systems provide parallel pathways for the processing of nociceptive information (Hunt and Rossi, 1985) and that both cell populations can play a role in the development of chronic pain states, maybe selectively in inflammatory conditions and neuropathic states, respectively (Snider and McMahon, 1998).

This schematic picture should not be considered a rigid and permanent one. Rather, we face a flexible and plastic structure, as evidenced in at least two major processes: development and injury. In both, neurotrophins perform crucial tasks. During embryogenesis and early postnatal life, for instance, the large majority of murine small diameter DRG cells expresses trkA and requires NGF for survival. But as the animal matures, many of these neurones change their trophic factor dependency, down-regulating trkA and up-regulating receptors for GDNF (Silos-Santiago et al., 1995; Molliver and Snider, 1997; Molliver at al., 1997). Likewise, after peripheral axotomy, primary sensory neurones modify neuropeptide expression, down-regulating substance P and CGRP and up-regulating tyrosine and galanin (Hokfeld et al., 1994). Indeed, a whole body of evidence points to the role of different neurotrophic factors in regulating short- and long-term changes in nociceptor sensitivity and dorsal horn excitability. NGF contribution has so far been the most studied: in many inflammatory conditions, its levels increase and its administration in the experimental setting (in animals and humans) provokes sensory abnormalities, like thermal hyperalgesia, which are prevented by anti-NGF antibodies (Lewin et al., 1993; Petty et al., 1994; Woolf et al., 1994; Mendell at al., 1999). Part of NGF effects could be mediated by the up-regulation of brain-derived neurotrophic factor, BDNF, expressed by the trkA and CGRP type of adult sensory neurones which, being released in an activity-dependent manner, can act as a central neuromodulator of pain (Michael et al., 1997; Thompson et al., 1999). Sciatic nerve transection also results in pronounced GDNF depletion and altered electrophysiological properties in non-peptidergic DRG cells, with the neurotrophin restoring control conditions (Jongen et al., 1999; Cummins et al., 1999). Neurotrophins effects are not limited to modulation and support of neuronal function in molecular terms; rather, they can even inhibit the anatomical rearrangement of sensory fibres which may follow nerve damage, preventing Aβ tactile fibres from sprouting and making connection with nociceptive pathways in the dorsal horn. This phenomenon is important in neuropathic states, where it can represent the basis of touch-evoked pain (mechanical allodynia; Woolf et al., 1995; Bennett et al., 1998).

Thus plasticity manifests itself already at the first sensory neuron, both at peripheral and central terminals. Two aspects are relevant, for which the terms auto- and heterosensitization have been suggested (Woolf and Salter, 2000). The first refers to activation-dependent plasticity. This is a progressive increase in the response of the system to repeated stimuli, and can be elegantly exemplified by the changes in activity of the receptor for capsaicin, a natural substance present in capsicum peppers (vanilloid receptor 1, VR1), which is a non-selective cation excitatory channel also activated by noxious heat and modulated by protons (Caterina et al., 1997; Caterina and Julius, 2001). Autosensitization may also involve other PAF receptors, such as the purinergic receptor for ATP, $P2X_3$, and acid-sensing ion channels (ASICs). The second term, heterosensitization (also defined as peripheral sensitization), refers to an increase in the excitability of the terminal membrane, which is brought about by sensitizing substances that do not themselves activate the transducer. Many of these are released by inflammatory cells (e.g. bradykinin, histamine, serotonin, prostaglandins); others come from axonal release (substance P) or autonomic endings (epinephrine) and exert their effects by activating cascades of second messengers, including intracellular kinases, leading to receptor and/or ion channels phosphorylation. The broad picture of the many transducers involved in the generation of trains of action potentials in nociceptive PAFs and of the modulation of the gain of the input channel is becoming richer and more complex every day and is currently the subject of intense study (Reichling and Levine, 1999). Molecular details of these processes will be given in subsequent chapters of this handbook.

Although much of the current knowledge on nociceptors is derived from cutaneous nerve terminals, it must be emphasized that important differences exist in the processing of nociceptive information from other tissues. Muscles, joints, teeth and most thoracic and abdominal organs are endowed with free nerve endings belonging to thinly myelinated Aδ and unmyelinated C fibres, which are excited by one or more of mechanical (pressure, stretch), chemical (inflammation, ischemia) and thermal stimuli. Generally, they are polymodal in character (Willis and Coggeshall, 1991; Meyer et al., 1994; Cervero, 1994).

The specificity theory, which considers pain as a separate modality encoded and transmitted along a specific channel, finds solid evidence in the existence of high-threshold somatic nociceptors, which are excited only by stimuli intense enough to threaten the integrity of the skin. However, the pattern theory, which postulates the existence of intensity receptors, still finds support for the visceral district. Here, both specific nociceptors and intensity-receptors have been found in different apparatus and even in the same organ (Cervero and Jänig, 1992; Sengupta and Gebhart, 1995). Afferent fibres travel along the sympathetic or parasympathetic nerves, have their cell bodies in the dorsal root ganglia, and innervate their targets much more sparsely, and with bigger receptive fields than their cutaneous counterparts. Pain sensations evoked from the viscera are often poorly localized and referred to other tissues. This is due to their convergence onto somatotopically organized second-order neurons receiving cutaneous input.

One last peculiar class of nociceptors is worth of mention: it was first described in cat joints, where units could be recorded, which did not respond in normal conditions, not even at potentially tissue damaging intensities, but could be recruited after inflammation-induced sensitisation (Schaible and Schmidt, 1988). These chemosensitive C-fibres were subsequently demonstrated in many other tissues, including skin and viscera, and were termed "silent" nociceptors (Michaelis et al., 1996). Their discharge could significantly contribute to the intense stream of activity which in pathological states underlies the phenomenon of central sensitisation.

To conclude, it must once again be emphasized that nociceptive PAFs do not belong to a single group whose defining characteristics are easily classifiable, but rather are a miscellaneous group widely differing in neurochemical features, in threshold of activation and in the qualities of the pain sensation they can evoke. Their role is not limited to afferent transmission of action potentials, but includes active axonal secretion of neurotransmitters and peptides (e.g. CGRP, substance P) whose role in amplifying the inflammatory response consequent to tissue damage is termed neurogenic inflammation. They can be the first target of a series of plastic events mediating the transition from acute to chronic pain.

THE DORSAL HORN

The central branches of the nociceptive DRG neurones are grouped in the lateral part of the dorsal root and upon entering the spinal cord typically bifurcate rostrally and caudally and extend a few segments in the Lissauer tract. Subsequently, their ramifications enter the dorsal horn and make synaptic contacts with second-order projecting neurones, interneurones or motoneurones (for spinal reflexes). The grey matter of the spinal cord is classically subdivided cytoarchitectonically into 10 laminae, numbered from I to X, where laminae I to VI make up the dorsal horn, VII to IX the ventral horn and lamina X is situated around the central canal (Rexed, 1952). Nociceptive input is mainly concentrated in laminae I, II, V, VI and X. Second-order projecting neurones belong to two classes: nociceptive-specific (NS) and wide-dynamic range (WDR) cells. The first class receives information only from Aδ and C fibres, whereas the second receives signals from nociceptive and Aβ fibres, thus encompassing a much wider range of stimulus intensities (Price and Dubner, 1977). Although a close correspondence between cell type, lamina localization and input from periphery cannot be rigorously established, a gross correlation may be made whereby NS cells are mostly located in lamina I (where they connect mainly with cutaneous Aδ fibres) and outer lamina II (where they receive input mainly from cutaneous C fibres), while WDR cells are situated chiefly in lamina V. Visceral and deep somatic pain is conveyed to laminae I, V, VI and X, converging with skin input on the same neurones and thus representing the anatomical substrate of the phenomenon of referred pain. Projecting neurones which receive information exclusively from non-nociceptive fibres (Aβ) are present, especially in laminae III and IV (Basbaum and Jessell, 2000; Millan, 1999; Yaksh, 1998). Nociceptive PAFs make synaptic contacts with interneurones as well. These belong to the NS and WDR types, and synaptic contacts are made by: 1) connecting PAFs with projecting neurones in different laminae; 2) connecting sensory and motor neurones for the production of propriospinal (intra- and intersegmental) reflexes; and 3) mediating the effects of descending pathways from brainstem centres, predominantly but not exclusively inhibitory. Morphologically, stalked (limiting) and islet (central) cells have been described in the substantia gelatinosa (Cajal, 1995) and it has been proposed that they correspond to excitatory and inhibitory interneurones, respectively (Gobel, 1978).

Since the mid-sixties, when the gate control theory of pain was first published (Melzack and Wall, 1965), the dorsal horn and its circuitry has become the subject of intense study and hot debate. As is well known, the theory put forward a model whereby pain impulses could be filtered and modified upon entering the spinal cord (the "gate"), so that, depending on the simultaneous arrival of nociceptive and non-nociceptive signals and the ensuing balance of activation/inhibition of inhibitory interneurones, noxious information could gain more or less access to ascending pathways. Islet inhibitory cells in lamina II could provide the crucial link, receiving peptidergic axons from PAFs on their dendrites and releasing GABA and/or glycine back on PAFs or on downstream nociceptive neurones (Hayes and Carlton, 1992). Although not confirmed, the theory had its most forceful and lasting impact in the emphasis it posed on the function of the CNS as an active dynamic modulator of incoming signals, both in the enhancing and suppressing directions (Melzack, 1999). The dorsal horn thus gained consideration as a state-dependent sensory processor, which could be set in different modes (or states), its output being drastically altered by pathological conditions (Woolf, 1994).

A significant augmentation of the nociceptive output from the dorsal horn (or from its craniocervical analog, the spinal tract of the trigeminal nerve) is observed in the phenomenon known as central sensitisation (Woolf, 1983). As in peripheral sensitisation, an exaggerated response to painful stimuli can be detected (hyperalgesia). However, whereas in peripheral sensitisation the pain threshold is decreased by the sensitised $A\delta$ and C high-threshold afferent fibres, in central sensitisation low intensity stimuli can attain the status of pain through the $A\beta$ mechanoreceptors in virtue of the processing at the dorsal horn level. Central sensitisation plays a conspicuous part in neuropathic pain, and understanding its mechanisms of action is therefore crucial for a successful therapy (Woolf and Mannion, 1999). Differences between the two conditions were first experimentally evidenced by peripheral studies employing capsaicin and intraneural microstimulation (Treede et al., 1992; LaMotte et al., 1991; Torebjörk et al., 1992). Subsequently, the anatomical and physiological substrate has been progressively elucidated and molecular details are being identified every day, making the dorsal horn, particularly the "first" synapse in the pain pathway, one of the hottest spot in pain physiology.

Excitatory amino acids (glutamate and aspartate) released from PAF small, clear vesicles act at N-methyl D-aspartate (NMDA) and non-NMDA receptors, such as α-amino-3-hydroxy-5-methyl-4-isoxazolepropionic acid (AMPA), kainate and metabotropic glutamate receptors. Neurokinins (substance P, neurokinin A) simultaneously released from PAFs large, dense-core vesicles act on neurokinin (NK) receptors. In physiological conditions, post-synaptic depolarisation is brought about by Na^+ influx at the AMPA receptors, while entrance of Na^+ and Ca^{2+} through NMDA channels is prevented by a Mg^{2+} voltage-dependent plug. Sustained nociceptive PAF activity, such as that present in neuropathic states, provokes a greater post-synaptic depolarisation and sets off a number of second messenger cascades through the activation of NK receptors, the final effect of which is to amplify the depolarisation to a degree sufficient to remove the Mg^{2+} block and call into action the NMDA channels.

NMDA channels play a key role in the altered excitability of the dorsal horn by inducing an inward Ca^{2+} current that triggers both short- and long-term responses. Among the first, there is the activation of phospholipase C with production of IP_3 and DAG, the activation of PKC, the production of cAMP, cGMP and nitric oxide. Among the second, there is the induction of translational changes, with activation of immediate early genes, such as those of the c-fos and c-jun families (Woolf and Costigan, 1999). Electrophysiologically, the short-time effect can be visualized in the phenomenon of "wind up", i.e. the progressive increase in discharge frequency of the second-order neuron, following a long duration, repetitive peripheral stimulation (Mendell, 1966; Davies and Lodge, 1987; Dickenson and Sullivan, 1987). In the long run, long-term potentiation (LTP), one of the mechanisms of associative learning and memory in many areas of the CNS (Collingridge and Singer, 1990), also comes into play. Its effects are proportional to the length of stimulation, coming to involve progressively more and more genes (Abraham et al., 1993), with final plastic transformation of cell phenotype and morphology. Thus the response to subsequent noxious inputs can be permanently altered.

In addition to NK and excitatory aminoacids receptors, a host of other receptors and channels can be expressed both pre- and postsynaptically in the dorsal horn, binding many endogenous or exogenous molecules with excitatory or inhibitory influence on the processing of nociceptive information. Among others, μ, δ and κ opioid, GABA, glycine, α_2 adrenergic, serotonin (5-HT) colecistokinin (CCK), adenosine receptors have been intensely studied. Their role is not necessarily the same in physiological and pathological conditions, and their up- or down-regulation can induce attenuation or intensification of their effects in modulating synaptic plasticity.

ASCENDING SYSTEMS

Spinal cord nociceptive projection neurones convey information upward to brainstem and diencephalic areas, and hence to the cortex. The ascending systems are grouped in two different sectors of the spinal cord, the anterolateral (or ventrolateral) and the posterior (or dorsal) quadrants. Experimental evidence comes mainly from studies in rats, cats and monkeys, but has also been attested in man by the results of therapeutic cordotomies. Methods employed include examination of chromatolytic reaction after spinal section, retrograde and anterograde labelling, electrophysiological recordings, observations of behavioural reactions to noxious stimuli before and after selective lesions (for an exhaustive description of pain pathways see Willis, 1985; Bonica, 1990; Willis and Coggeshall, 1991; Willis and Westlund, 1997; Yaksh, 1998 and references therein).

In the ventrolateral funiculus (VLF), the spinothalamic, spinoreticular and spinomesencephalic tracts are located. The spinothalamic tract has one part directed to the medial thalamus (also known as paleo-spinothalamic tract) and a second part, prominent in primates and humans, directed to the lateral thalamus (also known as neo-spinothalamic tract). In addition, direct spinohypothalamic and spinoamygdalar tracts have recently been described (Burstein et al., 1987; Burstein and Pontrebic, 1993).

In the dorsal funiculus (DF) two distinct tracts ascend, which have been implicated in pain transmission: the spinocervicothalamic and the postsynaptic dorsal column pathways. Their existence was postulated after the observation that the complete VLF section could not completely abolish pain sensation and that posterior midline myelotomy was of some efficacy in relieving human pelvic cancer pain (Hirshberg et al.,1996; Nauta et al., 2000).

Compared with the dorsal horn, much less is known about neurotransmitters in ascending tracts. In the thalamus, in immunohistochemical and electrophysiological studies a role of glutamate through the activation of ionotropic and metabotropic glutamate receptors is strongly suggested (Ericson et al., 1995; Salt and Eaton, 1996), and many neuropeptides, e.g. SP, CCK and dynorphin have been identified supraspinally and may play a facilitatory role on the upgoing nociceptive traffic (Li, 1999; Millan, 1999). Moreover, the same processes underlying sensitisation in the dorsal horn (see above) may also be active at the thalamic level: for example, NMDA receptors may modulate inflammation-produced hyperalgesia, suggesting that plastic modifications can occur not only in the dorsal horn but also in more cranial regions of the neuraxis (Kolhekar et al., 1997).

Spinothalamic Tract

The spinothalamic tract is the most important ascending pain system, especially in primates and humans, although its role is not exclusively devoted to the conduction of nociceptive information, carrying also temperature and proprioceptive signals. It is formed by fibres originating mainly in the contralateral side, crossing in the anterior commissure one to two segments from the cell body spinal level. An uncrossed, ipsilateral component has also been described. The fibres are somatotopically arranged, so that the caudal ones are located more laterally in the VLF and those from progressively more rostral segments join in medioventrally. This arrangement is maintained also in the brainstem.

Neurons forming the neo-spinothalamic tract, directed to the lateral thalamus, and those forming the paleo-spinothalamic tract, directed to the medial thalamus, are positioned in most of the laminae of the dorsal and ventral horn, and some also in lamina X surrounding the central canal, but their laminar prevalence differs significantly: cells from laminae I and IV-VI prevail in the neo-, and cells from deeper laminae (VI-VIII) form the bulk of the paleo-spinothalamic tract (Willis and Coggeshall, 1991).

In the lateral thalamus, the main projection target is the ventral posterior lateral nucleus (VPL), both in its caudal (VPL$_c$) and oral (VPL$_o$) parts. Somatotopic organization is maintained and most cells projecting here belong to the NS type, exhibiting small receptive fields with a larger surrounding region with higher threshold. Other projection sites include the ventral posterior inferior nucleus (VPI) and the medial part of posterior thalamus (POm). Nociceptive fibres coming from the trigeminal system originate in the caudal part of the trigeminal spinal nucleus where, similarly to the dorsal horn, NS and WDR neurones can be found. Many of them convey discriminative information to the thalamic ventral posterior medial nucleus (VPM), forming a neo-trigeminothalamic tract, equivalent to the neo-spinothalamic tract.

In the medial thalamus, fibres terminate in the intralaminar nuclear group, especially the central lateral (CL) and parafascicular (PF) nuclei, and in the medial dorsal nucleus (MD), without somatotopic organization. Most cells projecting in these areas are of the WDR type and display large receptive fields, often covering the whole body. Fibres from the caudal part of the trigeminal spinal nucleus also project to the medial thalamus, forming a paleo-trigeminothalamic tract.

The segregation into a lateral and a medial compartment is far from absolute. For example, a number of fibres directed to the VPL nucleus send collaterals to the CL nucleus, i.e. the same neuron projects in both compartments. However, the characteristics of the two components are sufficiently dissimilar to suggest a separate role, in the process of the sensory-discriminative and of the motivational-affective aspects of pain, respectively.

Spinoreticular and Spinomesencephalic Tracts

The spinoreticular and spinomesencephalic tracts carry nociceptive information from the spinal cord to the reticular formation and the midbrain. Because of their connections with the thalamus, these two systems are often included in the definition of paleo-spinothalamic tract, with which they have in common both origin (mainly from the spinal cord deep laminae) and destination (mainly the intralaminar nuclei of medial thalamus). Collaterals or terminals of ascending fibres contact neurones in the caudal medulla (n. retroambiguus, n. superspinalis and n. medullae oblongatae centralis), in the medial reticular formation (n. reticularis gigantocellularis, n. reticularis paragigantocellularis, n. reticularis pontis caudalis), and in the parabrachial region (locus coeruleus, Kölliker-Fuse and parabrachial nuclei). In the midbrain, relay stations include the periaqueductal gray (PAG), the cuneiform, intercolliculus, superior and inferior colliculi, Edinger-Westphal, Darkschewitsch and red nuclei. The majority of fibres follow a crossed path, passing contralaterally either at the spinal level or at the intertectal commissure, but ipsilateral tracings have also been reported.

These pathways supply anatomical substrate to circuits subserving general functions such as aversive behaviour, arousal, activation of autonomic reflexes. Such functions can be accomplished both by suprasegmental reflexes and in coordination with higher centres, in loops engaging diencephalic and telencephalic structures involved in motivational-affective responses. The recently described spinohypothalamic and spinoamygdalar tracts can also contribute, regulating hormonal secretion and behaviour in response to cutaneous and visceral noxious stimulation.

Spinocervicothalamic and Postsynaptic Dorsal Column Pathways

Some of the cells located in laminae I and III-V send their axons dorsally in the ipsilateral DF, up to the lateral cervical nucleus located at C1-C2 level. From here, cervical-thalamic fibres project to the contralateral VPL and the posterior complex. Only a few of the cells in this system respond to painful stimuli, the majority exhibiting tactile responses. Moreover, the lateral cervical nucleus is constantly present in cats and primates, but has only sporadically been discerned in humans.

Of more relevance to human pain transmission is the postsynaptic dorsal column pathway, which has recently been implicated in visceral nociception (Willis and Westlund, 2001). Cells of origin, positioned in laminae III-IV (which receives mainly tactile input) and lamina X, travel along the ipsilateral DF, together with the gracile and cuneatus fasciculi. From the homonymous nuclei, fibres decussate and join the medial lemniscus directed to the lateral thalamus. Thus visceral nociception appears to travel in both VLF and DF and to reach both lateral and medial thalamus.

FROM THALAMUS TO CORTEX

From the foregoing brief analysis of the ascending nociceptive tracts, the thalamus emerges as the target of all pathways, either directly or indirectly via one or more interposing stations (e.g. the reticular formation and the midbrain). The widely dissimilar characteristics of its many nuclei and its multiple connections make it a relay station apt to adequately transmit the temporal and spatial aspects of pain, its intensity, quality and its emotional meaning (Bushnell, 1995).

Historically, the neo-spinothalamic tract, the lateral thalamus and its cortical projections to the primary somatosensory area (SI) have been considered altogether as the most important pain transmitting system. Electrophysiological recordings and behavioural experiments performed in thalamic nuclei, in awake and anaesthetised monkeys, have shown that a variable percentage of VPL and VPM cells respond to noxious stimuli. These neurons belong to both NS and WDR types, are somatotopically ordered and have small contralateral receptive fields, as do the second-order dorsal horn neurones projecting to these nuclei (Kenshalo et al., 1980; Bushnell and Duncan, 1987; Apkarian and Shi, 1994). Many of them receive a dual visceral and low-threshold somatic input (Bruggemann et al., 1994). From VPL and VPM nuclei, fibres reach Brodmann cortical areas 1 (along the crest of postcentral gyrus) and 3b (in the depth of the central sulcus) in the ipsilateral primary somatosensory area (SI): here, arranged in clusters in layers III-V, NS and WDR neurones have been demonstrated in primates to have the same cellular properties as the thalamic neurons (Kenshalo and Isensee, 1983; Kenshalo and Douglass, 1995). The sensory-discriminative aspects of pain sensation can be efficaciously encoded and processed by this so-called "lateral system" (Treede at al., 1999). Support for the discriminative role of this lateral system comes also from more recent studies in humans, where standard electroencephalography, measures of brain electrical spectral activity, recording of brain evoked potentials, and imaging techniques such as PET and fMRI, have all been used to monitor and map clinical pain (Chen, 1993a,b).

Parallel and complementary to this main pain transmitting system, a "medial nociceptive system" exists (Treede at al., 1999), whose role is to provide the complex circuit generating the affective-emotional component of pain, i.e. those aspects regarding its unpleasantness, its negative hedonic quality and the negative emotions associated with it: in one word, the "suffering". Without it, the pain experience is incomplete and can hardly be defined as such.

The medial thalamus receiving input from the paleo-spinothalamic tract projects to several cortical areas: the secondary somatosensory area (SII), located in the parietal lobe, on the upper bank of the lateral (Sylvian) fissure; the parasylvian cortex, including the insula and the parietal operculum; the prefrontal, orbito-frontal and anterior cingulate cortices. Many of these areas are strongly connected with one another and with the limbic system, i.e. the ensemble of paleocortical and subcortical structures involved in the global processing of emotions (Papez, 1937; MacLean, 1990). In contrast to SI, somatotopic organization is generally lacking, suggesting a role in aspecific arousal in response to a noxious stimulus, rather than its precise spatial and temporal localization.

Once again, it must be emphasised that the two systems are not isolated pathways, cut off from one another; their separate delineation is especially useful in conceptual terms, but their interconnection at all levels contributes to give to the pain experience its character of whole perception, with simultaneous awareness of all its aspects. The attention focused in recent years on the cortical representation of pain and on the implications of motivational and emotional components for clinical pain therapy warrants some further discussion.

CORTICAL REPRESENTATION OF PAIN

The idea that the cerebral cortex is involved in the perception of pain is relatively recent. An early report by Head and Holmes (1911) attributed it only to the thalamus, because even extensive lesions of the cortex never appeared to be associated with changes in pain sensation, and electrical stimulation of somatosensory cortex during surgery had never been reported to elicit pain (Penfield and Boldrey, 1937). It was only in 1951 that a study by Marshall evidenced localized loss of pain sensation in patients with parietal lesions (Marshall, 1951). In the 80s, the first nociceptive neurones were recorded in the monkey SI area (Kenshalo and Isensee, 1983). Today, the role of the cortex in pain perception is not only well established, but new, non-invasive techniques, such as magnetoencephalography (MEG) allow in humans sophisticated measures of temporal activation. For example, in contrast to tactile sequential processing, SI and SII appear to be activated simultaneously by pain stimuli, suggesting a preserved direct access of information from thalamus to SII and hence to temporal lobe limbic structures involved in learning and memory. This may reflect the evolutionary importance of learning to avoid dangerous behaviour (Ploner et al., 1999; 2000). Moreover, the high correlation between stimulus intensity and activity in contralateral SI is not paralleled in SII, where bilateral sharp activation above threshold seems to reflect more the all-or-none recognition of the noxious stimulus rather than its discriminative evaluation (Timmermann et al., 2001).

The understanding of the cortical representation of pain must necessarily move from the multiple aspects of the pain experience: sensory-discriminative, affective-motivational and cognitive. As outlined above, these components are conveyed from the periphery in distinct pathways. But how are they processed and how do they emerge as a unique conscious experience from the many cortical areas engaged in pain perception? Although this remains largely a matter of debate and a field of active research for the future, a few tentative steps have been made.

Upon presentation of painful stimuli, human brain imaging studies show activation of different cortical regions: SI, SII, the anterior cingulate cortex (ACC), the insular cortex (IC), and the prefrontal cortex (Davis et al., 2000; Hudson, 2000). The role of SI in pain processing is controversial: activation increase (Talbot et al., 1991), no variation (Jones et al., 1991) or even activation decrease (Apkarian et al., 1992) have been reported. Discrepancies were not resolved by later studies (for a review see Bushnell et al., 1999). Beside differences in statistical analysis or technical approaches, an interesting explanation for such variation is suggested to be the influence of cognitive modulation in SI activity. In other words, attention directed toward or away from a painful stimulus could increase or decrease SI response, respectively (Bushnell et al., 1999). The somatosensory cortex is classically associated to the sensory-discriminative component of pain, encoding stimulus spatial, temporal and intensity information. Support for this role comes from electrophysiological studies (Kenshalo et al., 1988; Chudler et al., 1990; Dong at al., 1994), as well as from experiments employing hypnotic suggestions to manipulate the subject's perception of pain intensity (Hofbauer et al., 2001). However, in other studies, intensity coding in SI has been denied as being dependent more on touch than on nociception (Peyron et al., 1999).

The secondary somatosensory (SII) and the insular cortices (IC) have almost constantly been implicated in pain representation: parasylvian lesions can modify pain perception, parasylvian seizures can be painful, local activity can be altered in PET and MEG studies by delivering painful stimuli (Greenspan et al., 1999; Scholz et al., 1999; Svensson et al., 1997; Bromm and Lorenz, 1998). Stimulus intensity coding is here again matter of debate, with contradictory results being reported, i.e. positive correlation between hot stimuli and SII activity (Peyron et al., 1999) and between cold noxious stimuli and IC activity (Craig et al., 2000) or all-or-none activation in SII (Timmermann et al., 2001). By using single unit recordings, nociceptive neurones in these areas are more difficult to identify than tactile neurones, maybe because of the mechanical search criteria generally used (Dong at al., 1989). Also, recent fMRI data point toward an at least partial separation of tactile and nociceptive areas in the parietal operculum (Gelnar et al., 1999) and in anterior nociceptive and posterior tactile insula (Davis et al., 1998). A potential sensory-discriminative role for these areas is therefore still open to discussion.

Anatomical data in primates (Apkarian and Shi, 1994; Craig et al., 1994) and MEG data in humans (Ploner et al., 1999; 2000) are strongly in favour of direct access of nociceptive information to SII and IC, rather than indirect arrival via somatotopically arranged SI, as is the case of tactile input. These observations point to the participation of these structures in determining the arousal state of the individual, alerting him to the presence of a dangerous context. When arousal is eliminated by means of sedation or general anaesthesia, also parasylvian cortex activity is drastically reduced (Bromm et al., 2000). Thus, the role of the nociceptive area in the vicinity of the lateral sulcus would be a cognitive-evaluative one as well, possibly linked to generation of pain memory (Treede et al., 2000). Moreover, IC may also be part of circuits subserving pain affect. In the Schilder-Stengel syndrome, patients with insular lesions suffer from pain asymbolia: their pain sensation is normal, but their reaction is anomalous, with inadequate emotional responses and lack of withdrawal (Berthier et al., 1988). This should not be surprising, as the insula is part of the limbic system, the overall function of which is to give the sensory experience its emotional colours.

Another cortical area which is also part of the limbic system and which is constantly activated by painful stimuli is the anterior portion of the cingulate gyrus, which has been known for decades to take part in pain circuits. Following mid-century prefrontal lobotomies in psychotic patients, a reduction of the unbearable suffering often associated with the disease was observed, and subsequent surgical refinements, with lesions restricted to the anterior part of the cingulate cortex, were also applied to otherwise intractable neoplastic and neuropathic pain states (Freeman and Watts, 1950; LeBeau, 1954; Ballantine et al., 1987). The cingulate cortex has been proposed to be divided in two distinct regions, on the basis of different cytoarchitecture and connections: an anterior "executive" one, consisting of Brodmann areas

24, 25 and 33, engaged in multiple motor functions including those related to affect, and a posterior "evaluative" one, comprising areas 23, 29, 30 and 31, involved in visuospatial and mnestic functions (Vogt et al., 1992). The anterior region, extending around the rostrum of the corpus callosum, can be further subdivided into an "affect" and a "cognition" division. The first, extensively connected with the amygdala and the periaqueductal gray, is implicated in the assignment of the emotional content to stimuli and in the evaluation of their motivational value, and participates in the regulation of endocrine and autonomic functions. The second, with rich connections to the striatum, contributes to skeletomotor control and cognitive response selection, including appropriate pain responsiveness (Devinsky et al., 1995).

Imaging studies show that pain-related activity in ACC can be selectively modulated by cognitive factors (Petrovic and Ingvar, 2002), e.g. by altering hypnotically the unpleasantness of a nociceptive stimulus but not its intensity (Rainville et al., 1997). Moreover, an illusion of pain, such as the noxious cold produced by a thermal grid with alternated innocuous hot and cold bars, is sufficient to activate the ACC (Craig et al., 1996). Similarly, activity in ACC and other areas correlates with psychophysical pain assessment in patients with phantom-limb pain (Willoch et al., 2000). Attention/distraction, expectation, and placebo analgesia are further cognitive factors influencing ACC activity (Longe et al., 2001; Porro et al., 2002; Petrovic et al., 2002).

Thus, rather than being localized in a "pain center", pain appears to be a highly distributed system. Its global organization has so far been much less investigated than individual areas, but it seems likely that the awareness of the different pain components arise from the contribution of many regions, with information processed in a parallel rather than in a serial way (Coghill et al., 1999).

REFERENCES

Abraham WC, Mason SE, Demmer J, Williams JM, Richardson CL, Tate WP, Lawlor PA, Dragunow M. Correlations between immediate early gene induction and the persistence of long-term potentiation. *Neuroscience* 1993;56(3):717-727.

Apkarian AV, Shi T. Squirrel monkey lateral thalamus. I. Somatic nociresponsive neurons and their relation to spinothalamic terminals. *J Neurosci* 1994;14(11):6779-6795.

Apkarian AV, Stea RA, Manglos SH, Szeverenyi NM, King RB, Thomas FD. Persistent pain inhibits contralateral somatosensory cortical activity in humans. *Neurosci Lett* 1992;140(2):141-147.

Averill S, McMahon SB, Clary DO, Reichardt LF, Priestley JV. Immunocytochemical localization of trkA receptors in chemically identified subgroups of adult rat sensory neurons. *Eur J Neurosci* 1995;7(7):1484-1494.

Ballantine HT, Bouchoms AJ, Thomas EK, Giriunas IE. Treatment of psychiatric illness by stereotactic cingulotomy. *Biol Psychiat* 1987;22:807-819.

Basbaum AI, Jessel TM. The perception of pain. In: Kandel ER, Schwartz JH, Jessell TM, editors. Principles of neural science. 4th ed. *New York: McGraw Hill*, 2000, pp. 472-491.

Baumann TK, Simone DA, Shain CN, LaMotte RH. Neurogenic hyperalgesia: the search for the primary cutaneous afferent fibers that contribute to capsaicin-induced pain and hyperalgesia. *J Neurophysiol* 1991 Jul;66(1):212-227.

Belemonte C, Cervero F. Neurobiology of nociceptors. *Oxford: Oxford University Press*, 1996.

Bennett DL, Michael GJ, Ramachandran N, Munson JB, Averill S, Yan Q, McMahon SB, Priestley JV. A distinct subgroup of small DRG cells express GDNF receptor components and GDNF is protective for these neurons after nerve injury. *J Neurosci* 1998;18(8):3059-3072.

Berthier M, Starkstein S, Leiguarda R. Asymbolia for pain: a sensory-limbic disconnection syndrome. *Ann Neurol* 1988;24:41-49.

Besson JM, Chaouch A. Peripheral and spinal mechanisms of nociception. *Physiol Rev* 1987;67:67-186.

Besson JM, Guilbaud G, Ollat H. Forebrain areas involved in pain processing. *Paris: John Libbey Eurotext*, 1995.

Bonica, JJ. The management of pain. 2nd ed. *Philadelphia: Lea and Febiger*, 1990.

Bromm B, Lorenz J. Neurophysiological evaluation of pain. *Electroencephalogr Clin Neurophysiol* 1998;107(4):227-253.

Bromm B, Scharein E, Vahle-Hinz C. Cortex areas involved in the processing of normal and altered pain. In: Sandkuler J, Bromm B, Gebhart G, editors. Nervous system plasticity and chronic pain. *Amsterdam: Elsevier*, 2000.

Bruggemann J, Shi T, Apkarian AV. Squirrel monkey lateral thalamus. II. Viscerosomatic convergent representation of urinary bladder, colon, and esophagus. *J Neurosci* 1994;14(11):6796-6814.

Burstein R, Cliffer KD, Giesler GJ Jr. Direct somatosensory projections from the spinal cord to the hypothalamus and telencephalon. *J Neurosci* 1987;7(12):4159-4164.

Burstein R, Potrebic S. Retrograde labeling of neurons in the spinal cord that project directly to the amygdala or the orbital cortex in the rat. *J Comp Neurol* 1993;335(4):469-485.

Bushnell MC, Duncan GH, Hofbauer RK, Ha B, Chen JI, Carrier B. Pain perception: is there a role for primary somatosensory cortex? *Proc Natl Acad Sci U S A* 1999;96(14):7705-7709.

Bushnell MC, Duncan GH. Mechanical response properties of ventroposterior medial thalamic neurons in the alert monkey. *Exp Brain Res* 1987; 67 (3):603-614.

Bushnell MC. Thalamic processing of sensory-discriminative and affective-motivational dimensions of pain. In: Besson JM, Guilbaud G, Ollat H, editors. Forebrain areas involved in pain processing. *Paris: John Libbey Eurotext*, 1995, pp.63-78.

Cajal SR. Histology of the nervous system of man and vertebrates. Vol. 1. Swanson N, Swanson LW (Engl. Trans.), *New York: Oxford University Press*, 1995.

Campbell JN, LaMotte RH. Latency to detection of first pain. *Brain Res* 1983;266(2):203-208.

Caterina MJ, Julius D. The vanilloid receptor: a molecular gateway to the pain pathway. *Annu Rev Neurosci* 2001;24:487-517.

Caterina MJ, Schumacher MA, Tominaga M, Rosen TA, Levine JD, Julius D. The capsaicin receptor: a heat-activated ion channel in the pain pathway. *Nature* 1997; 389 (6653):816-824.

Cervero F, Jänig W. Visceral nociceptors: a new world order? *Trends Neurosci* 1992;15 (10):374-378.

Cervero F. Sensory innervation of the viscera: peripheral basis of visceral pain. *Physiol Rev* 1994; 74 (1):95-138.

Chen AC. Human brain measures of clinical pain: a review. I. Topographic mappings. *Pain* 1993a; 54 (2):115-132.

Chen AC. Human brain measures of clinical pain: a review. II. Tomographic imagings. *Pain* 1993b; 5 4(2):133-144.

Chudler EH, Anton F, Dubner R, Kenshalo DR Jr. Responses of nociceptive SI neurons in monkeys and pain sensation in humans elicited by noxious thermal stimulation: effect of interstimulus interval. *J Neurophysiol* 1990; 63 (3):559-569.

Coghill RC, Sang CN, Maisog JM, Iadarola MJ. Pain intensity processing within the human brain: a bilateral, distributed mechanism. *J Neurophysiol* 1999; 82 (4):1934-1943.

Collingridge GL, Singer W. Excitatory amino acid receptors and synaptic plasticity. Trends Pharmacol Sci 1990;11(7):290-296.

Craig AD, Bushnell MC, Zhang ET, Blomqvist A. A thalamic nucleus specific for pain and temperature sensation. *Nature* 1994;372:770-773.

Craig AD, Chen K, Bandy D, Reiman EM. Thermosensory activation of insular cortex. *Nat Neurosci* 2000;3:184-190.

Craig AD, Reiman EM, Evans A, Bushnell MC. Functional imaging of an illusion of pain. *Nature* 1996;384(6606):258-260.

Cummins TR, Black JA, Dib-Hajj SD, Waxman SG. Glial-derived neurotrophic factor upregulates expression of functional SNS and NaN sodium channels and their currents in axotomized dorsal root ganglion neurons. *J Neurosci* 2000;20(23):8754-8761.

Davies SN, Lodge D. Evidence for involvement of N-methylaspartate receptors in 'wind-up' of class 2 neurones in the dorsal horn of the rat. *Brain Res* 1987;424(2):402-406.

Davis KD, Kwan CL, Crawley AP, Mikulis DJ. Functional MRI study of thalamic and cortical activations evoked by cutaneous heat, cold, and tactile stimuli. *J.Neurophysiol* 1998;80:1533-1546.

Davis KD. The neural circuitry of pain as explored with functional MRI. *Neurol Res* 2000;22(3):313-317.

Devinsky O, Morrell MJ, Vogt BA. Contributions of anterior cingulate cortex to behaviour. *Brain* 1995;118:279-306.

Dickenson AH, Sullivan AF. Evidence for a role of the NMDA receptor in the frequency dependent potentiation of deep rat dorsal horn nociceptive neurones following C fibre stimulation. *Neuropharmacology* 1987;26(8):1235-1238.

Dong WK, Chudler EH, Sugiyama K, Roberts VJ, Hayashi T. Somatosensory, multisensory, and task-related neurons in cortical area 7b (PF) of unanesthetized monkeys. *J Neurophysiol* 1994;72(2):542-564.

Dubner R, Bennett GJ. Spinal and trigeminal mechanisms of nociception. *Annu Rev Neurosci* 1983;6:381-418.

Ericson AC, Blomqvist A, Craig AD, Ottersen OP, Broman J. Evidence for glutamate as neurotransmitter in trigemino-and spinothalamic tract terminals in the nucleus submedius of cats. *Eur J Neurosci* 1995;7(2):305-317.

Freeman W, Watts JW. Psychosurgery: intelligence, emotional and social behavior following prefrontal lobotomy for mental disorders. 2nd ed. *Springfield: Charles C Thomas*, 1950.

Gebhart GF. Visceral pain. *Seattle: IASP Press*, 1995.

Gelnar PA, Krauss BR, Sheehe PR, Szeverenyi NM, Apkarian AV. A comparative fMRI study of cortical representation for thermal painful, vibrotactile, and motor performance tasks. *Neuroimage 1999*;10:460-482.

Gobel S. Golgi studies of the neurons in layer II of the dorsal horn of the medulla (trigeminal nucleus caudalis). *J. Comp. Neurol.* 1978;180(2):395-413.

Greenspan JD, Lee RR, Lenz FA. Pain sensitivity alterations as a function of lesion location in the parasylvian cortex. *Pain* 1999;81(3):273-282.

Hayes ES, Carlton SM. Primary afferent interactions: analysis of calcitonin gene-related peptide-immunoreactive terminals in contact with unlabeled and GABA-immunoreactive profiles in the monkey dorsal horn. *Neuroscience* 1992;47(4):873-96.

Head H, Holmes G. Sensory disturbances from cerebral lesions. *Brain* 1911;34:102-254.

Hirshberg RM, Al-Chaer ED, Lawand NB, Westlund KN, Willis WD. Is there a pathway in the posterior funiculus that signals visceral pain? *Pain* 1996;67(2-3):291-305.

Hofbauer RK, Rainville P, Duncan GH, Bushnell MC. Cortical representation of the sensory dimension of pain. *J Neurophysiol* 2001;86(1):402-411.

Hokfelt T, Zhang X, Wiesenfeld-Hallin Z. Messenger plasticity in primary sensory neurons following axotomy and its functional implications. *Trends Neurosci* 1994;17(1):22-30.

Hudson AJ. Pain perception and response: central nervous system mechanisms. *Can J Neurol Sci* 2000;27(1):2-16.

Hunt SP, Rossi J. Peptide- and non-peptide-containing unmyelinated primary afferents: the parallel processing of nociceptive information. *Philos Trans R Soc Lond B Biol Sci* 1985;308(1136):283-289.

International Association for the Study of Pain. Pain terms: a list with definitions and notes on usage. *Pain* 1979;6:249-252.

Jones AK, Brown WD, Friston KJ, Qi LY, Frackowiak RS. Cortical and subcortical localization of response to pain in man using positron emission tomography. *Proc R Soc Lond B Biol Sci* 1991;244(1309):39-44.

Jongen JL, Dalm E, Vecht CJ, Holstege JC. Depletion of GDNF from primary afferents in adult rat dorsal horn following peripheral axotomy. *Neuroreport* 1999;10(4):867-871.

Kenshalo DR Jr, Chudler EH, Anton F, Dubner R. SI nociceptive neurons participate in the encoding process by which monkeys perceive the intensity of noxious thermal stimulation. *Brain Res* 1988;454(1-2):378-382.

Kenshalo DR Jr, Giesler GJ Jr, Leonard RB, Willis WD. Responses of neurons in primate ventral posterior lateral nucleus to noxious stimuli. *J Neurophysiol* 1980;43(6):1594-1614.

Kenshalo DR, Douglass DK. The role of the cerebral cortex in the experience of pain. In: Bromm B, Desmedt JE, editors. Pain and the brain: from nociception to cognition. *New York: Raven Press*, 1995, pp. 21-34.

Kenshalo DR, Isensee O. Responses of primate SI cortical neurons to noxious stimuli. *J Neurophysiol* 1983;50(6):1479-1496.

Klement W, Arndt JO. The role of nociceptors of cutaneous veins in the mediation of cold pain in man. *J Physiol* 1992;449:73-83.

Kolhekar R, Murphy S, Gebhart GF. Thalamic NMDA receptors modulate inflammation-produced hyperalgesia in the rat. *Pain* 1997;71(1):31-40.

LeBeau J. Psycho-chirurgie et fonctions mentales. *Paris: Masson*, 1954.

Lewin GR, Ritter AM, Mendell LM. Nerve growth factor-induced hyperalgesia in the neonatal and adult rat. *J Neurosci.* 1993; 13(5):2136-2148.

Li YQ. Substance P receptor-like immunoreactive neurons in the caudal spinal trigeminal nucleus send axons to the gelatinosus thalamic nucleus in the rat. *J Hirnforsch* 1999;39(3):277-282.

Longe SE, Wise R, Bantick S, Lloyd D, Johansen-Berg H, McGlone F, Tracey I. Counter-stimulatory effects on pain perception and processing are significantly altered by attention: an fMRI study. *Neuroreport* 2001;12(9):2021-2025.

MacLean PD. The triune brain in evolution: role in paleocerebral functions. *New York: Plenum Press*, 1990.

Marshall J. Sensory disturbances in cortical wounds with special reference to pain. *J Neurol Neurosurg Psychiatry* 1951;14:187-204.

Melzack R, Wall PD. Pain mechanisms: a new theory. *Science* 1965;150:971-979.

Melzack R. From the gate to the neuromatrix. *Pain* 1999;Suppl 6:S121-126.

Mendell LM, Albers KM, Davis BM. Neurotrophins, nociceptors, and pain. *Microsc Res Tech* 1999;45(4-5):252-261.

Mendell LM. Physiological properties of unmyelinated fiber projection to the spinal cord. *Exp Neurol* 1966;16(3):316-332.

Michael GJ, Averill S, Nitkunan A, Rattray M, Bennett DL, Yan Q, Priestley JV. Nerve growth factor treatment increases brain-derived neurotrophic factor selectively in TrkA-expressing dorsal root ganglion cells and in their central terminations within the spinal cord. *J Neurosci* 1997;17(21):8476-8490.

Michaelis M, Habler HJ, Jänig W. Silent afferents: a separate class of primary afferents? *Clin Exp Pharmacol Physiol* 1996;23(2):99-105.

Millan MJ. The induction of pain: an integrative review. *Prog Neurobiol* 1999;57:1-164.

Molliver DC, Snider WD. Nerve growth factor receptor TrkA is down-regulated during postnatal development by a subset of dorsal root ganglion neurons. *J Comp Neurol* 1997;381(4):428-438.

Molliver DC, Wright DE, Leitner ML, Parsadanian AS, Doster K, Wen D, Yan Q, Snider WD. IB4-binding DRG neurons switch from NGF to GDNF dependence in early postnatal life. *Neuron* 1997;19(4):849-861.

Nagy JI, Hunt SP. Fluoride-resistant acid phosphatase-containing neurones in dorsal root ganglia are separate from those containing substance P or somatostatin. *Neuroscience* 1982;7(1):89-97.

Nauta HJ, Soukup VM, Fabian RH, Lin JT, Grady JJ, Williams CG, Campbell GA, Westlund KN, Willis WD Jr. Punctate midline myelotomy for the relief of visceral cancer pain. *J Neurosurg* 2000;92(2 Suppl):125-130.

Papez JW. A proposed mechanism of emotions. Arch Neurol Psychol 1937;38:725-743.

Penfield W, Boldrey E. Somatic motor and sensory representation in cerebral cortex of man as studied by electrical stimulation. *Brain* 1937;60:389-443.

Petrovic P, Ingvar M. Imaging cognitive modulation of pain processing. *Pain* 2002;95(1-2):1-5.

Petrovic P, Kalso E, Petersson KM, Ingvar M. Placebo and opioid analgesia-- imaging a shared neuronal network. *Science* 2002;295(5560):1737-1740.

Petty BG, Cornblath DR, Adornato BT, Chaudhry V, Flexner C, Wachsman M, Sinicropi D, Burton LE, Peroutka SJ. The effect of systemically administered recombinant human nerve growth factor in healthy human subjects. *Ann Neurol* 1994;36(2):244-246.

Peyron R, Garcia-Larrea L, Gregoire MC, Costes N, Convers P, Lavenne F, Mauguiere F, Michel D, Laurent B. Haemodynamic brain responses to acute pain in humans: sensory and attentional networks. *Brain* 1999;122:1765-1780.

Ploner M, Schmitz F, Freund HJ, Schnitzler A. Differential organization of touch and pain in human primary somatosensory cortex. *J Neurophysiol* 2000;83(3):1770-1776.

Ploner M, Schmitz F, Freund HJ, Schnitzler A. Parallel activation of primary and secondary somatosensory cortices in human pain processing. *J Neurophysiol* 1999;81(6):3100-3104.

Porro CA, Baraldi P, Pagnoni G, Serafini M, Facchin P, Maieron M, Nichelli P. Does anticipation of pain affect cortical nociceptive systems? *J Neurosci* 2002;22(8):3206-3214.

Price DD, Dubner R. Neurons that subserve the sensory-discriminative aspects of pain. *Pain* 1977;3(4):307-338.

Rainville P, Duncan GH, Price DD, Carrier B, Bushnell MC. Pain affect encoded in human anterior cingulate but not somatosensory cortex. *Science* 1997;277(5328):968-971.

Raja SN, Meyer RA, Ringkamp M, Campbell JN. Peripheral neural mechanisms of nociception. In: Wall PD, Melzack R, editors. Textbook of pain. 4th ed. Edinburgh: *Churchill-Livingstone*, 1999, pp. 11-57.

Reichling DB, Levine JD. The primary afferent nociceptor as pattern generator. *Pain* 1999;Suppl 6:S103-109.

Rexed B. The cytoarchitectonic organization of the spinal cord in the rat. J. Comp. *Neurol.* 1952;96:415-466.

Salt TE, Eaton SA. Functions of ionotropic and metabotropic glutamate receptors in sensory transmission in the mammalian thalamus. *Prog Neurobiol* 1996;48(1):55-72.

Schaible HG, Schmidt RF. Time course of mechanosensitivity changes in articular afferents during a developing experimental arthritis. *J Neurophysiol* 1988;60(6):2180-2195.

Scholz J, Vieregge P, Moser A. Central pain as a manifestation of partial epileptic seizures. *Pain* 1999;80(1-2):445-450.

Sengupta JN, Gebhart GF. Mechanosensitive afferent fibers in the gastrointestinal and lower urinary tracts. In: Gebhart GF, editor. Visceral pain. Progress in pain research and management, vol.5, Seattle: *IASP Press*,1995, pp. 75-98.

Sherrington CS. The integrative action of the nervous system. New York, *Scribner*, 1906.

Silos-Santiago I, Molliver DC, Ozaki S, Smeyne RJ, Fagan AM, Barbacid M, Snider WD. Non-TrkA-expressing small DRG neurons are lost in TrkA deficient mice. *J Neurosci* 1995;15(9):5929-5942.

Silverman JD, Kruger L. Selective neuronal glycoconjugate expression in sensory and autonomic ganglia: relation of lectin reactivity to peptide and enzyme markers. *J Neurocytol* 1990;19(5):789-801

Snider WD, McMahon SB. Tackling pain at the source: new ideas about nociceptors. *Neuron* 1988;20:629-632.

Stucky CL, Lewin GR. Isolectin B(4)-positive and -negative nociceptors are functionally distinct. *J Neurosci* 1999;19(15):6497-6505.

Svensson P, Minoshima S, Beydoun A, Morrow TJ, Casey KL. Cerebral processing of acute skin and muscle pain in humans. *J Neurophysiol* 1997;78(1):450-460.

Talbot JD, Marrett S, Evans AC, Meyer E, Bushnell MC, Duncan GH. Multiple representations of pain in human cerebral cortex. *Science* 1991;251(4999):1355-1358.

Thompson SW, Bennett DL, Kerr BJ, Bradbury EJ, McMahon SB. Brain-derived neurotrophic factor is an endogenous modulator of nociceptive responses in the spinal cord. *Proc Natl Acad Sci U S A* 1999;96(14):7714-7718.

Timmermann L, Ploner M, Haucke K, Schmitz F, Baltissen R, Schnitzler A. Differential coding of pain intensity in the human primary and secondary somatosensory cortex. *J Neurophysiol* 2001;86(3):1499-1503.

Torebjörk HE, Lundberg LE, LaMotte RH. Central changes in processing of mechanoreceptive input in capsaicin-induced secondary hyperalgesia in humans. *J Physiol* 1992;448:765-780.

Treede RD, Apkarian AV, Bromm B, Greenspan JD, Lenz FA. Cortical representation of pain: functional characterization of nociceptive areas near the lateral sulcus. *Pain* 2000;87:113-119.

Treede RD, Kenshalo DR, Gracely RH, Jones AK. The cortical representation of pain. *Pain* 1999;79(2-3):105-111.

Treede RD, Meyer RA, Campbell JN. Classification of primate A-fibre nociceptors according to their heat response properties. *Pflügers Archives* 1991;(Suppl 1) 418:R42.

Treede RD, Meyer RA, Raja SN, Campbell JN. Evidence for two different heat transduction mechanisms in nociceptive primary afferents innervating monkey skin. *J Physiol* 1995;483:747-758.

Treede RD, Meyer RA, Raja SN, Campbell JN. Peripheral and central mechanisms of cutaneous hyperalgesia. *Prog Neurobiol* 1992;38(4):397-421.

Van Hees J, Gybels J. C nociceptor activity in human nerve during painful and non painful skin stimulation. *J Neurol Neurosurg Psychiatry* 1981;44(7):600-607.

Vogt BA, Finch DM, Olson CR. Functional heterogeneity in cingulate cortex: the anterior executive and posterior evaluative regions. *Cereb Cortex* 1992;2:435-443.

Vulchanova L, Olson TH, Stone LS, Riedl MS, Elde R, Honda CN. Cytotoxic targeting of isolectin IB4-binding sensory neurons. *Neuroscience* 2001;108(1):143-155.

Vulchanova L, Riedl MS, Shuster SJ, Stone LS, Hargreaves KM, Buell G, Surprenant A, North RA, Elde R. P2X3 is expressed by DRG neurons that terminate in inner lamina II. *Eur J Neurosci* 1998;10(11):3470-3478.

Wall PD, Melzack R. Textbook of pain. 4th ed. Edinburgh: Churchill-Livingstone, 1999.

Willis WD Jr, Westlund KN. The role of the dorsal column pathway in visceral nociception. *Curr Pain Headache Rep* 2001;5(11):20-26.

Willis WD, Coggeshall RE. Sensory mechanisms of the spinal cord. 2nd ed. New York: *Plenum Press*, 1991.

Willis WD, Westlund KN. Neuroanatomy of the pain system and of the pathways that modulate pain. *J Clin Neurophysiol* 1997;14(1):2-31.

Willis WD. The pain system. Basel: *Karger*, 1985.

Willis WD. The pain system: the neural basis of nociceptive transmission in the mammalian nervous system. Basel: *Karger*, 1985.

Willoch F, Rosen G, Tolle TR, Oye I, Wester HJ, Berner N, Schwaiger M, Bartenstein P. Phantom limb pain in the human brain: unraveling neural circuitries of phantom limb sensations using positron emission tomography. *Ann Neurol* 2000;48(6):842-849.

Woolf CJ, Costigan M. Transcriptional and posttranslational plasticity and the generation of inflammatory pain. *Proc Natl Acad Sci U S A* 1999;96(14):7723-7730.

Woolf CJ, Mannion RJ. Neuropathic pain: aetiology, symptoms, mechanisms, and management. *Lancet* 1999;353(9168):1959-1964.

Woolf CJ, Safieh-Garabedian B, Ma QP, Crilly P, Winter J. Nerve growth factor contributes to the generation of inflammatory sensory hypersensitivity. *Neuroscience* 1994;62(2):327-331.

Woolf CJ, Salter MW. Neuronal plasticity: increasing the gain in pain. *Science* 2000;288(5472):1765-1769.

Woolf CJ, Shortland P, Reynolds M, Ridings J, Doubell T, Coggeshall RE. Reorganization of central terminals of myelinated primary afferents in the rat dorsal horn following peripheral axotomy. *J Comp Neurol* 1995;360(1):121-134.

Woolf CJ. Evidence for a central component of post-injury pain hypersensitivity. *Nature* 1983;306(5944):686-688.

Woolf CJ. The dorsal horn: state-dependent sensory processing and the generation of pain. In: Wall PD, Melzack R, editors. Textbook of pain. 3rd ed. Edinburgh: *Churchill-Livingstone,* 1994, pp.101-112.

Yaksh TL. Physiologic and pharmacologic substrates of nociception and nerve injury. In: Cousins MJ, Bridenbaugh PO, editors. Neural blockade in clinical anesthesia and management of pain. 3rd ed. Philadelphia: *Lippincott-Raven Publishers*, 1998, pp.727-780.

In: The Handbook of Chronic Pain
Editors: S. Kreitler, D. Beltrutti, et al., pp. 25-40

ISBN 978-1-60021-044-0
© 2007 Nova Science Publishers, Inc.

Chapter 2

Biochemical Basis of Nociception - Roles of Cytokines

Emiko Senba, Hiroki Imbe and Hitoshi Kashiba

WHAT ARE CYTOKINES?

Cytokines can be defined as soluble factors that are involved in intercellular communication in various (immune, hematopoietic and nervous) systems through specific receptors expressed on the surface of target cells. Cytokines are produced and released by various kinds of cells, such as glial cells, fibroblasts, macrophages and neurons, in the primary afferent pathway. The pain transmission system is supported by these factors. Phenotype expression in sensory neurons, remodeling of sensory system associated with chronic pain and regeneration of injured sensory neurons are also regulated by these cytokines.

Cytokines are now classified into several families according to the structural homology of their receptors and downstream signal transduction mechanisms [1]. All the cytokine receptors, except those for chemokines (G-protein-coupled receptors with seven transmembrane), are single chains with one transmembrane region (Fig.1). Receptors for growth factors or neurotrophins have serine-threonine kinase, or tyrosine kinase in their cytoplasmic domains, respectively. But receptor components of interleukins (class I cytokines) and interferons (class II cytokines) do not have such enzymatic motifs in their structure. Instead they are associated with Janus kinase (JAK) family kinases. Receptors for class III cytokines, such as tumor necrosis factor (TNF), constitute the TNF receptor superfamily and are associated with proteins termed TRAF or TRADD. IL-1 receptor (IL-1R) is associated with adapter protein MyD88.

This chapter will highlight the roles of neurotrophins, GDNF, IL-6 family cytokines and their receptors in nociception. We have now growing evidence to show that these cytokines are essential for the formation and maintenance of the primary sensory system.

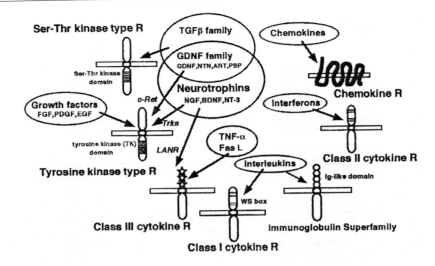

Figure 1. Cytokines are classified into several families according to the structure of receptors and downstream signal transduction mechanisms.

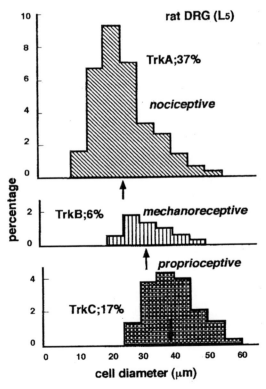

Figure 2. Cell diameter histogram of TrkA-, TrkB-, and TrkC- positive neurons in the rat DRG. TrkA-positive neurons are mainly small-, TrkB are medium-, and TrkC are large-sized.

NEUROTROPHINS

Nerve growth factor (NGF), brain-derived neurotrophic factor (BDNF) and neurotrophin-3 (NT-3) are members of neurotrophins, and TrkA, TrkB, TrkC are high affinity receptors for them, respectively. Trks possess tyrosine kinase (TK) domain in the cytoplasmic region, and are expressed in a non-overlapping manner by sensory neurons. About 35-40%, 5-10%, and 15-20% of the rat dorsal root ganglion (DRG) neurons are positive for TrkA, TrkB, and TrkC mRNAs, and these neurons are mainly small-, medium-, and large-sized, respectively [2] (Fig.2). All the Trk-positive neurons express low affinity neurotrophin receptor (LANR) [2], which is a member of Class III cytokine receptors (Fig. 1). Small TrkA-positive DRG neurons are dependent on NGF, involved in pain transmission and synthesize peptides, such as substance P (SP) or calcitonin gene-related peptide (CGRP) but not somatostatin (SOM) [3,4]. BDNF is also synthesized in these neurons [5] (Fig.3 A,B).

Gene targeting of these neurotrophins or their receptors have revealed that TrkA neurons are nociceptive, TrkB neurons are mechanoreceptive and TrkC neurons are proprioceptive. NGF or TrkA deficient mice completely lack small DRG neurons and insensitive to pain and temperature. Mutant mice of TrkC or NT-3 lack proprioceptive DRG neurons. Null mutation of BDNF in mice induces a loss of medium sized DRG neurons and slowly adapting tactile sensation [6]. TrkA-expressing neurons are essential for pain perception. Mutations in TrkA gene were identified in patients with congenital insensitivity to pain [7].

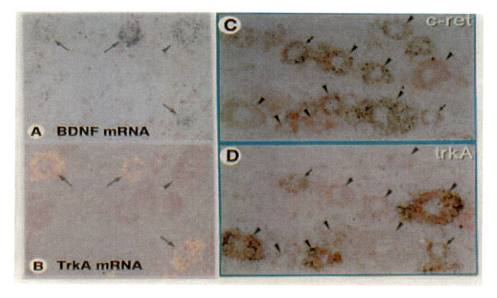

Figure 3. BDNF is synthesized in TrkA-positive neurons. Serial sections show that most of the BDNF mRNA expressing neurons (arrows in A) are TrkA mRNA-positive (B). C-Ret mRNA and TrkA mRNA are not colocalized (arrowheads in C,D). Neurons showing colocalization are indicated with arrows.

GLIAL CELL LINE-DERIVED NEUROTROPHIC FACTOR (GDNF)

Glial cell line-derived neurotrophic factor (GDNF), a novel neurotrophic factor for DRG neurons, was identified as a member of TGF-β family, but its signal transducer was found to be c-Ret with TK domain (Figs.1,4). The receptor for GDNF is a complex of GDNF receptor α-1 (GFRα-1), which is a GPI (glycosyl-phosphatidyl inositol)-linked (membrane-bound) ligand binding protein without intracellular domain, and c-Ret, which acts as the signal transducing domain (Fig.4). About 60% and 35% of the lumbar DRG neurons of rats expressed c-Ret and TrkA, respectively [8]. C-Ret-positive small DRG neurons are mostly devoid of TrkA (Fig.3 C,D), but 9 % of DRG neurons expressed both TrkA and c-Ret. Forty five percent of DRG neurons were positive for GFRα-1 mRNA and about 80 % of these neurons were labeled with c-ret mRNA signals. Not c-Ret but GFRα-1 mRNA expression was up-regulated in axotomized DRG neurons [8]. About 80% of small DRG neurons are TrkA-positive at prenatal stage (E15) in mice, but a half of them switches their dependence from NGF to GDNF after birth (P7) [9]. In GDNF-deficient mice a significant reduction (-23%) in the number of spinal sensory neurons was observed [10], while GFRα-1 deficient mice had a normal neuronal population in DRG [11]. Other members of GDNF family, neurturin (NTN), artemin (ART) and persephin (PSP) were discovered. GPI-linked ligand binding proteins, GFRα-2, GFRα-3 and GFRα-4, which are homologous to GFRα-1, were also identified and showed to bind preferentially NTN, ART and PSP, respectively. GFRα-1 and c-Ret mRNAs are also expressed by a significant number of large DRG neurons, most of which are origins of peritrichial A-fibers. GDNF receptor components are exclusively expressed by isolectin B4 (IB4) binding, c-Ret positive small neurons. Plant lectins are used to characterize the cell-surface carbohydrates expressed on DRG neurons. IB4-lectin is a galactose-binding plant lectin and widely used as a marker of a subset of small DRG neurons [12].

Expression of GDNF family receptor components by sensory neurons in addition to Trks adds some complexity to the classification of DRG neurons. GFRα-2 is expressed by about one third of DRG neurons, and also highly localized within the IB4 binding population of DRG neurons [13]. There is a high level of coexpression of different ligand binding domains such as GFRα-1 and GFRα-2. C-Ret/IB4 cells can be subdivided into four subpopulations based on their expression of the GFR subunits; GFRα-1 alone (20% of IB4 cells), GFRα-2 alone (30%), both GFRα-1 and GFRα-2 (30%) and neither GFRα-1 nor GFRα-2 (20%) [13]. Functional difference of these subgroups are not known, although a comparison of GDNF/GFRα-1 deficient and NTN/GFRα-2 deficient mice supports the hypothesis that GDNF and NTN exhibit a significant degree of functional specificity. In addition, ligand specificity of these GPI-linked proteins is still obscure. The fact that GDNF deficient mice suffer a more severe loss of DRG neurons, as compared with the GFRα-1 deficient mice [10,11] may suggest that survival effects of GDNF on DRG neurons are mediated by a second receptor. NTN-knockout animals demonstrate a 45% reduction in GFRα-2 expressing neurons in the DRG.

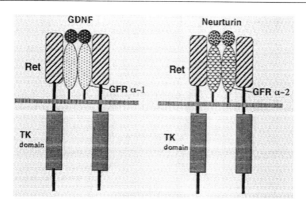

Figure 4. Receptor for GDNF is composed of GDNF binding protein GFR□-1 and signal transducing receptor c-Ret with TK domain. Other members of GDNF family, Neurturin, Artemin and Percephin bind to GFRα-2, GFRα-3, GFRα-4 domain, respectively.

CLASSIFICATION OF NOCICEPTORS (FIG.5)

Small DRG neurons are thus divided into at least two subgroups; one is NGF dependent and SP/CGRP positive and the other is dependent on GDNF family [14]. Central processes of these neurons differentially terminate in the dorsal horn, TrkA-positive and SP/CGRP containing C-fibers terminate in laminae I,IIo and considered to transmit inflammatory pain (see below). C-Ret-positive C-fibers terminate in lamina IIi, where protein kinase Cγ (PKCγ) containing dorsal horn neurons are packed. These fibers are considered to transmit neuropathic pain, since PKCγ knock-out mice do not exhibit neuropathic pain [15]. C-Ret-positive neurons are intensely labeled by IB4, but we found that more than 80% of TrkA-positive neurons are also labeled with IB4, although the staining intensity is weak [16] (Fig.5).

About 10% of DRG neurons synthesize SOM. We have shown that all the SOM-producing neurons are c-Ret-positive small ones [17], so they belong to the latter group. Roles of SOM in nociception are still obscure. The synthesis of SOM in DRG neurons starts ontogenetically very late (after 2 weeks postnatally) compared to that of SP, which is constantly seen from the prenatal stage. These findings coincide with the previous observation that GDNF dramatically increases SOM content in cultured DRG neurons from adult rats, but not in neonatal neurons [18].

It is well known that C-fibers are sensitive to capsaicin, the main pungent ingredient in "hot" chili peppers. Most of the SP-immunoreactive cells (more than 80%) were VR1 (vanilloid receptor 1)-positive, and 60~80% of IB4-labelled cells were also VR1-positive [19]. It should also be mentioned that most of the ATP-sensitive neurons expressing P2X3 receptor, a ligand-gated ion channel activated by ATP, are involved in the latter subgroup of small DRG neurons. P2X3 receptor immunoreactivity was observed in about 35% of the rat DRG neurons, virtually all small in diameter and labeled with IB4 [20]. In the dorsal horn, P2X3 receptor-immunoreactive terminals were restricted to lamina IIi. After sciatic nerve transection, P2X3 receptor expression dropped by more than 50% in L4,5 DRG and intrathecally delivered GDNF completely reversed axotomy-induced down-regulation of the

P2X3 receptor [20], confirming that small DRG neurons expressing P2X3 receptor are GDNF-dependent. P2X3 deficient mice have normal sensori-motor function, but showed enhanced thermal hyperalgesia in chronic inflammation and reduced pain-related behavior in formalin test [21]. Dorsal horn neurons of these animals were unable to respond to "warm" stimuli.

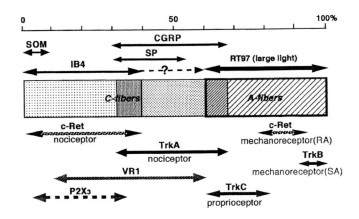

Figure 5. Schematic drawing to show chemically defined DRG neurons of the rat. About 60% of DRG neurons are small ones that give rise to C-fibers. They are divided into NGF-dependent (TrkA-positive) and GDNF family-dependent (c-Ret-positive) ones. IB4 lectin labels the latter group intensely, while it also labels the former weakly.

PHENOTYPIC CHANGES IN PATHOLOGICAL CONDITIONS

Peripheral inflammation increases the level of NGF in the tissue, which leads to up-regulation of synthesis of peptides and BDNF in TrkA-positive DRG neurons. Increased release of these substances in the dorsal horn may sensitize dorsal horn neurons, inducing spontaneous pain and hyperalgesia [22]. Systemic NGF treatment increases BDNF-immunoreactivity in DRG and in the dorsal horn [22].

On the other hand, nerve injury blocks the transport of NGF and down-regulates the production of these substances in small neurons, but the production of SP/CGRP/BDNF is up-regulated in large type A neurons [23,24,25]. Following nerve injury, large type A neurons acquire the ability to synthesize substances which are mainly expressed in small DRG neurons in normal condition. Preprotachykinin (PPT) mRNA is down-regulated in small neurons and up-regulated in large neurons [23]. These neurons project to the dorsal column nucleus (DCN) and transmit tactile or proprioceptive information. SP produced in large neurons is transported to the DCN. Therefore, SP-immunoreactive fibers are increased in the DCN of axotomized side. CGRP and BDNF mRNAs are also down-regulated in small neurons, and large neurons start to synthesize these substances after axotomy [24,25]. Electrical stimulation of injured nerve at C-fiber strength causes c-fos expression in the DCN of axotomized side, which is never seen in the DCN on the contralateral side or in control animals [23]. Peptides and BDNF released in the DCN may lead to activation of NMDA receptors and c-fos expression in DCN neurons. Thus, injured A-fibers obtain biochemical features of C-fibers, which may partly explain the symptom "allodynia" that characterizes peripheral neuropathic pain.

Nerve injury blocks the transport of NGF from the periphery, but on the other hand it may trigger the synthesis of various factors in injured peripheral nerve. These factors may up-regulate the production of peptides which are not expressed in intact DRG neurons such as vasoactive intestinal polypeptide (VIP), galanin and neuropeptide Y (NPY). Leukemia inhibitory factor (LIF) is one of the candidate factors responsible for these changes in neuropeptide phenotype. Intraneural injection of LIF into the intact sciatic nerve was shown to induce a significant increase in the number of galanin-immunoreactive neurons in the L4,5 DRG neurons [26]. Injection of IL-6 showed weaker but similar effects on DRG neurons. Moreover, the up-regulation of galanin-immunoreactivity in DRG neurons after axotomy was prevented by the treatment with antibody against gp130 at the proximal end of the transected nerve [26]. These findings indicate that IL-6 family cytokines, especially LIF and IL-6 may be responsible for the up-regulation of galanin in DRG neurons after axotomy.

Nerve injury causes marked increase of GFRα-1 (Fig.7) and GFRα-3 mRNAs in DRG neurons [8,27], while the expression of GFRα-2 was markedly reduced. The level of c-Ret mRNA was not changed. NTN and ART, novel members of the GDNF family bind to GFRα-2 and GFRα-3, respectively. Both GFRα-2 and GFRα-3 mRNAs are expressed principally in small DRG neurons [27]. ART may have trophic action on small diameter DRG neurons, particularly after nerve injury. Damaged sensory neurons are likely to become more sensitive to GDNF and ART and less sensitive to NTN.

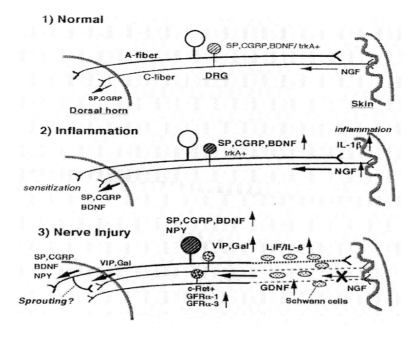

Figure 6. Schematic drawing to show the phenotype changes in DRG neurons in various pathological conditions, such as tissue inflammation and nerve injury.

DO Aβ-FIBERS SPROUT INTO LAMINA II AFTER NERVE INJURY?

The hypothesis that A-fibers sprout into lamina II after nerve injury is widely accepted as a pathogenetic mechanism of allodynia [28]. Cholera Toxin B (CTB) subunit is used as a marker of A-fibers, because it binds to GM1 ganglioside expressed on the surface of large DRG neurons [29]. When CTB is injected into the sciatic nerve of normal control rats, CTB-positive fibers are observed only in laminae III,IV and deeper layers of the dorsal horn. Lamina II is devoid of CTB staining, because it is occupied by CTB-negative C-fiber terminals. The application of CTB into the sciatic nerve axotomized 2~3 weeks before, CTB positive fibers are observed also in lamina II. Woolf et al. thought that nerve injury triggers the sprouting of A-fibers into lamina II [28].

However, there remains another possibility. If small neurons acquire the ability to take up CTB after nerve injury, it is reasonable to find CTB-positive fibers in the superficial laminae in axotomized animals. Recently Tong et al. [30] addressed this issue, and found that CTB is taken up by both small and large neurons after axotomy. We also looked at CTB staining in the DRG and confirmed the finding of the latter group; more numerous small neurons were labeled in axotomized DRG. Although the precise mechanism how small neurons obtain the ability to take up CTB after axotomy is not clear, we should be more cautious with the interpretation of CTB staining in the dorsal horn after nerve injury.

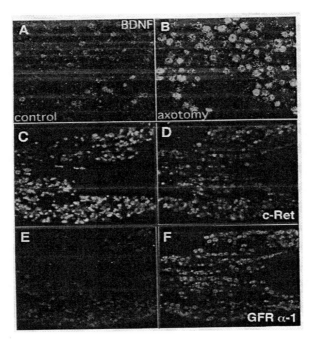

Figure 7. Photomicrographs showing expression of BDNF (A,B), c-Ret (C,D) and GFRα-1 (E,F) mRNAs in normal (A,C,E) and axotomized (B,D,F) DRG neurons. Note that axotomy markedly up-regulates BDNF mRNA expression in large neurons. Expression of c-Ret mRNA was not changed, while that of GFRα-1 mRNA was increased following axotomy.

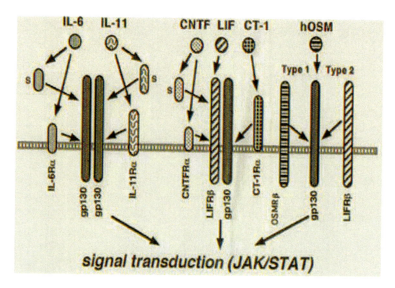

Figure 8. Receptors for IL-6 family cytokines (IL-6, IL-11, CNTF, LIF, CT-1, OSM) share a common signal transducer gp130 and LIFRβ. CNTF, ciliary neurotrophic factor; LIF, leukemia inhibitory factor; CT-1, cardiotrophin-1; hOSM, human oncostatin M; S, soluble form.

IL-6 FAMILY CYTOKINES

Receptors for IL-6 family cytokines, such as IL-6, IL-11, ciliary neurotrophic factor (CNTF), LIF, cardiotrophin-1(CT-1) and oncostatin M (OSM), share a common signal transducer gp130 [1]. Signal transduction of IL-6 and IL-11 requires homo-dimerization of gp130, and others such as LIF and CNTF require hetero-dimerization of LIFRβ with gp130 (Fig.8). IL-6 binds to IL-6R, and this IL-6/IL-6R complex then associates with gp130, allowing it to heterodimerize. LIF binds at low-affinity to LIFR. LIFR is then heterodimerized with gp130 to form the high affinity and signal transducing complex. The structures of LIFR and OSMR are closely related to gp130 and referred as the gp130-subfamily. These receptors do not have enzymatic motifs such as receptor tyrosine kinase in their structure, but their intracellular domains are associated with JAK family kinases such as JAK1, JAK2, Tyk2, phosphorylation of which then activate STAT3 (signal transducers and activators of transcription 3). Phosphorylation of other tyrosine residue of gp130 intracellular domain activates MAP kinase pathways. Class I (interleukins) and class II (interferons) cytokines bind to their receptors to activate specific kinds of JAK-STAT families. Most of DRG neurons express gp130 and LIFRβ mRNAs and small neurons are immunoreactive to JAK1, JAK2 and Tyk2 [31](Fig. 9). Probably through these signaling molecules, these cytokines, CNTF, LIF, OSM and CT-1, exert trophic effects on DRG neurons and support their survival [32].

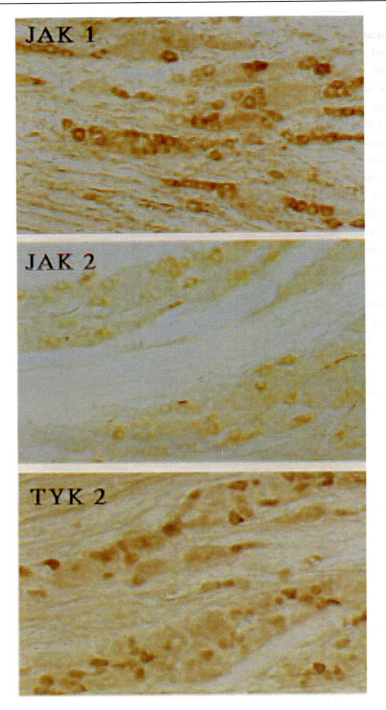

Figure 9. Photomicrographs showing that small DRG neurons are immunoreactive to JAK1, JAK2 and Tyk2.

There is contradictory evidence whether LIF is pro-inflammatory or anti-inflammatory. LIF is shown to serve as early anti-inflammatory and analgesic factor during peripheral inflammation [33]. LIF is synthesized by keratinocytes in response to TNF-α. On the other hand, null mutation of LIF impairs inflammatory response to injury, including recruitment of mast cells and macrophages, and injury-induced GFAP expression in Schwann cells [34], indicating that LIF plays important roles in the activation of inflammatory process. This discrepancy should be solved in future studies. When peripheral nerves are damaged, LIF is synthesized by Schwann cells in injured peripheral nerve and retrogradely transported to increase the synthesis of galanin in injured DRG neurons [26]. Since LIFRβ mRNA is up-regulated in axotomized DRG neurons (unpublished observation: E.S.), DRG neurons seem to become more sensitive to IL-6 family cytokines after nerve injury.

Injection of IL-6 into normal skin does not cause pain or hyperalgesia, because intact DRG neurons do not express IL-6R. Injection of IL-6 with soluble IL-6R causes hyperalgesia. Since IL-6 deficient mice show sensory impairments [35], IL-6 is assumed to be essential for the development and maintenance of sensory system. IL-6 is considered to stimulate the synthesis of galanin in DRG neurons and mediate hypersensitive responses, because induction of galanin after nerve injury was reduced in IL-6 knock-out mice [36]. It was also shown that IL-6 promotes the survival of DRG neurons and axonal regeneration of injured neurons. Nerve injury induces IL-6 mRNA in a subset of rat DRG neurons [37]. These findings suggest that IL-6 is essential to the maintenance of sensory functions and regeneration of axons after nerve injury.

We have recently demonstrated that OSMR is expressed in small DRG neurons which express both the VR1 and P2X3 receptors. OSM-deficient mice displayed significantly reduced responses to acute noxious stimuli, suggesting that OSM plays an essential role in the development of a subpopulation of nociceptive DRG neurons [38,39].

OTHER CYTOKINES

TNF-α, a member of class III cytokines, is also implicated in inflammatory and neuropathic pain [40,41]. Binding of TNF-α to TNFR1 activates various intracellular pathways, including 1) apoptotic pathway, 2) JNK (C-terminal kinase) and 3) NF-kB (Fig.10). Activation of NF-kB is considered to counteract the apoptotic pathway. TNF-α is synthesized by Schwann cells in injured nerve [42]. Application of TNF-α into the peripheral nerve causes hyperalgesia [41] and trapping TNF-α by antibodies can prevent the symptom. Since TNFR1 and R2 mRNAs are expressed by Schwann cells (unpublished observation: E.S.), TNF-α may exert its effects on primary afferent fibers probably through the activation of Schwann cells.

It is well known that IL-1β activates sensory nerve terminals and induces hyperalgesia [43,44]. IL-1α,β and IL-1ra (receptor antagonist) are ligands for IL-1R. IL-1 binds to IL-1R to form IL-1-Il-1R complex, which then activates signal transduction in the presence of IL-1R accessory protein (AcP). Both IL-1R and IL-1R-AcP do not possess intracellular domain with kinase activity. Association of MyD88 is necessary for signal transduction (Fig.10).

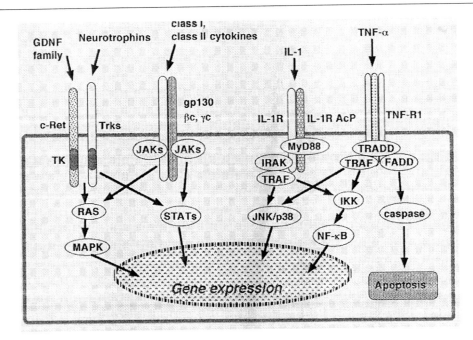

Figure 10. Schematic drawing showing cytokine receptors and signal transduction pathways. Receptors for neurotrophins and GDNF family have TK domain in their intracellular domain, while other receptors need the association of kinases or adapter proteins for further signal transduction. βc, common β chain; γc, common γ chain.

CONCLUDING REMARKS

Recent advances in our understanding of cytokine-mediated signal transduction and their effects on pain transmission system were discussed. There are many other cytokines, such as IL-2 and interferon-γ [45] that might be involved in pain mechanisms. Further studies focusing on the roles of cytokines in pain transmission system may provide us new tools for the treatment of chronic pain based on the molecular mechanisms.

REFERENCES

[1]   Kishimoto T., Taga T. and Akira S., Cytokine signal transduction. *Cell* 76:253-262, 1994.

[2]   Kashiba H., Noguchi K., Ueda Y. and Senba E., Coexpression of trk family members and low-affinity neurotrophin receptors in rat dorsal root ganglion neurons. *Mol. Brain Res.* 30:158-164, 1995.

[3]   Senba E and Kashiba H: Sensory afferent processing in multi-responsive DRG neurons, *Prog.Brain Res.* 113:387-410, 1996.

[4]   Kashiba H., Ueda Y. and Senba E., Coexpression of preprotachykinin A (PPTA), a-calcitonin gene related peptide (α-CGRP), somatostatin (SOM) and neurotrophin

receptor family mRNAs in rat dorsal root ganglion neurons. *Neuroscience* 70:179-189, 1996.

[5] Kashiba H., Nemoto K., Ueyama T. and Senba E., Relationship between BDNF- and Trk-expressing neurons in rat dorsal root ganglion: an analysis by in situ hybridization. *Neuroreport*, 8:1229-1234, 1997.

[6] Caroll P., Lewin G.R., Kolzenburg M., Toyka K.V. and Thoenen H., A role for BDNF in mechanosensation. *Nature Neurosci.* 1:42-46, 1998.

[7] Indo Y., Tsuruta M., Hayashida Y., Azharul Karim M., Ohta K., Kawano T., Mitsubuchi H., Tonoki H., Awaya Y. and Matsuda I., Mutations in the TRKA/NGF receptor gene in patients with congenital insensitivity to pain with anhidrosis. *Nature Genet.*13:485-488, 1996.

[8] Kashiba H., Hyon B. and Senba E., Glial cell line-derived neurotrophic factor and nerve growth factor receptor mRNAs are expressed in distinct subgroups of dorsal root ganglion neurons and are differentially regulated by peripheral axotomy in the rat. *Neurosci. Lett.* 252:107-110, 1998.

[9] Molliver D.C., Wright D.E., Leitner M.L., Parsadanian A.S., Doster K., Wen D., Yan Q. and Snider W.D., IB4-binding DRG neurons switch from NGF to GDNF dependence in early postnatal life. *Neuron* 19:849-861, 1997.

[10] Moore M.W., Klein R.D., Farinas I., Sauer H., Armanini M., Phillips H., Reichardt L.F., Ryan A.M., Carver-Moore K. and Rosenthal A., Renal and Neuronal abnormalities in mice lacking GDNF. *Nature* 382:76-79, 1996.

[11] Cacalano G., Farinas I., Wang L-C., Hagler K., Forgie A., Moore M., Armanini M., Phillips H., Ryan A.M., Reichardt L.F., Hynes M., Davies A. and Rosenthal A., GFRα-1 is an essential receptor component for GDNF in the developing nervous system and kidney. *Neuron* 21:53-62, 1998.

[12] Silverman J.D. and Kruger L., Selective neuronal glycoconjugate expression and autonomic ganglia: relation of lectin reactivity to peptide and enzyme markers. *J. Neurocytol.* 19:789-801, 1990.

[13] Bennett D.L.H., Michael G.J., Ramachandran N. Munson J.B., Averill S. Yan Q., McMahon S.B. and Priestley J.V., A distinct subgroup of small DRG cells express GDNF receptor components and GDNF is protective for these neurons after nerve injury. *J. Neurosci.* 18:3059-3072, 1998.

[14] Snider W.D. and McMahon S.B.: Tackling pain at the source: new ideas about nociceptors. *Neuron* 20: 629-632, 1998.

[15] Malmberg A.B., Chen C., Tonegawa S. and Basbaum A.I., Preserved acute pain and reduced neuropathic pain in mice lacking PKCgamma. *Science* 278:279-283, 1997.

[16] Kashiba H., Uchida Y. and Senba E., Difference in binding by isolectin B4 to trkA and c-ret mRNA-expressing neurons in rat sensoty ganglia. *Mol. Brain Res.* 95:18-26, 2001.

[17] Kashiba H. and Senba E., Delayed expression of somatostatin mRNA in GDNFs-dependent rat sensory neurons during postnatal development. Develop. *Brain Res.* 125:147-152, 2000.

[18] Adler J.E., Age-dependent differential regulation of sensory neuropeptides by glial cell line-derived neurotrophic factor. *J. Neurochem.* 71:170-177, 1998.

[19] Tominaga M., Caterina M.J., Malmberg A.B., Rosen T.A., Gilbert H., Skinner K., Raumann B.E., Basbaum A.I. and Julius D., The cloned capsaicin receptor integrates multiple pain-producing stimuli. *Neuron* 21:531-543, 1998.

[20] Bradbury E.J., Burnstock G. and McMahon S.B., The expression of P2X3 purinoreceptors in sensory neurons: effects of axotomy and glial-derived neurotrophic factor. Mol. Cell. *Neurosci.* 12:256-68, 1998.

[21] Souslova V., Cesare P., Ding Y., Akopian A.N., Stanfa L., Suzuki R., Carpenter K., Dickenson A., Boyce S., Hill R., Nebenius-Oosthuizen D., Smith A.J.H., Kidd E.J. and Wood J.N., Warm-coding deficits and aberrant inflammatory pain in mice lacking P2X3 receptors. *Nature* 407:1015-1017,2000.

[22] Thompson S.W.N., Bennett D.L.H., Kerr B.J., Bradbury E.J. and McMahon S.B., Brain-derived neurotrophic factor is an endogenous modulator of nociceptive responses in the spinal cord. Proc. *Natl. Acad. Sci.* USA 96:7714-7718, 1999.

[23] Noguchi K., Kawai Y., Fukuoka T., Senba E. and Miki K., Substance P induced by peripheral nerve injury in primary afferent sensory neurons and its effect on dorsal column nucleus neurons. *J. Neurosci.* 15:7633-7643, 1995.

[24] Miki K., Fukuoka T., Tokunaga A. and Noguchi K., Calcitonin gene-related peptide increase in the rat spinal dorsal horn and dorsal column nucleus following peripheral nerve injury: Up-regulation in a subpopulation of primary afferent sensory neurons. *Neuroscience* 82:1243-1252, 1998.

[25] Kashiba H and Senba E: Up- and down-regulation of BDNF mRNA in distinct subgroups of rat sensory neurons after axotomy. *Neuroreport* 10:3561-3565, 1999.

[26] Thompson S.W.N, Priestley J.V. and Southall A: GP130 cytokines, leukemia inhibitory factor and interleukin-6, induce neuropeptide expression in intact adult rat sensory neurons in vivo: Time-course, specificity and comparison with sciatic nerve axotomy. *Neuroscience* 84: 1247-1255, 1998.

[27] Bennett D.L.H., Boucher T.J., Armanini M.P., Poulsen K.T., Michael G.J., Priestley J.V., Phillips H.S., McMahon S.B. and Shelton D.L., The glial cell line-derived neurotrophic factor family receptor components are differentially regulated within sensory neurons after nerve injury. *J. Neurosci.* 20:427-437, 2000.

[28] Woolf C.J., Shortland P., Reynolds M., Ridings J., Doubell T. and Coggeshall R.E., Reorganization of central terminals of myelinated primary afferents in the rat dorsal horn following peripheral axotomy. J. Comp. *Neurol.* 360:121-134, 1995.

[29] Robertson B. and Grant G., Immunocytochemical evidence for the localization of the GM1 ganglioside in carbonic anhydrase-containing and RT 97-immunoreactive rat primary sensory neurons. *J. Neurocytol.* 18:77-86, 1989.

[30] Tong Y-G., Wang H.F., Ju G., Grant G., Hokfelt T. and Zhang X., Increased uptake and transport of cholera toxin B-subunit in dorsal root ganglion neurons after peripheral axotomy: Possible implications for sensory sprouting. *J.Comp. Neurol.* 404:143-158, 1999.

[31] Mizuno M., Kondo E., Nishimura M., Ueda Y., Yoshiya I., Tohyama M. and Kiyama H., Localization of molecules involved in cytokine receptor signaling in the rat trigeminal ganglion. *Mol Brain Res* 44: 163-166, 1997.

[32] Thier M, Hall M, Heath J.K., Pennica, D. and Weis J., Trophic effects of cardiotrophin-1 and interleukin-11 on rat dorsal root ganglion neurons in vitro. *Mol Brain Res* 64:80-84, 1999.

[33] Banner L.R., Patterson P.H, Allchorne A., Poole S. and Woolf C.J., Leukemia inhibitory factor is an anti-inflammatory and analgesic cytokine. *J Neurosci* 18:5456-5462, 1998.

[34] Sugiura S., Lahav R., Han J., Kou S.Y., Banner L.R., de Pablo F., Patterson P.H.. Leukaemia inhibitory factor is required for normal inflammatory responses to injury in the peripheral and central nervous systems in vivo and is chemotactic for macrophages in vitro.Eur. *J. Neurosci.* 12:457-466, 2000.

[35] Zhong J., Dietzel I.D., Wahle P., Kopf M. and Heumann R., Sensory impairments and delayed regeneration of sensory axons in interleukin-6-deficient mice. *J. Neurosci.* 19:4305-4313, 1999.

[36] Murphy P.G., Pamer M.S., Borthwick L., Gauldie J., Richardson P.M. and Bisby M.A.: Endogenous interleukin-6 contributes to hypersensitivity to cutaneous stimuli and changes in neuropeptides associated with chronic nerve constriction in mice. Eur. *J. Neurosci.* 11:2243-2253, 1999.

[37] Tamura S., Morikawa Y. Miyajima A. and Senba E., Expression of oncostatin M receptor β in a specific subset of nociceptive sensory neurons. Eur. *J. Neurosci.* 17:2287-2298, 2003.

[38] Morikawa Y., Tamura S., Minehata K., Donovan P.J., Miyajima A. and Senba E. Essential function of oncostatin M in nociceptive neurons of dorsal root ganglia. *J. Neurosci.* 24:1941-1947, 2004.

[39] Murphy P.G., Grondin J., Altares M. and Richardson P.M., Induction of interleukin-6 in axotomized sensory neurons. *J. Neurosci.*, 15:5130-5138, 1995.

[40] Woolf C.J., Allchorne A., Safieh-Garabedian B. and Poole S., Cytokines, nerve growth factor and inflammatory hyperalgesia: the contribution of tumor necrosis factor alpha. Brit. *J. Pharmacol.* 121:417-24, 1997.*Neuroscience* 73:625-629, 1996.

[41] Wagner R. and Myers R.R., Endoneurial injection of TNF-α produces neuropathic pain behaviors. *Neuroreport* 7:2897-2901, 1996.

[42] Wagner R. and Myers R.R., Schwann cells produce tumor necrosis factor alpha: expression in injured and non-injured nerves.

[43] Fukuoka H., Kawatani M. Hisamitsu T. and Takeshige C., Cutaneous hyperalgesia induced by peripheral injection of interleukin-1 beta in the rat. *Brain Res.* 657:133-140, 1994.

[44] Watkins L.R., Maier S.F. and Goehler L.E., Immune activation: the role of pro-inflammatory cytokines in inflammation, illness responses and pathological pain states. *Pain* 63:289-302, 1995.

[45] Robertson B., Xu X.-J. Hao J.-X., Wiesenfeld-Hallin Z., Mhlanga J., Grant G. and Kristensson K., Interferon-γ receptors in nociceptive pathways: role in neuropathic pain-related behavior. *Neuroreport* 8:1311-1316, 1997.

In: The Handbook of Chronic Pain
Editors: S. Kreitler, D. Beltrutti, et al., pp. 41-56

ISBN 978-1-60021-044-0
© 2007 Nova Science Publishers, Inc.

Chapter 3

Taxonomy and Classification of Pain

P. Prithvi Raj

Taxonomy means "taxis", and nomon means "rules" in Greek. It defines classification of living and extinct organisms. In clinical practice the word taxonomy means the "systematic classification of subjects", sorted into groups to reflect similarity, with generally broader groups residing over those that are more restricted. An orderly arrangement in chronic pain is an immense task, and many systems have been proposed. Whatever system is created needs to have a wide enough application to cover both clinical practice and research and not just some bureaucratic regulations. It is reasonable to ask why taxonomy is necessary. The reason is that physicians face problems in dealing with complex and chronic pain, and a clear understanding of pain syndromes is needed in order to treat them effectively and reliably. Some of the problems faced with pain include: 1) Inexact definition of pain, 2) Difficult and unreliable method to measure or quantify pain,and 3)Observer bias in assessing a patient's behavior, which quantifies the intensity of pain.

THE NEED FOR STANDARDIZATION OF PAIN NOMENCLATURE

Pain, as a presenting problem for symptom, remains one of the most common reasons patients seek help form health care professionals. Frequently, this pain is identified and treated, although for a significant number of patients the pain never goes away. Some persistent pains have identifiable causes, but in quite a few cases there is no known etiology. Persistent pain may affect the elderly, the worker, the housewife, the cancer patient, the stroke patient, and sometimes even the paraplegic. These difficult pain syndromes are managed daily by almost all medical specialists, ranging from general practitioners to neurologists, from neurosurgeons to orthopedists, from physiatrists to psychiatrists and anesthesiologists. Different specialists treat pain problems in different ways depending on their particular discipline. What is needed is a common body of knowledge about pain that helps define the problem, standardizes or verifies different treatments, allows measurements and enables comparing treatment outcomes for both clinicians and clinical researchers.

The need for a common language was realized by John Bonica quite early in his career. He expressed it eloquently in an editorial in the journal, *Pain*. [3] There he described the contemporary condition of pain medicine as a "Tower of Babel." Harold Merskey, who chaired the International Association of Study of Pain (IASP) subcommittee on taxonomy, emphasized the importance of taxonomy to clinicians and highlighted the important benefits of effectively classifying pain syndromes. [4]

Wilson [5] wrote in an editorial that the time has surely arrived when the collective ingenuity of algologists could devise a classification system that could accurately describe the pain syndrome in terms useful for diagnosis and relevant for therapy.

Today, with the widespread use of the Internet and World Wide Web, as well as the penetration of managed care and the insistence on outcome data, this need for pain classification has taken on a new meaning. Physicians treating pain symptoms, specialists coping with complex pain problems, patients suffering from intractable pain, insurers, workmen's compensation agencies, and pain researchers are constantly reviewing classification systems looking for solutions to their pain problems. Well-defined terminologies and clearly stated categories of pain syndromes will go a long way to help them. Classifications are also an essential part of the "language of health" that is being created for the electronic clinical record.[6]

HISTORY OF CLASSIFICATIONS IN MEDICAL DISCIPLINES

Syndenham in 1676 is credited with the introduction of classification in medicine. At that time the objective was to identify the disease in order to predict the prognosis. Later, with the progress in clinical pathology and technology, the framework of classification changed, but the main purpose remained the same. Unlike chemistry and biology, where impressive natural and phylogenetic classifications exist, medical classifications are far from perfect. Ideally, classes of a satisfactory taxonomy must be mutually exclusive and jointly exhaustive. Complete consistency is beyond the hope of any medical system of classification. [4] In clinical practice and in planning services the need exists for a disease-specific classification. [7]

The historical fluxes in medical understanding are reflected by the inconsistency in taxonomies. In medical classification, one finds, side by side, diagnostic categories based on pathology (cancer), pathophysiology (diabetes), nosology (fibromyalgia), functional complaints (constipation), symptom diagnosis (abdominal pain), and problem behaviors (drug abuse). [8] Maltred [1] described this unstructured approach as a sign of the pragmatic attitudes in clinical medicine, which are not always compatible with the image of medicine as a scientific and strictly logical discipline. Before discussing pain classification, some of the major classifications in medicine are briefly described.

DEFINITION OF PAIN

The International Association for the Study of Pain (IASP) defines pain is "an unpleasant sensory and emotional experience associated with actual or potential tissue damage or described in terms of such damage." [1-3] In this definition, it is important to emphasize that pain is always subjective, a sensation, and unpleasant; and we are urged to evaluate both the physical and the nonphysical components of the experience called *pain*. Pain is actually a construct or concept. [2] It is a function of the personal theoretic orientation of the health professional. For instance, a neurosurgeon who sees pain only as a neuroanatomic or neurophysiologic event will not see the psychologic aspects of pain as significant. On the other hand, the psychologist will understand pain to be an integration of physical, psychologic, and social factors and will apply emotional, environmental, and psycho-physiologic questions to patients in search of variations within these realms. Thus two qualified specialists can come up with very different impressions of a patient's pain.

Chronic pain really means that the pain is not acute. [3] This is pain that persists in spite of good therapy and sometimes extraordinary treatment. The problem with chronic pain is that it can interfere with the patient's attitude concerning health and recovery, behaviors, and lifestyle. Furthermore, these patients suffer. In fact, the emotional/psychosocial influence on pain has been highlighted by Twycross. [4] He assessed factors that affected the pain threshold (the point at which a given stimulus provokes the report of pain from a patient) in hospice patients in England. He listed conditions, such as discomfort, insomnia, fatigue, anxiety, fear, anger, and depression as factors that would tend to lower a patient's threshold. On the other hand, the threshold could be raised by relief of pain, restful sleep, relaxation, sympathy and understanding, elevation of mood, and diversion from the pain.

Pain is clearly a multidimensional experience. It is neurophysiologic, biochemical, psychological, ethnocultural, religious, cognitive, affective, and environmental. Thus its classification can be understandably complex and its management elusive at worst and difficult at best. It results in physiologic, anatomic, and behavioral changes that persist even when the original pathology is removed.

ACUTE VERSUS CHRONIC PAIN

Table 1 characterizes the differences between acute and chronic pain based upon clinical features. These two entities are different diseases; each is characterized by the knowledge base required to evaluate and manage them. The knowledge is derived from the clinical experience gained by healthcare professionals who choose to deal with pain patients. They consider the extent of the patient's body involvement with pain and the time it takes for the chronic pain syndrome to develop; the nervous system responses to either the acute or the ongoing pain; the possibility that adverse behavioral consequences will develop; and that all treatments done for acute pain may make chronic pain worse.

Table 1. Acute versus chronic pain

Acute pain	Chronic pain
Ample training and opportunity	Less so
Evaluation and R_x takes less time	Time consuming
Pain is a useful signal	Pain is a disease affecting attitudes, lifestyles and behavior
Pain plus anxiety	Pain plus frustration
Usually self-limiting/short R_x	Persists/long R_x
Individual problem	Pain is more than the patient
Priority of R_x options	Different than for acute
Patient *needs* to be in tune with R_x goals	Less so
Likelihood of success with proper R_x	Less so
Expectations of R_x are high	Less so

CHRONIC PAIN

Feuerstein presented the components of an operational definition for chronic pain. [2] In this categorization, he found the following components important:

1. Pain sensation
2. Pain behavior
3. Functional status at work (this basically involves the traditional ergonomic considerations)
4. Functional status at home (this includes not just the physical environment, but evaluation of the family interaction system based upon roles that each member plays, the communications that occur, and the problem-solving skills that are available to individuals and within the family unit)
5. The emotional state of the patient (this plays a significant role in the initiation, exacerbation, and maintenance of chronic pain; again, pain is not all physical and this important component must be evaluated)
6. Somatic preoccupation (this reflects the patient's ability to focus on bodily symptoms, almost to the exclusion of the ability to function)

TAXONOMY AND CLASSIFICATION OF PAIN

Single axis classification systems based on the previous components merely distinguish acute from chronic pain or describe cancer pain syndromes. These systems generally become inadequate when descriptors and qualifiers are needed beyond the simple, primary designation for purposes of exacting exchange of information. [5,6] The IASP subcommittee on Taxonomy created the first multiaxial system, based upon the region of the body involved in chronic pain, the organ systems affected, the temporal characteristics and pattern of the pain, the duration and intensity, and the etiology. [1,3,5,6]

Table 2 presents the five-axis pain taxonomy. Axis I deals with the regions where the pain occurs (Table 3). Axis II details the systems of the body, which are involved in the pain (Table 4). Axis III describes the temporal characteristics of the pain with attention to the pattern of occurrence (Table 5). Axis IV is based on statements of intensity provided by the patient, which indicate the time since onset of the pain (Table 6). Table 7 demonstrates the components of Axis V, which is based on the etiology of the patient's pain.

Table 2. The IASP Five-Pain Taxonomy: Overview

Axis I	Region
Axis II	System
Axis III	Temporal characteristics of pain: pattern of occurrence
Axis IV	Patient's statement of intensity: time since onset of pain
Axis V	Etiology

Table 3. Axis I: Regions*

Region	Code
Head, face, and mouth	000
Cervical region	100
Upper shoulder and upper limbs	200
Thoracic region	300
Abdominal region	400
Lower back, lumbar spine, sacrum, and coccyx	500
Lower limbs	600
Pelvic region	700
Anal, perineal, and genital region	800
More than three major sites	900

From Merskey H: classification of chronic pain, Descriptions of chronic pain syndromes and definitions of pain terms. *Pain Supp* 3:S10, 1986.

* Record main site first. If there are two important regions, record separately. If there is more than one site of pain, separate coding will be necessary.

Table 4. Axis II: Systems

System	Code
Nervous system (central, peripheral, and autonomic)	00
And special senses; physical disturbance or dysfunction Nervous system (psychological and social)	10
Respiratory and cardiovascular systems	20
Musculoskeletal system and connective tissue	30
Cutaneous and subcutaneous, and associated glands (breast, apocrine, etc.)	40
Gastrointestinal system	50
Genitourinary system	60
Other organs or viscera (e.g., thyroid, lymphatic, hemopoietic)	70
More than one system	80

From Merskey H: Classification of chronic pain. Descriptions of chronic pain syndromes and definitions of pain terms. *Pain Suppl* 3:S10, 1986.

Table 5. Axis III: Temporal characteristics of pain

Pattern of occurrence	Code
Not recorded, not applicable, or not known	0
Single episode, limited duration (e.g., ruptured aneurysm, sprained ankle)	1
Continuous or nearly continuous, nonfluctuating (e.g., low back pain)	2
Continuous or nearly continuous, fluctuating severity (e.g., ruptured intervertebral	3
disk)	4
Recurring, irregularly (e.g., headache, mixed type)	5
Recurring, regularly (e.g., premenstrual pain)	6
Paroxysmal (e.g. tic douloureux)	7
Sustained with superimposed paroxysms)	8
Other combinations	9
None of the above	

From Merskey H: Classification of chronic pain. Descriptions of chronic pain syndromes and definitions of pain terms. *Pain Suppl* 3:S10, 1986.

Table 6. Axis IV: Statement of intensity: Time since onset of pain

Time		Code
Not recorded, not applicable, or not known		.0
Mild		
	1 month or less	.1
	1 month to 6 months	.2
Medium:	More than 6 months	.3
	1 month or less	.4
	1 month to 6 months	.5
Severe:	More than 6 months	.6
	1 month or less	.7
	1 month to 6 months	.8
	More than 6 months	.9

From Merskey H: Classification of chronic pain. Descriptions of chronic pain syndromes and definitions of pain terms. *Pain Suppl* 3:S10, 1986.

Table 7. Axis V: Etiology

Etiology	Code
Genetic or congenital disorders (e.g., congenital dislocation)	.00
Trauma, operation, burns.	.01
Infective, parasitic.	.02
Inflammatory (no known infective agent) immune reactions	.03
NeoplasmToxic, metabolic (e.g., alcoholic neuropathy, anoxia,	.04
vascular, nutritional, endocrine) radiation	.05
Degenerative, mechanical Dysfunctional (including	.06
psychophysiological)	.07
Unknown or other Origin is psychological* (e.g., conversion hysteria,	.08
Depressive hallucination)	.09

From Merskey H: Classification of chronic pain. Descriptions of chronic pain syndromes and definitions of pain terms. *Pain Suppl* 3:S10, 1986. *No physical cause should be held to be present nor any pathophysiologic mechanism.

Advantages

The advantages of the IASP five region system are: [1,3]

1. This was developed by a multidisciplinary association that is widely diversified in geography and expertise.
2. IASP publishes a respected and well-circulated journal so taxonomy is well distributed.
3. The system should be easy to adopt because it is based on five axes already used in medicine.
4. It is a starting point for a complex task.

The IASP system is provisional, yet it is a framework and a place to begin. Using the system should improve spoken and written communication by standardizing the recording of symptoms, complaints, and observations; the reporting of research; and the exchange of information. As a result there would be improvement in the relevance of research and in the management of pain throughout the world.

Disadvantages

It is clearly hard to be mutually exclusive and completely exhaustive with any system. The IASP system uses some natural breakouts and some that are artificial but convenient.

Ventafridda and Caraceni criticized the IASP system for shedding little light on the classification issue. They felt that the system was just a list of diseases and lesions that cause pain. [7] They cautioned that physicians should beware of using terms that deny the physical component of pain, and would thereby influence treatment choices.

Procacci and Maresca noted that in trying to deal with international populations of patients linguistic and philological issues, and the operative applicability of the taxonomy would need to be addressed. [8] There would also be epistemological issues. One of their fundamental points is that the physician needs to be able to use the system, and their criticism of the IASP system was that it was too elaborate and difficult for the ordinary physician to use.

CONTROVERSY

Turk and Rudy suggested that the lack of a universally accepted classification system has resulted in a lot of confusion, and that investigators and physicians are unable to compare observations and results of research. [9] They noted that an infinite number of classification systems can be developed deductively, depending upon the rationale behind common factors believed to differentiate diagnoses. Their data suggested that the psychosocial and behavioral responses associated with chronic pain are common to a diverse sample of pain patients despite the differences in demographic characteristics and medical diagnoses. They have proved that taxonomy is still an issue and that so far there does not exist a universal system.

International Classification of Diseases (Icd)

IDC is published by the World Health Organization (WHO) and is used primarily for the statistical purpose of documenting mortality and morbidity worldwide. [9] At present, in the United States, ICD-9C is widely used, even though ICD-10 was published in 1992. [10] In the term ICD-9CM, CM stands for "clinical modification." This modification is published by national governments to provide the additional data required by clinicians, researchers, epidemiologists, medical record librarians, and administrators of inpatient and outpatient community programs. The coding system consists of three volumes: volume 1 is a tabular list of numeric codes; volume 2 is an alphabetical index of diseases; and volume 3 is a list of procedural codes. Volumes 1 and 2 are needed to determine the appropriate code for the patient's condition, whereas volume 3 is used mainly by hospitals. [11]

Pain specialists require a more detailed framework of classification than the general systems available, so it may be said that in ICD-9, insofar as pain is concerned, the classification is in a state of disarray. [11] With regard to chronic pain, it is very important to establish a system of classification that goes beyond general international classification systems like the ICD.

Diagnostic and Statistical Manual of Mental Disorders (DSM) [12]

The need to classify mental disorders has been clear throughout the history of medicine, but there has been little agreement concerning which disorders should be included and about t the optimal method to organize them.

The initial impetus for developing a classification of mental disorders was the need to collect statistical information for a general census. Out of this need grew the *Diagnostic and Statistical Manual of Mental Disorder (DSM)* published by the American Psychiatric Association. DSM-1 was developed as a variant of the ICD-6 in 1952. Since then the developers of the DSM have worked closely with ICD developers and have improved and modified this classification to make it compatible with the ICD. The codes and terms provided in the latest version, DSM-IV (1994), are fully compatible with ICD-9CM and ICD-10. This type of cooperation is very useful and mutually beneficial. It may serve as a model of collaboration for other medical disciplines.

The Basic Divisions of the DSM-IV are as follows:

Axis I	Clinical Psychiatric Diagnosis
Axis II	Personality Disorders/Mental Retardation
Axis III	General Medical Condition
Axis IV	Psychosocial and Environmental Problems
Axis V	Global Assessment of Functioning

Another attractive feature of the DSM-IV classification is its usefulness in multi-axial assessment, which allows for evaluation on several axes, each of which refers to a different domain of information that may help the clinical plan treatment and predict outcome. A multi-axial system provides a convenient format for organizing and communicating clinical information, for capturing the complexity of clinical situations, and for describing the heterogeneity of individuals presenting with the same diagnosis.

A drawback of the DSM-IV with regard to pain is that it emphasizes the assessment of mental functioning and psychopathology, which is not suitable for the majority of patients with chronic pain. [13]

EMORY PAIN ESTIMATE MODEL (EPEM)

Probably the first attempt at evidence-based integration of the multi-axial assessment of pain was proposed by Brena and Koch [25] in the form of the EPEM. [26] Brena developed a two-dimensional strategy where the presence of pathology and behavior were the axes. Then, using the median division of these dimensions, four classes of chronic pain were created. These classes have proved useful in established triage and prognosis in certain groups of pain patients, specifically those with chronic low back pain and chronic headache.

Turk and Rudy [23] highlight some of the basic theoretical and quantitative problems of this model and recommend that the EPEM be viewed as a conceptual model rather than an adequately operationized empirical one. They feel that this model of establishing classification may lead to erroneous or nonindependent patient assignment, since it is derived from external mathematical criteria rather than from divisions or clustering occurring within patient groups.

MULTI-AXIAL ASSESSMENT OF PAIN (MAP)

Psychologists play an important role in the delivery of clinical services to chronic pain patients. Their involvement is based on evidence supporting the important cognitive [27] and affective, [28] contributions to the perception and reporting of pain. To address this aspect, in 1987 Turk and Rudy [30] proposed a classification system for chronic pain patients based on the empirical integration of psychosocial and behavioral data that they label the Multi-axial Assessment of Pain (MAP). Turk and Rudy [31] identified three unique subgroups of chronic pain patient and labeled them (1) dysfunctional, (2) interpersonally distressed, and (3) minimizers/ adaptive copers. Their primary hypothesis was that certain modal psychosocial and behavioral response patterns recur in chronic pain patients and that these patterns represent somewhat homogeneous subgroups of chronic pain patients, independent of medical diagnosis. In their study, they cross-validate and confirm the uniqueness and accuracy of the taxonomy.

The instrument they used to collect data is the Multidimensional Pain Inventory (MPI). [31] MPI has the advantage of having been standardized on a population of patients with chronic pain.

The MAP classification system seems to have good reliability and external validity. Its robustness was tested on three common but diverse groups of chronic pain patients. The data suggested, that despite differences in demographic characteristics and medical diagnosis among patients with chronic low back pain, headache, and temporomandibular disorders, the psychosocial and behavioral responses associated with chronic pain are common. [32]

A polydiagnostic approach was suggested in the hope that it would serve to encourage the clinicians and researchers to think concurrently in terms of two different diagnostic systems - biomedical and psychosocial-behavioral - that may prove complementary for the pain patient.

CLASSIFICATION IN PAIN MEDICINE

Because of its subjective nature, pain is very difficult to classify, especially chronic pain. Turk and Rudy [23] address classification strategies in chronic pain. Conceptually, two important considerations are (1) the approach to classification and (2) the dimensions of a classification.

The theoretical approach to classification involves testing predetermined theoretical formulations in the classification, whereas the empirical approach is inductive and tries to identify naturally occurring sets of variables that characterize various sub-groups. The other systematic input comes from various pain specialists. Emphasis was placed on the description of each pain syndrome in a detailed format. Each description is detailed enough to allow the pain practitioner to identify the pain syndrome encountered in practice and to help codify it. IASP was instrumental in changing the name of the condition recognized as *reflex sympathetic dystrophy* to *complex regional pain syndromes*. [4] IASP definition of pain and other pain-related terms are widely accepted by the general medical community, but the coding system is not used frequently.

In 1988 Vervest [21] reported numerous overlap problems with the first classification. In the second edition he helped to correct them. [4]

Turk [22] did a preliminary assessment of reliability of the IASP taxonomy. He found overall axis I reliability was excellent, although several subcategories were not found to be very reliable. For axis V, overall observed agreement was 68%, in contrast to the 38% agreement rate expected by chance. The other criticism of the IASP classification [23] is in the emphasis placed on pain site to the exclusion of psychosocial and behavioral factors; in addition, the system has limited use in identifying patients who have problems managing their pain. Siddall [24] notes that no attempt was made in the revised edition (1994) to define or categorize pain that occurs after spinal cord injury. Despite these limitations, criticisms, or even omissions, [24] the IASP classification remains a monumental international effort that should be used more extensively. Periodic revision or even alterations so as to render it more comprehensive may also be helpful.

An important consideration in classification systems is the dimension,that is, the nature of the information that will be used in assigning categories. Merksey states that classification systems in medicine (especially pain) must be comprehensive but cannot always be consistent. The most important requirement is that they should be practical. [11]

Various attempts have been made to classify pain, but many pertain to a particular category only. Some of the most common categories are described here, followed by classifications (Table 8). Editor: insert here table 8 which is typed now on pp. 16-17 below.

Table 8. Some Commonly Used Categories of Pain

1) Neurophysiologic Mechanism
    a) Nociceptive
    b) Somatic
    c) Visceral
    d) Neuropathic (nonnociceptive)
        i)   Neuropathic
        ii) Central
        iii) Peripheral
    e) Psychogenic
2) Temporal (time-related)
    a) Acute
    b) Chronic

3) Etiological
    a) Cancer pain
    b) Post-herpatic Neuralgia
    c) Pain of Sickle Cell Disease
    d) Pain of Arthritis
4) Regional Pain
    a) Headache
    b) Profacial pain
    c) Low back pain

NOCICEPTIVE CATEGORY

The nociceptive category describes a laboratory prototype pain and can be seen mainly as an unpleasant sensation. Nociceptors have been identified in all tissues and organs except the nervous system. Nociceptors are stimulated by noxious stimuli, which are transmitted via pain fibers to the spinal cord and from there are projected to the thalamus and ultimately perceived as pain by the cerebral cortex. Traditionally these pain pathways have been discussed using the most restrictive definition of pain. [14] However, this is more or less a laboratory or experimental condition that is hard to duplicate fully in clinical situations.

The nociceptive category is subdivided into somatic and visceral pain. The fundamental difference between them is that somatic pain is carried along the sensory fibers, while visceral pain may be carried by autonomic (sympathetic) fibers.

It is very difficult to determine the relative contribution of the somatic and visceral systems to a particular pain. It is likely that there is an autonomic component to every pain. [15]

Somatic pain is more intense and discrete, whereas visceral pain is diffuse and poorly localized; the phenomenon of referred pain often causes difficulty in evaluation. Overall, the nociceptive category of pain is relatively easy to diagnose and manage.

NEUROPATHIC CATEGORY

Commonly accepted terminology for nonnociceptive pain is neuropathic pain. As already mentioned, nociceptors are not found in the central nervous system. Neuropathic pain is defined as pain produced by an alteration of neurological structure and/or function. The main difference separating neuropathic from nociceptive pain is the absence of continuous nociceptive input. Patrick Wall [16] described four possible mechanisms of peripheral neuropathic pain, as follows:

1. The "gate" might be caused to malfunction.
2. The nerve might become mechanically sensitive and generate an ectopic impulse.
3. There might be a cross talk between large and small fibers.
4. There might be damage in the central processing function.

Central Neuropathic Pain Category

Pain caused by a lesion in the central nervous system, such as thalamic pain, post-stroke pain, post-paraplegia pain, or post-quadriplegia pain. These pain syndromes are among the most therapeutically challenging categories to manage.

Peripheral Neuropathic Pain Category

Lesions in the peripheral nervous system may be responsible for a persistent pain state, that is, CRPS II (causalgia), post-herpatic neuralgia, or painful neuropathies (i.e., diabetic), fall into this pain category.

Psychogentic Pain Category

Before diagnosing psychogenic pain, a very careful search to exclude all somatic pathology and a thorough assessment by an experienced psychiatrist are essential. The diagnosis should not be made solely on the basis of a diagnostic or differential nerve block.

DSM-IV lists a number of psychological or psychiatric conditions in which pain may be a significant factor. This listing may be useful, but should not constitute the sole guide for diagnosis.

ETIOLOGICAL CATEGORY

The most important category in pain is pain associated with cancer. Usually the pain is caused directly by the cancer or its treatment, but the pain may also result from a noncancerous preexisting or coexisting condition.

REGIONAL CATEGORY

Pain is described by the patient the way it most commonly occurs. The physician, on the other hand, describes it according to an anatomic classification, such as *headache* or *low back pain*.

SUMMARY

Chronic pain is recognized as a complex condition influenced by various factors, including biological, physiological, behavioral, environmental, and social aspects. [16] Classification systems are devices for sorting the complex elements of reality into logical entities. [1] The IASP classification provides a deductive multi-axial approach to pain when physical descriptions of pain are detailed, but operates to some extent at the expense of psychosocial and behavioral aspects of chronic pain. The Multi-axial Assessment of Pain (MAP) provides good reliability and external validity, and in addition it has the advantage of having been tested on diverse groups of chronic pain patients. A polydiagnostic approach as proposed by Turk may prove complementary. Currently existing pain classifications with refinement, modification, and improvement may lead to their acceptance for wider use.

REFERENCES

[1] Merskey H: Classification of chronic pain. Descriptions of chronic pain syndromes and definitions of pain terms. *Pain Suppl* 3, 1986.

[2] Feuerstein M: Definitions of pain. In Tollison CD editor: *Handbook of Chronic Pain Management.* Baltimore, Williams and Wilkins, 1989.

[3] Bonica JJ: Definitions and taxonomy of pain, In Bonica JJ, editor: *The Management of Pain.* Philadelphia, Lea and Febiger, 1990.

[4] Twycross RG: The relief of pain in far-advanced cancer. *Reg Anesth* 5(3):2-11, 1980.

[5] Boyd DB: Taxonomy and classification of pain. In Tollison CD, editor: *Handbook of Chronic Pain Management.* Baltimore, Williams and Wilkins, 1989.

[6] Longmire DR: Tutorial 7: The classification of pain and pain syndromes. *Pain Digest* 2:229-233, 1992.

[7] Ventafridda V, Caraceni A: Cancer pain classification: A controversial issue. *Pain* 46:1-2, 1991.

[8] Procacci P, Maresca M: Considerations on taxonomy of pain. *Pain* 45:332-333, 1991.

[9] Turk DC, Rudy TE: The robustness of an empirically derived taxonomy of chronic pain patients. *Pain* 43:27-35, 1990.

[10] Malterud K, Hollnagel H: The magic influence of classification systems in clinical practice, *Scandanvin Journal of Primary Health Care* 15:55-6, 1997.

[11] Engum B, Solheim BG: Medical coding and classification systems (Norwegian), *Tidssknift for Den Norske Laegeforening* 114(6):695-494, 1994.

[12] Bonica JJ; The need of taxonomy, *Pain* 6:247-252, 1979.

[13] Merskey H, Bogduk N: *Classification of chronic pain,* ed. 2, Seattle, 1994, IASP Press.

[14] Wilson P: Taxonomy? Never again. *Clinical Journal of Pain,* 13:281-282m 1997.

[15] Stuart-Buttle C, Read J, Sanderson H: *A language if health in action; read codes, classifications and groupings,* Proceedings/AMIA Annual Fall Symposium, NHS Centre for Coding and Classification, 75-79, England, 1992.

[16] Harper A: Symptoms of impairment, disability and handicap in low back pain: a taxonomy, *Pain* 50:189-195, 1992.

[17] Lamberts H, Woods M: international primary care classifications: the effect of fifteen years evolution, *Fam Practice* 9:330-339,1992.

[18] International Classification of Diseases, 9th Revision, WHO, *Geneva,* 1978.

[19] *ICD-10 (International Statistical Classification of Disease and related Health Problems 10th revision),* vol 1, Geneva, 1992, WHO.

[20] Merskey H: *Development of a universal language of pain syndromes: advances in pain research and therapy,* vol 5, New York< 1983, Raven Press.

[21] *DSM-IV: Diagnostic and Statistical Manual of Mental Disorders.* American Psychiatric Association, 1994, Washington DC.

[22] Jamison R, et al: Cognitive behavioral classifications of chronic pain; replication and extension of empirically derived patient profiles, *Pain* 57:277-292,1994.

[23] Yaksh TL: *Neurologic mechanisms of pain, In Cousins MJ, Bridenbaugh PO, eds: Clinical anesthesia and management of pain,* ed. 2, Philadelphia, 1988, J.B. Lippincott.

[24] Wilson PR: *Sympathetically maintained pain.* In Stanton-Hicks M (ed.): *Pain and sympathetic nervous system,* Boston, 1990, Kluwer Academic Publishers.

[25] Wall PD: *Introduction.* In: Wall PD, Melzak R. (ed.): *Textbook of pain,* ed. 2, Edinburgh, 1989, Churchill Livingstone.

[26] Bonica JJ: *The management of pain,* ed. 2, Philadelphia, 1990 Lea and Febiger.

[27] Pilowsky I: Abnormal illness behavior (dysnosognosia), *Psychother Psychosom* 46: 76-84, 1986.

[28] Turk DC, Rudy TE: *A cognitive behavioral perspective on chronic pain management,* Baltimore, 1989, Williams and Wilkins.

[29] Hempel C: *Introduction to the problem of taxonomy.* In Zubin J (ed): *Fields studies in the mental disorders,* pp. 3-22, New York, 1961, Grune and Stratton.

[30] Vervest A, Schimmer G: Letter to the editor, taxonomy of pain of the iasp, *Pain* 34:318-321, 1988.

[31] Turk DC, Rudy TE: IASP taxonomy of chronic pain syndromes, preliminary assessment of reliability. *Pain* 30:177-189, 1987.

[32] Turk DC, Rudy TE: *Classification logic and strategies in chronic pain.* In Turk DC, Melzak R, (ed): *Handbook of pain assessment,* New York, 1992, The Guilford Press.

[33] Sidall PJ, Taylor DA, Cousins MJ: Classification of pain following spinal cord injury, *Spinal Cord* 35:35-75, 1997.

[34] Brena SF, Koch DL: The pan estimate model for the quantification and classification of chronic pain states, *Anesthesiology Review* 2:8-13,1975

[35] Brena SF: Chronic pain states: a model classification, *Psychiatric Annals* 14:778-782, 1984.

[36] Turk DC, Rudy TE: Assessment of cognitive factors in chronic pain; a worthwhile enterprise. *Journal of Consulting and Clinical Psychology,* 54:760-768, 1986.

[37] Melzak R, Casey KL: *Sensory, motivation and central control determinants in pain; a new conceptual model.* In Kenshalo D. (ed): *The skin senses,* pp. 137-153, Springfield, IL, 1968, Charles C. Thomas.

[38] Fordyce WE: *Behavioral methods for chronic pain and illness.* St Louis, 1976, Mosby.

[39] Turk DC, Rudy TE: Towards a comprehensive assessment of chronic pain patients; a multi-axial approach. *Behavioral Research and Therapy,* 25:237-239, 1987.

[40] Turk DC, Rudy TE: Towards an empirically derived taxonomy of chronic pain patients: integration of psychological assessment data. *Journal of Consulting and Clinical Psychology,* 56(2):233-238, 1988.

[41] Kern RD, Turk DC, Rudy TE: The West Haven-Yale Multidimensional Plan Inventory (WHYMPI). *Pain* 23:345-356, 1985.

[42] Turk DC, Rudy TE: The robustness of an empirically derived taxonomy of chronic pain patients, *Pain* 43:27-35, 1990.

[43] Altman D, et al: Is there a case for an international medical press council? *JAMA* 272(2) 166-167, 1994.

[44] Boelen C: Prospect for changes in medical education in the twenty-first century, *Academic Medicine* 70(7) S21-31, 1995.

[45] Garfinkd P, et al: Views on classification and diagnosing eating disorders, *Canadian Journal of Psych,* 40(8); 445-456, 1995.

[46] Jones A: Utilizing Peplau's psychodynamic theory for stroke patient care, *J Clinical Nursing* 4(1) 49-54, 1995.

[47] Flaming D: Patient suffering; a taxonomy from the nurses perspective, *J Adv Nursing* 22(6)1120-1127, 1995.

[48] Farquhar M: Definitions of quality of life: a taxonomy, *Journal of Nursing Administration* 26(11):29-35, 1996.

[49] Marlatt GA: Taxonomy of high-risk situation for alcohol relapse, evolution development of a cognitive behavioral model, *Addiction* 91S:S37-49, 1996.

[50] Micek W, Berry L, Gilski D: Patient outcomes; the link between nursing diagnosis and interventions, *Journal of Nursing Administration* 272(2) 166-167, 1994.

[51] Nouwen A, Gingras J, et al: The Development of an Empirical Psychosocial Taxonomy for Patients with Diabetes. Health Psychology. 16(3):263-271, 1997.

[52] Loser J: A taxonomy of pain, *Pain* 1:81-84, 1975.

[53] Agnew D: A taxonomy for diagnosis and information storage in chronic pain, *Bulletin of Los Angeles Neurological Society* 44:84-86, 1976.

[54] Oleson J: International headache society of classification and diagnostic criteria for headache disorders, cranial neuralgias and facial pain, *Cephalgia* 8:s7, 1988.

[55] Twycross R: Cancer Pain classification, *ACTA Anesth Scandanavia* 41:141-145, 1997.

[56] Cherny N, Coyle N, Foley K: Suffering in the advanced cancer patient: a definition and taxonomy, *Journal of Palliative Care* 10:2, 57-70, 1994.

[57] Wastell D, Gray R: The numerical approach to classification: a medical application to develop a typology for facial pain, *Statistics in Medicine* 6:137-146, 1987.

[58] MacFarlane G, et al: Widespread pain: is an improved classification possible? *J Rheumatology* 23(9):1628-1632, 1996.

[59] Weber F, Rust M: Diagnosis and therapy of tumor pain 1: classification of tumor pain (German), Fortschritte des Medizin 112(30):429-432, 1994.

[60] Stanton-Hicks M, et al: Reflex sympathetic dystrophy: changing concepts and taxonomy, *Pain* 63:127-133, 1995.

[61] Elliott K: Taxonomy and mechanism of neuropathic pain, *Seminars in Neurology* 14(3): 195-205, 1994.

In: The Handbook of Chronic Pain
Editors: S. Kreitler, D. Beltrutti, et al., pp. 57-74

ISBN 978-1-60021-044-0
© 2007 Nova Science Publishers, Inc.

Chapter 4

Chronic Non Cancer Pain

G. Savoia and M. Loreto

EPIDEMIOLOGY

Chronic pain is commonly defined as pain that persists for longer than the expected time frame for healing or pain associated with progressive, non malignant disease. Chronic non-cancer pain is a common problem and there have been many attempts to estimate its prevalence in the general population (Table I) [1, 2, 3]. Zagari et al. [1] reviewed some of these studies and concluded that chronic pain affected 8-30% of the general adult population. Common causes of chronic pain included back and neck pain, myofascial/fibromyalgia syndromes, headaches, arthritis and neuropathic syndromes. In order to estimate the magnitude of this problem Latham and Davis [4] examined studies from the USA and the UK, and reported estimates of 40-70 million people affected by chronic pain.

Table I. The magnitude of the chronic-pain problems

Condition	General population suffering pain (%)	Source
Chronic pain	8-30	Zagari et al, 1996
Back and/or neck pain	43-47	Zagari et al, 1996; Hitchcock 1994
Headache	8-19	Zagari et al, 1996; Hitchcock 1994
Severe pain in disabled people	30	Astin et al, 1996

Epidemiological surveys investigate the amount of pain and the adequacy of its management. Quality of health care has five components: effectiveness, efficacy, efficiency, humanity and equity. Effectiveness analyses whether a therapy works in general conditions, whereas efficacy analyses whether a therapy has been tested in ideal conditions, usually a randomised controlled trial. The key recommendations of the American Society of Anesthesiologists (ASA) practice guidelines for chronic pain management are: A comprehensive history and physical examination of the patient with chronic pain; a through diagnostic evaluation; counseling and coordination of care; periodic monitoring and measurement of clinical outcomes; multidisciplinary and multimodality pain management [5]. Data derived from metanalysis of trials on chronic pain treatment are often contradictory and do not support any evidence on long-term (> 90 days) outcome. Chronic pain causes intense physical suffering and may severely affect a person's quality of life by increasing levels of depression, anxiety, sleep disturbance and fatigue. The goal of therapy is to control pain and to rehabilitate the patients so that they can function as well as possible.

Gender Differences in Pain

Epidemiological studies have shown that women suffer more often than men from severe and chronic painful clinical conditions, in more regions of the body. These conditions include migraine headaches as well as facial, oral, back and musculoskeletal pain. Furthermore, from adolescence on, the genders differ in the way in which they perceive, describe and cope with pain. It is therefore possible that increased pain reporting by women may be due to their being more sensitive "detectors" of pain. Gender differences in pain experience may arise from:

1. different sex role expectations, greater health awareness or more interest in symptoms in women;
2. differences in the neuronal systems that detect, transmit and modify pain signals;
3. sex-determined influences on function, for example through sex hormones;
4. stimulation method in the experimental setting [6].

CLASSIFICATION

Etiologies of chronic pain can be delineated by the inciting pathological process, namely, inflammatory, neuropathic, or mixed. Mechanisms of inflammatory pain can be classified according to the various effects of inflammation. Mechanisms of neuropathic pain can be classified according to the region of the nervous system in which the predominant pathophysiological change occurs (central/spinal).

The IASP (International Association for the Study of Pain) [7] classified the common causes of chronic pain syndromes on the basis of etiologic criteria and involved sites (Table II).

Table II. Classification of chronic non-malignant pain

Relatively Generalized Syndromes	
Peripheral neuropathy	203.X2a (arms, infective) 203.X3a (arms, inflammatory or immunoreactions) 203.X5a (arms, toxic, metabolic) 203.X8a (arms, unknown or other) 603.X2a (legs, infective) 603.X3a (legs, inflammatory or immunoreactions) 603.X5a (legs, toxic, metabolic, etc) 603.X8a (arms, unknown or other) X03.X4d (Von Reckling-hausen's disease)
Stump Pain	203.X1a (arms) 603.X1a (legs)
Phantom Pain	203.X7a (arms) 603.X7a (legs)
Complex Regional Pain Syndrome, Type I (Reflex Sympathetic Dystrophy)	203.X1h (arms) 603.X1h (legs)
Complex Regional Pain Syndrome, Type II (Causalgia)	207.X1h (arms) 607.X1h (legs)
Central Pain If three or more sites are involved, code first digit as 9 : If only one or two sites are involved, code according to specific site or sites (e.g., for head or face, code 003.X5c, etc)	903.X5c (vascular) 903.X1c (trauma) 903.X2c (infection) 903.X3c (inflammatory) 903.X4c (neoplasm) 903.X8c (unknown)
Syndrome of Syringomyelia (when affecting head or limb; code additional entries for other areas)	007.X0 (face) 207.X0 (arm) 607.X0 (leg)
Polymyalgia Rheumatica	X32.X3a
Fibromyalgia (Fibrositis)	X33.X8a
Rheumatoid Arthritis	X34.X3a
Osteoarthritis	X38.X6a
Calcium Pyrophosphate Dihydrate Deposition Disease (CPPD)	X38.X0 or X38.X5a
Gout	X38.X5b
Hemophilic Arthropathy	X34.X0a
Burns	X42.X1 or X82.X1

Table II. Continued

Relatively Generalized Syndromes	
Pain of psychological origin muscle tension delusional or hallucinatory hysterical, conversion, or hypochondriacal associated with depression	X33.X7b X1X.X9a X1X.X9b X1X.X9d
Factitious illness and malingering	No code: see note in text
Regional Sprains or Strains (code only)	X33.X1d
Sickle Cell Arthropathy (code only)	X34.X0c
Purpuric Arthropathy (code only)	X34.X0d
Stiff Man Syndrome (code only)	934.X8
Paralysis Agitans (code only)	902.X7
Epilepsy (code only)	X04.X7
Polyarteritis Nodosa (code only)	X5X.X3
Psoriatic Arthropathy and other Secondary Arthropathies (code only)	X34.X8c
Paiful Scar (code only)	X4X.X1b
Systematic Lupus Erythematosis, Systemic Sclerosis and Fibrosclerosis, Polymyositis and Dermatomyositis (code only)	X33.X3b
Infective Arthropathies (code only)	X33.X3c
Traumatic Arthropathy (code only)	X33.X1a
Osteomyelitis (code only)	X32.X2f
Osteitis deformnas (code only)	X32.X5b
Osteochondritis (code only)	X32.X5b
Osteoporosis (code only)	X32.X5c
Muscle spasm (code only)	X32.X2d
Local Pain, no cause Specified (code only)	X7X.Xxa or X3X.X8e
Guillam-Barré Syndrome	901.X3

Major Pain Mechanisms

The history of the last century reviewed by Melzack and Wall [8] is marked by a persistent search for pain fibers and pathways and a pain center in the brain. The specificity theory proposed that injury activates specific pain receptors and fibers, which in turn project pain impulses through a spinal pain pathway to a pain center in the brain. The psychological experience of pain, therefore, was virtually equated with peripheral injury. There was no room for psychological contributions to pain, such as attention, past experience, and the meaning of the situation. The major opponent to the specificity approach was labeled "pattern theory". The different pattern theories that were developed were generally vague and inadequate and shared the assumption that the brain was merely a passive receiver of messages [9]. According to the new gate control theory the major emphasis was placed on the modulation of inputs in the spinal dorsal horns and the dynamic role of the brain in pain processes. Psychological factors, which were previously dismissed as "reactions to pain", were now considered as an integral part of pain processing, and new avenues for pain control were opened. The gate control theory forced the medical and biologic sciences to accept the brain as an active system that filters, selects, and modulates inputs. The dorsal horns, too, were not merely passive transmission stations but sites at which occurred the dynamic activites of inhibition, excitation, and modulation.

The revolution introduced by the gate control theory consisted in highlighting the central nervous system as an essential component in pain processes. The brain mechanism that underlies the experience of the body as a unit also comprises a unified system that acts as a whole and produces a neurosignature pattern of a whole body. The conceptualization of this unified brain mechanism lies at the heart of a new theory, and neuromatrix best characterizes it. Matrix is defied as "something within which something else originates, takes form or develops" [10]. The neuromatrix is the origin of the neurosignature; the neurosignature originates and takes form in neuromatrix. Though the neurosignature may be triggered or modulated by input, the input is only a "trigger" and does not produce the neurosignature itself. The array of neurons in a neuromatrix is genetically programmed to perform the specific function of producing the signature pattern. The final, integrated neurosignature pattern for the body-self ultimately produces awareness and action. The neuromatrix, distributed throughout many areas of the brain, comprises a widespread network of neurons that generates patterns, processes information that flows through it, and ultimately produces the pattern that is felt as a whole body. The stream of neurosignature output produces the feelings of the whole body with constantly changing qualities. When all sensory systems are intact, inputs modulate the continuous neuromatrix output to produce the wide variety of experiences we feel. The experience of the body-self involves multiple dimensions - sensory, affective, evaluative, postural, and many others. The sensory dimension is subserved by portions of the neuromatrix that lies in the sensory projection areas of the brain; the affective dimension is subserved by areas in the brain near to the limbic system. Each major psychological dimension or quality of experience is subserved by a particular portion of the neuromatrix - a neuromodule- which contributes a distinct portion of the total neurosignature.

Thirty years after the publication of Melzack and Wall's gate control theory [11], the pathophysiology underlying the chronic pain is still a major theme of research. Basic proposed mechanisms for the processing of sensory information that is interpreted as pain of a chronic nature have led to the study of neural plasticity and a multitude of cellular substances (tissue autocoids or inflammatory mediators). Tissue damage can provoke the liberation of autocoids, such as nitric oxide, serotonin, histamine, bradykinin, prostaglandins, substance P, kinin and leukotrienes which have excitatory effects on peripheral nociceptors. The presence of reactive oxygen species induced genetic expression of the immediate early genes c-fos and c-jun, which are responsible for forming the protein dimers Fos and Jun. These proteins are involved in the tissue healing and repair processes. The chemical signals are interpreted by the dorsal horn neurons as noxious inputs and cause release of excitatory neurotransmitters from afferent C-fibers and A-delta nociceptors (glutamate and substance P, which acts synergistically with N-methyl D-aspartae NMDA). The neurotransmitter release increases postsynaptic neuronal calcium ions, provoking a rapid change in gene expression in the postsynaptic dorsal horn neurons (laminae 1, 2 and 5) of the spinal cord [12, 13]. This gene expression involves the transcription of the immediate early gene c-fos by its messenger RNA, which initiates formation of the protein Fos. Fos is a part of the transcription factor complex AP-1, which may be partially responsible for the development of chronic changes in neuronal excitability. Another probable mechanism involves the spinal processing of information. An afferent barrage from C-fibers causes an increase in the excitability of central neurons, which is mediated by excitatory amino acids at the NMDA receptor. Once the changes become established, they may become independent of the peripheral input necessary to initiate them. In addition, one must consider the role of nerve growth factor as a mediator of persistent visceral pain, since it causes sensitization of sensory neurons. Nerve growth factor upregulates the expression of sensory neuropeptides calcitonin gene-related peptide and substance P, and these in turn contribute to central sensitization of sensory neurons. These processes cause the long-term changes in neural circuitry (table III) that give rise to the phenomenon of chronic pain, or especially in neuropathic pain, to the phenomenon of the "central pain" [14].

Table III. Possible mechanisms for chronic pain

Peripheral nervous system
sensitization of peripheral neurons
unmasking of silent nociceptors
collateral sprouting
increased activity of damaged axons and their sprouts
invasion of dorsal root ganglia by sympathetic postganglionic neurons
Central nervous system
hyperexcitability of central neurons
reorganisation of synaptic connectivity in spinal cord and elsewhere within the central nervous system
disinhibition-removal of tonic descending inhibitory activity and other mechanisms

Phantom Limb Pain

The new theory of brain function provides an explanation for phantom limb pain. An excellent series of studies found that 72% of amputees had phantom limb pain a week after amputation, and 60% had pain 6 months later [15, 16]. Even 7 years after amputation, 60% still continued to suffer phantom limb pain, which means that only about 10% to 12% of amputated obtain pain relief. The active body neuromatrix, in the absence of modulating inputs from the limbs or body, produces a signature pattern that is transduced in the sentient neural hub (SNH) into a hot or burning quality. The cramping pain may be due to messages from the action neuromodule to move muscles in order to produce movement. The origin of these pains, then, lies in the brain.

Back Pains and Myofascial Pains

Because the action-neuromatrix maintains specific tensions on all muscles at all times, it is possible that sudden minor accidents may produce stresses and strains on muscles in a localized part of the body, which then send abnormal messages to the body neuromatrix. The action-neuromatrix, in order to mantain posture and balance, may then change the tension on more distant muscles and ultimately produce a vicious circle of abnormal feedback and output for action. The traditional trigger-points and physical therapies could produce changes in inputs, which sometimes help, but the major cause may be the abnormal messages from the brain that maintain abnormal tensions on a large part of the body musculature.

Myofascial syndromes such as fibromyalgia also remain a mystery and are difficult to understand. It is well known that fibromyalgia is associated with a characteristic distribution of trigger points and sleep disorders, and is usually found in tense, hard-working, younger people. The underlying mechanism is usually sought in long-term activities in the spinal cord, but the cause may be in the brain, and an abnormal output thus maintains an abnormal pattern of tension on musculature throughout a widespread portion of the body. The therapy may require re-education of the muscles of a large part of the body [7, 8].

Referred Pain

Referred pain is a complex phenomenon that must be examined at many levels. It is usually due to a combination of peripheral and central causes. Most commonly, the mechanisms are obvious and can be understood on the basis of the anatomy of the spinal cord. The physiologic mechanism in these cases is known to involve spinal cells at the first central synapse. Dorsal horn cells in lamina V that belong to the "wide dynamic range" (WDR) category are innervated by small diameter fibers from the viscera as well as large diameter fibers (with low threshold) from the skin [7]. These WDR cells provide the mechanism for referred pain in which pathology of a deep structure seems to come from a cutaneous area that is often tender. The tenderness, however, is due to central summation, not to peripheral injury or inflammation. Sometimes the mechanisms involve the brain and are complex. Even when referred pain involves trigger points that can be associated with muscles in spasm, it is likely that a spinal (viz. trigger points) or brain (e.g. phantom limb pain) mechanism is involved.

Categories of Pain

In general, pain falls into three main categories: acute, chronic and cancer-related pain. There are three categories of pain which differ in various properties: duration, biological value, nerve conduction, autonomic nervous system involvement, associated pathology, prognosis, associated problems, social effects and treatments.

Transient pain: it refers to the response to a noxious stimulus which does not produce long term sequelae (e.g. a pin prick); it requires nociceptor specialization.

Tissue injury pain: primary afferent (sensitization, recruitment of silent nociceptors, alteration in phenotype, hyperinnervation) and CNS mediated (central sensitization recruitment, summation, amplification);

Nervous system injury pain: primary afferent (acquisition of spontaneous and stimulus-evoked activity by nociceptor axons and somata at loci other than peripheral terminals, phenotype change) and CNS mediated (central sensitization, deafferentation of 2nd order neurons, disinhibition, structural reorganization)[17].

COMMON CHRONIC SYNDROM

Peripheral Neuropathy

It refers to constant or intermittent burning, aching, or lancinating limb pains due to generalized or focal diseases of peripheral nerves. It is usually distal (especially in the feet) with burning pain, but often more proximal and deep with aching, constant or sharp lancinating "tabetic" and intermittent pain, especially nocturnal and in the legs. It is focal with mononeuropathies, concentrated in the territory of the affected nerve (e.g. meralgia paresthetica). This type of pain is common in neuropathies, diabetes, amyloid, alcoholism, polyarteritis, Guillam-barré Syndrome, neuralgic amyotrophy, and Fabry's disease. the age of onset is variable, usually after second decade. The symptoms include sensory loss, especially to pinprick and temperature; sometimes reflex loss; sometimes signs of loss of sympathetic function; smooth, fine skin; and hair loss. Laboratory. findings include features of primary disease and features of neuropathy: reduced or absent sensory potentials, slowing of motor and sensory conduction velocities, and EMG evidence of muscle denervation. The usual course of the syndrome includes distal burning and deep aching pains which are often longlasting and the disease processes are relatively unresponsive to therapy. The pain resolves spontaneously weeks or months in self-limited conditions, such as Guillain-Barré syndrome or neuralgic amyotrophy. There is nerve fiber damage, and usually axonal degeneration. Pain occurs especially when there is small fiber damage (sensory fibers). Nerve biopsy may reveal the above, plus features of the specific disease process. The criteria for peripheral neuropathy are : chronic distal burning or deep aching pain with signs of sensory loss with or without muscle weakness, atrophy and reflex loss. The differential diagnosis should be made with spinal cord and muscle disease [18,19].

Phantom Limb Pain

The term "phantom limb pain" refers to pain in a part of the body that has been deafferented or amputated. Both peripheral and central factors have been considered as determinants of phantom limb pain. New insights into phantom limb pain have come from studies that examined functional and structural changes in the primary sensory and motor areas that occur after injury or stimulation and learning. A comprehensive model of the development of phantom limbs should include both peripheral and central factors, and should assume that pain memories established before and during the amputation may be powerful elicitors of phantom limb pain [20]. These data suggest that long-lasting noxious input may lead to long term changes that manifest themselves as cortical pain memory. Huse et al showed that the best predictor of later phantom limb pain is not only acute pain in the perioperative phase, but also the duration and intensity of chronic pain before the amputation.. Pain before the amputation significantly increases the incidence of phantom limb and stump pain.

Up to 70% of amputees suffer from phantom limb pain. Phantom limb pain is difficult to treat and prevention may now yield to more effective methods. There are strong indications that regional anaesthesia started preoperatively, generally 24-72 hours before surgery and continued for some days postoperatively, is effective in preventing phantom limb pain.

Use of myoelectric prosthesis might be one method to influence phantom limb pain. It was recently shown that intensive use of a myoelectric prosthesis was positively correlated with both reduced phantom limb pain and reduced cortical reorganization. An alternative approach in patients for whom prosthesis use is not viable is the application of behaviourally relevant stimulation. The demonstration that motor cortex stimulation can lead to the experience of a painful phantom sensation supported the assumption that the joint activation of the motor and parietal cortex may have created that painful phantom limb. The pharmacological interventions might also be appropriate either for treatments of chronic phantom limb pain or for prevention of the occurrence of phantom limb pain after surgery. Agents, such as NMDA antagonists or GABA agonists are effective in reducing phantom limb pain in at least some of the patients. Pre-emptive analgesia has not consistently been efficacious in preventing the onset of phantom limb pain [21].

Herpetic and Post-Herpetic Neuralgia

Herpes zoster is acute viral disease caused by the varicella virus. This virus belongs to the DNA group of diseases and primarily affects the posterior root ganglion of spinal nerves. Herpes zoster is characterized by the development of a vesicular rash which develops along a specific dermatomal pattern. These vesicles usually begin to dry up after one week and may heal in about a month. This condition is usually associated with an intense necrotizing reaction in the dorsal root ganglion and also in the dorsal horn of the spinal cord. Thus, although cutaneous manifestation is the portion of this condition that is worrying, a more sinister change may take place in some patients in the spinal cord. It is the resulting neuronal injury at the dorsal root ganglion level and at the dorsal horn level of the spinal cord which produces the self-perpetuating and excruciating pain long after the vesicular rash has healed.

The pathophysiology of nociception in patients with herpes zoster is not well understood. It is postulated that activation of nociceptive primary afferents by direct viral attack produces inflammatory changes not only in the skin and peripheral nerves but also in the posterior root ganglion, nerve roots, leptomeninges, and dorsal horn of the spinal cord itself.

Postherpetic neuralgia is described as dermatomal pain occurring after the vesicular rash of herpes zoster has healed, and it is characterized by a constant aching, burning pain and paroxysms of sharp stabbing pain. In many patients, there are no pain–free intervals. The affected skin usually shows significant scarring with pigmentation changes, and there may be alterations in sensation of pain, temperature, and light touch. Postherpetic neuralgia may involve both peripheral and central mechanisms. It is postulated that the dorsal root ganglion and dorsal horn of the spinal cord neuronal injury may initiate a self perpetuating series of changes which may result in pain of postherpetic neuralgia. Impairment of segmental pain-modulating systems and diminished large-fiber function may contribute to increased transmission of nociception through the dorsal horn of the spinal cord. These central mechanisms may be the reason why proximal ablative procedures usually fail to provide sustained pain relief. The dysesthetic pain in these lesions may also be due to damaged or regenerating nociceptive fibers, whereas the stabbing pain may relate to activation of nociceptive nervi nervorum.

Fibromyalgia

Fibromyalgia is a disorder of unknown aetiology, characterized by chronic widespread pain and the presence of tender points, often accompanied by several non-specific symptoms, such as fatigue, depressive mood, and sleep disturbances. Its central characteristics is chronic, generalized pain in the joints, muscles and spine, although the pain originates from ligaments and insertions of muscles and is not articular. The patients often have morning stiffness but there are no signs of inflammation and ESR (erythrocyte sedimentation rate) is normal [22]. Fibromyalgia is characterized by several symptoms: fatigue (90% of patients), early morning stiffness (80%), sleep disturbances (70%), paraesthesias (60%), headache (50%), anxiety (50%) and irritable bowel (40%). Another characteristic of fibromyalgia is that, in contrast to articular rheumatic conditions, pain responds badly to pain medication. Physical examination reveals no abnormalities except for the presence of tender points,. Also laboratory investigation yields normal results. There are no diagnostic criteria for fibromyalgia but the American College of Rheumatology criteria for the classification are as follows [23]:\

> chronic (over 3 months) widespread pain (axial plus upper and lower sement plus left and right sided), in combination with pain in 11 or more of 18 specific tender points sites at palpation with an approximate force of 4 Kg; the presence of a second clinical disorder does not exclude the diagnosis of fibromyalgia.

Fibromyalgia is often considered as one of the functional somatic syndromes because it shares with these syndromes many of its symptoms as well as the lack of knowledge of the pathogenesis. It is now supposed that afferent central pain amplification, and perhaps also the impairment of dorsal descending pain inhibiting systems underlie widespread allodynia and hyperalgesia. In addition, neuroendocrine perturbations, physical deconditioning, sleep disturbance, health beliefs, and mood disorder are all supposed to play a role in the modulation of pain via the amplification or inhibition of the sensory or affective component of pain and in other symptoms (in which NMDA receptor appears to be hyperexcitable). A uniform and satisfactory treatment strategy for fibromyalgia is lacking. Management should be tailored to symptoms, functioning and the well-being of individual patients. Essential in the management of fibromyalgia are the enhancement of functional capacities and quality of life [24,25,26]:

1. Graded daily physical exercise is the key therapy to prevent the progression of physical deconditioning, to enhance functional capacities, and to manage fibromyalgia symptoms;

2. adherence to physical exercise will probably be improved if treatment is embedded in educational packages aimed at maladaptive cognitions and motivation for change;

3. cognitive behavioural therapy may be considered to help patients in setting up individualized realistic goals in life and ways of coping with the consequences of fibromyalgia, such as depressive mood, activies of daily living, sleep disturbances, depressive self-statements, and physical deconditioning;

4. for symptomatic treatment pharmacological medication may be considered for individual patients. Analgesics may provide some benefit. Tricyclic antidepressants may have a moderate modulating effect on pain, mood and sleep. For subgroups of patients with severely invalidating pain, some other pharmaceutical agents may need to be evaluated in future, for instance, NMDA or 5-hydroxytryptamine 3 receptor antagonists.

Stump Pain

Stump pain is focused at the site of amputation of an upper or lower extremity. The . pain is not referred to the absent body part but is perceived in the stump itself, usually in the region of a transected nerve. It is experienced as a sharp, often jabbing pain in the stump, and is usually aggravated by pressure on, or infection in the stump. Pain is often elicited by tapping or percussion over the neuroma in the transected nerve or nerves. Stump pain develops several weeks to months after amputations and persists indefinitely if untreated. After prosthesis to avoid pressure or neuromata, it is advisable to resect neuromata so that they no longer lie in pressure areas and utilize for this purpose neurosurgical procedures, such as rhizotomy and ganglionectomy or spinal cord or peripheral nerve stimulation in properly selected patients. In cases of stumpt pain differential diagnoses with phantom limb pain and radiculopathy are important.

Complex Regional Pain Syndrome (CPRS)

This title is being introduced to cover the painful syndromes which formerly were described under the headings of "Reflex Sympathetic Dystrophy" and "Causalgia". There has been dissatisfaction with the term "reflex sympathetic dystrophy" because not all the cases seem to have sympathetically maintained pain, and not all were dystrophic. The syndrome broadly corresponding to what has formerly been described as reflex sympathetic dystrophy is now termed CRPS Type I and Causalgia is described as CPRS Type II.

CPRS remains a troublesome disorder. Some progress has been made to refine the diagnostic criteria so as to render the diagnosis more specific. The diagnosis can be made clinically by applying a checklist that clusters features into separate categories of sensory, vasomotor, sudomotor, and motor/trophic changes (Table IV).

Diagnostic criteria for CRPS proposed by the IASP [27] are:

(a) the presence of an initiating noxious event or a cause of immobilization;
(b) continuing pain, allodynia, or hyperalgesia in which the pain is disproportionate to any inciting event;
(c) evidence at some time of oedema, change in skin blood flow, or abnormal sudomotor activity in the region of pain;
(d) and exclusion of this diagnosis by the existence of conditions that would otherwise account for the degree of pain and dysfunction

Table IV. Checklist for the diagnosis of CPRS [28]

History		No	Yes
	burning pain skin sensitivity to touch skin sensitivity to cold abnormal swelling abnormal hair growth abnormal nail growth abnormal sweating abnormal skin colour changes abnormal skin temperature changes limited movement		
examination	mechanical allodynia hyperalgesia to single pinprick summation multiple pinprick cold allodynia abnormal swelling abnormal hair growth abnormal skin colour changes abnormal skin temperature (>1.°C) limited range of movement motor neglect		

The pathophysiological mechanisms of the symptoms and signs still remain obscure, and some authorities maintain that they are psychogenic. Stellate ganglion blocks appear to be effective in reducing the recurrence of CPRS in patients needing to undergo surgery on a previously affected limb. Vitamin C appears to reduce the incidence of CPRS after fractures of the radius. Physiotherapy offers little advantage over social work attention. Biphosphonates appear to be promising both as a means of reducing pain and of reversing osteoporosis. Spinal cord stimulation has been proved to relieve pain but it does not improve function [29].

CRPS Type I

CRPS Type I is a syndrome that usually develops after an initiating noxious event, is not limited to the distribution of a single peripheral nerve , and is apparently disproportionate to the inciting event. It is associated at some point with evidence of oedema, changes in skin blood flow, abnormal sudomotor activity in the region of the pain, or allodynia or hyperalgesia. Pain often follows a trauma, which is usually mild and is not associated with significant nerve injury, such as a fracture, a soft tissue lesion, or immobilization related to visceral disease. The onset of symptoms usually occurs within one month of the inciting event. The pain is described as burning and continuos and is exacerbated by movement. The intensity of pain fluctuates over time, and allodynia or hyperalgesia may be found which are not limited to the territory of a single peripheral nerve. The symptoms and signs may spread proximally or involve other extremities. Impairment of motor function is frequently seen. Associated symptoms and signs are atrophy of the skin, nails and other soft tissues, as well as alterations in hair growth and loss of joint mobility, which may however fluctuate at times. Sympathetically maintained pain may be present and may be demonstrated with pharmacological blocking or provocation techniques. Laboratory findings include skin temperature asymmetry over 1°C, with asymmetry of sudomotor function test. The bone uptake phase with three-phase bone scan reveals a characteristic pattern of subcutaneous blood pool changes. Radiographic examination may demonstrate patchy bone demineralization. In cases with sympathetically maintained pain, sympatholytic interventions may provide temporary or permanent pain relief. The diagnostic criteria are:

1. the presence of an initiating noxious event, or a cause of immobilization;
2. continuing pain, allodynia or hyperalgesia in which the pain is disproportionate to any inciting event;
3. evidence at some time of oedema, changes in skin blood flow, or abnormal sudomotor activity in the region of pain;
4. exclusion of this diagnosis by the existence of conditions that would otherwise account for the degree of pain and dysfunction.

Differential diagnosis: CRPS II (causalgia), traumatic vasospasm, cellulitis, Raynaud's disease, thromboangioitis obliterans, thrombosis.

CRPS Type II

This diagnosis refers to burning pain, allodynia and hyperpathia, usually in the hand or foot, after partial injury of a nerve or one of its major branches. The onset occurs immediately after partial nerve injury but may be delayed for months. The most commonly involved nerves are the median, the sciatic, the tibial and the ulnar. Spontaneous pain occurs which is described as constant and burning, and is exacerbated by light touch, stress, temperature changes or movement of the involved limb, visual and auditory stimuli and emotional disturbances. The intensity of pain may fluctuate over time. Other signs are: changes in skin temperature, oedema, hyper or hypohidrosis and impairment of motor function. The associated symptoms and signs resemble those of CRPS I. In addition, affective disorders may occur.

Laboratory findings include asymmetry of skin temperature, and side to side asymmetry of sudomotor test. The bone uptake phase with three-phase bone scan reveals a characteristic pattern of periarticular uptake. Radiographic examination may demonstrate patchy bone demineralization. As in CRPS I, the social and physical impairments are inability to perform activities of daily living as well as occupational and recreational activities.

Diagnostic criteria are:

1. the presence of continuing pain, allodynia, or hyperalgesia after a nerve injury, not necessarily limited to the distribution of the injured nerve;
2. evidence at some time of oedema, changes in skin blood flow, or abnormal sudomotor activity in the region of the pain;
3. the exclusion of this diagnosis by the existence of conditions that would otherwise account for the degree of pain and dysfunction.

Osteoarthritis

Ostheoarthritis (OA) is the most common joint condition and one the most frequent causes of disability in the developed world. OA pain is of multifactorial origin, and is only partly related to inflammatory mechanisms. It has been shown that there is a relatively poor correlation between clinical problems and structural changes. Pain may be generated by a number of mechanisms [30]. In bone tissue, pain may be generated by periosteal elevation by osteophytes, trabecular microfractures pressure on the subchondral bone, or by raised intraosseos pressure. In articular tissue, pain may be caused by inflammatory synovitis, pinching of synovial villi, or joint capsule distinction. Periarticular pain can be generated by ligament damage, muscle spasm or bursitis. Perceived pain may also be increased through neural plasticity, by psychosocial factors, physical demands and neuromuscular problems.

There is currently no causative treatment of OA, and therefore all treatment modalities in OA must be considered symptomatic, in other words, pain killing.

The choice of analgesic treatment in OA must be highly individual; no guidelines can rigidly define a treatment regimen for a condition such as OA [31]. All current therapeutic options can be divided into two symptom-modifying groups and into structure-modifying drugs. The first symptom-modifying group includes fast-acting agents, such as analgesics (including paracetamol and opioids), NSAIDs and also corticosteroids. Many concerns have been voiced about the safety of NSAIDs [32] and the significant gastrointestinal and renal toxicities of NSAIDs are well known. Selective COX-2 inhibitors appear to be safer than traditional NSAIDs. However, they are currently expensive and their safety profile will only emerge as more data from clinical practice become available [33]. The second group of symptom-modifying drugs are the SYSADOAs (symptomatic slow-acting drugs in OA), such as hyaluronic acid, glucosamine sulphate, chondroitin sulphate and diacerein [34]. Their advantages are a persistent effect and a lack of gastrointestinal toxicity. Their disadvantages are that they have a relatively small, delayed effect, that they are currently expensive, and that some have troublesome adverse reactions. Hyaluronic acid also has the disadvantage that it must be injected into the affected joint, an inconvenient procedure that also limits the number of sites that can be treated. It is not known whether they are cost-effective, and whether it is best to administer them continuously or periodically [35]. The American College of Rheumatology (ACR) guidelines recommend starting therapy with non-pharmacological modalities and then progressing to paracetamol, to low and then high doses of NSAIDs, and finally to joint surgery, if the condition does not respond. In case of inflammation, the use of corticosteroids is also recommended [36, 37]. These guidelines are simple but they cannot be used for all patients in every phase of their disease. There are patients with moderate to severe pain, who do not obtain sufficient pain relief with paracetamol or NSAIDs, or who cannot tolerate these drugs because of adverse reactions. For patients with moderate to severe pain, who do not obtain sufficient pain relief with paracetamol and non-steroidal inflammatory drugs (NSAIDs) or do not tolerate them, the remaining options are opioids. The strong adverse reactions of traditional opioids, may disadvantage the use of these drugs in OA patients. At present, accumulating data indicate that tramadol may be suitable for OA pain.

Recently, at the EULAR (European League Against Rheumatism) 2000 Conference an update of the ACR Guidelines was announced which now accepts tramadol as one option for the treatment of OA (Figure 1). Tramadol is an alternative symptomatic treatment of moderate to severe OA pain. It can be combined with NSAIDs to either increase the level of analgesia, without increasing NSAID-related toxicity, or to reduce such toxicity by decreasing the NSAID dose. Tramadol causes neither adverse reactions related to prostaglandin inhibitions nor permanent organ damage. It also has no effect on chondrocytes, and has fewer opioid-related problems, including dependence. In fact, tramadol has no extreme abuse potential and tolerance development is minimal. The adverse reactions that tramadol does commonly induce, such as nausea and dizziness, generally occur at the beginning of therapy, and attenuate with continued treatment. Tramadol should also be tested further in other conditions involving pain, such as rheumatoid arthritis, ankylosing spondylitis, fibromyalgia, and soft-tissue rheumatism, including back pain.

Central Pain

Central pain is caused by a primary lesion or dysfunction in the central nervous system, and is usually associated with abnormal sensibility to temperature and to noxious stimulation. The onset may be instantaneous but it usually occurs after a delay of weeks or months and the pain increases gradually.The regional distribution of the pain correlates neuroanatomically with the location of the lesion in the brain and spinal cord. It may also be restricted simply to the face or part of one extremity. Many different qualities of pain occur (e.g., burning, aching, pricking, lancinating) and dysesthesias are common. Some patients have no pain at rest but suffer from evoked pain, paresthesias and dysesthesias. The pain may be superficial or deep. Associated symptoms and signs include monoparesis, hemiparesis or paraparesis together with somatosensory abnormalities in the affected areas. Impaired sensibility for temperature and noxious stimulation are leading signs. The threshold for tactile, vibration and kinesthetic sensibility may be increased or normal. MRI or CT may show a relevant lesion. TENS may give relief, and anticonvulsivant drugs help in some instances (especially carbamazepine). Certain antidepressants (amitryptiline) seem to give the best relief and some think that phenotiazines may be helpful.

Cerebrovascular lesions (infarcts, hemorrages), multiple sclerosis and spinal cord injuries are the most common causes. Central pain is also common in syringomyelia, syringobulbia, spinal vascular malformation and after operations like cordotomy. The central pain occurs in patients who have lesions affecting the spino-thalamocortical pathways. The lesions may sometimes involve the medial leminiscal pathways.

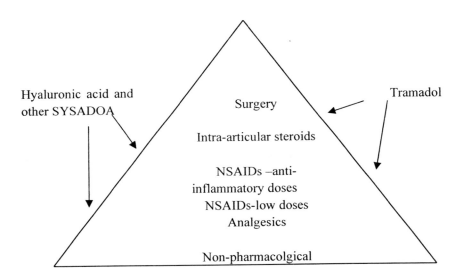

Figure 1. The therapeutic pyramid in osteoarthritis

REFERENCES

[1]   Zagari MJ, Mazonson PD, Longton WC. Pharmacoeconomics of chronic non-malignant pain. Pharmacoeconomics 1996; 10: 356-77.

[2]   Astin M, Lawton D, Hirst M. The prevalence of pain in disabled population. Soc Sci Med 1996; 42: 1457-64.

[3]   Hitchcock LS, Ferrell BR, McCafferty M. The experience of chronic non-malignant pain. J Pain Symptom Manage 1994; 9: 312-18.

[4]   Latham J, Davis BD. The socioeconpmic impact of chronic pain. Disabil Rehab 1994; 16: 39-44 - World Health Organization. Cancer pain relief and palliative care. report of

a WHO expert committee. World Health Organization Technical Report Series, 2nd ed. Geneva, Swizerland: WHO 1996).

[5]   A Report by the American Society of Anaesthesiologists Task Force on Pain Management, Chronic Pain Section. Practice Guidelines. Anaesthesiology 1997; 86: 995-1004.

[6]   Giles BE, Walker JS. Gender differences in pain. Current opinion in Anaesthesiology 1999; 12, 5:591-595.

[7]   International Association for the Study of Pain. Classification of chronic pain. In: Merskey H, Bogduk N. Task Force on taxonomy. IASP Press, Seattle.1994; Part I: 6, 7.

[8]   Melzack R, Wall PD. Pain mechanisms: a new theory. Science 150: 971-979, 1965.

[9]   Livingston WK. Pain mechanisms. New York: MacMillan, 1943.; Noordenbos W. Pain. Amsterdam. Elsevier, 1959.

[10] Webster's Seventh New collegiate Dictionary, Springfield MA. G and C Merriam Co, 1967, 522.

[11] Devor M. The pathophisiology of damaged peripheral nerves. In Wall PD, Melzack R (eds): Texbook of Pain, ed.3. Edinburgh, Churchill-Livingstone, 1994: 79-100.

[12] Sheng M, McFadden G, Greenberg ME. Membrane depolarization and calcium induce c-fos transcription via phosphorylation of transcription factor CREB. Neuron 1990; 4: 571-582.

[13] Chiu R, Boyle WJ, Meek J et al. The c-Fos protein interacts with c-Jun/AP1 to stimulate the transcription of AP-1 responsive genes. Cell 1988; 54: 541-552.

[14] Johnson BW. Tutorial 23: Mechanisms of chronic pain. Pain Digest 1996; 6: 97-108.

[15] Krebs B, Jensen TS, Kroner K. Phantom limb phenomena in amputees 7 years after limb amputation. Pain suppl 2: S85, 1984.

[16] Jensen TS, Krebs B, Nielsen J, Rasmussen P. Immediate and long-term phantom limb pain in amputees: incidence, clinical characteristics and relationship to pre-amputation limb pain. Pain 21: 267-78, 1985.

[17] Woolf CJ, Bennet GJ, Doherty M, Ducker R, Kidd B, Koltzenburg M, Lipton R, Loeser JD, Payne R and Torebjork E. Towards a mechanism-based classification of pain? Pain 1998; 77: 227-229.

[18] Thomas PK. Pain in peripheral neuropathy: clinical and morphological aspects. In: J. Ochoa and W. Culp (eds). Abnormal Nerves and Muscles as Impulse Generators, Oxford universityPress, New Yoprk 1982.

[19] Asburn AK, Fields HL. Pain due to peripheral nerve damage: an hypothesis. Neurology 1984; 34: 1587-590.

[20] Flor H, Braun C, Helbert T, Birbaumer N. Extensive reorganization of primary somatosensory cortex in chronic back pain patients. Neurosci lett 1997; 224: 5-8.

[21] Nikolajsen L, Illkjaer S, Christensen JH. Randomised trial of epidural bupivacaine and morphine in prevention of stump and phantom pain in lower limb amputation. Lancet 1997; 350: 1353-1357.

[22] Geenen R, Jacobs JWG. Fibromyalgia: diagnosis, pathogenesis, and treatment. Current Opinion in Anaesthesiology 2001; 14: 533-39.

[23] Wolfe F, Smythe HA, Yunus MB. The American College of Rheumatology 1990 criteria for the classification of fibromyalgia. Report of the Multicenter Committee. Arthritis Rheum 1990; 33: 160-72.

[24] Lautenschlager J. Present stae of medication therapy in fibromyalgia syndrome. Scand J rheumatol 2000; 29 Suppl.113: 32-36.

[25] Richards S, Cleare A. treating fibromyalgia. rheumatology 2000; 39: 343-46.

[26] Hadhazy VA, Ezzo J, Creamer P, Berman BM. Mind-body therapies for the treatment of fibromyalgia. a systematic review. J Rheumatol 2000; 27: 2911-2918.:

[27] Merskey H, Bogduk N. Classification of chronic pain. Desciptions of chronic pain syndromes and definitions of pain terms. 2nd edn. Seattle: IASP Press 1994.

[28] Galer BS, Bruehl S, Harden RN. IASP diagnostic criteria for complex regional pain syndrome: a preliminary empirical validation study. Clin J Pain 1998; 14: 48-54.

[29] Bogduk N. Complex regional pain syndrome. Current opinion in Anaesthesiology 2001; 14: 541-546.

[30] Pinals RS. Mechanisms of joints destruction pain disability in osteoarthritis. Drugs 1996; 52 (Suppl 3): 14-20.

[31] Pavelka K. Treatment of pain in osteoarthritis. European Journal of Pain 2000; 4 Suppl A: 23-30.

[32] Brandt KD. Osteoarthritis. In: Fauci AS, Braunwald E, Isselbacher KJ, eds. Harrison's Principles of Internal Medicine, Interantional Edition, 14th edn. New York: McGraw Hill, 1998;1935-1941.

[33] Bensen WG, Fiechtner JJ, McMillen JI, Zhao WW, Yu SS, Woods EM, Hubbard RC, Isakson PC, Verburg KM, Geis GS. Treatment of osteoarthritis with celecoxib, a cyclooxigenase-2 inhibitor: a randomized, controlled, trial. Mayo Clin Proc 1999; 74: 1095-1105.

[34] Wollheim FA. Current pharmacological treatment of osteoarthritis. Drugs 1996; 52 (Suppl 3): 27-38.

[35] Altman R, Howell DS. Disease-modifying osteoarthritis drugs. In: Brandt K, Doherty M, Lohmander S, eds. Osteoarthritis. Oxford: Oxford University Press, 1998; 417-428.

[36] Hochberg MC, Altman RD, Brandt KD, Clark BM, Dieppe PA, Griffin MR, Moskowitz RW, Schnitzer TJ. Guidelines for the medical management of osteoarthritis. Part I. Osteoarthritis of the hip. Arthritis and Rheumatism 1995a; 38: 1535-1540.

[37] Hochberg MC, Altman RD, Brandt KD, Clark BM, Dieppe PA, Griffin MR, Moskowitz RW, Schnitzer TJ. Guidelines for the medical management of osteoarthritis. Part II. Osteoarthritis of the knee. Arthritis and Rheumatism 1995b; 38: 1541-1546.

Part II: Psychological and Psychosocial Considerations

In: The Handbook of Chronic Pain
Editors: S. Kreitler, D. Beltrutti, et al., pp. 77-99

ISBN 978-1-60021-044-0
© 2007 Nova Science Publishers, Inc.

Chapter 5

Quality of Life and Coping in Chronic Pain Patients

Shulamith Kreitler and David Niv

INTRODUCING QUALITY OF LIFE INTO THE CONTEXT OF PAIN

Pain is a comprehensive bio-socio-psychological event. When this conclusion came to be generally accepted by those who deal with the treatment, management and investigation of pain, it was first understood in terms of the factors producing and affecting pain. However, gradually this conclusion came to be applied also in regard to the effects of pain. It became increasingly evident that chronic pain affects much more than the damaged tissues and the neuronal channels transmitting the pain sensation. Pain may dominate attention, impair concentration, lower interest in the world, evoke anxiety and fear, produce depression, instigate conflicts within one's family, lower one's ability to work, even reduce one's will to live, to mention just a few of the more salient effects. All this has been evident to clinicians and relatives of chronic pain patients (CPPs) for a long time, but has come to be identified as a legitimate domain of inquiry only fairly recently, with the introduction of the concept of quality of life (QOL). The application of QOL in regard to pain may have been delayed relative to other domains of medicine because pain is commonly considered as an integral part of QOL itself (Portenoy, 1990). Hence it had to be abstracted from the complex of QOL before the issue of the impact of pain on QOL could be addressed. But with over 8000 items elicited in the MedLine by the combination 'pain and QOL' little doubt is left about the central role of QOL in regard to the understanding, assessment and management of pain. Introducing QOL into the context of pain represents the culmination of the development from nociception, in the narrow sense of the term, to the whole person, in the broad sense of the term.

DEFINITION OF QOL

QOL is usually defined as the individuals' perception of their functioning and well-being in different domains of life (Fayers and Machin, 2000) or in more specific terms, the individuals' evaluation of their position in life, in the context of the culture and value systems in which they live, and in relation to their goals, expectations, standards and concerns (WHOQOL Group, 1995). 'Health related QOL' (HRQOL) is QOL as it is assumed to be affected by some health disorder, medical procedure or treatment (Schipper, 1991).

The standard definitions highlight the following characteristics of QOL:

a) QOL is a *subjective* construct, reflecting the individual's view of one's well-being and functioning. This view may differ both from the evaluation of the patient's performance status, which assesses the pain's objective effects on the patient's functioning, and from the evaluation of the patient's actual state by others, including family members and health professionals (Chaitchik, Kreitler, Rapoport et al., 1992; Sprangers and Aaronson, 1992);

b) QOL is a *phenomenological* construct, which provides a surface image of the situation without explaining why and how it arose;

c) QOL is an *experiential or evaluative* construct, which presents a judgment without any attempt to relate the judgments to any objectively verifiable facts;

d) QOL is a *dynamic* construct, which is expected to be sensitive to any significant changes in the individual's state;

e) QOL is a *multidimensional* construct, which is based not merely on a single global measure but on evaluations of QOL in several specific domains that have been identified as major constituents of QOL;

f) QOL is *quantifiable* construct, which may be assessed so that it provides scores comparable from one individual to another as well as from one state to another in the same individual.

TOOLS OF ASSESSMENT OF QOL

Most tools for assessing QOL rely on the individuals' self-reports and provide scores comparable across participants. They include items to which one is requested to respond by checking one of the presented alternatives. The items refer to a set of domains or facets, and mostly also to a general evaluation of QOL. The following scales are reliable and valid assessment tools of QOL, often used in pain studies:

a) **World Health Organization Quality of Life (WHOQOL)** is a multidimensional, multilingual questionnaire designed for cross-cultural assessments, which includes 276 items, referring to 29 facets constituting 6 domains: the physical (e.g., sleep, sex); social relationships; psychological (e.g., emotions, cognition); level of independence (e.g., mobility, work capability); health and social care (e.g., availability and quality of services); spirituality, religion and personal beliefs (WHOQOL Group, 1995).

b) **MOS 36 Item Short Form Health Survey (SF-36)** is a general health questionnaire assessing the spiritual, social and mental aspects of QOL. It includes 8 subscales (with scores in the range of 0 – 100): physical functioning; role functioning – physical; bodily pain; social functioning; mental health; role functioning – emotional; vitality; and general health perceptions (Stewart, Hays and Ware, 1988).

c) **The Psychological General Well-Being Scale (PGWB)** is a 22 item inventory with 6 subscales: anxiety, depression, vitality, positive well-being, self-control and general health. Each subscale has 3 to 5 items whose scores range from 0 to 15 or 20 or 25. The total index score ranges from 0 to 110 (Dimenaes, Gliesse, Hallerbaeck et al., 1993).

d) **The Nottingham Health Profile (NHP)** is a measure of perceived health with 38 items referring to 6 domains (i.e., energy, sleep, emotional reaction, social isolation, physical mobility and pain) and to the frequency of health-related problems in regard to paid employment, housework, hobbies, family life, social life, sex life and holidays (Wicklund, 1990).

e) **Migraine Specific Quality of Life Questionnaire (MSQOL)** is a disease specific scale, assessing the global subjective impact of migraine (Wagner, Patrick, Galer et al., 1996).

EFFECT OF PAIN ON QOL

A great number of studies in different countries with hundreds of pain patients suffering from pain due to different causes and diagnoses show that pain causes a significant decrease in QOL (Becker, Thomsen, Olsen et al., 1997; Garratt, Ruta, Abdala et al., 1993; Hagen, Kvien and Bjorndal, 1997; Skevington, 1998). The scores of pain patients on the QOL measures SF-36 and PGWB are lower than those of patients suffering from other diverse diseases, such as gastrointestinal symptoms, hypertension, cardiopulmonary diseases or major depression (Arnold, Witzeman, Swank et al., 2000; Becker et al., 1997; Stewart et al., 1988; Ware, Gandek, and IOQLA Project Group, 1994; Well, Stewart, Hays et al., 1989). In fact, the QOL of chronic non-malignant pain patients is among the lowest observed for any medical condition (Becker et al., 1997).

EFFECTS OF PAIN ON SPECIFIC DIMENSIONS OF QOL

A closer analysis shows that pain affects adversely not only the overall level of QOL, but also most of its more specific dimensions. Thus, pain was correlated negatively with 5 of the 6 domains of QOL assessed by the WHOQOL scale – all except spirituality, religion and personal beliefs (Becker et al., 1997), in the following descending order: the physical domain (mainly the facets of discomfort, energy and fatigue, sexual activity and sleep), psychological well-being (mainly positive feelings, cognitive activities and self-esteem), level of independence (mainly mobility, activities of daily life and dependence on medications) and environmental health and services (mainly physical safety and security, availability of social care, and work satisfaction) (Skevington, 1998). On the PGWB the most badly affected domains were the negative feelings of anxiety and depression, followed by social functioning and by psychological well-being. Similarly, on the SF-36 the most affected domains were role functioning – physical, and role functioning – emotional (Becker et al., 1997). In women with recurrent breast or gynecological cancers pain was correlated mainly with decrease in physical and social functioning (Rummans, Frost, Suman et al., 1998). In cancer patients with advanced metastatic disease, pain affected mainly interpersonal relations in contrast to physical symptoms which affected mainly functioning focused on oneself (Kovner, Kreitler, Inbar, in press).

In general, the most strongly affected domains are the physical, followed by the emotional, social and cognitive. The most strongly affected facets of QOL (according to the WHOQOL) are the availability of health and social care, mobility, working capacity, activity of daily living, negative mood, sleep, dependence on medication and physical safety. The least affected facets include communication capacity, perception of home environment, information and skills, and religious beliefs (Stewart et al., 1988).

Accordingly, pain reduces well-being and functioning in the most diverse domains of QOL, but it does not affect all domains to the same degree, so that some domains are affected only minimally. This implies, first, that a pain patient experiences many important aspects of life differently than a non-pain patient. Second, treating a pain patient requires addressing, in addition to the pain itself, diverse domains of life affected by pain, primarily those affected most strongly by pain (e.g., physical functioning, social relations). And thirdly, helping the pain patient to focus on the domains of QOL least affected by pain (e.g., religious beliefs, perception of home environment) may improve the patient's QOL and thus promote his or her ability to cope with the pain and moderate the overall effects of pain on QOL.

EFFECTS OF SPECIFIC CHARACTERISTICS OF PAIN ON QOL.

The following are pain characteristics that contribute to lowering the pain patient's QOL:

a) **Pain intensity.** The more intense the pain, the lower is the level of QOL (Rummans et al., 1998; Skevington, 1998). This holds for chronic pain as well as acute pain in the two weeks prior to assessment, and even when disease severity, treatment setting, fatigue and depression are considered. However, it requires larger changes in intensity to effectuate smaller changes in QOL (Latru, Fontaine and Colleau, 1997; Skevington, 1998).

b) **Extent of the body area** affected by pain. The decrease in QOL is larger when the area is extensive than when pain is regional (Croft, Rigby, Boswell et al., 1993), or when there are two different kinds of pain than when there is only one kind (Dartigues, Michel, Lindoulsi et al., 1998).

c) **Co-morbidity.** QOL decreases more when the patient has more than one disease, even if the additional one may not even be related to pain (Cuijpers, van Lammern, and Duzijn, 1999).

d) **Pain duration.** The adverse effect of pain on QOL increases the longer the pain has lasted (the compared durations were up to 1 month, 2-12 months, or 12 months or more; Skevington, 1998).

e) **Pain components.** QOL is affected adversely by the emotional and evaluative components of pain but not by the sensory one (Passchier, de Boo, Quaak et al., 1996).

THE EFFECT OF PAIN ON QOL IN SPECIFIC DISEASES

The disease context of the pain may modulate the effect of pain on QOL. This may occur through symptoms produced by the disease. For example, if the pain limits physical mobility or functioning, as in osteoporosis or rheumatoid arthritis, pain reduces QOL more than when there is no or less physical disability (Hagen et al., 1997; Leidig-Bruckner, Minne, Scleich et al., 1997). In cancer patients with pain, problems in breathing and appetite were predictors of lower QOL (Allison, Locker, Wood-Dauphinee et al., 1998). Even the sheer burden of symptoms that pain patients may have, decreases their level of QOL (Desbiens, Mueller-Rizner, Connors et al., 1999). In some diseases the effect of pain on QOL is particularly salient in a specific domain. For example, in cancer patients pain affected social functioning and interpersonal relations (Haythornwaite, Raja, Fisher et al., 1998; Strang and Qvarner, 1990) whereas physical symptoms affected mainly functioning focused on oneself (Kovner et al., in press).

In some diseases the effect of pain on QOL is modulated significantly by the patient's expectations. For example, due to the frequency of migraine attacks, migraine patients report a decrease in QOL also during the pain-free periods because they feel the constant threat of another attack (Blau, 1984). In orthopedic patients, following an accident, even severe pain which reduces the functional status, does not seriously lower QOL if it is expected to be temporary (Kreitler, Chaitchik, Rapaport et al., 1993).

THE EFFECT OF TREATMENTS OF PAIN ON QOL

Many studies show that effective pain treatments lead to positive effects on QOL (e.g., Zhao, Dedhiya, Bocanegra et al., 1999; Aparasu, McCoy, Weber et al., 1999). However, QOL assessments are often more responsive to changes in clinical conditions than even pain measures are (Linton, Bradley, Jensen et al., 1989; Skevington, 1998). For example, the superiority of oxaprozin treatment (1200 mg once a day for 6 weeks) over placebo in patients with osteoarthritis of the knee was evident sooner in measures of QOL than in measures reflecting pain reduction (Zhao et al., 1999).

Sometimes two treatments may be equally effective in reducing pain but one may still have better effects on QOL, as for example, an internally powered spinal cord stimulation system over the externally powered because it produces more improvements in physical functions (Stultz, 1999). Similarly, coupling pharmacological treatment with a psychosocial intervention (no matter which) produces greater improvement in QOL than drugs alone (Mantovani, Astara, Lampis et al., 1996).

Forms of administering drugs do not always affect QOL. Thus, neither pain reduction nor QOL differ for different forms of administering morphine, e.g., by suspension or tablets (Boureau, Saudubray, D'Arnouz et al., 1992), in continuous infusion or intermittent bolus doses (Gourlay, Plummer, Cherry et al., 1991). However, sometimes two treatments equally effective in reducing pain may differ in QOL effects because one of them produces more unpleasant side effects or its prescribing is interpreted by many patients as signifying disease deterioration (e.g., morphine as compared to transdermal fentanyl) (Ahmedzai, Allan, Fallon et al., 1996; Coyle, Adelhardt, Portenoy et al., 1990; Stein, 1995). Notably, even an invasive technique like celiac plexus block was superior to morphine in pancreatic cancer patients because by providing a long-lasting analgesic effect, it reduced morphine consumption and thus prevented deterioration in QOL for a longer period of time (Kawamata, Ishitani, Ishikawa et al., 1996).

Hence, in addition to reducing pain, pain treatment also improves QOL. There are three possibilities to account for this effect. First, pain reduction may reduce negative emotions, such as anxiety and depression, contingent upon the pain, which affect adversely QOL, for example, by limiting physical and social activities. Accordingly, weakening pain may weaken anxiety and depression which in themselves are potent factors dampening QOL directly and indirectly. Thus, in metastatic cancer patients who got palliative radiotherapy, reduction in pain was attended by reduction in depression and anxiety and increases in vigor and curiosity, as well as in QOL domains, such as functioning in the family and communication with friends (Kovner et al., in press).

Second, pain reduction may improve the patient's functional state and symptoms. In most disorders the pain affects adversely at least to some extent the patient's functional capacity, e.g., lifting objects, even walking. These physical limitations reduce QOL. Reducing pain improves the functional ability and may thus contribute to improving the patient's QOL. For example, in prostate cancer patients with painful bone metastases intravenous clodronate for 10 days led to reduction of pain which brought about increases in QOL when it enabled improvement in the activity score (Cresswell, English, Hall et al., 1995).

Third, pain reduction is often interpreted by patients in a positive way, for example, as improvement in health or at least as a chance for improvement, or as a sign that they are not yet beyond being helped or even fully recovering. Hence, it may improve the patient's mood and energy level in a way that may result in more activities contributing to raising one's QOL (Kovner et al., in press).

INDIVIDUAL DIFFERENCES MODERATING THE EFFECTS OF PAIN ON QOL

Several demographic characteristics affect the impact of pain on QOL. For example, lower educational level, older age, being a female and unemployment tended to increase the impact of pain on QOL. Age and gender also played a role in regard to the domains in which the deterioration became manifest, for example, in older male patients - physical function and vitality, whereas in older females – emotional relations (Allison et al., 1998; Redigor, Barrio, de la Fuente et al., 1999).

Meanings assigned to pain are another important factor modulating the impact of pain on QOL. If pain is viewed as a punishment and expiation for sins, or as an integral aspect of human existence, it is likely to be accepted to a greater degree and to affect QOL less than if it is viewed as injustice, preventable accident or as failure on the part of health professionals (Morris, 1999). Further, when back pain is interpreted as disabling, as is often the case in the US, it affects QOL more than when it is interpreted as merely impairing function, as is often the case in Japan (Brena, Sanders and Motoyama, 1990).

The meaning of pain may differ also in line with the underlying disorder. For example, in HIV patients who considered pain as a sign of progression in the disease, pain produced more reduction in QOL than in those who did not consider pain as a threat of this kind (Payne, Jacobsen, Breitbart et al., 1994). Also for cancer patients, the initiation of even mild pain may signify a deterioration of the disease and thus affect appreciably QOL, disproportionally to the increase in pain (Portenoy, 1990; Strang, 1997). However, when pain was considered merely as a side-effect of treatment (viz., bone marrow transplantation), it did not reduce QOL even when it was severe (Bush, Donaldson and Sullivan, 1995). .

PAIN IS NOT IDENTICAL WITH QOL

The reviewed studies show that pain affects QOL. The effect was shown for different types of pain, diseases, cultures and individuals. It is strong and pervasive, manifested in many domains of life, including the physical, emotional, social and cognitive. However, it is no less evident that pain and QOL are distinct constructs, neither one of which can be considered as a component of the other. Indeed, changes in pain are often attended by corresponding changes in QOL, even though the changes may not be matched in pace and timing. But this is not always the case: sometimes pain worsens while QOL does not change or even improves (Portenoy, 1990); at other times pain remains constant while QOL deteriorates. Discrepancies of this kind are not really surprising or novel for pain clinicians. They have known for long that disability and even suffering have relatively little to do with tissue damage per se as well as with the pain experience, but they have much to do with how patients and those around them cope with the pain. This insight has gradually established itself on the scene of pain research. Hence, coping on the part of the individual came to be generally considered as a major factor intervening between pain and its effects on QOL.

Thus, pain is no doubt a co-determinant of QOL but coping is the intervening factor which has to be considered if we are to understand the impact of pain on QOL and help to minimize or limit its deleterious effects.

COPING AND THE PAIN CONTEXT

Coping is a kind of response subserving adaptation that is evoked when there is a gap in the appraisal of resources by the individual: those appraised as required by the situation far exceed those appraised as available to him or her. This specific gap is identified as defining stress for the individual. Hence, it is attended by characteristic physiological and psychological correlates, such as respiratory reactions or emotional distress, and it is experienced as unpleasant, endangering well-being and disrupting adaptation. Coping is designed to help the individual react in a way that enables restoring adaptation.

Thus, according to this transactional model (Lazarus and Folkman, 1984), coping is a function of the appraisals of the situation in relation to oneself. When the gap in the appraisals is nil or very small, there is a state of adaptation. When the gap is medium, the situation is experienced as challenging. When the gap is very-large, the individual experiences despair and hopelessness. Coping is the response that sets in when the gap is large, that is, above medium (which is challenging) and below very large (which is despair evoking). Accordingly, coping is situation-bound insofar as it depends on a certain situation that evokes the gap in resource appraisals. But, it is individual-bound insofar as the appraisals are subjective and the evoked coping responses depend to some extent on the individual's disposition (Holahan, Moos and Schaefer, 1996).

Pain often calls forth coping responses because in addition to being itself a highly unpleasant and difficult experience it has further characteristics that enhance its difficulty for the individual: it often limits physical functioning and thus reduces one's independence and other pleasurable activities; it is a lonely experience that is hard to share with others and may not always be credible to others; it is often bound with uncertainty about underlying medical conditions and future developments. In short, pain is a real hazard for QOL. As such, it requires coping and often elicits it.

ASSESSING COPING IN PAIN PATIENTS

Most coping inventories request the patient to describe their thoughts, feelings or actions in response to a major stressor, which may be left for the patient to identify or is specified as the pain. Specifying the stressor is preferable in that it reduces ambiguities but provides the same results when the patient identifies pain as the major stressor. The following are the main instruments used for assessing coping:

a) **The Ways of Coping Checklist (WCC)** has several versions. The original one with 67 items asks the patient to specify the stressor and rate the frequency with which he/she uses specific responses, grouped into two broad scales: one assessing problem-focused coping (i.e., efforts to change the situation, e.g., gathering information, planning action), the other assessing emotion-focused coping (i.e., efforts to change one's internal state, e.g., getting support, distancing, avoidance) (Lazarus and Folkman, 1984).

b) **Vanderbilt Pain Management Inventory (VPMI)** is a 27 items questionnaire requesting patients to indicate on a 5-point rating scale the frequency with which they react to pain of at least moderate intensity with cognitive or behavioral responses (e.g., praying for relief, depending on others for help), grouped into two broad scales labeled active coping and passive coping (Brown and Nicassio, 1987).

c) **The Coping Strategies Questionnaire (CSQ)** is a 44-item questionnaire asking the patients to indicate on a 7-point rating scale the extent to which they use 6 cognitive and 2 behavioral strategies when experiencing pain: diverting attention, reinterpreting pain, self-statements of strengthening, ignoring the pain, praying or hoping, catastrophizing (worrying whether it will end), increasing activity level, increasing treatments of pain (Rosenstiel and Keefe, 1983) (see also Chapter 11, section 'Appraisal of Beliefs, Perceived Self-Efficacy and Coping Styles').

d) **Coping with Health Injuries and Problems Scale (CHIP)** is a 32 item questionnaire asking the patients to rate on a 5-point scale how often they use in response to pain or any other illness or injury different responses, grouped into 4 coping scales: palliative coping (self-help responses designed to alleviate the unpleasantness of the situation), instrumental coping (task-oriented responses, e.g., seeking medical information), distraction coping (thinking or doing other things), and emotional preoccupation (focusing on the emotional results of the problem) (Endler, Parker and Summerfeldt, 1998).

e) **The Pain-Related Self-Statements Scale (PRSS)** includes 35 item questionnaire that requests the patients to rate on a 6-point scale how often they engage in response to pain in different characteristic pain-related cognitions, such as "it will never stop", "I can help myself" (Flor, Behle and Birbaumer, 1993).

STRATEGIES USED IN COPING WITH PAIN

According to the "composite measures" approach it is customary to refer to coping in terms of general coping strategies, each of which consists of more specific responses. The main advantages of these measures are that they provide general information, their relation to adjustment was examined empirically, they were used in a great many studies, they enable easy comparison across samples and studies, and they are easy to describe and communicate. Their main shortcoming is that they are too general, are based on sets of responses that often are not correlated, and are of little use in interventions with pain patients.

One of the best known composite measures is emotion-focused (attempts to reduce the stress and the negative emotions) versus problem-focused (attempts to reduce the pain per se) (Lazarus and Folkman, 1984). Another common composite measure is passive coping (withdrawal or giving up control to someone or something other than the individual, e.g., wishful thinking, praying, restricting activities, taking medication, calling a doctor) versus active coping (initiating some activity in order to control the pain, e.g., deliberate distraction, engaging in leisure or physical activity) (Brown and Nicassio, 1987). Sometimes the pair of illness-focused (e.g., attempts to overcome the pain, getting medical information) versus wellness-focused (e.g., relaxing, distraction) coping strategies is used (Jensen, Turner, Romano and Strom, 1995). A further classification is based on distinguishing between cognitive coping strategies (e.g., counting, distraction, imagery) and behavioral (actions designed to control pain, e.g., resting in bed, seeking social support, taking analgesics) (Fernandez, 1986). Sometimes a distinction is made between attentional coping strategies (focusing attention directly on the source of the pain in an attempt to manage it, e.g., exercising the painful area, seeking information) and avoidant (avoiding thinking or acting on the source of pain, e.g. denying pain sensations, distraction) (Suls and Fletcher, 1985).

According to the "individual measures" approach, coping is described in terms of specific responses, such as catastrophizing or distraction. The advantages of this approach are that the responses are conceptually purer, describe the actual actions of the patients and are useful in intervention studies. Studies based on individual coping responses provide a reliable and valid assessment of coping with pain by specific individuals in the framework of specific diseases. The main shortcoming is that this approach yields results that may be difficult to generalize and compare across samples and studies. Examples of individual coping strategies that have been identified in pain patients include catastrophizing, praying/hoping, reinterpreting pain sensations, ignoring pain, diverting attention from the pain, or facing pain as a challenge (Boothby, Thorn, Stroud et al., 1999).

MALADAPTIVE STRATEGIES OF COPING WITH PAIN

A landmark review of studies up to 1991 as well as later studies showed that passive coping strategies, such as praying, hoping, wishful thinking, withdrawal, resting and use of medication (assessed by the CSQ, VPMI), are associated with increased pain, depression, distress, lower positive affect, disability and poorer psychological adjustment (Jensen, Turner, Romano and Karoly, 1991; Zautra, Burleson, Smith et al., 1995).

Further CSQ-based composite measures labeled Helplessness and Avoidance were associated with higher levels of disability (Lenhart and Ashby, 1996). A composite measure of Helplessness (withdrawal and catastrophizing) was positively associated with psychological distress and negatively with activity level, and a composite measure of Medical Remedies (e.g., guarding, applying heat or cold, using medication) was negatively associated with activity level (Kleinke, 1992).

Studies based on individual coping strategies usually used one or more of the following outcome measures to assess maladjustment: higher levels of psychological distress, more negative affect and less positive affect, less uptime, higher rates of analgesic use, more pain-related physician visits, more frequent and longer hospitalizations, poorer physical functioning and greater disability, higher ratings of pain intensity, more reports of pain interference in daily activities, lower levels of general activity, more psychosocial dysfunction, and reduced ability to work as well as lower rate of return to work. The coping strategies that were found to be maladaptive in regard to pain include the following:

a) **Catastrophizing**: It denotes the excessive use of negative statements concerning the pain at present and in the future, such as 'it's awful', 'I expect the worst', 'I am overwhelmed". This seems to be the most widely researched strategy. A large body of studies demonstrated almost unanimously its maladaptive nature in regard to different categories of pain patients (e.g., Geisser, Robinson, Keefe et al., 1994; Hill, 1993; Robinson et al., 1997). However, two controversial issues remain unresolved. It has been suggested that catastrophizing may be an appraisal mechanism reflecting the threat of pain to one's well-being rather than a coping strategy (Jensen et al., 1991). Further, since catastrophizing is a salient feature in depressive cognition in general, it has been debated whether it may not assess vulnerability to depression so that depression is the mediating factor between catastrophizing and adjustment to pain (Sullivan and D'Eon, 1990).

b) **Praying/Hoping**: Sometimes it is called Escape Avoidance (Vitaliano, Russo, Carr et al., 1985) or Wishful Thinking (Jensen et al., 1991). It denotes an attitude of waiting for a miracle to happen or relying on doctors to find one day a cure for one's ailment. Many studies showed the positive correlations of this strategy with dysfunction and negative with adaptation. Yet, it should be noted that in this context praying seems to have more to do with passive wishful thinking than with religiosity that could have positive contributions to adaptation (Pargament, 1997), as indicated by at least one study (Blalock, DeVellis and Giorgino, 1995).

c) **Avoidance**: It denotes a strategy that consists in reducing the frequency of different activities, designed to decrease ongoing pain as well as anticipated increases in pain in the future. Some of these reduced activities – especially physical activities and exercise – may indeed reduce ongoing pain, especially in the early stages of recovery. But this would not hold for other activities from which the patient may withdraw, such as social activities, entertainment and work (Philips, 1987). Moreover, it does not hold for withdrawal from all types of activities in the long term. Coping by means of avoidance often serves the patient to avoid various unpleasant tasks and obligations (e.g., household chores, marital strife, duties at work). With time, though pain severity remains unchanged, the avoidance leads to reduced sense of control over the pain, increased physical disability and increased psychological distress (Holmes and Stevenson, 1990; Jaspers, Heuvel, Stegenga et al., 1993; Vitaliano et al., 1985).

d) **Social support seeking**: It denotes seeking out relations with others that could help the patient instrumentally and emotionally. Satisfaction with one's social support is related to more intense pain, more pain behaviors (e.g., sighing, grimacing, groaning, limping, guarding, rubbing, taking pain medication) and lower adjustment. The reason for this unexpected finding may be that solicitous spouses and other family members may facilitate expression of pain sensations and suffering through their sympathy and attention to the patient's pain behaviors and complaints. Further, while feeling helpless to alleviate the pain, they may encourage the patient to avoid the performance of various duties, especially the unpleasant ones, thus enhancing the patient's disability (Flor, Kerns and Turk, 1987; Romano, Turner, Friedman et al., 1992). Finally, patients may feel that the support they get from others is contingent on pain, so that maintaining the support requires keeping up the pain (Portenoy, 1990). Only in one study 'seeking emotional support from others' was associated negatively with distress and positively with activity level (Kleinke, 1992).

e) **Asking for help**: It denotes an attitude of growing dependence on other people, both relatives or friends as well as health professionals, and a concomitant growing withdrawal from doing things for oneself and in general. It was found to be detrimental for adjustment (Jensen et al., 1995)

f) **Comforting thinking**: It denotes minimizing the pain and its effects (e.g., "it will pass, don't worry"). It was found to be related negatively to adjustment (Jaspers et al., 1993).

g) **Palliative coping**: It denotes coping designed mainly to attain palliation, e.g., comforting, calming down. It was found to contribute to lower adjustment (Jaspers et al., 1993).

h) **Sedative hypnotic medication**: It denotes an increasing use of different types of medication designed not only to control pain but mainly to relax and overcome the negative emotions of tension, anxiety and depression. This strategy was found to be negatively correlated with adjustment (Jensen et al., 1995).

i) **Pacing**: It denotes adapting one's level of activity to the pain, namely, slowing down, resting, etc. It is negatively associated with adjustment (Van Lankveld, Pad Bosch, de Putte, et al., 1994)

j) **Guarding**: It denotes not moving specific painful body parts, being cautious in whatever one does. This strategy was found to be detrimental for adjustment (Jensen et al., 1995).

ADAPTIVE STRATEGIES OF COPING WITH PAIN

There is considerable evidence that active coping (e.g., problem solving, information seeking, exercise, activity) is negatively correlated with depression, negative affect and physical disability, and positively with activity level, namely, with overall better psychological and physical functioning (Jensen et al., 1991; Zautra et al., 1995).

A composite measure labeled Coping Attempts (based on the CSQ and including the subscales of Calming or Coping Self-Statements, Reinterpreting Pain Sensations, Ignoring Pain Sensations, Increasing Activity Level and Diverting Attention) was associated in several studies weakly with less activity reduction, fewer emergency room visits, and lower levels of psychosocial disability (though not of physical disability) (Gil, Williams, Thompson et al., 1991; Gil, Thompson, Keith et al., 1993; Martin, Bradley, Alexander et al., 1996).

Another composite factor labeled Self-Management (comprising Coping self-statements, Distracting activities, and Exercise) was associated negatively with distress and positively with activity level (Kleinke, 1992). Similarly, a factor labeled Pain Control and Rational Thinking (based on the CSQ) was related to lower levels of pain, depression, physical impairment and psychological disability (Beckham, Keefe, Caldwell, et al., 1991; Keefe, Caldwell, Martinez et al., 1991).

The following are the major individual coping strategies that were found to be adaptive in regard to chronic pain:

a) **Problem-focused coping.** It denotes attempts to overcome the pain by solving the medical or psychological problem that brought it about and sustains it. It may be assessed by low scores on Avoidance on the CSQ (Blalock et al., 1995).

b) **Regular exercise** It denotes engaging in systematic motor exercises designed to solve the physical problem that has generated the pain. The exercises are often orthopedically prescribed and supervised (Jensen et al. 1995)..

c) **Positive self-statements**: It denotes coping by saying to oneself statements, such as "I see it as a challenge and don't let it bother me", "I will deal with the pain", "It will get better in the near future". There is some evidence for positive effects on pain severity, psychological distress and general activity (Hill, 1993; Robinson et al., 1997; Van Lankveld et al., 1994). But the majority of studies did not find that this strategy was related to adjustment (Geisser et al., 1994; Robinson et al., 1997).

d) **Social comparison**: It denotes a strategy that consists in viewing oneself as better off than others. Studies suggest that it sometimes acts as adaptive to pain (Jensen et al., 1991).

COPING STRATEGIES NOT RELATED TO ADJUSTING TO PAIN

The following coping strategies were found in the majority of studies not to be related significantly to adjustment to chronic pain:

a) **Ignoring pain**: It denotes the approach of "I tell myself it doesn't hurt", or "I behave as if there were no pain". The majority of studies showed it had little influence on adjustment for most chronic pain patients (Geisser et al., 1994). According to some studies this strategy was related to lower ratings of pain (e.g., Robinson et al., 1997). Hence, it could perhaps be useful in coping with acute pain.

b) **Distraction/Diverting attention**: It is sometimes called Cognitive Refocusing (Varni, Waldron, Gragg et al., 1996) or Increasing Activity (Geisser et al., 1994). It denotes the use of activities designed to direct one's attention away from the pain, for example, reading a book, watching TV, going for a walk. It was found to be related to lower sensation of pain and sometimes to more positive mood (Varni et al., 1996) but not to better adjustment. Like Ignoring Pain it could be useful for handling acute pain, especially when weak or moderate. Notably, in CPPs it was related to higher pain severity and more interference of pain in daily activities (Robinson et al., 1997).

c) **Reinterpreting pain**: It is sometimes called Distancing from Pain. It denotes the use of cognitive mechanisms for transforming pain sensations from, say, pain to warm feeling or shooting pain to tingling. This strategy was not related to most measures of functional or psychological adjustment. It was even found to be related to higher rates of psychosocial dysfunction (Hill et al., 1995). But since it was found to be related to reducing acute pain (ter Kuile, Spinhoven and Linssen, 1995), it could be helpful in regard to acute pain.

d) **Keeping busy**: It denotes coping by getting absorbed in action, particularly of the routine kind, despite the pain. It was not found to be related to adjustment (Jensen et al., 1995).

e) **Emotional expression**: It denotes coping by means of expressing the pain-related affect one experiences. It was found not to affect adjustment to chronic pain (Blalock et al., 1995).

f) **Self-blame:** It is sometimes called also Self-Criticism (Blalock et al., 1995), It denotes assuming responsibility for negative events, including the pain. It was not found to play a role in adjusting to chronic pain (Jensen et al., 1991).

FUNCTIONING OF THE COPING STRATEGIES

The above sections presented three classes of coping strategies in line with their relation to adjustment to chronic pain. This distinction is based on empirical evidence, part of which is correlational. Hence, it is still unclear whether the coping strategies merely covary with adaptation or actually determine it. With this caveat in mind, the tripartite distinction is useful for the clinician because it provides indications which coping strategies are to be promoted, which are to be discouraged and which ones may be overlooked. In applying this approach several considerations about the functioning and determinants of coping strategies are in order.

First, most CPPs apply more than one strategy at any one time or in different phases of their coping. Hence, in assessing coping strategies of a certain CPP it is necessary to look for a set of strategies rather than rely on one or more dominant strategies. The adaptive strategies may not be the most salient one in the patient's repertory.

Second, the effectiveness of a coping strategy for adaptation may vary with pain characteristics, such as its intensity and duration. For example, avoidance coping may be useful in the initial stages, but when pain persists for longer periods this strategy may increasingly lead to maladjustment (Philips, 1987). Again, when pain is of high intensity, reinterpreting pain (or cognitive restructuring) may be used for moderating pain, even if only partly and only temporarily, and thus enable applying other strategies that have a larger adaptation impact.

Third, coping strategies may interact, so that they can be applied in conjunction. For example, catastrophizing has been consistently shown to be maladaptive. Hence it is important to attempt weakening it. This may prove more difficult when catastrophizing is particularly strong, that is, when the pain is of high intensity and poorly localized (Hadjitavropoulos and Craig, 1994). Cognitive restructuring may be applied for moderating pain to a certain extent and perhaps localizing it too so that the patient gains some sense of control over the situation and may thus become more susceptible to an intervention designed to decrease catastrophizing.

Fourth, coping strategies may have different aspects, so that even a basically maladaptive strategy may have beneficial aspects or may be applied in a manner that contributes to adaptation. One example is seeking social support. Some CPPs may be so depressed and entrenched in their lonely suffering that they are not responsive to an intervention designed to promote adaptation. Social support, especially with its comforting and emotion-sharing aspects, may serve to help them become more responsive to adaptive interventions. Another example is taking medication. It is often considered as part of passive coping insofar as it consists in relying on some external agent for managing one's pain. But it can also be used within the framework of active coping when emphasis is placed on the aspect of free choice by the patient of a means designed to promote the problem-solving approach to one's pain.

Finally, in order to understand and apply coping for promoting the patient's welfare, it is important to consider the dependence of coping strategies on the individual's dispositions. These include both personality traits and beliefs. There is evidence that some coping strategies may be used more frequently by individuals with particular personality traits. Thus, CPPs with higher external locus of control relied more heavily on maladaptive pain coping strategies (hoping and praying but not problem-focused coping) than those with low external locus of control, and also reported more psychological distress (Crisson and Keefe, 1988). Similarly, due to their tendencies to focus on the external world and on social activities, extraverts tend to apply coping strategies, such as seeking social support, or diversion through social activities (Phillips and Gatchel, 2000). Finally, CPPs high in optimism did not use catastrophizing, but rather one of the following two sets of coping strategies: either active coping strategies, which were associated with the perception of an ability to control pain, or hoping and praying, which was associated with the perception of inability to control pain (Novy, Nelson, Hetzel et al., 1998).

The example of optimism underscores the importance of beliefs in addition to personality traits as determinants of coping strategies. This conclusion is reinforced by findings showing that pain treatments may change beliefs but not coping strategies (Jensen, Turner, and Romano, 1994) and that beliefs may determine other components of adjustment than coping strategies (Turner, Jensen and Romano, 2000).

Thus, beliefs may affect the choice of coping strategies. For example, beliefs about self-efficacy in control of pain may be related to the more active coping strategies, such as exercise and problem-focused coping that may affect also persistence in cognitive-behavioral treatment (Kerns and Rosenberg, 1997). Patients who believed that their pain is stable and enduring as well as mysterious and defying any explanation (as assessed by the Pain Beliefs and Perceptions Inventory) had a stronger tendency to catastrophizing about their pain and employed fewer cognitive coping strategies as compared to patients who believed that their pain was of short duration and could be explained (Williams and Keefe, 1991).

Beliefs affect adjustment not only via coping strategies but also directly. For example, patients who believed that they were disabled (as assessed by The Survey of Pain Attitudes) had lower adjustment 1 to 7 years after completing pain treatment (Jensen and Karoly, 1991). Similarly, arthritis patients who had high scores on self-efficacy for pain had higher activity levels, namely, were better adjusted (DeGood and Shutty, 1992). In line with the cognitive orientation theory, beliefs are considered as guiding behaviors (Kreitler and Kreitler, 1982). This thesis has been demonstrated in a body of research that showed the interrelations between beliefs and behaviors, when the beliefs are relevant in contents and form. Since adjustment is often the product of specific behaviors of the patient, it is to be expected that beliefs would predict adjustment (Kreitler and Kreitler, 1991).

COPING AND QUALITY OF LIFE

Adjustment and QOL are interrelated concepts. Both denote states of the individual, within the context of external and internal circumstances, which may be difficult. Both refer to the overall state of the individual as manifested in various domains, rather than one domain or aspect. Both are subject to homeostatic striving toward an optimal level: adjustment is commonly considered as dependent on various behaviors or attitudes of the individual. QOL too evidences stabilization on some optimal level, drawing on positive components in a broad range of domains when major mainstays, such as health or employment are impaired (see compensatory model of QOL in Kreitler, Chaitchik, Rapoport et al., 1993). The main differences between adjustment and QOL are in range (adjustment is more limited) and assessment (adjustment is assessed objectively, QOL subjectively). Thus, the coping strategies identified in the literature as conducive to adjustment or impairing it are relevant for QOL.

Research on coping with pain identified several coping strategies related to adjustment to pain. Most notable are the consistent findings about the maladaptive function of the strategies of catastrophizing, hoping/praying, wishful thinking, pain-contingent rest, guarding, avoidance of activities, using sedative-hypnotic medication, seeking of social support, comforting thinking and palliative coping. The list of adaptive strategies is shorter. It includes mainly problem-focused coping, regular exercise, and possibly positive coping self-statements and positive social comparisons. It is of interest to note that most of the evidence points to coping strategies responsible for maladjustment. Accordingly, it seems that at present the safest recommendation for adjustment is simply to keep at bay the maladaptive strategies.

Analyzing the coping strategies from the point of view of their relation to the gap between available and required resources shows that none of the maladaptive strategies decreases the gap. Except for catastrophizing that may even increase the gap, the maladaptive strategies express in different forms acceptance of the gap as an immutable "given". The fantasy-based strategies (i.e., hoping/praying, wishful thinking) indicate that only extraordinary interventions, like miracles, could help; rest, guarding and avoidance of actions indicate that the individual has accepted the situation and acts accordingly, namely, reduces activities; finally, using sedatives, support seeking, comforting and palliative thinking indicate awareness on the part of the individual that nothing much can be done to change the situation.

In contrast, the adaptive coping strategies target reduction of the gap in two ways. The main one seems to be overcoming the pain by solving the problem that generated the pain (e.g., treatment, exercising) and the secondary seems to be strengthening one's self confidence and assurance (e.g., by positive coping self-statements and positive social comparisons) so that one is better able to attack the main target of overcoming the pain.

Accordingly, it seems that the maladaptive or adaptive nature of the strategies depends on how they relate to the appraisals of the resources that produce the stressful gap. Appraisals are cognitive contents and as such reflect the beliefs of the individual about the situation, the pain, and oneself. The implication thereof is that in order to harness adaptive coping in the service of promoting the patients' QOL, the main emphasis is to be placed on changing the patients' beliefs so that they consider the pain as a phenomenon that may be reduced or overcome, and themselves as capable of bringing this about, if they get the adequate medical and psychological help.

REFERENCES

Ahmedzai, S., Allan, E., Fallon, M., et al. (1994) Transdermal fentanyl in cancer pain. *Journal of Drug Development, 6*, 93-97.

Allison, P. J., Locker, D., Wood-Dauphinee, S., Black, M., and Feine, J. S. (1998). Correlates of health-related quality of life in upper aerodigestive tract cancer patients. *Quality of Life Research, 7*, 713-722.

Aparasu, R., McCoy, R. A., Weber, C., Mair, D., and Parasuraman TV (1999) Opioid-induced emesis among hospitalized nonsurgical patients: Effect on pain and quality of life. *Journal of Pain and Symptom Management, 18*, 280-288.

Arnold L. M., Witzeman, K. A., Swank, M. L., McElroy, S. L., and Keck P. E. Jr. (2000). Health-related quality of life using the SF-36 in patients with bipolar disorder compared with patients with chronic back pain and the general population. *Journal of Affective Disorders, 57*, 235-239.

Becker, N., Thomsen, A. B., Olsen, A. K., Sjorgen, P., Bech, P., Eriksen, J. (1997). Pain epidemiology and health related quality of life in chronic non-malignant pain patients referred to a Danish multidisciplinary pain center. *Pain, 73*, 393-400

Beckham, J. C., Keefe, F. J., Caldwell, D.S., and Roodman, A. A. (1991). Pain coping strategies in rheumatoid arthritis: Relationships to pain, disability, depression, and daily hassles. *Behavior Therapy, 22*, 113-124.

Blalock, S. J., DeVellis, B.M., and Giorgino, K. B. (1995). The relaionship between coping and psychological well-being among people with osteoarthritis: A problem-specific approach. *Annals of Behavioral Medicine, 17*, 107-115.

Blau, J. N. (1984). Fears aroused in patients by migraine. *British Medical Journal, 288*, 1126.

Brena S. F., Sanders, S. H., and Motoyama, H. (1990). American and Japanese low back pain patients: cross cultural similarities and differences. *Clinical Journal of Pain, 6*, 118-124.

Boothby, J. L., Thorn, B. E., Stroud, M. W., and Jensen, M. P. (1999). Coping with pain. In R. J. Gatchel and D.C. Turk (Eds.), *Psychosocial factors in pain: Critical perspectives* (pp. 343- 359). New York: Guilford.

Boureau, F., Saudubray, F., D'Arnoux, C., Vedrenne, J., Esteve, M., Roquefeuil, B., Siou, D. K., Brunet, R., Ranchere, J.Y., and Roussel, P. (1992). A comparative study of controlled- release morphine (CRM) suspension and CRM tablets in chronic cancer pain. *Journal of Pain and Symptom Management, 7*, 393-399.

Brown, G. K., and Nicassio, P. M. (1987). Development of a questionnaire for the assessment of active and passive coping strategies in chronic pain patients. *Pain, 31,* 53-63.

Bush, N. E., Donaldson, G., and Sullivan, K. (1995). Quality of life of 125 adults surviving 6-28 years after bone marrow transplantation. *Social Science and Medicine, 40,* 479-490.

Chaitchik, S., Kreitler, S., Rapoport, Y., and Algor, R. (1992). What do cancer patient spouses know about the patients? *Cancer Nursing, 15,* 353-362.

Coyle, N., Adelhardt, J., Portenoy, R. K., and Foley, K. M. (1990). Characters of terminal illness: Longitudinal assessment of patients with advanced cancer. *Journal of Pain and Symptom Management, 5,* 83-90.

Cresswell, S. M., English, P. J., Hall, R. R., Roberts, J.T., and Marsh, M. M. (1995). Pain relief and quality-of-life assessment following intravenous and oral clodronate in hormone- escaped metastatic prostate cancer. *British Journal of Urology, 76,* 360-365.

Crisson, J. E., and Keefe, F. J. (1988). Relationship of locus of control to pain coping strategies and psychological distress in chronic pain patients. *Pain, 35,* 147-154.

Croft, P., Rigby, A. S., Boswell, R., Schollum, J., and Silman, A. (1993). The prevalence of chronic widespread pain in the general poulation. *Journal of Rheumatology, 20,* 710-713.

Cuijpers, P., van Lammern, P., and Duzijn, B. (1999). Relation between quality of life and chronic illnesses in elderly living in residential homes: A prospective study. *International Psychogeriatrics, 11,* 445-454.

Dartigues, J. F., Michel, P., Lindoulsi, A., Duvrca, B., and Henry, P. (1998). Comparative view of the socioeconomic impact of migraine versus low back pain. *Cephalagia,_18* (supp 21), 26-29.

Desbiens, N. A., Mueller-Rizner, N., Connors, A. F. Jr., Wenger, N. S., and Lynn, J. (1999). The symptom burden of seriously ill hospitalized patients. *Journal of Pain and Symptom Management, 17,* 248-255.

DeGood, D. E., and Shutty, M. S. (1992). Assessment of pain beliefs, coping and self-efficacy. In D. C. Turk and R. Melzack (Eds.), *Handbook of pain assessment* (pp. 214-234). New York: Guilford.

Dimenaes, E., Gliese, H., Hallerbaeck, H., Svedlund, J., and Wiklund, I. (1993). Quality of life in patients with upper gastrointestinal symptoms. *Scandinavian Journal of Gastroenterology, 28,* 681-687.

Endler, N. S., Parker, J. D. A., and Summerfeldt, L. J. (1998). Coping with health problems: Developing a reliable and valid multidimensional measure. *Psychological Assessment, 10,* 195-205.

Fayers, P. M., and Machin, D. (2000). *Quality of life: Assessment, analysis and interpretation.* Surry, UK: Wiley.

Fernandez, E. (1986). A classification system of cognitive coping strategies for pain. *Pain, 26,* 141-151.

Flor, H., Behle, D. J., and Birbaumer, N. (1993). Assessment of pain-related cognitions in chronic pain patients. *Behavior Research and Therapy, 31,* 63-73.

Flor, H., Kerns, R. D., and Turk, D. C. (1987). The role of spouse reinforcement, perceived pain, and activity levels of chronic pain patients. *Journal of Psychosomatic Research, 31,* 251-259.

Garratt, A. M., Ruta, D. A., Abdala, M. I., Buckingham, J. K., and Russell, I. T. (1993). The SF- 36 health survey questionnaire: an outcome measure suitable for routine use within the NHS? *British Medical Journal, 306,* 1440-1444.

Geisser, M. E., Robinson, M. E., Keefe, F.J., and Weiner, M. L. (1994). Catastrophizing, depression, and the sensory, affective, and evaluative aspects of chronic pain. *Pain, 59,* 79-83.

Gil, K. M., Thompson, R. J. Jr., Keith, B. R., Tota-Faucette, M., Noll, S., and Kinney, T. R. (1993). Sickle cell disease pain in children and adolescents: Change in pain frequency and coping strategies over time. *Journal of Pediatric Psychology, 18,* 621-637.

Gil, K. M., Williams, D. A., Thompson, R. J., and Kinney, T. R. (1991). Sickle cell disease in children and adolescents: The relation of child and parentpain coping strategies to adjustment. *Journal of Pediatric Psychology, 16,* 643-663.

Gourlay, G. K., Plummer, J. L., Cherry, D.A., Onley, M. M., Parish, K. A., Wood, M. M., and Cousins, M. J. (1991). Comparison of intermittent bolus with continuous infusion of epidural morphine in the treatment of severe cancer pain. *Pain, 47,*135-140.

Hadjitavropoulos, H. D., and Craig, K. D. (1994). Acute and chronic low-back pain: Cognitive, affective and behavioral dimensions. *Journal of Consulting and Clinical Psychology, 62,* 341-349.

Hagen, K. B., Kvien, T. K., and Bjorndal, A. (1997). Muskoskeletal pain and quality of life in patients with noninflammatory joint pain compared to rheumatoid arthritis: A population survey. *Journal of Rheumatology, 24,* 1703-1709.

Haythornthwaite, J. A., Raja, S. N., Fisher, B., Frank, S. M., Brendler, C. B., and Shir, Y. (1998). Pain and quality of life following radical retropubic prostatectomy. *Journal of Urology, 160,* 1761-1764.

Hill, A. (1993). The use of pain coping strategies by patients with phantom limb pain. *Pain, 55,* 347-353.

Hill, A., Niven, C. A., and Knussen, C. (1995). The role of coping in adjustment of phantom limb pain. *Pain, 62,* 79-86.

Holahan, C.J., Moos, R.H., and Schaefer, J.A. (1996). Coping, stress esistance and growth: Conceptualizing adaptive functioning. In M. Zeidner and N. S. Endler (Eds.), *Handbook of coping: Theory, research, applications* (pp. 24-43). New York: Wiley.

Holmes, J. A., and Stevenson, C. A. Z. (1990). Differential effects of avoidant and attentional coping strategies on adaptation to chronic and recent-onset pain. *Health Psychology, 9,* 577-584.

Jaspers, J. P.C., Heuvel, F., Stegenga, B., and de Bont, L.G.M. (1993). Strategies for coping with pain and psychological distress associated with temporomandibular joint osteoarthrosis and internal derangement. *Clinical Journal of Pain, 9,* 94-103

Jensen, M. P., and Karoly, P. (1991). Control beliefs, coping efforts, and adjustment to chronic pain. *Journal of Consulting and Clinical Psychology, 59,* 431-438.

Jensen, M. P., Turner, J. A., and Romano, J. M. (1994). Correlates of improvement in multidisciplinary treatment of chronic pain. *Journal of Consulting and Clinical Psychology, 62,* 172-179.

Jensen, M. P., Turner, J. A., Romano, J. M., and Karoly, P. (1991). Coping with chronic pain: A critical review of the literature. *Pain, 47,* 249-283.

Jensen, M. P., Turner, J.A., Romano, J. M., and Strom, S. E. (1995). The Chronic Pain Coping Inventory: Development and preliminary validation. *Pain, 60,* 203-216.

Kawamata,M., Ishitani, K., Ishikawa, K., Sasaki, H., Ota, K., Omote, K., and Namiki, A. (1996).Comparison between celiac plexus block and morphine treatment on quality of life in patients with pancreatic cancer pain. *Pain, 64,* 597-602.

Keefe, F. J., Caldwell, D. S., Martinez, J., Nunley, J., Beckham, J., and Williams, D. A. (1991). Analyzing pain in rheumatoid arthritis patients. Pain coping strategies in patients who have had knee replacement surgery. *Pain, 46,* 153-160.

Kerns, R. D., and Rosenberg, R. (1997). *Pain stages of pain as predictors of pain treatment outcome.* Paper presented at the Annual Meeting of the American Pain Society, New Orleans.

Kleinke, C. L. (1992). How chronic pain patients cope with pain: Relation to treatment outcome in a multidisciplinary pain clinic. *Cognitive Therapy and Research, 16,* 669-685.

Kovner, F., Kreitler, S., and Inbar, M. (in press) The effect of palliative radiotherapy on the emotional state and psychological quality of life in advanced cancer patients. *Annals of Oncology.*

Kreitler, S., Chaitchik, S., Rapaport, Y., Kreitler, H., Algor, R. (1993). Life satisfaction and health in cancer patients, orthopedic patients and healthy individuals. *Social Science and Health, 36,* 547-556.

Kreitler, H., and Kreitler, S. (1982). The theory of cognitive orientation: Widening the scope of behavior prediction. In B. Maher and W. B. Maher (Eds.), *Progress in Experimental Pesonality Research, Vol. 11,* pp. 101-169. New York: Academic Press

Kreitler, S., and Kreitler, H.(1991). Cognitive orientation and physical disease or health. *European Journal of Personality, 5,* 109-129.

Latru, F., Fontaine, A., and Colleau, S. (1997). Unestimation and undertreatment of pain in HIV disease multicenter study. *British Medical Journal, 314,* 23-28.

Lazarus, R.S., and Folkman, S. (1984). *Stress, appraisal, and coping.* New York: Springer.

Leidig-Bruckner, G., Minne, H. W., Schlaich, C., Wagner, G., Scheidt-Nave, C., Bruckner, T.,Gebest, T., Gebest, H. J., and Ziegler, R. (1997). Clinical grading of spinal osteoporosis: quality of life components and spinal deformity in women with chronic low back pain and women with vertebral osteoporosis. *Journal of Bone and Minerals Research, 12,* 663-675.

Lenhart, R. S., and Ashby, J. S. (1996). Cognitive coping strategies and coping modes in relation to chronic pain disability. *Journal of Applied Rehabilitation Counseling, 27,* 15-18.

Linton, S. J., Bradley, L. A., Jensen, I., Sprangforth, E., and Sundell, L. (1989). The secondary prevention of low back pain: a controlled study with follow-up. *Pain, 36,* 137-207.

Mantovani, G., Astara, G., Lampis, B., et al. (1996). Impact of psychosocial intervention on the quality of life of elderly cancer patients. *Psycho-Oncology, 15,* 127-135.

Martin, M. Y., Bradley, L. A., Alexander, R. W., Alarcon, G.S., Triana-Alexander, M., Aaron, L. A. AND Albers K. R. (1996). Coping strategies predict disability in patients with primary fibromyalgia. *Pain, 68,* 45-53

Morris, D. B. (1999). Sociocultural and religious meanings of pain. In R. J. Gatchel and D. C. Turk (Eds.), *Psychosocial factors in pain: Clinical perspectives* (pp. 118-131). New York: Guilford.

Novy, D. M., Nelson, D. V., Hetzel, R. D., Squitieri, P., and Kennington, M. (1998). Coping with chronic pain: Sources of intrinsic and contextual variability. *Journal of Behavioral Medicine, 21*, 19-34.

Pargament, K. I. 1997). *The psychology of religion and coping.* New York: Guilford.

Passchier, J., de Boo, M., Quaak, H. Z. A., and Brienen, J. A. (1996). Health-related quality of life of chronic headache patients as predicted by the emotional component of their pain. *Headache, 36,*556-560.

Payne, D., Jacobsen, P., Breitbart, W., Passik, S., Rosenfeld, B., and McDonald, M. (1994). *Negative thoughts associated to pain are associated with greater pain, distress and disability in AIDS pain.* Abstract presented at the Annual Meeting of the American Pain Society, Miami, FL.

Philips, H. C. (1987). Avoidance behavior and its role in sustaining chronic pain. *Behavior Research and Therapy, 25,* 273-279.

Phillips, J. M., and Gatchel, R. J. (2000). Extraversion-introversion and chronic pain. In R. J. Gatchel and J. N. Weisberg (Eds.), *Personality characteristics of patients with pain* (pp. 181-202). Washington, DC: American Psychological Association.

Portenoy, R. K. (1990) Pain and quality of life: Clinical issues and implications for research. *Oncology, 4,* 172-178.

Regidor, E., Barrio, G., de la Fuente, L., Domingo, A., Rodriguez, C., and Alonzo, J. (1999).Association between educational level and health-related quality of life in Spanish adults. *Journal of Epidemiology and Community Health, 53,* 75-82.

Robinson, M. E., Riley, J. L., Myers, C. D., Sadler, I. J., Kvaal, S. A., Geisser, M. E., and Keefe, F. J. (1997). Coping Strategies Questionnaire: A large sample, item level factor analysis. *Clinical Journal of Pain, 13,* 43-49.

Romano, J.M., Turner, J. A., Friedman, L. S., Bulcroft, R. A., Jensen, M. P., Hops, H. and Wright, S.F. (1992). Sequential analysis of chronic pain behaviors and spouses responses. *Journal of Consulting and Clinical Psychology, 60,* 777-782.

Rosenstiel, A. K., and Keefe, F. J. (1983). The use of coping strategies in low-back pain patients: Relationship to patient characteristics and current adjustment. *Pain, 17,* 33-40

Rummans, T. A., Frost, M., Suman, V. J., Taylor, M., Novotny, P., Gendron, T., Johnson, R.,Hartmann, L., and Evans, R. W. (1998). Quality of life and pain in patients with recurrent breast and gynecologic cancer. *Psychosomatics, 39,* 437-445.

Schipper, H. (1990). Guidelines and caveats for quality of life measurement in clinical practice and research. *Oncology (Huntington), 4,* 51-57.

Skevington, S. M. (1998). Investigating the relationship between pain and discomfort and quality of life, using the WHOQOL. *Pain, 76,* 395-406.

Sprangers, M. A. G., and Aaronson, N. K. (1992). The role of health care providers and significant others in evaluating the quality of life of patients with chronic disease: A review. *Journal of Clinical Epidemiology, 45,* 743-760.

Stein, C. (1995). The control of pain in peripheral tissues by opioids. *New England Journal of Medicine, 332,* 1685-1690.

Stewart, A. L., Hays, R. D., and Ware, J. E. (1988). The MOS short form general health survey. Reliability and validity in a patient population. *Medical Care, 26*, 724-735.

Strang, P. (1997). Existential consequences of unrelieved cancer pain. *Palliative Medicine, 11*, 299-305

Strang, P., and Qvarner, H. (1990). Cancer-related pain and its influence on quality of life. *Anti Cancer Research, 10*, 109-112.

Sullivan, M. J. L., and D'Eon, M. J. (1990). Relation between catastrophizing and depression in chronic pain patients. *Journal of Abnormal Psychology, 99*, 260-263.

Suls, J., and Fletcher, E. (1985). The relative efficacy of avoidant and non-avoidant coping strategies: A meta-analysis. *Health Psychology, 4*, 249-288.

ter Kuile, M.M., Spinhoven, P., and Linssen, A.C.G. (1995). Responders and nonresponders to autogenic training and cognitive self-hypnosis: Prediction of short- and long-term success in tension-type headache patients. *Headache, 35*, 630-636.

Turner, J. A., Jensen, M. P., and Romano, J. M. (2000). Do beliefs, coping and catastrophizing independently predict functioning in patients with chronic pain? *Pain, 85*, 115-125.

Van Lankveld, W., Van't Pad Bosch, P., Van de Putte, L., Naring, G., Van der Staak, C. (1994). Disease-specific stressors in rheumatoid arthritis: Coping and well-being. *British Journal of Rheumatology, 33*, 1067-1073.

Varni, J. W., Waldron, S. A., Gragg, R. A., Rappoff, M. A., Bernstein, B. H., Lindsley, C. B., and Newcomb, M. D. (1996). Development of the Waldron/VarniPediatric Pain Coping Inventory. *Pain, 67*, 141-150.

Vitaliano, P. P., Russo, J., Carr, J. E., Maiuro, R. D., and Becker, J. (1985). The Ways of Coping Checklist: Revision and psychometric properties. *Multivariate Behavioral Research, 20*, 3-26.

Ware, J. E., Gandek, B., and the IQOLA Project Group. (1994). The SF-36 Health Survey: Development and use in mental health research and the IQOLA Project. *International Journal of Mental Health, 23*, 49-73.

Wells, K., Stewart, A., Hays, R. D., Burnam, M. A., Rogers W., Daniels, M., Berry, S., Greenfield, S., and Ware, J. (1989). The functioning and well-being of depressed patients. *Journal of the American Medical Association, 262*, 914-919.

WHOQOL Group. (1995). The World Health Organization Quality of Life assessment (WHOQOL): Position paper from the World Health Organization. *Social Science and Medicine, 41*,1403-1409.

Wiklund, I. (1990). The Nottingham Health Profile - a measure of health-related quality of life. *Scandinavian Journal of Primary Health Care Supplement, 1*, 15-18.

Williams, D. A., and Keefe, F. J. (1991). Pain beliefs and the use of cognitive-behavioral coping strategies. *Pain, 46*, 185-190.

Zautra, A. J., Burleson, M. H., Smith, C. A., Blalock, S. J., Wallston, K. A., DeVellis, R. F., DeVellisB.M., and Smith, T. W. (1995). Arthritis and perceptions of quality of life: An examination of positive and negative affect in rheumatoid arthritis patients. *Health Psychology, 14*, 399-408.

Zhao, S. Z., Dedhiya, S. D., Bocanegra, T.S., Fort, J. G., Kuss, M. E., Rush, S.M. (1999). Health related quality of life effects of Oxaprozin and Nabumetone in patients with osteoarthritis of the knee. *Clinical Therapy, 21,* 205-217.

In: The Handbook of Chronic Pain   ISBN 978-1-60021-044-0
Editors: S. Kreitler, D. Beltrutti, et al., pp. 101-114   © 2007 Nova Science Publishers, Inc.

Chapter 6

Patient and Family in the Context of Chronic Pain

Shulamith Kreitler and Michal M. Kreitler

Pain is a highly personal and subjective experience. The protagonist as well as the victim is the individual patient. Yet, in recent years there is a growing awareness of the involvement of the family in many of the aspects and phases of the phenomenon of pain. This awareness is grounded in two complementary approaches: first, the approach that considers the primary role of the family in regard to health and disease in general (Litman, 1979); and second, the approach that considers pain as dependent on psychosocial factors in addition to the nociceptive stimuli (Chapter 17, this book). Among the psychosocial factors the family may be expected to be of primary relevance and importance. Accordingly, a body of data has accumulated demonstrating the crucial role that the family plays in the antecedents, development, maintenance, effects, treatment and recovery of the pain patient. This chapter will highlight the major forms and manifestations of family involvement in pain so that its harmful effects can be minimized and its positive effects can be harnessed and mobilized for the patient's benefit. The role of the family differs in regard to each aspect and phase.

ANTECEDENTS OF PAIN IN THE CONTEXT OF THE FAMILY

The findings showed an increased frequency of pain problems in the families of origin of chronic pain patients (Payne and Norfleet, 1986; Turk, Flor and Rudy, 1987). According to an epidemiological survey 40%-50% of those reporting pain also reported that a parent had a pain problem (Crook et al., 1984). In psychiatric patients those with hypochondriachal symptoms as compared to those with no such symptoms reported more similarity between their own symptoms and those of their mothers but also more often a poor relationship with the mother (Kreitman et al., 1965). Similarly, psychiatric patients with pain reported about more pain in their parents and siblings than those without pain (Merskey, 1965). Again, depressed patients with pain reported more pain problems in their families than patients without pain (Mohamed et al, 1978). Comparing the family histories of pain patients and psychiatric patients showed that in each group about a third had a positive family history of pain, but in the families of pain patients there were more often cases of chronic pain, psychosomatic disorders and alcoholism (Chaturvedi, 1978).

Not only is the incidence of pain higher in the families of pain patients than in the families of other patients, but there is also similarity in specific features of the pain between the pain patients and the family members.. A comparison of patients suffering of non-organic abdominal pain with patients suffering of abdominal pain with known organic etiology showed that in 51.6% of the former group one or both parents suffered from abdominal pain as compared with 18.5% in the latter group (Hill and Blendis, 1967). Also Mohamed et al. (1978) found a relationship between the location of pain in the patients and the location in the patient's family members. Notably, a correlation was reported between reports of intermittent pain and number of familial pain models in a population of students (Edwards et al., 1985).

The findings about increased incidence of pain in the families of chronic pain patients are open to several interpretations. It is possible to view the findings as suggestive of a genetic background for chronic pain, although at present the issue of the genetics of chronic pain is still unclear. An alternative interpretation would be in terms of social learning theory, according to which children learn from their parents how to become a chronic pain patient. The similarity in pain location between parents and children provides strong support for the social learning interpretation. Thus, Christensen and Mortensen (1975) found that children were likely to have the same pain symptoms as their parents at present but less likely to have those the parents had as they were themselves children. The learning could take place directly through parents who use specific responses that act as reinforcement schedules for pain behaviors (Violon, 1985) or by modeling. However, the shortcoming of this interpretation is that it does not account for the fact that not all parents with chronic pain transmit the problem to their children, or rather, that not all children of chronic pain parents become themselves chronic pain patients. Thus, in the best case social learning would be a risk factor or necessary factor but not a sufficient one.

Finally, a third interpretation would endorse the psychodynamic view. Accordingly, individuals may develop a pain problem because of certain family characteristics that may include chronic pain but also alcoholism, physical health problems, bodily deformity, or depression, to mention just a few. Problems of this type in the families of origin may create an atmosphere that breeds aggression, guilt, and vulnerability to physical symptomatology that could render the option of chronic pain a viable one for the individual in later life under circumstances of crisis or other difficulties. Several studies are often cited as supportive evidence for this interpretation. Thus, Blumer and Heilbronn (1982) showed that 63% of chronic pain patients had a family member or close friend with a physical handicap or deformity; Violon (1985) found that early emotional deprivation, battering and abandonment were frequent in patients with atypical facial pain or cluster headaches; Hudgens (1979) found that 41% of the treated pain patients reported that their parents were harsh, distant and demanding; Gross et al. (1980-81) showed that 80% of patients with pelvic pain came from dysfunctional families, with an abundance of violence and passive-dependent relationships, and scarcity of maternal warmth and support. Some observations have even suggested the possibility of incest in the early history of pain patients (Gross et al., 1980-81; Roy, 1982). In sum, diverse findings that have accumulated indicate that early family relationships could set the stage for chronic pain later in life.

THE STATE OF THE PAIN PATIENT'S CURRENT FAMILY

The impact of the current family of the pain patient on pain is so significant that it has been identified as playing a more important role than medical factors in the transition from acute to chronic pain in low back pain (Valat, Goupille and Vedere, 1997). An accumulating set of data shows that in many cases the current families of chronic pain patients tend to be dysfunctional. Hudgens (1977) reported that in the majority of families in a treatment program for chronic pain the patient was highly dependent on the spouse or on a significant other, communication between family members was indirect, family members were incapable of handling anger, and social contacts were narrow. Ratings of pretreatment characteristics of families of pain patients showed that in 68-87% of the families family members had poor communication habits (e.g., withholding emotions, avoiding emotional topics, not resolving conflicts), the pain patient was meeting dependency needs indirectly, and the family roles were rigid (i.e., inability or unwillingness to change roles so as to adapt to the new circumstances) (Payne, 1982). Similarly, Waring (1983) found in the families of pain patients a passive approach to the marriage relationship on the part of both partners, disagreements between them on social contacts with others, lack of closeness and intimacy, and absence of communication about personal matters.

Furthermore, associations were found between family relations and pain. A comparison of chronic low back pain patients and healthy controls on the Family Environment Scale detected greater psychological distress and more conflicts in the pain patients. Within the group of the patients, more conflicts were related to higher depression and anxiety (Feuerstein et al., 1985). Again, a study with neuromuscular pain patients showed that patients' reports of greater family significance, less impact of pain on the family and more routine and meaningful rituals in family life were associated with a better state of the patients and their positive mood (Greene and Pargament, 1997).

Findings of the kind reported in this section are difficult to interpret. One possibility is that the structure and functioning of families of chronic pain patients have been faulty from the very start, even before the pain problem showed up. In that case, the family may have played a role in the emergence of the symptom, at least in the sense of a risk factor. Another possibility is that the families of pain patients have become faulty in their structure and functioning as a consequence of the emergence of the pain problem (see section on "The effects of pain on the family"). This may be the case in particular in regard to families that have been vulnerable from the start. However it may be, dysfunctional families may be expected not to be able to provide too much help and support to the chronic pain patient.

EFFECTS OF PAIN ON THE FAMILY

It could be expected that a continuous health problem, such as chronic pain of one family member would affect the whole family. Several studies show that spouses and family members of chronic pain patients suffer psychologically and report significantly more health problems than spouses of healthy partners (Rowat and Knafl, 1985). One reason may be due to the financial impact of chronic pain. Since the chronic pain patient may work fewer hours and the treatments may also cost money, spouses of pain patients were found to invest more time in housekeeping and household maintenance, which resulted in less time for personal needs and leisure activities (Kemler and Furnee, 2002). Further, chronic pain in the family tends to increase role tension between patients and spouses and to reduce their work activity (Klein, Dean and Bogdanoff, 1967). Adverse effects were reported in families and children of mothers with chronic pain as compared to healthy or diabetic mothers (Dura and Beck, 1988). Increased prevalence of sexual dysfunction and of psychophysiological disorders were found in the families of chronic pain patients (Flor et al., 1987; Maruta et al., 1981). A study of the spouses of chronic pain patients showed that 20% were clinically depressed, and 35% were maritally dissatisfied, whereby the marital dissatisfaction correlated significantly with the patient's functional impairment (Ahern, Adams and Follick, 1985). Also in the case of female low-back sufferers a correlation was found between the pain patient's level of disability and of psychological distress and marital dissatisfaction of the spouse (Saarijärvi et al., 1990). Some studies showed that one of the most difficult problems faced by the spouses of chronic pain patients was their uncertainty about the disease of their partner, their sense of being unable to control it and the difficulty of assigning meaning to it (Flor, Turk and Scholz, 1987; Rowat and Knafl, 1985). However, other studies did not find evidence for distress or dysfunction in chronic pain families (Deyo, 1986; Revenson and Majerovitz, 1990).

Some effects of pain on the family may be mediated by the manipulative behavior of the pain patients themselves. A factor analysis of pain measures and personality data of chronic pain patients yielded a factor of interpersonal alienation and manipulativeness that accounted for a significant proportion of the variance (Timmermans and Sternbach, 1974). This factor indicated a tendency to project blame and responsibility away from oneself onto others, outwardly directed anger and hostility, interpersonal conflict, and a sense of alienation from others. These tendencies suggest the possibility of "pain games" and using pain in order to gain benefits from others in the family setup.

It may be expected that a family that suffers a lot because of one of its members who is a pain patient, may affect adversely the pain patient himself or herself. The adverse effect may be due to the fact that a suffering family may not be able to provide the patient the help and support he or she may need. Another kind of adverse effect may be due to the patients' reactions to the suffering of the family. The patients' distress may be deepened through their inability to help their families and the guilt they may feel because of all the trouble they are causing.

In this context it is appropriate to mention the possibility that chronic pain of one family member may act as a stabilizing factor in specific family systems. Several scenarios may be described. One scenario is that the family has been at the point of disintegrating but holds off in order to help the suffering family member and provide him or her a steady framework.

Another scenario is that the family has been loaded with negative feelings which its members were incapable of expressing openly or of suppressing any longer. The illness of one family member may help all parties to control the expression of the negative feelings, a fact that contributes to the survival of the family as a unit. Finally, a third scenario is a family that suffers from a conflict of power between two of its members. By turning into a pain patient one of the members becomes "weaker", thereby contributing to resolving the conflict (e.g., Delvey and Hopkins, 1982; Swanson and Maruta, 1980; Waring, 1977). One study with headache patients is of particular interest in this context (Basolo-Kunzer et al., 1991). It showed that the patient's headache frequency and severity correlated positively with family cohesion and adaptability, and that headache severity correlated positively with marital affection, spouses' marital cohesion and spouses' affection.

However, the contribution of the pain problem to stabilizing the family is difficult to investigate empirically, because research tools are mostly inadequate for studying systems and because due to social desirability it is to be expected that family members will be reluctant to admit the positive contribution of the pain.

EFFECTS OF THE FAMILY ON PAIN

The effects of the family on pain are diverse. They may be manifested in different domains - mainly in the experiential, emotional, cognitive or behavioral domains, and they may be mediated by diverse means.

Experiential and Emotional Effects

Although pain is a subjective experience, its particular quality may be affected by the reactions of the people closest to the pain patient. There is evidence that the manner in which individuals define their symptoms is largely based on consultation with members of their families (Turk and Kerns, 1985). The family may contribute to defining the pain as an alien element that did not belong to the family or to the patient. They may thus turn it into a dissociated neutral or hostile component. In that case, the private character of the pain is intensified for the patient. In contrast, the family may treat the pain as a quasi "family member", as a phenomenon that is being considered, discussed, "spoiled", reported about. In that case, the pain stops being a completely private experience and is being shared by the patient with his or her family.

Also other attitudes may be observed. Family members may simply ignore the patient's pain, they may behave as if the pain did not exist or they may suggest to the patient directly or indirectly that they do not quite believe the pain is as serious as the patient makes them believe. In that case, the family delegitimizes the pain. This attitude not only leaves the patient alone in the battle field but adds frustration and anger to the experience of pain (Darling, 1983). Notably, family delegitimation of the patient's pain was identified as one of the strongest predictors of developing chronicity in low back pain (Reis et al., 1999).

If, on the other hand, the family overdramatizes the situation, the patient has indeed gained partners in his or her fight with the pain but may also feel more anxiety about the pain (e.g., the patient may conclude, as it were, "if it is indeed that serious, then I may be really very sick and in a hopeless situation"). Another possible result in such cases is that the patient may, so to say, "fall in love" with the pain and cherish it as the source of one's special focus of attention in regard to the family.

Notably, correlations were detected between specific aspects of family functioning (assessed by the Family Environment Scale) and quality of pain (assessed by the McGill Pain Questionnaire). In a group of low back chronic pain patients, more family conflicts were related to higher affective pain ratings whereas increased family organization was related to higher evaluative pain ratings (Feuerstein et al., 1985).

There are further emotional effects of the family on the patient's pain. Some of them are positive. Positive effects on the patient's pain include alleviating the suffering and speeding up the process of recovery. Family support was found to be one of the most important resources that contribute to the chronic patient's well-being and ability to withstand the multiple stresses of chronic pain (Hallberg and Carlsson, 1998). Support is manifested primarily in the emotional domain. It includes encouragement and positive reinforcement for the patient's efficacious attempts at controlling pain. Depressive symptom severity and affective distress have been found to be positively related to the frequency of negative pain-related responding on the part of the spouse (Kerns et al., 1990, 1991) and inversely related to the presence of support on the part of the spouse (Brown et al., 1989).

In contrast, a negative emotional impact may be exerted not only by ignoring the patient and providing no support or encouragement but also through more direct means. If family members experience and express their fear and anxiety concerning the pain, the patient's anxiety may be enhanced, which in turn is likely to intensify the pain (Al Absi and Rokke, 1991) and increase pain behavior (Lethern et al., 1983). A further negative impact may be exerted by an outright negative attitude on the part of the family. Family members may complain how hard it is for them to go on with their routine without the patient's help, or how difficult it is for them to go on with their daily life and in addition take care of the patient. In some cases the patient is even blamed directly for letting the situation get that bad. Negative and punishing attitudes of this kind evoke and intensify guilt on the part of the patient. The result is intensified suffering of the patients.

Cognitive Effects

Also in the cognitive domain the effects of the family on the patient's pain may be positive or negative. Positive effects mediated by cognitive means may consist in providing the patient role models for successful coping with chronic pain. In addition to role models the family also provides cognitive beliefs and schemas that may help the patient devise useful coping strategies and attitudes to the pain, for example, optimism, or emphasizing progress even if minor (Thomas, 2000).

Negative effects mediated by cognitive means may consist in promoting dysfunctional thinking in the patient, providing information about the difficulty of overcoming chronic pain and the improbability of recovery, as well as emphasizing the hopelessness of the patient's overall state.

Behavioral Effects

The family plays a most important role by affecting the patient's pain-related behavior. This aspect has been emphasized in particular by the operant behavior perspective on chronic pain (Fordyce, 1976). The basic claim is that expressions of pain, including complaints of pain and incapacity, moaning or sighing, withdrawal and inactivity are maintained by the attention of significant others, contingent on their expression, even when nociception has stopped. Many studies provided support for the claim that the family affects the external manifestations of pain. Over-solicitous spouses may bring about an increase in the exhibition of pain behavior in comparison to partners who react less to the behavioral manifestations of pain (Flor, Kerns and Turk, 1987). Several studies demonstrated the relation between perceived spouse solicitousness and reports of pain intensity (Kerns et al., 1990; Turk et al., 1992), reports of pain behavior frequency (Kerns et al., 1991), observed frequency of pain behavior (Paulsen and Altmaier, 1995) and reports of behavioral interference, inactivity and disability (Flor, Kerns and Turk, 1987). One study found specifically statistical relationships between reported disability and observed solicitous spousal behavior contingent upon the patients' demonstrations of pain (Romano et al., 1992, 2000). Conversely, more punishing responses from the significant other to pain are related to less intense pain in arthritis patients (Faucett and Levine, 1991).

One of the more interesting studies in this domain compared pain patients who described their spouses as non-solicitous and those who described them as solicitous. The former had pain of shorter duration and reported a lower level of pain when they believed their spouses were observing them than when they believed a neutral person was observing (Block et al., 1980). The authors concluded that spouses may become discriminative cues for pain behavior and if they do not leave the marriage at an earlier stage of the pain, they turn into solicitous partners, thus contributing to the maintenance of the pain.

In sum, the findings suggest that the spouse (or, for that matter, also other close persons) may increase pain behavior and intensify the pain experience of the patient by a "caring" approach that reinforces directly and indirectly expressions of distress and suffering. However, it is the patient's *perception* of the solicitous or punishing response of the spouse that is related to the patient's pain experience and behavior more than what the spouse says he or she does (Flor et al., 1987).

Conclusion

The above observations demonstrate the strong impact that the family may have on pain. These effects may become manifest in various domains, may be mediated by emotional, cognitive, and behavioral means, and may be of a positive, negative or mixed kind. Furthermore, some of the effects may be specific, for example, they may relate to the patient's readiness to work, whereas other effects may be of a more global nature, say, overall mood, depression or generalized dependency.

However, it is to be considered that the mentioned particular effects seem to be moderated by the effect of the global atmosphere in the family. Pain-relevant support is more reinforcing when it is delivered by a spouse who is generally reinforcing and supportive (Kerns and Weiss, 1994). The relation of negative responding to pain and depressive symptoms in the pain patient will be intensified when the whole relationship is distressing. Further, a globally satisfying relationship may moderate the otherwise deleterious effects of pain-specific negative responding, thus exerting a buffering effect on the development of depression (Kerns et al., 1990; Goldberg, Kerns and Rosenberg, 1993).

Models of Family Involvement in Chronic Pain

The complexity and multi-directionality of the effects of family on chronic pain have prompted the formation of various models attempting to integrate the variety of involved interactions. Perhaps the best known is the cognitive-behavioral transactional model of family functioning (Kerns and Payne, 1996). Its major tenets are that the family is the basic unit of analysis and consideration, that the family and its members actively interact with the environment evaluating information about sources of stress (e.g., disease) and resources of coping with the stress, forming and evaluating various alternative responses to the stress. The cognitions and response options are shared by the family members and affect the problem solving attempts within the family unit.

The "family adjustment and adaptation response" (FAAR) is another model grounded in the cognitive-behavioral transactional approach, which attempts to account for the effects of the role of the family in chronic pain (Patterson and Garwick, 1994). The model is based on three assumptions. One is that the family tries to keep a balance in functioning between its resources and stresses in handling the issues of chronic pain. Another is that the balance of functioning is affected by the meanings the family members assign to the illness and to the family's resources. And the third is that the balance in functioning is the outcome of a prolonged dynamic process of adjustments. The goal of the whole process is to maintain the old balance, and if this proves impossible to create a new balance by developing new resources and coping strategies, reducing the stresses of the situation and changing the assigned meanings.

Basic to both and similar models is the emphasis on cognitions and interactions within the family and between the family and the broader environment. Models of this kind have been useful in guiding research into the role of the family in chronic pain and in devising therapeutic approaches involving the family in the treatment of pain.

The Role of the Family in Recovery from Pain

The family plays a complex role also in the treatment and recovery from chronic pain. One important aspect concerns the handling of information. The family often acts as the provider of information. High agreement was found between patients and spouses in evaluating the severity and impact of the pain (Swanson and Maruta, 1980). Sternbach (1986) has emphasized the importance of interviewing the partner of the pain patient in order to learn as fast as possible about the patient's attitudes and how these affect the patient's illness behavior. However, the family serves also as a channel for communicating information to the patient. It was found that family members absorb better than the patient information about the pain and its causes, and this may help in correcting the patient's faulty attributions about the causes of the pain (Violon, 1992).

Further, it is evident that the family may also be an important factor encouraging the patient to undergo treatment and to persevere in the efforts for overcoming chronic pain despite difficulties, setbacks and slow progress.

There is evidence that personality characteristics of family members, such as hysteria or hypochondriasis of spouses, predict treatment failures of chronic pain patients (Roberts and Reinhart, 1980). An intact family was found to be the most important factor for predicting maintenance and even improvement of good treatment results in pain patients after a multimodal program (Wooley et al., 1978). In chronic pain patients (aged 18-83) a 1-year rehabilitation program led to better results in terms of pain intensity, activity level, and reliance on medication if their families were perceived as supportive and free of conflicts (Jamison and Virts, 1990). Further, a review showed that an intact family or support system improved the results of pain management (Payne and Norfleet, 1986).

Family Therapy in the Treatment of Pain

In view of the close involvement of the family in the pain patient's pain, it is not surprising that various models of family therapy have been developed for treatment of chronic pain. In all types of family therapy the participants include beside the patient one or more of the close family members, mostly the spouse. Three major treatment approaches have been developed: the cognitive-behavioral, the transactional and the systems approach of structural family therapy. Variants combining two or three of these approaches are common. The behavioral approach teaches family members to ignore dysfunctional pain behaviors and to reinforce the functional ones. The transactional approach promotes awareness of ways patients may use to get psychological benefits from their pain and supports participants' attempts to overcome and discontinue these attempts. The systems approach focuses on changing the whole family organization so that a new functional system emerges whose stability and functioning do not require the patient to assume the sick role.

Family therapy has been applied in a great number of studies with pain patients (see reviews in Kerns, 1999; Kerns and Payne, 1996; Payne and Norfleet, 1986). There are a fair number of studies reporting positive results of family therapy, in a multimodal and rarely as a single therapeutic agent. For example, Hudgens (1979) reported positive results of family therapy as a single agent in regard to pain level, activity level, family relationships and use of medication, with maintenance of the gains for 6 to 24 months by 75% of the families (18 of 24). Yet, there are also quite a number of studies showing no clear superiority of couples treatment as compared with treatment of the patient alone (e.g., Radojevic et al., 1992; Saarijarvi, 1991).

It should however be noted that it is difficult to assess the contribution of family therapy to the patients' recovery because of several reasons. First, in the majority of cases family therapy has been applied as part of a multimodal comprehensive treatment program, conjoined with other therapeutic components. Secondly, in many cases there is a large dropout of patients in the course of treatment, which renders assessment difficult. Thirdly, there is hardly ever an attempt to evaluate the extent to which family members actually followed the instructions provided in the treatment. And, fourthly, family therapy by its nature is difficult to evaluate because due to its interactional character it involves a multiplicity of perspectives and a variety of viewpoints of different participants which render its impact elusive (e.g., a change in the family organization may affect some of the family members who in turn cause change in the patient, whose change affects the family functioning etc.) (Lemmens et al., 2003).

Some General Conclusions

The evidence concerning the relations of family and chronic pain serve to highlight the fact that pain or rather the patient with pain do not exist in a void but rather in an environment. A major component in that environment is the family that may play a crucial role in the onset of pain, its maintenance, coping with it, and eventual recovery from it or no recovery. This insight is probably responsible for the increased attention that is being assigned to family members in the diagnosis and treatment of chronic pain in pain clinics in many countries. Factors that may enhance or mitigate the effect of the family on a patient's pain may be the degree to which the patient considers the pain as a private affair that is to be handled independently of the family, and the family's pressure to be part of the pain diagnosis and treatment. Attention to factors of this kind may help in future research on the potential contribution of the family to the pain patient's well-being.

REFERENCES

Ahern, D., Adams, A., and Follick, M. (1985). Emotional and marital disturbance in spouses of chronic low back pain patients. *Clinical Journal of Pain, 1*, 69-74.

Al Absi, M., and Rokke, P. D.(1991). Can anxiety help us tolerate pain? *Pain, 46,* 43-51.

Basolo-Kunzer, M., Diamond, S., Maliszewski, M., Weyermann, L. et al. (1991). Chronic headache patients' marital adn family adjustment. *Issues in Mental Health Nursing, 12,* 133-148.

Block, A., Kremer, E., and Gaylor, M. (1980). Behavioral treatment of chronic pain: the spouse as a discriminative cue for pain behavior. *Pain, 9,* 243-252.

Blumer, D., and Heilbronn, M. (1982). Chronic pain as a variant of depressive disease. *Journal of Nervous and Mental Disease, 170,* 381-406.

Brown, G. K., Wallston, K. A., and Nicassio, P. M. (1989). Social support and depression inrheumatoid arthritis. *Journal of Applied Social Psychology, 19,* 1164-1181.

Chaturvedi, S. K. (1987). Family morbidity in chronic pain patients. *Pain, 30,* 159-168.

Christensen, M. F., and Mortensen, O. (1975). Long-term prognosis in children with recurrent abdominal pain. *Archives of Diseases in Childhood, 50,* 110-114.

Crook, J., Rideout, E., and Browne, G. (1984). The prevalence of pain complaints in the general population. *Pain, 18,* 299-314.

Darling, R. B. (1983). Parent-professional interaction: The roots of misunderstanding. In M. Seligman (Ed.), *The Family with a handicapped child.* New York: Grune and Stratton.

Delvey, J., and Hopkins, L. (1982). Pain patients and their partners: The role of collusion in chronic pain. *Journal of Marital and Family Therapy, 8,* 135-142.

Deyo, R. A. (1986). The early diagnostic evaluation of patients with low back pain. *Journal of General Internal Medicine, 1,* 328-338.

Dura, J. R., and Beck, S. J. (1988). A comparison of family functioning when mothers have chronic pain. *Pain, 35,* 79-89.

Edwards, P., Zeichner, A., Kuczmierczyk, A., and Broczkowski, J. (1985). Familial pain models: the relationship between family history of pain and current pain experience. *Pain, 21,* 379-384.

Faucett, J., and Levine, J. D. (1991). The contributions of interpersonal conflict to chronic pain in the presence or absence of organic pathology. *Pain, 44,* 35-43.

Feuerstein, M., Sult, S., and Houle, M. (1985). Environmental stressors and chronic low back pain: life events, family and work environment. *Pain, 22,* 295-307.

Flor, H., Kerns, R. D., and Turk, D. C. (1987). The role of spouse reinforcement, perceived pain, and activity levels of chronic pain patients. *Journal of Psychosomatic Research, 31,* 251-259.

Flor, H., Turk, D. C., and Scholz, O. B. (1987). Impact of chronic pain on the spouse: Marital, emotional and physical consequences. *Journal of Psychosomatic Research, 31,* 63-71.

Fordyce, W. E. (1976). *Behavioral methods for chronic pain and illness.* St. Louis, MO: C. V. Mosby.

Goldberg, G. M., Kerns, R. D., and Rosenberg, R. (1993). Pain relevant support as a buffer from depression among chronic pain patients low in instrumental activity. *Clinical Journal of Pain, 9,* 34-40.

Greene, B. E., and Pargament, K. I. (1997). Family coping with chronic pain. *Families, Systems and Health, 15,* 147-160.

Gross, R., Doerr, H., Caldirola, G., and Ripley, H. (1980-1). Borderline syndrome and incest in chronic pelvic pain patients. *International Journal of Psychiatry and Medicine, 10,* 79-96.

Hallberg, L. R., and Carlsson, S. G. (1998). Psychosocial vulnerability and maintaining forces related to fibromyalgia. In-depth interviews with twenty-two female patients. *Scandinavian Journal of Caring Sciences, 12,* 95-103.

Hill, L., and Blendis, L. (1967). Physical and psychological evaluation of 'non-organic' abdominal pain. *Gut, 8,* 221-229.

Hudgens, A. (1977). The social worker's role in a behavior management approach to chronic pain. *Social Work Health Care, 3,* 77-85.

Hudgens, A. J. (1979). Family-oriented treatment of chronic pain. *Journal of Marital and Family Therapy, 5,* 67-78.

Jamison, R. N., and Virts, K. L. (1990). The influence of family support on chronic pain. *Behavior Research and Therapy, 28,* 283-287.

Kemler, M. A., and Furnee, C. A. (2002).The impact of chronic pain on life in the houseold. *Journal of Pain and Symtom Management, 23,* 433-441.

Kerns, R. (1999). Family therapy for adults with chronic pain. In R. J. Gatchel and D. C. Turk (Eds.), *Psychosocial factors in pain* (pp. 445-456). New York: Guilford

Kerns, R. D., Haythornwaie, J., Southwick, S., and Giller, E. L. (1990). The role of marital interaction in chronic painand depressive symptom severity. *Journal of Psychosomatic Research, 34,* 401-408.

Kerns, R. D., and Payne, A. (1996). Treating families of chronic pain patients. In R. J. Gatchel and D. C. Turk (Eds.) *Psychological approaches to pain management: A practioner's handbook* (pp. 283-304). New York: Guilford.

Kerns, R. D., Southwick, S., Giller, E. L., Haythornthwaite, J., Jacob, M. C., and Rosenberg, R. (1991). The relationship between reports of pain-related social interactionsand expressions of pain and affective distress. *Behavior Therapy, 22,* 101-111.

Kerns, R. D., and Weiss, L. H. (1994). Family influences in the courseof chronic illness: A cognitive-behavioral trasactional model. *Annals of Behavioral Medicine, 16,* 116-121.

Klein, R. F., Dean, A., and Bogdanoff, M. D. (1967). The impact of illness upon the spouse. *Journal of Chronic Diseases, 20,* 241-248.

Kreitman, N., Sainsbury, P., Pearce, K., and Costain, W. (1965). Hypochondriasis and depression in outpatients in a general hospital. *British Journal of Psychiatry, 3,* 607-615.

Lemmens, G., Verdegem, S., Heireman, M., Lietaer, G., Van-Houdenhove, B., Sabbe, B., Eisler, I. (2003). Helpful events in family discussion groups with chronic pain patients: A qualitative study of differences in perception between therapists/observers and patients/family members. *Families, Systems and Health, 21,* 37-52.

Lethern, J., Slade, P. D., Troup, J. D. G., and Bentley, G. (1983). Outline of a fear avoidance model of exaggerated pain perception –I. *Behavior Research and Therapy, 21,* 401-408.

Maruta, T., Osborne, D., Swanson, D., and Halling, J. (1981). Chronic pain patients and spouss: Marital and sexual adjustment. *Mayo Clinic Proceedings, 56,* 307-310.

Merskey, H. (1965). Psychiatric patients with persistent pain. *Psychosomatic Research, 9,* 299-309.

Mohamed, S. N., Weisz, G. M., and Waring, E. M. (1978). The relationship of chronic pain to depression, marital adjustment, and family dynamics. *Pain, 5*, 285-292.

Patterson, J. M., and Garwick, A. W. (1994). The impact of chronic illness on families: A family systems perspective. *Annals of Behavioral Medicine, 16*,131-142.

Paulsen, J. S., and Altmaier, E. M. (1995). The effects of perceived versus enacted social support on the discriminative cue function of spouses for pain behaviors. *Pain, 60,* 103-110.

Payne, B. A. (1982). *A transpersonal family treatment program for chronic pain patients.* Unpublished doctoral dissertation, California Institute of Transpersonal Psychology, Menlo Park, CA.

Payne, B., and Norfleet, M.A. (1986). Chronic pain and the family: a review. *Pain, 26*, 1-22.

Radojevic, V., Nicassio, P. M., and Weisman, M. H. (1992). Behavioral intervention with and without family support for rheumatoid arthritis. *Behavior Therapy, 23*, 13-30.

Reis, S., Hermoni, D., Borkan, J. M., Biderman, A., Tabenkin, C., and Porat, A. (1999). A new look at low back pain in primary care: A Rambam Israeli Family Practice Network study. *Journal of Family Practice, 48*, 299-303.

Revenson, T. A., and Majerovitz, S. D. (1990). Spouses' support provision to chronically ill patients. *Journal of Social and Personal Relationships, 7*, 575-586.

Roberts, A. H., and Reinhart, L. (1980). The behavioral management of chronic pain: Long term follow-up with comparison groups. *Pain, 8*, 151-162.

Romano, J. M., Jensen, M. P., Turner, J. A., Good, A. B., Hops, H. (2000). Chronic pain patient-partner interactions: Further support for a behavioral model of chronic pain. *Behavior Therapy, 31*, 415-440.

Romano, J. M., Turner, J. A., Friedman, L. S., Bulcroft, R. A., Jensen, M. P., Hops, H., and Wright, S. F. (1992). Sequential analysis of chronic pain behaviors and spouse responses. *Journal of Consulting and Clinical Psychology, 60*, 777-782.

Rowat, K. M., and Knafl, K. L. (1985). Living with chronic pain: The spouse's perspective. *Pain, 23*, 259-271.

Roy, R. (1982). Marital and family issues in patients with chronic pain: a review. *Psychotherapy and Psychosomatics, 37*, 1-12.

Saarijärvi, S., Ryteköski, U., and Karpi, S-L. (1990). Marital satisfaction and distress in chronic low-back pain patients and their spouses. *Clinical Journal of Pain, 6*, 148-152.

Saarijärvi, S. (1991). A controlled study of couple therapy in low back pain patients: Effects on marital satisfaction, and health attitudes. *Journal of Psychosomatic Research, 35*, 265-272.

Sternbach, R. A. (Ed.), (1986). *The psychology of pain* (2nd ed). New York: Raven Press

Swanson, D. W., and Maruta, T. (1980). The family viewpoint of chronic pain. *Pain, 8*, 163-166.

Thomas, V. (2000). Cognitive behavioral therapy in pain management for sickle cell disease. *International Journal of Palliative Nursing, 6*, 434-442.

Timmermans, G., and Sternbach, R. A. (1974). Factors of human chronic pain: an analysis of personality and pain reaction variables. *Science, 184*, 806-808.

Turk, D. C., Flor, H., and Rudy, T. E. (1987). Pain and families: I. Etiology, maintenance, and psychosocial impact. *Pain, 30*, 3-27.

Turk, D. C. and Kerns, R. D. (1985). The family in health and illness. In D.C. Turk and R. D. Kerns (Eds.), *Health, illness and families: A life span perspective* (pp. 1-22). New York: Wiley.

Turk, D. C., Kerns, R. D., and Rosenberg, R. (1992). Effects of marital interaction on chronic painand disability: Examining the down side of social support. *Rehabilitation Psychology, 37,* 259-274.

Valat, J. P., Goupille, P., and Vedere, V. (1997). Low back pain: risk factors for chronicity. *Revue du Rhumatisme (English Edition), 64,* 189-194.

Violon, A. (1985). Family etiology of chronic pain. International *Journal of Family Therapy,* 7, 235-246.

Violon, A. (1992). *A douleur rebelle.* Desclée de Brouwer (pp. 69-86). Paris.

Waring, E. (1977). The role of the family in symptom selection and perpetuation in psychosomatic illness. *Psychotherapy and Psychosomatics, 28,* 253-259.

Waring, E. (1983). Marriages of patients with psychosomatic illnesses. *General Hospital Psychiatry, 5,* 49-53.

Wooley, S., Blackwell, G., and Winger, C. (1978). A learning theory model of chronic illness behavior: theory, treatment and research. *Psychosomatic Medicine, 40,* 379-400.

In: The Handbook of Chronic Pain
Editors: S. Kreitler, D. Beltrutti, et al., pp. 115-134

ISBN 978-1-60021-044-0
© 2007 Nova Science Publishers, Inc.

Chapter 7

Psychological and Psychopathological Characteristics of Patients with Pain

Shulamith Kreitler and David Niv

INTRODUCTION

In the last decades the linear causal model of pain as a sensory event gave way to the conception of pain as a multi-dimensional phenomenon. The commonly identified four basic dimensions of pain are: (a) the sensory, reflecting the underlying physical harm or problem (viz. nociception), (b) the affective, reflecting the negative emotions evoked by the pain sensation and the physical harm (e.g., unpleasantness, distress, annoyance, fear), (c) the cognitive, reflecting the evaluation of the problem and the whole situation at present and the expectations for the future, and (d) the behavioral, reflecting overt behavioral expression of pain and the more general sickness behaviors including functional disability (Loeser and Egan, 1989; Wade and Price, 2001). These four dimensions interact and affect one another. For example, the cognitive evaluation of the seriousness of the physical harm may intensify the affectively-based suffering, whereas stoic behavior may attenuate the intensity of the pain sensations. The interaction among the four dimensions is probably the reason for the low interrelations observed between physical harm and pain sensation or disability, as well as between pain sensation and psychological distress or disability (Magora and Schwartz, 1980; Waddell and Main, 1984). All four dimensions of pain are psychological and all four are affected by the personality of the individual with pain. Hence, it has become generally accepted that understanding, management and treatment of pain require consideration of psychological aspects.

The focus of this chapter is the chronic pain patient (CPP), namely, the patient whose pain lasts more than 6 months after the initial injury. We will review factors that are primarily psychological or psychiatric, have been assessed by reliable and valid instruments, and their relation to pain has been established empirically. Two problems overshadow this field of study. The first is basically methodological and consists in the difficulty to distinguish between psychological aspects that are the effects of pain and those that are personality characteristics of the CPP essentially independent of the pain, though sometimes even affecting it or appearing as a response to it. The second problem is the unclarity whether there is or even whether we should theoretically expect a personality type or a set of personality traits characteristic of the CPP. Some researchers doubt it (e.g., Turk and Salovey, 1984). Hence, few studies examined general personality characteristics of the CPP whereas many more studies dealt with psychological reactions to pain.

The approach we adopted in this review is that even psychological responses to pain are considered as being determined to some extent by the personality of the CPP, defined broadly to include traits, behavioral tendencies, beliefs, attitudes and meanings assigned to pain and other stressors. Hence, it is assumed that even the responses to pain reflect also more constant tendencies and not just temporary context- or situation-bound reactions, especially if we deal with responses that do not refer directly to the pain itself (e.g., descriptions of the pain).

PSYCHIATRIC CORRELATES OF CHRONIC PAIN

It is commonly accepted that chronic pain (CP) has psychiatric correlates. The Task Force on Taxonomy (Merskey and Bogduk, 1994) has identified several pain syndromes on a psychological basis (i.e., muscle tension pain; delusional or hallucinatory; hysterical, conversion or hypochondriacal pain; or pain associated with depression) which may affect any part of the body (e.g., chest, lower back), and are defined as pain in the absence of any organic basis, with a psychological etiology and often accompanied by additional psychopathology.

Several studies used DSM criteria for identifying psychiatric problems in CPPs. Estimates of Axis I diagnoses (major clinical disorders, e.g. schizophrenia, mood disorders) in CPPs range from 86.5% (Katon, Egan and Miller, 1985) to 90% (Large, 1986). Of all CPPs 60% (Fishbain, Goldberg, Meagher, Steele and Rosomoff, 1986) to 69% (Reich, Rosenblatt and Tupin, 1983) meet criteria for more than one Axis I disorder. Of these patients, 31% (Weisberg et al., 1996) to 59% (Fishbain et al., 1986) have an Axis II disorder (i.e., personality disorders - obsessive-compulsive, antisocial). In addition, 77% of CPPs meet criteria for psychopathological disorders before the onset of pain. All these percentages are higher than the base rates for the general population.

In line with DSM criteria, the main psychiatric diagnoses for CPPs were found to be major depression, addictive disorders and anxiety disorders (Polatin, Kinney, Gatchel, Lillo and Mayer, 1993). The addictive disorders include substance abuse mainly of analgesics (12.6%), alcohol (9.7%) and sedatives (7%) (Hoffman, Olofsson, Salen and Wickstrom, 1995).

The most frequent Axis II disorders observed in CPPs are of the paranoid (range 2% to 33%, Polatin et al., 1993; Weisberg et al., 1996), dependent (range 3% to 17%, Fishbain et al., 1986; Polatin et al., 1993), histrionic (range 4% to 14%, Polatin et al., 1993; Reich et al., 1983) and borderline kinds (range 7% to 15%, Polatin et al., 1993; Reich et al., 1983).

In men Axis I disorders are of an intermittent explosive nature, adjustment disorders (viz., not working) and alcohol and drug abuse, whereas in women depression and somatization predominate; Axis II disorders are in men mainly of the paranoid and narcissistic kind, and in women mainly histrionic (Fishbain et al., 1986).

Concerning patients with a positive lifetime history for psychopathology, 54% of those with major depression, 94% of those with substance abuse and 95% of those with anxiety disorders, had had these syndromes before the onset of their CP. Hence, it seems that certain disorders (viz. substance abuse and anxiety disorders) precede the onset of pain, whereas others (mainly depression) develop in about half the cases before the CP and in about half the cases after the CP (Polatin et al., 1993). It is of importance to note that 29.7% CPPs have at least one first-degree blood relative suffering from an affective disorder, and 37.8% have at least one suffering from alcohol abuse (Katon, Egan and Miller, 1985).

According to the common psychiatric assessment tool SCL-90 (Symptom Check List-90), about 39% of CPPs had at least moderately high scores on 6 of the 9 clinical scales, especially somatization, depression, obsession-compulsion, anxiety and hostility (in men) or phobia (in women). The higher the scores the more psychological distress there was. The main diagnoses in the patients with higher scores were major depression (11.3%), dysthymia (9%), personality disorders (7.7%) and adjustment disorders (2.7%) (Williams, Urban, Keefe, Shutty and France, 1995).

Notably, somatization is the SCL scale on which CPPs score highest. In recent years there is a growing body of data showing that CPPs tend toward somatization, defined as the tendency for reporting numerous physical symptoms and excessive health care seeking, reflecting a lowered threshold for perceiving and reporting bodily symptoms and amplification or misinterpretation of these symptoms (Dworkin, 1994; Saarijarvi, Hyyppa, Lehtinen and Alanen, 1990). The majority of low back CPPs reported a lifetime history of multiple somatic symptoms (25.8% over 12 symptoms, 51.5% 7-11 symptoms, as compared with 4.1% and 8.2% respectively in controls) (Bacon, Bacon, Atkinson, Slater et al., 1994). Patients high on somatization report more bodily sensations than controls both after physical exercise (treadmill test) and after a rest period (Schmidt, Gierlings and Peters, 1989), have high levels of autonomic arousal, tend to experience an almost total body response, often manifest emotional disturbances and maladaptive styles on the MMPI (Iezzi, Stokes, Adams and Pilon, 1994), as well as major depression, and alcohol dependency (Bacon et al., 1994).

Studies using the Millon Behavioral Health Inventory showed that anxiety (specifically, somatic anxiety) and depression are the commonest problems in CPPs and that the scores decline with improvement in pain (Labbe, Goldberg, Fishbain, Rosomoff and Steele-Rosomoff, 1989). When compared to nonclinical controls, CPPs scored higher though still in the normal range on obsessive-compulsive, dependent and schizoid personality disorders, but their highest scores were on the histrionic, passive-aggressive and narcissistic scales (Baggi et al., 1995).

Studies using the MMPI showed that four clusters of results (coded as P-A-I-N) were typical for CPPs (Costello, Hulsey, Schoenfeld and Ramamurthy, 1987). These clusters (the same for men and women) are unique for CPPs and differ from those identified for example in cardiac patients (Robinson, Greene and Geissner, 1993). The 'P' cluster (15%) consists in elevated scores on most psychopathological scales, reaching into the clinical range. This cluster is typical of patients reporting most intense pain that affects a broad range of domains and is of longest duration, and are characterized by low SES, restricted daily activities, unemployment, deterioration of social relations, and sleep disorder. The 'A' cluster (20%) consists of the 'conversion V' pattern (i.e., elevated scores on Hypochondriasis and Hysteria and low on Depression). The 'I' cluster (30%) consists of elevated scores on three scales (Hopochondriasis, Depression and Hysteria) and is often called the "neurotic triad" since it is common in neurotic individuals experiencing a lot of anxiety. These scores are higher in CPPs than in acute pain patients (e.g., Sternbach, Wolf, Murphy and Akeson, 1973) and may decline to normal after a successful rehabilitation program (Barnes, Gatchel, Mayer and Barnett, 1990). 'I' patients are the physically most infirm with multiple surgeries and hospitalizations. The 'N' cluster (25%) is 'normal' in that no MMPI scale is elevated and it characterizes patients with the shortest pain duration, moderate claims of ill health, who often have better education and employment, and good response to treatment The major axis is defined by the P and N clusters, with A and I clusters located in-between on the continuum of pathology.

These findings suggest that only a minority of the CPPs suffer from severe psychopathology (15%) whereas about half (50%) suffer from personality disorders along the so-called neurotic lines. At least in two studies CPPs scored higher than controls on measures of neuroticism (Chaturverdi, 1986; Magni, de-Bertolini, Dodi and Infantino, 1986).

The salience of hysteria and hypochondriasis in the findings based on the MMPI lends support to Freud's (1955) claim that CP is a result of a conversion neurosis, serving as a compromise between the fulfillment of a forbidden wish and its punishment (Van-Houdenhove, 1988). It also conforms to the early findings by Engel (1959) who diagnosed most of his CPPs as hysteric or hypochondriac. However, the elevated scores on the Hysteria scale reflect mainly high scores on Bodily Concern items but low on Psychological Denial (Ornduff, Brennan and Barratt, 1988).

Depression is by far the most salient of the psychiatric correlates detected in CPPs and has been studied more than all other psychiatric aspects of CP. The reported prevalence of depression in CPPs has varied from 10% to 100% (Romano and Turner, 1985) due to variability in assessment methods of depression and of pain and selection of samples. Most studies that used only RDC (Research Diagnostic Criteria) and DSM criteria reported current prevalence rates of 30-54%, and lifetime prevalence rates of 32%, which are higher than the respective rates in the general population (5% and 17%) or in other diseases (e.g., cancer: 4% and 23%, cardiac disease: 14% and 27%) (Banks and Kerns, 1996). The depression in CP consists mainly of somatic symptoms rather than emotional (Estlander, Takala and Verkasalo, 1995), a fact that may cause problems in regard to differential diagnosis between CP and depression, which share quite a number of manifestations (e.g., fatigue, insomnia) (France and Krishnan, 1988a). The temporal sequence of pain and depression is that pain precedes depression in about 46% of the cases, appears together with depression in about 50% of the cases, and follows depression in about 4% (range 0% to 12%) of the cases (Atkinson, Slater, Patterson, Grant and Garfin, 1991; Bradley, 1963; Lindsay and Wyckoff, 1981). The high rate of depression in CPPs may be related to the high suicide rate observed in CPPs, which is higher than in other medically ill persons (Pilowsky, 1984).

In general, the nature of the relation between pain and depression remains unsettled. Most investigators assume they are related and only a minority claims that they are not related but merely appear to be so because each is so common in the general population

(Tauschke, Merskey and Helmes, 1990). There are four major hypotheses about the pain-depression interrelation. The first is that *pain is the cause of the depression* (Tauschke et al., 1990), so that depression is merely a reaction to the pain, mediated by cognitive and behavioral factors characteristic of CPPs (Rudy, Kerns and Turk, 1988). Thus, Beck (1976) argues that pain activates the vulnerability for depression which consists in negative schemata and the negative cognitive triad (i.e., negative thoughts about the self, the world and the future (the "cognitive distortion model"). Seligman (1975) claims that pain causes depression because it constitutes the uncontrollable negative event for individuals who tend to make internal, stable and global attributions (i.e., the depressive attributional style or the "learned helplessness model"). In contrast, Fordyce (1976) argues that pain activates depression by reducing rewards as a result of restricting the range of activities due to impairement or fear of pain. A large body of data supports the view that depression is a reaction to pain. Thus, for example, studies showed that depression develops mainly when there are conflicts with significant others about pain and little social support (Faucett, 1994) and that depression does not occur immediately when pain shows up but later, after exposure to suffering, disability and frustrations (Gatchel, 1996). On the other hand, however, the intensity of pain may (Turk, Okifuji and Scharff, 1995) or may not (Bishop, Eagley, Fisher and Sullivan, 1993) be related to depression.

The second hypothesis is that *depression is a risk factor for pain*, so that a person with depression tends more than others to become a CPP. The rationale is that depression often precedes pain, increases pain sensitivity and lowers pain tolerance thresholds. The evidence is based on mood induction studies showing that inducing a depressive mood increases self focusing of attention and reporting of pain (Salovey, 1992) and decreases pain tolerance (Zelman, Howland, Nichols and Cleeland, 1991). Further, a depressed individual tends to see things in negative terms and begins to view the acute pain negatively. When these tendencies are coupled with the depressive attributional style (Seligman, 1975), they may lead to increase in the severity of the pain and giving up of attempts to control it - all of which result in the acute pain turning into chronic pain (Gatchel, 1996). A recent modified variant of this hypothesis is the diathesis-stress thesis which argues that CP is the result of certain premorbid psychological predispositions toward depression, which in the face of the challenge of pain and disability, evolve into the syndrome of clinical depression (Banks and Kerns, 1996).

The third hypothesis is that *pain and depression co-occur because they are similar psychologically,* namely, they share a common psychodynamic core (e.g., aggression turned inward, against the self). Accordingly, one can replace the other, i.e., chronic pain may be the equivalent of a depressive disorder, masked depression or a variant of depression (Lopez-Ibor, 1972; von-Knorring, 1989) whereas depression may present as CP (Chaturverdi, 1987a). This thesis is weakened by studies which show that antidepressants may reduce or cancel depression but not pain (e.g., Turner and Denny, 1993) or that analgesic drugs may reduce pain but not depression (Nilsson and von Knorring, 1989).

Finally, the fourth hypothesis is that *pain and depression co-occur because they are similar biologically,* namely, the same central nervous biogenic amines (e.g., serotonin and norepinephrine) play a role in both (Walker, Katon, Harrop-Griffiths, Holm, Russo and Hickok, 1988; Ward, Bloom, Dworkin, Fawcett, Narasimhachari and Friedel, 1982).

In addition to studies that dealt with identifying common psychiatric labels in CPPs, there are investigations that focus on psychodynamic aspects relevant for the mental health of CPPs. One such aspect concerns the childhood background of CPPs. The findings are inconclusive. Engel (1959) observed in pain patients suffering, defeat, neglect and abuse in childhood. Walker et al. (1988) found sexual victimization in childhood in women with chronic pelvic pain, and Carlsson (1986) observed in CPPs more negative childhood experiences. Pilowsky et al. (1982) found that pain patients had more hospitalizations in later childhood in contrast to depressives who had more in earlier childhood, but Merskey et al., (1987) found that they did not differ in childhood experiences from patients in general practice and Tauschke et al. (1990) found that they had more normal childhoods than psychiatric patients with no pain.

The use of defense mechanisms is another aspect of relevance for mental health. The evidence indicates that CPPs use preferentially the more mature defenses such as, Reversal (negation, denial, reaction-formation and repression) and Turning Against the Self and less Turning Against the Object and Projection (Mendelson, 1984; Passchier et al., 1988; Tauschke et al., 1990). Hence, it may be concluded that the preferred defense mechanisms by CPPs do not promote serious psychopathology.

A complementary view of the role of psychiatry in CP may be gained by considering, even briefly, that pain is a common symptom in psychiatric patients, especially in those suffering from major depression (40% to 84% according to different estimates), dysthymia, general anxiety disorders, somatoform disorders, alcohol and opioid dependencies, hypochondriasis and conversion disorder. In some disorders (e.g., somatoform) pain is common even as a primary complaint (it is the major symptom in 18.6% of psychiatric patients, Chaturverdi, 1987b). In schizophrenics it is often denied. CP in psychiatric patients is often transient, is usually of insidous onset, occurs in multiple sites - more often in the head and trunk than the limbs - and may migrate from one site to another (France and Krishnan, 1988b).

In sum, the prevalence of psychiatric disorders in CPPs is high, and higher than in other medical conditions or in the general population. A CPP often has more than one disorder. The most common disorders are depression, which is at least partly reactive, anxiety disorders, addiction disorders, somatoform disorder, hysteria and hypochondriasis. There is evidence that in CP the depression, the anxiety and the hysteria differ from the regular forms in being mainly somatic. Childhood experiences, defense mechanisms and the nature and frequency of the disorders indicate that the rate of serious psychopathology is low.

EMOTIONAL CORRELATES OF CHRONIC PAIN

Pain is an intense experience with a salient affective dimension in addition to the sensory one (Melzack and Casey, 1968). A great number of studies dealing with descriptions of pain in terms of the McGill Pain Questionnaire or similar descriptors yielded by means of factor analysis factors of a clear emotional nature, labelled as affective-evaluative, immediate anxiety, emotional distress, angry depression, etc. (Fernandez and Turk, 1992; Kinsman, Dirks, Wunder, Carbaugh and Stieg, 1989). The sensory and affective components of pain are considered by some to be inseparable (Merskey and Spear, 1967), by others as distinguishable, with the sensory preceding the emotional (Beecher, 1957) or both components proceeding in parallel (Leventhal and Everhart, 1979). In any event, it is likely that the two components interact reciprocally, so that the sensation of pain evokes emotional distress and the distress in turn affects the perception of pain. However, a carefully designed study with chronic headache patients showed only that increased headache activity was associated weakly with increases in affect (anxiety, anger, depression) on the same day (isomorphic relation) but not that the one actually preceded the other (Arena, Blanchard and Andrasik, 1984).

Beyond the descriptions of pain itself, there are emotions identified as characteristic of CPPs. Studies showed that as compared to controls, CPPs tend to experience more social isolation, empathy with others experiencing pain (Bowman, 1994), tension, worry and irritability (Sofaer and Walker, 1994), guilt due to the pain (Saarijarvi et al., 1990) especially in men (Tauschke, Merskey and Helmes, 1990), frustration, anxiety (Wade, Price, Hamer, Schwartz and Hart, 1990), with a special emphasis on the five clusters of anxiety: restlessness, embarrassment, sensitivity, physiological anxiety and low self-confidence (Moore, Kinsman and Dirks, 1984), and feelings of despair and hopelessness (Hitchcock, Ferrell, Betty and McCaffery, 1994). As noted earlier ("Psychiatric Correlates of CP"), the commonness of depression in CP testifies to the prevalence of sadness in CPPs, sometimes due to premorbid depression or tendencies to depression, triggered by the pain itself. As expected, the positive or neutral emotions (surprise, interest and joy) were correlated negatively with pain-related affective distress, whereas the negative emotions (anger, fear and sadness) were related positively to the affective component of pain evaluation and hence form a triad of important negative emotions constituting the affective distress in CPPs (Fernandez and Milburn, 1994).

Anger and its different manifestations (hostility, aggression, hatred, and resentment) is an emotion that plays an important role in CP. Several studies using different assessment tools found higher scores or frequency of anger in CPPs than in controls (Carlsson, 1987; Hatch, Schoenfeld, Boutros, Seleshi, Moore and Cyr-Provost, 1991; Schwartz, Slater, Birchler and Atkinson, 1991; Taylor, Lorentzen and Blank, 1990; Wade et al., 1990) as well as more externalized aggression (Egle, Schwab, Rudolf, Schoefer, Bassler and Hoffman, 1987), less inhibition of aggression (Carlsson, 1986) and increased external resentment (Merskey, 1965). Spear's (1967) study which did not find increase in covert or overt hostility in CP is an exception.

In men the scores of anger are higher than in women, in whom anxiety is more prominent (Kinder, Curtiss and Kalichman, 1986; Sternbach, Wolf, Murphy and Akeson, 1973). Yet, in a subgroup of CPPs anger played a unique role: in females the anger was externalized, in males it was suppressed (Curtiss, Kinder, Kalichman and Spana, 1988).

Anger is related to the experiencing of pain. In a study with the Profile of Mood States, anger accounted for 33% of the variance in pain severity, whereby anxiety and depression did not add to the variance accounted for by anger (Summers, Rapoff, Varghese, Porter and Palmer, 1992).

However, there is also evidence that CPPs tend to deny their anger for reasons of society's norms and social desirability, and confess to it only in an indirect way (Corbishley,

Hendrickson and Beutler, 1990; Franz, Paul, Bautz, Choroba and Hildebradt, 1986) or have "bottled-up anger" (Pilowsky and Spence, 1976). CPPs who deny anger and aggressivenss were found to be better adapted to their immediate social environment (Franz et al., 1986). The denial is manifested also in their reduced awareness of anger around them (Drysdale, 1989). Not surprisingly, CPPs also have difficulty in expressing anger, even as compared to other medical patients (e.g., surgical patients, Braha and Catchlove, 1986-87), apply reaction formation against aggression (Sivik and Hosterey, 1992) and are characterized by an inability to express intense anger (Kerns, Rosenberg and Jacob, 1991). It seems that most of the anger in CPPs is internalized rather than expressed (Tschannen, Duckro, Margolis, and Tomazic, 1992). Internalized anger in contrast to expressed anger accounted for a large portion of the variance in measures of pain intensity and interference (Kerns, Rosenberg and Jacob, 1991). The prevalence of anger in CPPs is especially important because it may be related to depression in a psychodynamic sense (depression is considered as anger turned in, Rosenzweig, 1976) or as a predictor (Tschannen et al., 1992) and may affect adversely the immune system (Beutler, Engle, Oro'-Beutler, Daldrup and Meredith, 1986).

Anger is probably not the only emotion whose expression or maybe even full internal deployment is inhibited. About emotionality in general in CPPs there are some contradictory findings. Some found that CPPs had stronger emotionality (Hadjstavropoulous and Craig, 1994) or less emotional repression (Gamsa and Vikis-Freibergs, 1991) and lower level of emotional control (Carlsson, 1987) whereas others found that they expressed a smaller range of positive as well as negative affect and viewed emotional expression as dangerous (Corbishley et al., 1990).

The latter finding is supported by the body of research on alexithymia in CPPs. Alexithymia is a disposition or disorder denoting an inability to label or express affect coupled with an impoverished fantasy life and a tendency to respond to emotional situations predominantly with physical responses. It has been associated with a number of illnesses and is considered to play a role in psychosomatic disorders. There is evidence that blocking the expression of affect in general (Beutler, Engle, Oro'-Beutler, Daldrup and Meredith, 1986) and alexithymia in particular (Dewaraja, Tanigawa, Araki, Nakata, Kawamura, Ago and Sasaki, 1997) affect adversly the immune system.

A large number of studies (e.g., Postpone, 1986) shows that CPPs with pain in various sites score on alexithymia (as assessed by different tools) higher than normal controls, psychotherapy patients, depressed patients, and medical patients with gastrointestinal, dermatological and other disorders (see review by Kreitler and Niv, 2001). Applying a within-group design showed that CPPs with higher alexithymia scored higher on anxiety and inhibited anger than those with low alexithymia. This means that at least in CPPs alexithymia denotes a linguistic-cognitive impairment which consists in responding emotionally but suppressing the emotions (especially anxiety and anger) or not labelling them adequately rather than an affective impairment of not responding emotionally (Kreitler, Gohar, Eldar, Ezer and Niv, 1995).

In sum, affect is an intrinsic aspect of the pain experience. A range of affects, mostly negative (i.e., anxiety, sadness/despair, and anger, especially inhibited anger) were found to be common in CPPs. It is still unknown to what extent these affects manifest premorbid tendencies and to what degree they are reactions to pain. Most characteristic of CPPs is alexithymia, which seems to denote inadequate labelling and expression of emotions rather than affective dearth.

PERSONALITY CORRELATES OF CHRONIC PAIN

In line with psychoanalytic practice some authors provided the general outlines of the personality of the CPP that has inspired some of the research in the field (Blumer and Heibronn, 1982; Engel, 1959).The major characteristics they attributed to the CPP were guilt feelings, because of some unconscious intense aggressive or forbidden sexual desire or deed, for which pain serves as a punishment; high tolerance for pain and masochistic tendencies; turning anger against oneself so that one is depressed, pessimistic, with self-deprecating attitudes and fragile self-esteem; dependence on others; poor sexual adjustment with sadomasochistic sexual fantasies; life histories revealing physical abuse by one's parents, poor tolerance of success and repeated episodes of suffering and defeat; moral uprightness and difficulty to acknowledge negative affects; tendency to be "solid citizens", namely, workaholism, relentless activity, denial of conflicts, and idealization of self and family relations. Thus, the pain-prone individual was described as suffering mainly from guilt and self-directed hostility, whereby the pain functions as self-punishment and has symbolic meanings related to the underlying conflicts (Merskey, 2000).

Empirical studies provided support for many of these tendencies. Thus, CPPs were found to be higher than controls in achievement motivation (Passchier, Goudswaard, Orlebeke and Verhage, 1988), ergomania (excessive work), and the tendency to be active throughout their life (Gamsa and Vikis-Freibergs, 1991), so much so (up to 70% reported hyperactivity, Van-Houdenhove, 1986) that a link between pain-proneness and action-proneness was suggested (Van-Houdenhove, Stans and Verstraeten, 1987). Younger CPPs score high on Type A (a pattern of variables representing presumably risk factors for coronary heart disease) which includes tendencies, such as achievement motivation, competitiveness, and pressing oneself for attaining more in a shorter time (high scores especially on the subscales Hard-Driving and Job Involvement of the Jenkins Activity Survey, Jenkins, Zysanski, and Rosenman, 1979) (Martin, Nathan and Milech, 1987; Workman and la-Via, 1988). Females with CP were found to be compliant, conscientious, passive, and rule-bound; concerned with being good and using passiveness and avoidance as their only response to life; avoiding conflict and risk, denying their own emotional needs, and considering life and emotional expression as dangerous (Corbishley et al., 1990). The tendency for denial is evident also in their attitude toward life problems: CPPs characteristically either disclaim having any life problems (only somatic ones) or if they admit to having some these are considered to be unrelated to their pain (Spence, Pilowsky and Minniti, 1985-6). Applying DSM criteria revealed that the traits of dependence and compulsiveness were common in CPPs (Large, 1986). Other studies showed that CPPs were rigid (Passchier et al., 1988) and adopted the passive-aggressive style more than healthy persons (Jay, Grove and Grove, 1987). In the same vein, a questionnaire study showed that CPPs avoid affective terms, and that they have assumed responsibility and were adjusted in the academic, occupational and social domain at a relatively young age (Swanson, 1984).

Particularly salient is the finding that CPPs are characterized by the internal control style rather than the external control one, namely, they consider themselves as active agents and feel responsible for what has happened to them in life (McCreary and Turner, 1984; Saarijarvi et al., 1990), especially those who are male (Tait, DeGood and Carron, 1982) and younger (Buckelew, Shutty, Hewett, Landon et al., 1990).

Several studies showed that CPPs score higher than controls on the personality factor of introversion, namely, they are focused on their internal world, adhere to strict standards, are sensitive and limit their social contacts (Phillips and Gatchel, 2000).

The general outlook of CPPs on life is pessimism and "future despair" (Labbe et al., 1989). Accordingly, they tend to overestimate adverse consequences, avoid discomfort at the expense of a long-range objective, over-generalize and denigrate themselves and their worth (Ciccone and Grzesiak, 1984). They have low self-esteem, a negative self-concept, and tend to expect failure. Thus, when engaged in physical activity they overrate the amount of required effort and persist less than controls, and in the absence of external feedback they have a lower performance level (Schmidt, 1985). Poor persistence of CPPs was observed also on the cold pressor test (Schmidt and Brands, 1986).

A finding that may be relevant in regard to the pain tolerance of CPPs is that the tendency to be tough and overoptimistic about potentially painful stimuli (viz. underprediction of pain in a lab setup) was identified as a risk factor for development and maintenance of CP (Arntz and Peters, 1995).

In regard to interpersonal behavior, CPPs were found to be sensitive, irritable (Swanson, 1984), less cooperative than healthy controls, as well as less sociable (Labbe et al., 1989). Their Rorschach protocols showed they had poor capacity to form positive human relations (Carlsson, 1987). Further, they experienced more stress in the family (scored much lower than controls on Cohesion, Independence and Organization of The Family Environmental Scale) (Naidoo and Pillay, 1994). Notably, CPPs associated pain with "being sensitive to others", Drysdale, 1989) and also were more vulnerable to interpersonal stress: after a maritally-focused stress interview CPPs terminated a physical activity task sooner than controls (Schwartz, Slater and Birchler, 1994).

Important information about the personality of CPPs may be gleaned from findings about typical coping mechanisms of CPPs in regard to pain. Most typical is the endorsement of cognitions supporting passivity and avoidance behaviors (e.g., avoiding stimulation, activity, social interactions, leisure pursuits) coupled with low expectations of controlling pain (assessed by The Cognitive Evaluations Questionnaire; Phillips, 1984). Coping by means of withdrawal, avoidance behaviors and catastrophizing (i.e., constant worrying, thoughts of catastrophe, negative attitudes to self) is so common that this triad gained the label of the "adversarialness factor" (Crook, Tunks, Kalaher and Roberts, 1988). Further, characteristics associated with severe pain are low self-efficacy beliefs (i.e., only weak conviction that one can successfully execute an action or attain a specific outcome) (Council, Ahern, Follick and Kline, 1988; Dolce, 1987), feelings of hopelessness and helplessness (assessed by the Pain Cognitions Questionnaire; Boston, Pearce and Richardson, 1990), passive coping strategies (Brown and Nicassio, 1987; Klapow, Slater, Patterson, Atkinson et al., 1995), coping strategies based on ignoring the pain, attention diversion, prayer and hoping (Keefe, Brown, Wallaston and Caldwell, 1989), catastrophizing (Estlander and Harkapaa, 1989; Geisser,

Robinson, Keefe, Weiner, et al., 1994), low satisfaction with social and support networks (Klapow et al., 1995), and an ego-synthonic approach to the pain (viz. accepting the pain as an integral constituent of oneself) as opposed to an ego-alien approach which considers it as distinct and alien to the self (Carasso and Kreitler, 1989).

In sum, the emerging image of the CPP is of an over-conscientious individual, who assumes responsibility and tries to behave inwardly and outwardly in conformity with requirements; is self-punitive and pessimistic; and copes mainly by means of avoidance, denial (especially in regard to negative emotions), and passivity.

A broader and more comprehensive view of the personality and motivational dynamics of the CPP may be obtained from a study performed in the framework of the cognitive orientation theory. The major tenet of the theory is that cognitive contents and processes provide motivational directionlity. In its original form the theory referred to molar human behaviors and provided the theoretical constructs and methodological tools for predicting behaviors, such as achievement, coming on time or being late, reactions to success and failure, conformity, cheating, quitting smoking or overeating, as well as for changing behaviors in the desired direction, such as impulsivity or aggressiveness in children (Kreitler and Kreitler, 1982). A more recent version of the cognitive orientation theory deals with the impact of cognitive contents and processes on physiological processes relevant for disease and health (Kreitler and Kreitler, 1991). These health relevant cognitive contents and processes are considered as an integral part of the background conditions promoting disease and health and are disease specific. A body of studies showed specific sets of cognitive themes and even conflicts characteristic for particular disorders, such as coronary heart disease or diabetes mellitus (Drechsler, Bruner and Kreitler, 1987; Kreitler, Weissler and Nurymberg, 2004). Preliminary findings with CPPs showed several themes and conflicts characteristic for CPPs. Here are some examples of conflicts: Giving to others and helping others versus doing for oneself and taking care of one's own interests; doing for yourself and taking care of oneself versus letting others take care of you; fulfilling one's duties toward others, undertaking commitments versus being free to enjoy, have fun, focus on oneself; being active versus not doing anything; experiencing feelings versus controlling them and not feeling at all the negative emotions (Kreitler and Niv, submitted). As will be noted, the mentioned themes resemble some of those found in other studies. The major addition of the cognitive orientation study is that it specifies the exact nature of some of the tendencies and highlights the conflicts in which they are embedded for the CPP. Thus, while former studies showed that the CPP tends to conform and behave in a rule-bound way, the present study shows first, that the conformity refers mainly to the behaviors of giving to others and doing things for others, and second, that the CPP is conflicted about conformity and would like instead also do things for oneself and be free to focus on one's needs and pleasures. The identified conflicts refer to basic and recurrent tendencies in daily life and may impair regular functioning. Thus, the conflict about giving to others or to oneself may result in frustration of satisfying basic needs and thus promote the pessimistic attitude and depressive mood of CPPs. Likewise, the conflict about being active or nonactive may promote withdrawal from action and the passivity noted so often in CPPs. It should be emphasized that the themes characteristic for CPPs differ from those identified as characteristic for CPPs who respond well to treatment (Kreitler, Kreitler and Carasso, 1987; Kreitler, Carasso and Kreitler, 1989).

SUMMING UP AND SOME CONCLUSIONS

Our review has revealed several psychological and psychiatric correlates characteristic of CP. The major ones are: (a) Specific psychiatric disorders, mainly depression, anxiety disorders, somatoform disorders and addiction disorders, and especially personality disorders, predominantly neurotic rather than psychotic in nature, reflecting partly premorbid tendencies and partly reactions to the pain itself; (b) Specific emotional tendencies, mainly increased anger and hostility, coupled with a tendency of emotional denial and suppression, assuming the general form of alexithymia; (c) Specific personality tendencies, mainly conflicts concerning activity versus non-activity, giving to others versus focusing on oneself, as well as tendencies for achievement, workaholism and coping by means of denial, passivity and avoidance.

In sum, the emerging image is of a complex personality type, including affective, motivational, personality, cognitive and behavioral tendencies, specific to chronic pain, contrary to the views which challenge the existence of such a type (e.g., Turk and Salovey, 1984).

Another conclusion is that chronic pain is a multi-facetted psychological-psychiatric-physiological phenomenon whose understanding and successful treatment depend on considering the interactions between the motivational, emotional and medical aspects.

REFERENCES

Arena, J. G., Blanchard, E. B. and Andrasik, F., The role of affect in the etiology of chronic headache, *J. of Psychosom. Res., 28* (1984) 79-86.

Arntz, A. and Peters, M., Chronic low back pain and inaccurate predictions of pain: Is being too tough a risk factor for the development and maintenance of chronic pain? *Behav. Res. and Therap.,33* (1995) 49-53.

Atkinson, J. H., Slater, M. A., Patterson, T. L., Grant, I. and Garfin, S. R., Prevalence, onset and risk of psychiatric disorders in men with low back pain: a controlled study, *Pain, 45* (1991) 111-121.

Bacon, N. M. K., Bacon, S. F., Atkinson, J. H., Slater, M. A., et al., Somatization symptoms in chronic low back pain patients, *Psychosom. Med., 45* (1994) 118-127.

Baggi, L., Rubino, I. A., Zanna, V. and Martignoni, M., Personality disordrs and regulative styles of patients with temporo-mandibular joint pain dysfunction syndrome, *Percept Motor Skills, 80* (1995) 267-273.

Banks, S. M. and Kerns, R. D., Explaining high rates of depression in chronic pain: A diathesis-stress framework, Psych. Bull., 119 (1996) 95-110.

Barnes, B., Gatchel, R. J., Mayer, T. G. and Barnett, J., Changes in MMPI profiles of chronic low back pain patients following successsful treatment, *J. of Spinal Disorders, 3* (1990) 353-355.

Beck, A. T., *Cognitive Therapy and the Emotional Disorders*, International Universities Press, NY, 1976.

Beecher, H. K., The measurement of pain: Prototype for the quantitative study of subjective responses, *Pharmacological Reviews, 9* (1957) 59-209.

Beutler, L., Engle, D., Oro'-Beutler, M., Daldrup, R. and Meredith, K., Inability to express intense affect: a common link between depression and pain? *J. Counsel. Clin. Psychol., 54* (1986) 752-759.

Bishop, S. R., Edgley, K., Fisher, R. and Sullivan, M. J. L., Screening for depression in chronic low back pain with the Beck Depression Inventory, *Canad. J. Rehab., 7* (1993) 143-148.

Blumer, D. and Heilbronn, M., Chronic pain as a variant of depressive disease, *J. Nerv. Ment. Dis., 170* (1982) 381-406.

Bowman, J. M., Reactions to chronic low back pain, *Issues in Ment. Health Nurs., 15* (1994) 445-453.

Bradley, J. J., Severe localized pain associated with the depressive syndrome, *Br. J. of Psychiatr., 109* (1963) 741-745.

Braha, R. E. and Catchlove, R. E., Pain and anger: inadequate expression in chronic pain patients, *Pain Clinic, 1* (1986-87) 125-129.

Brown, G. K. and Nicassio, P. M., The development of a questionnaire for the assessment of active and passive coping strategies in chronic pain patients, *Pain, 31* (1987) 53-65.

Boston, K., Pearce, S. A. and Richardson, P. H., The Pain Cognitions Questionnaire, *J. Psychosom. Res., 34* (1990) 103-109.

Buckelew, S. P., Shutty, M. S., Hewett, J., Landon, T., et al., Health locus of control, gender differences and adjustment to persistent pain, *Pain, 42* (1990) 287-294.

Carasso, R. and Kreitler, S., *Ego-syntonic and ego-alien pain*, Presented at the Intern. Conference on Pain, Tel-Aviv, Sept., 1989.

Carlsson, A.M., Personality characteristics of patients with chronic pain in comparison with normal controls and depressed patients, *Pain, 25* (1986) 373-382.

Carlsson, A.M., Personality analysis using the Rorschach test in patients with chronic non-malignant pain, *Br. J. Proj. Psychol., 32* (1987) 34-52.

Chaturverdi, S. K., Chronic idiopathic pain disorder, *J. Psychosom. Res., 30* (1986) 199-203.

Chaturverdi, S. K., Depressive psychosis presenting as chronic pain disorder, *Indian J. of Psychiat., 29* (1987a) 235-238.

Chaturverdi, S. K., Prevalence of chronic pain in psychiatric patients, *Pain, 29* (1987b) 231-237.

Ciccone, D. S. and Grzesiak, R. C., Cognitive dimensions of chronic pain, *Soc. Sci. Med., 19* (1984) 1339-1345.

Corbishley, M., Hendrickson, R., and Beutler, L., Behavior, affect and cognition among psychogenic pain patients in group expressive psychotherapy, *J. Pain Sympt. Manag., 5* (1990) 241-248.

Costello, R. M., Hulsey, T. L., Schoenfeld, L. S. and Ramammurthy, S., P-A-I-N: A four-cluster MMPI typology for chronic pain, *Pain, 30* (1987) 199-209.

Council, J. R., Ahern, D. K., Follick, M. J. nd Kline, C. L., Expectancies and functional impairment in chronic lowback pain, *Pain, 38* (1988) 323-331.

Crook, J., Tunks, E., Kalaher, S. and Roberts, J., Coping with persistent pain: A comparison of persistent pain sufferers in a specialty pain clinic and in a family practice clinic, *Pain, 34* (1988) 175-184.

Curtiss, G., Kinder, B., Kalichman, S. and Spana, R., Affective differences among subgroups of chronic pain patients, *Anx. Res., 1* (1988) 65-73.

Dewaraja, R., Tanigawa, T., Araki, S., Nakata, A., Kawamura, N., Ago, Y. and Sasaki, Y., Decreased cytotoxic lymphocyte counts in alexithymia, *Psychoth. and Psychosom., 66* (1997) 83-86.

Dolce, J. J., Self-efficacy and disability beliefs in behavioral treatment of pain, *Behav. Res. Therap., 25* (1987) 289-299.

Drechsler, I., Bruner, D. and Kreitler, S., Cognitive antecedents of coronary heart disease, *Soc. Sci. Med., 24* (1987) 581-588.

Drysdale, B., The construing of pain: A comparison of acute and chronic low back pain patients using the Repertory Grid technique, *Intern. J. of Personal Construct Psychol., 2* (1989) 271-286.

Dworkin, S. F., Somatization, distress and chronic pain, *Quality of Life Res., 3* (Suppl 1) (1994) S77-S83.

Egle, U. T., Schwab, R., Rudolf, M. L., Schoefer, M., Bassler, M., and Hoffman, S. O., *Illness behavior and defense mechanisms of patients with psychogenic pain, rheumatoid arthritis and fibrositis syndrome*, Presented at 5th World Cong. Pain, Hamburg, 1987.

Engel, G. E., 'Psychogenic' pain and the pain-prone patient, *Am. J. of Med., 26* (1959) 899-918.

Estlander, A. M. and Harkapaa, K., Relationship between coping strategies, disability and pain levels in patients with chronic low back pain, *Scand. J. Behav. Therap., 18* (1989) 59-69.

Estlander, A. M., Takala, E. P. and Verkasalo, M., Assessment of depresssion in chronic musculoskeletal pain patients, *Clin. J. of Pain, 11* (1995) 194-200.

Faucett, J. A., Depression in painful chronic disorders: The role of pain and conflict about pain, *J. Pain and Symp. Manag., 9* (1994) 520-526.

France, R. D. and Krishnana, K. R. R., Depression as a psychopathological disorder in chronic pain, In: R.D. France and K.R.R. Krishnan (Eds.), *Chronic Pain*, American Psychiatric Press, Washington DC, 1988a, pp. 194-219.

France, R. D. and Krishnana, K. R. R., Pain in psychiatric disorders, In: R.D. France and K.R.R. Krishnana (Eds.), *Chronic Pain*, American Psychiatric Press, Washington DC, 1988b, pp. 116-141.

Fernandez, E. and Milburn, T. W. Sensory and affective predictors of overall pain, and emotions associated with affective pain, *Clin. J. Pain, 10* (1994) 3-9.

Fernandez, E. and Turk, D. C., Sensory and affective components of pain: Separation and synthesis, *Psychol. Bull., 112* (1992) 205-217.

Fernandez, E. and Turk, D. C., The scope and significance of anger in the experience of chronic pain, *Pain, 61* (1995) 165-175.

Fishbain, D. A., Goldberg, M., Meagher, B. R., Steele, R. and Rosomoff, H., Male and female chronic pain patients catagorized by DSM-III psychiatric diagnostic criteria, *Pain, 26* (1986) 181-197.

Fordyce, W. E., *Behavioral Methods for Chronic Pain and Illness*, Mosby, St Louis, MO.,1976.

Franz, C., Paul, R., Bautz, M., Choroba, B., and Hildebrandt, J., Psychosomatic aspects of chronic pain: a new way of description based on MMPI item analysis, *Pain, 26* (1986) 33-43.

Freud, S., Studies of hysteria, In: S. Freud (J. Strachey Translator and Ed.), *Complete Psychological Works of ..., Vol. 2*, Hogarth Press, London, (1986) 1955.

Gamsa, A. and Vikis-Freibergs, V., Psychological events as both risk factors in, and consequences of, chronic pain, *Pain, 44* (1991) 271-277.

Gatchel, R. J., Psychological disorders and chronic pain: Cause-and-effect relationships, In: R.J. Gatchel and D.C. Turk (Eds.), *Psychological Approaches to Pain Management*, Guilford Press, NewYork, 1996, pp. 33-51.

Geisser, M. E., Robinson, M. E., Keefe, F. J., Weiner, M. L.et al., Catastrophizing, depression, and the sensory, affective and evaluative aspects of chronic pain, *Pain, 59* (1994) 79-83.

Hadjistavropoulos, H. D. and Craig, K. D., Acute and chronic low back pain: Cognitive, affective and behavioral dimensions, *J. Consult. Clin. Psychol., 62* (1994) 341-349.

Hatch, J., Schoenfeld, L., Boutros, N. N., Seleshi, E., Moore, P. and Cyr-Provost, M., Anger and hostilityin tension-type headache, *Headache, 31* (1991) 302-304.

Hitchcock, L. S., Ferrell, B. R. and McCaffery, M., The experience of chronic nonmalignanat pain, *J. Pain and Symp. Manag. 9* (1994) 312-318.

Hoffmann, N. G., Olofsson, O., Salen, B. and Wickstrom, L., Prevalence of abuse and dependency in chronic pain patients, *International J. of the Addictions, 30* (1995) 919-927.

Iezzi, A., Stokes, G. S., Adams, H. E. and Pilon, R. N., Somatothymia in chronic pain patients, *Psychosomatics, 35* (1994) 460-468.

Jay, G. W., Grove, R. N. and Grove, K. S., Differentiation of chronic headache from non-headache pain patients with the Millon Clinical Multiaxial Inventory (MCMI), *Headache, 27* (1987) 124-129.

Jenkins, C. D., Zysanski, S. J. and Rosenman, R. H., *The Jenkins Activity Survey*, New York, Psychological Corp., 1979.

Katon, W., Egan, K. and Miller, D., Chronic pain: Lifetime psychiatric diagnoses and family history, *Am. J. Psychiat.,142* (1985) 1156-1160.

Keefe, F. J., Brown, G. K., Wallston, K. A. and Caldwell, D. S., Coping with rheumatoid arthritis pain: Catastrophizing as a maladaptive strategy, *Pain, 37* (1989) 51-56.

Kerns, R. D., Rosenberg, R. and Jacob, M. C., *Anger expression and chronic pain*, Presented at the 10th Annual Scientific Meeting of the American Pain Society, 1991.

Kinder, B., Curtiss, G., and Kalichman, S., Anxiety and anger as predictors of MMPI elevations in chronic pain patients, *J. Pers. Assess., 50* (1986) 651-661.

Kinsman, R., Dirks, J. F., Wunder, J., Carbaugh, R. and Stieg, R., Multidimensional analysis of peak pain symptoms and experiences, *Psychoth. Psychosom., 51* (1989) 101-112.

Klapow, J. C., Slater, M. A., Patterson, T. L., Atkinson, J. H. et al., Psychosocial factors discriminating multidimensional clinical groups of chronic low back pain patients, *Pain, 62* (1995) 349-355.

Kreitler, S., Carasso, R. and Kreitler, H., Cognitive styles and personality traits as predictors of response to therapy in pain patients, *Pers., Individ. Diff., 10* (1989) 313-322.

Kreitler, S., Gohar, H., Eldar, A., Ezer, T. and Niv, D., Alexithymia in pain patients, *The Pain Clinic, 8* (1995) 205-306.

Kreitler, H. and Kreitler, S., The theory of cognitive orientation:Widening the scope of behavior prediction, In: B. Maher and W. B. Maher (Eds.), *Progress in Experimental Personality Research, Vol. 9*, New York, Academic Press, 1982, pp. 101-169.

Kreitler, S. and Kreitler, H., Cognitive orientation and physical disease or health, *Europ. J. Pers., 5* (1991) 109-129.

Kreitler, S., Kreitler, H. and Carasso, R., Cognitive orientation as predictor of pain relief following acupuncture, *Pain, 28* (1987) 323-341.

Kreitler, S. and Niv, D., The cognitive orientation of chronic pain (submitted)

Kreitler, S. and Niv, D. Pain and alexithymia: The nature of a relation, *The Pain Clinic, 13* (2001) 13-38.

Kreitler, S., Weissler, K. and Nurymberg, K., The cognitive orientation of Type II diabetes mellitus, *Patient Education and Counseling, 53* (2004) 257-267.

Leventhal, H. and Everhart, D, Emotion, pain and physical illness, In: C.E. Izard (Ed.), *Emotions in Personality and Psychopathology*, Plenum Press, New York, 1979, pp. 263-279.

Labbe, E. E., Goldberg, M., Fishbain, D., Rosomoff, H., and Steele-Rosomoff, R., Millon Behavioral Health norms for chronic pain patients, *J. of Clin. Psychol., 45* (1989) 383-390.

Large, R.G., DSM-III diagnosis in chronic pain: Confusion or clarity? *J. of Nerv. and Ment. Dis., 174* (1986) 295-303.

Lindsay, P. and Wyckofff, M., The depression-pain syndrome and its response to antidepressants, *Psychosomatics, 22* (1981) 511-577.

Loeser, J. D. and Egan, K. J., History and organization of the University of Washington Multidisciplinary Pain Center. In: J.D. Loeser and K. J. Egan (Eds.), *Managing the Chronic Pain Patient*, Raven Press, New York, 1989, pp. 3-20.

Lopez-Ibor, T. J., Masked depression, *Br. J. Psychiat., 120* (1972) 245-258.

McCreary, P. C. and Turner, J. A., Locus of control, repression-sensitization, and psychological disorder in chronic pain patients, *J. of Clin. Psychol., 40* (1984) 847-901.

Magni, G., de-Bertolini, C., Dodi, G. and Infantino, A., Psychological findings in chronic anal pain, *Psychopath., 19* (1986) 170-174.

Magora, A. and Schwartz, A., Relation between the low back pain syndrome and X-ray findings, *Scand. J. of Rehab. Med., 12* (1980) 9-15.

Martin, P. R., Nathan, P. R. and Milech, D., Type A behavior pattern and chronic headaches, *Behav. Change, 4* (1987) 33-39.

Melzack, R. and Casey, K. L., Sensory, motivational and central control determinants of pain: A new conceptual model, In: D.R. Kenshalo (Ed.), *The Skin Senses,* Charles C Thomas, Springfield, IL, 1968, pp. 423-443.

Mendelson, G., *The use of psychological defense mechanisms by chronic pain patients*, Presented at 4th World Congress of Pain, Seattle, WA, 1984.

Merskey, H., Psychiatric patients with persistent pain, *J. Psychosom. Res., 9* (1965) 299-309.

Merskey, H., History of psychoanalytic ideas concerning pain. In: R. J. Gatchel, J. N. Weisberg (Eds.), *Personality characteristics of patients with pain*, Washington, DC, American Psychological Association, 2000, pp. 25-35.

Merskey, H. and Bogduk, N. (Eds.) *Classification of Chronic Pain*, (2nd ed.), Seattle, WA, IASP Press,,1994.

Merskey, H. and Spear, F. G., The concept of pain, *J. of Psychosom. Res., 11* (1967) 59-67.

Moore, P. M., Kinsman, R. K. and Dirks, J. F., Subscales to the Taylor Manifest Anxiety Scale in three chronically ill populations, *J. of Clin. Psychol., 40* (1984) 1431-1433.

Naidoo, P. and Pillay, Y. G., Correlations among general stress, family environment, psychological distress, and pain experience, *Percep. and Motor Skills, 78* (3, Pt 2) (1994) 1291-1296.

Nilsson, H. L. and Von-Knorring, L., Clomipramine in acute and chronic pain syndromes (review), *Nordisk Psykiatrisk Tidsskrift, 43* (Suppl. 20) (1989) 101-113.

Ornduff, S. R., Brennan, A. F. and Barrett, C. L., The Minnesota Multiphasic Personality Inventory (MMPI) Hysteria (Hy) Scale: Scoring Bodily Concern and Psychological Denial subscales in chronic back pain patients, *J. of Behavior Med., 11* (1988) 131-146.

Passchier, J., Goudswaard, P., Orlebeke, J. F. and Verhage, F., Migraine and defense mechanisms: psychological relationship in young females, *Soc. Sci. Med., 26* (1988) 343-350.

Phillips, H. C., Avoidance behavior and its role in sustaining chronic pain. *Behav. Res. and Therap., 25* (1987) 273-279.

Phillips, J. M. and Gatchel, R. J., Extraversion-introversion and chronic pain. In: R. J. Gatchel, J. N. Weisberg (Eds.), *Personality characteristics of patients with pain*, Washington, DC, American Psychological Association, 2000, pp. 181-202.

Pilowsky, I., Pain and illness behavior assessment and management, In: P. D. Wall and R. Melzack (Eds.), *Textbook of Pain*, Churchill Livingston, London, 1984.

Pilowsky, I., Bassett, D. L., Begg, M. W., and Thomas, P. G., Childhood hospitalization and chronic intractable pain in a adults: a controlled retrospective study, *Int. J. Psychiat. Med., 12* (1982) 75-84.

Pilowsky, I. and Spence, N., Pain, anger, and illness behaviour, *J. Psychosom. Res., 20* (1976) 411-416.

Polatin, P. B., Kinney, R. K., Gatchel, R. J., Lillo, E., and Mayer, T. G., Psychiatric illness and chronic low back pain, *Spine, 18* (1993) 66-71.

Postpone, N., Alexithymia in chronic pain patients, *Gen. Hospital Psychiat., 8* (1986) 163-167.

Reich, J., Rosenblatt, R. M., and Tupin, J., DSM-III: A new nomenclature for classifying patients with chronic pain, *Pain, 16* (1983) 201-206.

Robinson, M. E., Greene, A. F., and Geissner, M. E., Specificity of MMPI cluster types to chronic illness, *Psychol. and Health, 8* (1993) 285-294.

Romano, J. M. and Turner, J.A., Chronic pain and depression: Does the evidence support a relationship? *Psychol. Bull., 47* (1985) 18-34.

Rosenzweig, S., Aggressive behavior and the Rosenzweig picture frustration study, *J. Clin. Psychol., 32* (1976) 885-891.

Rudy, T. E., Kerns, R. D. and Turk, D. C., Chronic pain and depression: Toward a cognitive-behavioral mediation model, *Pain, 35* (1988) 129-140.

Saarijarvi, S., Hyyppa, M. T., Lehtinen, V., and Alanen, E., Chronic low back pain patient and spouse, *J. of Psychosom. Res., 34* (1990) 117-122.

Salovey, P., Mood induced self-focused attention, *Journal of Person. and Soc. Psychol., 62* (1992) 699-707.

Schwartz, L., Slater, M. A. and Birchler, G. R., Interpersonal stress and pain behaviors in patients with chronic pain, *J. of Consult. and Clin. Psychol., 62* (1994) 861-864.

Schwartz, L., Slater, M., Birchler, G. and Atkinson, J. Depression in spouses of chronic pain patients: the role of pain and anger and marital satisfaction, *Pain, 44* (1991) 61-67.

Schmidt, A. J., Cognitive factors in the performance level of chronic low back pain patients, *J. of Psychosom. Res., 29* (1985) 183-189.

Schmidt, A. J. and Brands, A. M. E., Persistence behavior of chronic low back pain patients in an acute pain situation, *J. Psychosom. Res., 30* (1986) 339-346.

Schmidt, A. J., Gierlings, R. E. and Peters, M. L., Environmental and interoceptive influences on chronic low back pain behavior, *Pain, 38* (1989) 137-143.

Seligman, M. E. P., *Helplessness: On Depression, Development, and Death,* Freeman, San Francisco, 1975.

Sivik, T. and Hosterey, U., The Thematic Apperception Test as an aid in understanding the psychodynamics of development of chronic idiopathic pain syndrome, *Psychother. Psychosom., 57* (1992) 57-60.

Sofaer, B. and Walker, J., Mood assessment in chronic pain patients, *Disability and Rehabilitation, 16* (1994) 35-38.

Spear, F. G., Pain in psychiatric patients, *J. Psychosom. Res., 11* (1967) 187-193.

Spence, N.D., Pilowsky, I. and Minniti, R., The attribution of affect in pain clinic patients: a psychophysiological study of the conversion process, *Intern. J. Psychiat. Med., 15* (1985-6) 1-11.

Sternbach, R. A., Wolf, S. R., Murphy, R. W., and Akeson, W. H., Traits of pain patients: the low back 'loser', *Psychosom., 14* (1973) 226-229.

Summers, J. D., Rapoff, M. A., Varghese, G., Porter, K. and Palmer, P., Psychological factors in chronic spinal cord injury pain, *Pain, 47* (1992) 183-189.

Swanson, D. W., Some psychological observations on the chronic pain patient, *Psychiat. Annals, 14* (1984) 783-786.

Tait, R., DeGood, D. and Carron, H., A comparison of health locus of control beliefs in low-back patients in the U.S. and New Zealand, *Pain, 14* (1982) 53-61.

Tauschke, E., Merskey, H. and Helmes, E., Psychological defense mechanisms in patients with pain, *Pain, 40* (1990) 161-170.

Taylor, A., Lorentzen, L. and Blank, M., Psychologic distress of chronic pain sufferers and their spouses, *J. Pain Sympt. Manag., 5* (1990) 6-10.

Tschannen, T. A., Duckro, P. N., Margolis, R. B. and Tomazic, T. J. The relationship of anger, depression and perceived disability among headache patients, *Headache, 32* (1992) 501-503.

Turner, J.A. and Denny, M. C., Do antidepressant medications relieve chronic low back pain? *J. of Fam. Pratice, 37* (1993) 545-553.

Turk, D. C., Okifuji, A. and Scharff, L., Chronic pain and depression: Role of perceived impact and perceived control in different age cohorts, *Pain, 61* (1995) 93-101.

Turk, D. C. and Rudy, T. E. Toward an empirically derived taxonomy of chronic pain patients: Integration of psychological assessment data, *J. of Consult. and Clin. Psychol., 56* (1988) 233-238.

Turk, D. C. and Salovey, P., "Chronic pain as a variant of depressive disease": A critical reappraisal, *J. of Nerv. Ment. Dis., 172* (1984) 398-404.

Van-Houdenhove, B., Prevalence and psychodynamic interpretation of premorbid hyperactivity in patients with chronic pain, *Psychother. Psychosom., 45* (1986) 195-200.

Van-Houdenhove, B., Hysteria, depression and the nosological problem of chronic pain, *Acta Psychiatrica Belgica, 88* (1988) 419-430.

Van-Houdenhove, B., Stans, L and Verstraeten, D., Is there a link between "pain-pronenesss" and "action- proneness"? *Pain, 29* (1987) 113-117.

Von-Knorring, L., Perris, C., Eisemann, I., Eriksson, U. and Perris, H., Pain as a symptom in depressive disorders: Relationship to personality traits as assessed by means of KSP, *Pain, 17* (1983) 377-384.

von-Knorring, L., The pathogenesis of chronic pain syndromes, *Nordisk Psykiatrisk Tidsskrift, 43* (Suppl 20) (1989) 35-41.

Waddell, G. and Main, C. J., Assessment of severity in low back disorders, *Spine 9* (1984) 204-208.

Wade, J. B., and Price, D. D., Nonpathological factors in chronic pain: Implications for assessment and treatment. In: R. J. Gatchel, J. N. Weisberg (Eds.), *Personality characteristics of patients with pain*, Washington, DC, American Psychological Association, 2000, pp. 89-107

Wade, J. B., Price, D. D., Hamer, R. M., Schwartz, S. M., R. P., and Hart, R. P., An emotional component analysis of chronic pain, *Pain, 40* (1990) 303-310.

Walker, E., Katon, W., Harrop-Griffiths, J., Holm, L., Russo, J., and Hickok, L. R., Relationship of chronic pain to psychiatric diagnoses and childhood sexual abuse, *Amer. J. Psychiat., 145* (1988) 75-80.

Ward, N. G., Bloom, V. L., Dworkin, S., Fawcett, J., Narasimhachari, N. and Friedel, R. O., Psychobiological markers in co-existing pain and depression: Toward a unified theory, *J. of Clin. Psychiat., 43* (8, Sec. 2) (1982) 32-41.

Weisberg, J. N., Gallagher, R. M. and Gorin, A. *Personality disorder in chronic pain: A longitudinal approach to validation of diagnosis*. Paper presented at the 15th Annual Scientific Meeting of the American Pain Society, Washington, DC, Nov. 1996.

Williams, D. A., Urban, B., Keefe, F. J., Shutty, M. S. and France, R., Cluster analyses of pain patients' responses to the SCL-90R, *Pain, 61* (1995) 81-91.

Workman, E. A. and la-Via, M. F., Chronic pain, physical symptoms, and Type A behavior in young adults, *Psychol. Rep., 62* (1988) 333-334.

Zelman, D. C., Howland, E. W., Nichols, S. N., and Cleeland, C. S., The effects of induced mood on laboratory pain, *Pain, 46* (1991) 105-111.

In: The Handbook of Chronic Pain
Editors: S. Kreitler, D. Beltrutti, et al., pp. 135-141

ISBN 978-1-60021-044-0

Chapter 8

The Anthropology of Pain

Antonio Guerci

WHY STUDY THE ANTHROPOLOGY OF PAIN?

The main reasons for considering the anthropology of pain are the following:

(a) In order to understand why under the same conditions of pain, individuals and societies react differently; (b) In order to understand why some tendencies of individuals and societies, such as passivity or introversion are related in sick persons to higher pain resistance than other tendencies; (c) In order to explain how the pain threshold is an evolutionary mechanism of environmental adaptation that is influenced by biological and nonbiological factors; (d) In order to help account for phenomena, such as combat anesthesia; (e) In order to understand why many cultures have little appreciation for Western approaches to pharmacology and medicine, relying for pain treatment mainly on traditional analgesics or anesthetics; and (f) Because pain represents a moment of interaction between biology and culture.

Pain can be considered an instrument of communication and knowledge since it has always provided a cross-cultural basis for both the classification of disease and for drug research. While experimental physiologists consider pain a tangible sensorial experience to be analyzed and quantified, to the suffering person it is an affective experience that interweaves both the emotions and physical sensations.

Therefore, within the anthropological context, it is possible to analyze pain from two different perspectives. The first considers pain as an interaction (and sometimes as a clash) between biological and cultural conditions. The second takes into consideration the different "traditional" or "local" modalities that are universally requested to relieve the pain. As a result, it becomes evident that there is an increasing necessity for a deeper dialogue between biology and culture in evaluating and treating pain.

Biology and Culture: Competition or Synergism in Pain Perception?

Every human society integrates the concept of pain into its own worldview by assigning it a meaning or a value. Thus, many cultures consider the body as a mutable reality whose physiology is not exclusively explained on a purely biological basis, but rather is placed in a precise historical and social context (Guerci, 1998).

The pain threshold, when considered as a sophisticated evolutionary mechanism of adaptation, does not appear to differ to a great extent across individuals under artificial laboratory conditions. However, in the real world pain is subjective, and may be associated with precise biological, historical, and social conditions. Many factors contribute to the perception of pain and the level of the pain threshold: environment, age, gender, morphological and physiological components, ethnicity, social status, religious views, working activity, diet, etc. In addition, many different types of pain have been described: acute, chronic, self-inflicted, inflicted, anticipatory, spontaneous, accepted, experienced, related, or remembered. These adjectives reflect not merely different pain intensities but also different emotional thresholds and cultural relationships.

When medicine tries to separate pain from cultural attitudes, it often finds it difficult (and sometimes impossible) to treat various debilitating pains. Further, there is a decrease in the tolerance threshold as analgesics become increasingly available and the demand for anesthesia increases in relation to the disappearance of cultural values associated with personal resistance.

Medicine is relative by nature. It develops from the attempt to interpret and integrate in a scientific manner the secular culture that permeates the attitudes and influences the judgment of patients. This duality between the scientific and the secular provides a potential source for the development of misunderstandings. A consultation is an informal deliberation between a physician trying to understand what may not necessarily be obvious, and a patient who experiences difficulty in making himself or herself understood by a person who seems to take a pedantic view of things that are obvious to the patient. A mutually satisfactory explanation often takes negotiation, understanding, and compromise by both the physician and the patient (Sapir, 1921).

In this patient-physician relationship, the respective attitudes toward pain play a crucial role, especially when the physician feels that the patient may be exaggerating his or her pain or when the patient feels that the physician is minimizing his or her suffering. This determines the approach to analgesic treatment and initiates a series of reciprocal behaviors that could potentially have a negative impact on therapy.

The prescription of analgesics may also reflect more accurately the physician's attitudes toward pain rather than toward the suffering of the patient. Physicians of the Catholic tradition have long shown the tendency to prescribe small doses of morphine to alleviate chronic or terminal pain. Nevertheless, the rate of morphine utilization in 1987 was 20-fold higher in the Scandinavian countries compared to the rest of Europe. Likewise, the British have organized a movement with the purpose of alleviating terminal pain by prescribing considerably higher dosages of morphine compared to French physicians (Le Breton, 1995).

In contrast, the per capita use of analgesics in Japan is considerably lower compared with Western countries (Fields, 1988).

Other factors, in addition to interpersonal relationships and attitudes, can be important. The environment, even the physical setup, can contribute to a patient's perception of his or her condition and can influence treatment and recovery, as shown in a study by Ulrich (1984) of patients who underwent cholecystectomy. In this study, consumption of analgesics was 50% lower in patients whose room in the hospital faced a park with trees as compared with patients whose room faced a brick wall. Furthermore, the latter group had a longer mean post-operative hospital stay than the former group.

Emotional factors also play a fundamental role. An example is what some researchers have referred to as "combat anesthesia" (Beecher, 1975; Le Breton, 1995). This term refers to the fact that during battle, many soldiers do not immediately feel or suffer from the wounds that they had received. Of the soldiers wounded on the Italian Front in the Second World War, only one-third of those evacuated from the battlefield asked for morphine. Although they were seriously wounded these soldiers reported that they felt well, even after a period of time (Beecher, 1975). Additionally, wounded soldiers in frontline hospitals requested less analgesia than those in backline hospitals

Cultural and religious factors can have a decisive influence on the behaviors and values related to the tolerance and treatment of pain (Le Breton, 1995). A small study carried out on Sherpas and Americans trekking in Nepal showed a similarity in the liminal tolerance of pain perception, but the Sherpas had a higher stimulation tolerance threshold (Clark and Clark, 1980). A study of Italian and Irish patients in Boston hospitals also demonstrated cultural differences in dealing with pain (Zola, 1996).

Lambert et al. (1960) studied the pain threshold as a function of religious beliefs among Jewish and Protestant students. When evaluated as students, the Protestant group had a higher pain threshold. However, when told that the study was designed to evaluate religious differences, the Jewish students demonstrated a significant increase in their pain threshold.

Patient attitudes and psychological factors are also important determinants. Introverts feel pain sooner than extroverts (Haslam, 1967). Furthermore, while anxiety generally lowers the perception threshold of pain, relaxation techniques can increase the pain tolerance. In another study, Barber and Hahn demonstrated the role of will power and concentration on changes in the pain resistance threshold by suggesting to patients, whose hands were immersed in ice-cold water, that they imagine pleasant or unpleasant situations (Barber and Hahn 1962). When pleasant situations were imagined, a higher resistance to pain was obtained; when unpleasant situations were imagined, there was a decrease in the pain threshold, accompanied by increases in the heartbeat, muscular tension, and galvanic response in the skin.

The presence of supporting factors can mask or neutralize peripheral nociceptive impulses. For example, the maintenance of stoic behavior can result in activation of inhibitor impulses descending from the superior cortical areas of the nervous system. About 20% of patients undergoing surgery do not feel post-operative pain, and 65% of soldiers seriously wounded in battle do not feel pain at the moment of injury or in subsequent hours or days (Melzack, 1973).

Habituation also influences pain perception. Traditional societies that have rites of initiation almost always include painful trials that habituate the initiates to pain through circumcision, scarification, filing or removal of teeth, tattoos, or burning. Similarly, there are many cultural approaches to analgesia and the treatment of pain. Ultimately, most of them rely on physiologic mechanisms.

CULTURAL APPROACHES TO PAIN RELIEF: A PHYSIOLOGIC BASIS

It has been known for a long time that a stress or a shock cause secretion in the blood of numerous substances—ACTH, prolactin, beta-endorphins, enkephalins—that inhibit the transmission of pain, and in cases of stress, help the secretion of the hormones noradrenaline and adrenaline. Repeated stimulation of low intensity pain facilitates the emission of cerebral opioids to a greater extent than a single intense stimulation. Similar results can be obtained with stressful rather than painful stimulation, such as provoking unpleasant emotions or by a fright. A decrease in painful sensations following a stress (Stress Induced Analgesia; SIA), or anesthesia caused by pain, reveal different mechanisms than those that involve secretion of endorphins and/or enkephalins. Intermittent shocks implicitly contain a message of short duration, so that they suggest to the patient the idea that they could be avoided. However, the concept of inevitability and resignation would enable better tolerance of the pain (Renaud, 1982). This is probably what happens in populations that must continuously deal with painful and emotional stresses.

Humans and animals experimentally habituated to pain deal better with it than those not habituated. However, they bear the pain only if it is of short duration or if they know that it is unavoidable. Repeated shocks result in release of endorphins in the brain, and the opioid receptors become saturated thereby, acting like an injection of opioids during new painful stimulation. This anesthetic effect has been confirmed by using opioid antagonists, such as naloxone to abrogate the response.

There is also a parallel between learning to accept stress and the ability not to suffer from a painful stimulation. In Western culture we learn either to avoid stressful/painful situations, or to believe that we can avoid them. Therefore, there is a lower response of the endorphin-associated mechanism that results in habituation (Renaud, 1982). In contrast, habits have often become the morphine of the poor and, paradoxically, the resistance to pain is higher in developing countries than in developed countries (Scarpa, 1988).

In the biochemistry of pain, calcium plays an important role. Calcium deficiency was found to result in a congenital indifference to pain and self-mutilation observed in European children (Scarpa, 1980). This should be considered especially in light of the fact that according to the World Health Organization (WHO), calcium deficiency is common in many developing countries (FAO-OMS, 1962).

Even before psychoanalysis, human beings have found ways of tapping into their own subconscious. In the course of many traditional or religious rites, it is the preordained stresses, shocks, and pains that have primary importance. During these rites, besides the psychological tension that is present, environmental conditions can also help alter pain perception and thresholds. Factors such as temperature, humidity, atmospheric charge, the amount of carbonic anhydride-saturated air resulting from the presence of many people, as well as the use of candles, incense, hymns, or colors can contribute to the overall effect. In addition, the intense excitement or activity that often accompany certain rituals, such as pilgrimages or dances can result in a greater rate of perspiration, thereby affecting electrolyte and water homeostasis.

Religious beliefs themselves should also be considered. The religious fervor of a believer who is asking for healing can provoke cerebral impulses which affect the endocrine system via the hypothalamus, releasing chemical messengers, such as catecholamines (adrenaline, noradrenaline, and dopamine), serotonin, and endorphins. These compounds have an analgesic drug-like action and could be assumed to have the effect of "opening the barriers" between the conscious and the subconscious (Scarpa, 1988).

Notably, it was observed in France that women coming from Africa had a lower threshold of pain during menarche and/or their first sexual experience than women in Africa. It was hypothesized that the new environment and life conditions lowered the individual pain threshold, whereas in Africa the women's condition did not allow them to feel pain (Scarpa, 1988).

Some shamanistic practices are characterized by analgesia, euphoria, and amnesia. These effects could be caused by hypnotic induction. However, during endogenous analgesia, one of two factors may be responsible for the effect. The first is a psychogenic factor called "faith analgesia" which can be defined as an unconditional trust in the analgesic action of objects or practices. This probably has a placebo effect. The second may be attributed to the production of endorphins; it could be hypothesized to be the mechanism involved in acupuncture and in ritualistic phenomena of the type known as drum and dance.

The placebo effect appears to be different in the treatment of clinical and experimental pain. Beecher observed that placebo is ten times more efficient in alleviating clinical pain than experimental pain (Beecher, 1975); further, it has been reported that placebo was able to reduce pain in about 35% of tested patients (Evans, 1974; Beecher, 1975).

In human society, pain, like some other physiological phenomena, has gained a particular social and cultural meaning. Zborowski (1969) distinguished among self-inflicted pain (deliberately provoked for specific cultural reasons, such as the acquisition of a particular status within a society), pain caused by others (such as, in fights, wars or sports) and spontaneous pain (incurred through illness or injury). One can also define and distinguish between expected pain and accepted pain, with different variations that provide a continuum, somewhat like the following: experienced pain, reported pain, remembered pain with relative emotional thresholds, apprehension of the pain (with implicit tendency to avoid it), and anxiety of pain (paying special attention to the causes and consequences of the pain).

Two attitudes or behaviors relating to pain can also be characterized: fear of immediate pain and fear of the implications of the pain. For example, Zborowski (1952) compared two ethnic or cultural groups and found that the Italians fear mainly the pain itself, whereas Jewish people fear mainly the practical consequences of the pain, such as the effect on their work and its economic implications.

In the ethnomedical database of the Department of Anthropology of the University of Genova there is an inventory of thousands of substances and methods used by various populations and cultures (including Western industrial countries) for the purpose of alleviating pain. Prevalence analysis shows that the "drug" most often used throughout the world is prayer (*oracion, ensalmo, benzadura, mantra, price,* etc.), followed by chicken and salicylates. There are also many drugs empirically utilized by traditional cultures, and these drugs are often considered by Western medicine to be of questionable value. However, within the rationale of a particular culture, the choice of drugs or methods for pain relief is not questioned or doubted in any way. Indeed, it should be noted that many of the indigenous plants used against pain do contain active agents, such as coumarin, capsaicin (the active ingredient in chili peppers), and salicylates.

Minerals, plants and animals, chanting, dancing or music, scents and colors represent the tools of traditional medicine to lessen pain. While some of these may have a physiological basis for their impact, many also have a strong psychological component.

Dances can provide prophylactic healing or analgesic action. Often, by the purely symbolic act real effects can be achieved. A physical action increases the formation of endorphins and adrenaline. While the former can provide an analgesic effect, an excess of adrenaline beyond certain limits may collectively provoke excitability and aggresiveness. This explains the utility of dancing before a war attack, a hunting expedition, a fight, or even surgery (Scarpa, 1988).

Since early times, human beings obtained remedies from what was readily available, based on climate, soil, flora and fauna, and the development of cultural and social structures. Ethnomedicine and its subdivisions of magic, religion, and empirical treatments based on mineral, plant and animal therapies, may be associated with strange beliefs and unusual therapies. However, recent biomedical research has justified the use of some of these practices, which merit further study and scientific confirmation. The ultimate importance, though, is the ability of these agents and practices to alleviate human suffering.

SUMMARY

It is evident that there is a close correlation between culture and biology in the characterization and management of pain. While the medical establishment is still skeptical in regard to adopting a cultural approach to pain, it is hoped that the examples and discussion provided in this chapter will stimulate further research and debate. Such debate can open up new avenues of exploration for the understanding and treatment of the universal problem of pain. The newly developed discipline of ethnomedicine is one approach that can be investigated using standard scientific methods, thereby bridging the gap between science and culture.

REFERENCES

Barber T.X., Hahn K.W. (1962) Physiological and subjective responses to pain producing stimulation under hypnotically suggested and waking-imagined "analgesia". *Journal of Abnormal and Social Psychology* 65: 411-418

Beecher H.K. (1975) Quantification of the subjective pain. In: Weisenberg M. (ed), *Pain: Clinical and Experimental Perspectives*. St. Louis, MO: Mosby; 1975.

Clark W.C., Clark S.B. (1980) Pain responses in nepalese porters. «Science» 209: 410-412

Evans FJ. (1974) The placebo response in pain reduction. In: Bonica J.J. (ed), *Advances in neurology*. New York: Raven Press, 1974.

FAO-OMS (1962) *Besoin en calcium*. Genève: Organisation mondiale de la santé.

Fields H. (1988) Sources of variability in the sensation of pain. «Pain» 33 (2): 195-200.

Guerci A. (1998) An anthropological approach to pain. *Revista de la Sociedad Espanola del Dolor*, Vol. 5 Supplement 1, 19-27).

Haslam D.R. (1967) Individual differences in pain threshold and level of arousal. *British Journal of Psychology* 58(1):139-42

Lambert W.E., Libman E., Poser E.G., (1960) The effect of increased salience of membership group on pain tolerance. «Journal of Personality 28: 350-357.

Le Breton D. (1995) *Anthropologie de la douleur*. Paris: Métailié, 1995.

Melzack, R. (1973) *The puzzle of pain*. Penguin, Hardmonsworth: Basic Books Inc., 1973

Renaud, J. (1982) La soumission diminue la douleur. *Science et Vie* CXXXI: 74-77

Sapir, E. (1921) *Anthropologie. Tome 1: Culture et personnalité*. Paris : Les Éditions de Minuit, 1967.

Scarpa A. (1980) *Etnomedicina*. Milano: Lucisano, 1980

Scarpa A. (1988) *Etnomedicina*. I fattori psicosomatici nei sistemi medici tradizionali. Como: Red, 1988.

Ulrich R.S. (1984) View through a window may influence recovery from surgery. *Science* 224 (4647): 420-21.

Zborowski M (1952) Cultural components in response to pain. *Journal of Social Issues* 8 (4): 16-32

Zborowski M (1969) People in pain. Jossey-Bass, San Francisco

Zola I.K. (1996) Culture and symptoms. An analysis of patients' presenting complaints. *American Sociological Review* 31: 615-630.

Part III: Pain Evaluation

In: The Handbook of Chronic Pain   ISBN 978-1-60021-044-0
Editors: S. Kreitler, D. Beltrutti, et al., pp. 145-151   © 2007 Nova Science Publishers, Inc.

Chapter 9

The Medical Evaluation of Pain

Amnon Mosek

INTRODUCTION

The description and the evaluation of the mechanisms that induce pain are difficult and complex. This chapter is designed to delineate the basic principles of the evaluation of the patient in pain. The clinical approach and the laboratory modalities that may be of help in the diagnostic procedure of the patient in pain, will be described.

Often a patient suffering form pain arrives at the clinic after having seen several physicians and having undergone various unsuccessful treatments. While some patients may have high hopes, trusting that they have arrived to *the best* institution of pain treatment that will instantly relieve their pain, others have low expectations, assuming that another physician with additional treatments will also be of no help. It is therefore of great importance to establish good patient-physician rapport during the first visit, reassuring the patient that after an accurate diagnostic procedure, all that can be done to help him or her to diminish the pain, will be tried. This can bring about full cooperation of the patient, which is an important step for a successful treatment. The first visit of the patient in the clinic is therefore of longer duration than the rest. In this visit the history of the pain, the past treatments and previous evaluations have to be obtained and a physical and a pain-oriented examination have to be performed. Accordingly, laboratory and imaging modalities that may be of help in establishing the diagnosis will be prescribed. It is advisable that a treatment plan is established and presented to the patient, with the understanding that the plan will be carried out during the successive visits of the patient to the clinic, according to the patient's progression.

The next paragraphs will focus on the following three important aspects:

- Taking the history of the patient in pain.
- The clinical examination of the patients in pain.

- Laboratory testing of patients with pain.

TAKING THE HISTORY OF THE PATIENT IN PAIN

This is the first and the most important step in the evaluation of the patient. Since pain can be a symptom of many diseases, obtaining the full medical history is essential for understanding whether the pain is a primary condition or secondary to another disease. For example, diabetes mellitus may be complicated with painful radiculoneuropathy; a metastatic malignant disease may cause localized or diffused pain, and abdominal disorders may refer pain to the lower back. Obtaining general information on the patient's condition is therefore required, regarding weight loss, anorexia, the relation of the pain to meals, etc. In these cases, the primary disease has to be treated in addition to the treatment of pain.

Taking the history of the pain condition is focused on four main characteristics of pain:

(a) The localization and the distribution of the pain; (b) The time course and the duration of the pain; (c) The quality of the pain; and (d) The intensity of the pain.

The Localization and the Distribution of the Pain

Pain can be diffused or localized to a certain region of the body; its distribution varies according to the underlying pathological process.

Localized pain: The pain is confined to a certain region of the body. The area where the pain is felt may be small and well confined, but in other cases it may involve larger body areas. Localized pain may imply that a pathological process underlies the painful area. For example: tendonitis, bursitis, arthritis, bone fracture, muscle spasm, abscess, or other causes. Another type of localized pain is the radiating pain. In these cases the pain usually covers a larger area, which represents the area of distribution of a nerve or a muscle. An injury to a peripheral nerve may cause pain that will be distributed depending on the site of the injury. In a distal nerve injury, the pain will usually be felt distal to the lesion, in the area supplied by this nerve. When the injury is proximal, as in an injury to the root of the nerve at the level of the spinal cord (radiculopathy), the pain can radiate along the course of all the nerves that originate from this root. In case of a lesion to the lumbar roots, for example, the pain may radiate from the lower back down to the toes on one side. The distribution of the pain in these cases is along the defined dermatomes supplied by these roots, and their recognition is important for arriving at the proper diagnosis. One type of localized pain, which should always be kept in mind, is the pain that is referred from a remote area. This is the case of a lower back pain referred from pathology in the upper abdominal organs, or pain in the shoulder that is referred from a peptic ulcer. The physical examination of the patient, has to be oriented towards the possible diagnoses raised in the differential workout.

Diffuse pain: This type of pain is identified as affecting several regions of the body and sometimes the patient will state that every part of the body is painful. Diffuse pain tends to be of longer duration, its cause is not always known, and it is more difficult to treat. Diffuse pain is seen in patients with severe arthritis, severe osteoporosis, in advanced stages of a malignant disease and in fibromyalgia and depression. Taking the history in these patients should include the evaluation of depression, and to uncover a possible malignant disease.

The Time Course and the Duration of The Pain

The time course of the pain may reveal a pattern of occurrence that will be helpful in making the diagnosis.

Acute versus a long standing pain condition: New onset of acute pain is always of unknown cause, signifying that a recent change has occurred in the function of a certain organ. It therefore deserves a prompt medical evaluation to expose the source of the pain. Other patients may describe many years of recurrent, similar, acute pain episodes. In these patients the similarity of the episodes and their pattern of occurrence are important in defining the pain condition, as in the case of migraine, lower back pain or colic pain. It is important to note that in patients who suffer from a recurrent pain condition, a new episode of pain, different from their "regular" pain, needs to be evaluated as a new onset pain.

Stable versus a progressive pain condition: Worsening of a pain condition has to signify the progression of an underlying disease such as diabetes mellitus, malignancy, or others. In a patient with progressive pain symptoms, including those with a controlled pain condition, there is in need of a renewed evaluation of his or her medical condition.

A short versus a long duration pain episode: Short pain paroxysms (seconds) can occur from a variety of causes that involve, for example, the peripheral or central nervous system (trigeminal and other neuralgias, certain types of headaches), spasm or compression of a blood vessel, a joint lesion or muscle cramps. Other types of pain may last for hours before remitting (acute episode of lower back pain), while others may last without remission (chronic headache, arthritis, fibromyalgia).

The Quality of the Pain

It is not unusual that the pain is vague and hardly described by the patient. However, questioning the patient on the presence of certain types of sensations, may be of importance in making the correct diagnosis. A continuous, constant ache in the involved area, with further burning or pressure sensation may indicate a neuropathic pain. In these cases sharp paroxysms of pain may also appear. Paresthesias (the sensation of pins and needles on the skin) may indicate a nerve lesion and such a sensation will be felt in the area supplied by this nerve (carpal tunnel syndrome, radiculopathy). A pulsating type of pain is commonly ascribed to the involvement of blood vessels in the pathological process (migraine) or to a localized process such an abscess. Allodynia is a term used to describe a sensation of pain that is felt when a normal, non-painful stimulus is applied to the skin. Allodynia is commonly found in patients with post herpetic neuralgia and sympathetic maintained pain syndrome.

The Intensity of the Pain

This aspect of the pain is difficult to evaluate. The manner in which pain is expressed varies across people and depends on many factors. The psychological state of the patient at the time of evaluation, the patient's personality and environmental factors, all affect the way one will express the pain. Admittedly, pain has features beyond intensity that need to be assessed and are being assessed (see chapter 11). The importance of assessing the intensity of the pain is in providing both the patient and the physician a simple, immediately accessible and minimally intrusive measure of the success of the treatment.

The methods used for assessing the intensity of pain include verbal rating scales (VRSs), numerical rating scles (NRSs) and visual analogue scales (VASs). VRSs consist of a series of verbal descriptions of pain ordered from the least to the most intense (e.g., no pain, mild, moderate, severe) (Jensen and Karoly, 1992). The patient is requested to choose one of the words as describing best the pain he or she experience at that moment or in general. The descriptors are scored by assigning to them serial numbers, so that no pain is scored as zero, the next higher intensity is scored as 1 and so on up to the highest level of intensity in the series. NRSs typically consist of a series of numbers ranging from 0 to 10 or to 100, with the indication that the lowest number represents the lowest level of pain or "no pain" and the highest the worst possible or extreme level of pain. The patient is requested to choose the number that best represents his or her degree of pain at that moment or in general. The score is equal to the numerical value selected. The VAS mostly consists of a horizontal or vertical line 10 cm long, whose end-points are labeled by descriptors, such as "no pain" and "extreme pain" (Huskisson, 1983). The patient is requested to place a mark at the point that best represents his or her pain at the moment or in general. The distance in centimeters from the low end to the mark represents the numerical measure of the degree of pain. VASs were shown to be reliable measures of pain sensitive to various treatments of pain, and correlate highly with VRSs and NRSs (Choinière et al., 1990; Ekblom and Hansson, 1988). In order to facilitate and standardize the use of VASs, a visual analogue thermometer (VAT) has been developed (Choinière and Amsel, 1996). The VAT consists of a plasticized cardboard of white color with a horizontal black opening (10x2 cm), whose ends are labeled "no pain" and "unbearable pain", respectively. The opening is covered by a red opaque band that may be moved across the opening to the point the patient indicates as representing his or her pain intensity. The numerical value may be read on the back of the slide.

Alternately, one may establish a functional scale that measures the level of functioning of the patient, in relation to the degree of her or his pain.

Special Aspects

Once the above information was obtained and a general outline of the pain syndrome has been made, collecting further information on particular aspects of the pain syndrome may be of help in making the correct diagnosis. This type of information may include the timing of the pain (morning pain and stiffness as in rheumatoid arthritis, nocturnal pain as in cluster headache); the relation of the pain to gait (intermittent claudication in cases of peripheral vascular disorders); the different statures that provoke the pain (climbing or descending stairs, lying down or standing); avoiding behavior (as in trigeminal neuralgia or sympathetic maintained pain syndrome), etc.

Taking the history of the patient in pain has to be completed by obtaining further information on the influence of the pain on other aspects of the patient's life. This includes the evaluation of the mood of the patient, asking about the quality of sleep, appetite, thoughts, social relations etc. The effect of the pain on daily activities has to be evaluated in regard to its affect on working, functioning at home and social life. The success of the treatment has to be measured in relation to the changes that occur in these aspects.

The Physical Examination of the Patient with Pain

The patient is requested to remove his or her clothes and the medical examination has to include the following three components: I. A general physical examination; II. A neurological examination; and III. An evaluation of the area in pain.

I. The General Physical Examination
This includes three main aspects:

a) Inspection of skin: The color, the density and distribution of the hair, signs of dystrophy and signs of infection;
b) The posture: The level of the shoulders and of the pelvis, the presence of scoliosis or lordosis, and the length of the limbs;
c) The degree of movement: Of the head, shoulders, upper limbs, flexion and extension of the spine, the hip, knees and feet.

II. The Neurological Examination
This is a valuable examination that can be performed with the use of simple instruments. The aim of this examination is to evaluate whether there is a lesion in a muscle, a peripheral nerve or its root, or in the central nervous system. It is important to compare the findings between the left to the right sides of the patient. It includes:

a) The cranial nerves: The 12 pairs of cranial nerves are tested according to their function (the olfactory nerve is rarely tested): The visual acuity (the optic nerve, no. 2); The movements of the eyes (the oculomotor, the trochlear and the abdusence nerves, no. 3, 4, 6); The facial sensation (the trigeminal nerve, no. 5); The musculature of the face (the trigeminal and facial nerves, no. 5, 7); The hearing and equilibrium (the acoustic nerve, no. 8); The swallowing (glossopharyngeal and vagus nerves, no. 9, 10); The elevation of the shoulders and head rotation (the accessory nerve, no. 11); The movements of the tongue (the hypoglossal nerve, no. 12).
b) The muscle testing: The testing physician looks for signs of muscle atrophy and tests the tone of the muscle. Then, each muscle is evaluated by asking the patient to

activate the tested muscle against an antagonizing movement performed by the examiner.

c) The sensibility: This is tested for light touch (with a piece of cotton), pain (with the use of gentle needle), vibration (with the use of a tuning fork) and temperature (by applying a tube of cold and hot water to the skin).

d) The tendon reflexes: The brachioradialis, the biceps and the triceps in the upper limb The heel and the knee reflex in the lower limb, and the plantar response..

e) The cerebellar function: By performing the finger-nose and the heal-knee test and the tandem gait.

f) The gait: The patient is asked to walk few steps and the quality of the gait is evaluated. Features of gait that are of significance are, for example, antalgic gait (abnormal gait due to pain) , a limp, unsteadiness, or varying length of strides.

III. Examination of the Painful Area

This area should be tested last since the examination might be painful. Nevertheless, gently performed, the painful area can be thoroughly examined despite the unpleasantness it may cause. The scope of this examination is to refine our conceptions about the source of the pain made while taking the medical history of patient. At this point, we have to finally decide, for example, whether a lower back pain results from muscular spasm, a degenerative joint disease, or nerve compression, etc.

LABORATORY TESTS IN USE FOR THE EVALUATION OF THE PATIENT IN PAIN

The aim of these tests is to help in establishing the presumed diagnosis and to rule out other possible causes. Some of these tests are used to study the anatomy of the area suspected to cause the pain. Other tests are used to assess the function of certain systems.

The following are the commonly used laboratory aids:

a) *Plain X-ray films:* These are mainly used to image the texture of the bones and joints. Flexion and extension studies may also be used to study the function of the skeleton.

b) *Computed tomography (CT) or magnetic resonance imaging (MRI):* These studies are useful to image the gross anatomy of the bones, joints and the soft tissues of the body, including the central nervous system.

c) *Electromyography (EMG):* Used to study the function of the peripheral nervous system by evaluating nerve conduction and muscle function. This test does not evaluate the function of the small nerve fibers that carry pain.

d) *Bone scan:* Used in the study of bones and joints.

e) *Other tests:* Somatosensory Evoked potentials (SEP) can be used to assess the sensory function of the peripheral and central nervous system. Autonomic nervous system studies may be of aid in the evaluation of patients with sympathetic maintained pain syndrome.

REFERENCES

Choinière, M. and Amsel, R. (1996). A visual analogue thermometer for measuring pain intensity. *Journal of Pain and Symptom Management, 11,* 299-311.

Choinière, M., Melzack, R., Girard, N., Rondeau, J., and Paquin, M. J. (1990). Comparisons between patients' and nurses' assessments of pain and medication efficacies in severe burn injuries. *Pain, 40,* 143-152.

Ekblom, A. and Hansson, P. (1988). Pain intensity measurements in patients with acute pain receiving afferent stimulation. *Journal of Neurology, Neurosurgery and Psychiatry, 51,* 481-486.

Evaluation of function and disability. Robinson JP. In: *Bonica's management of pain.* Loeser JD, Butler SH, Chapman CR, Turk DG, eds.

Huskisson, . C. (1983). Visual analogue scale. In Melzack R (Ed)., *Pain measurement and assessment* (pp. 30-37). New York: Raven Press

Jensen, M. P. and Karoly, P. (1992). Self report scales and procedures for assessing pain in adults. In Turk, D. C. and Melzack, R. (Eds.) *Handbook of pain assessment* (pp. 135-151). New York: Guilford Press.

Lippincott Williams and Wilkins publ., Philadelphia USA. 2001, pp. 267-278.

Lippincott Williams and Wilkins publ., Philadelphia USA. 2001, pp. 342-362.

Medical evaluation of the patient with pain. Loeser JD. In: *Bonica's management of pain.* Loeser JD, Butler SH, Chapman CR, Turk DG, eds.

Special techniques for neurologic diagnosis. In: *Principles of neurology.*Victor M, Roper AH, eds. McGraw-Hill, USA. Seventh edition, 2001, pages 12-41.

The clinical method of neurology. In: *Principles of neurology.* Victor M,Roper AH, eds. McGraw-Hill, USA. Seventh edition, 2001, pages 3-11.

In: The Handbook of Chronic Pain
Editors: S. Kreitler, D. Beltrutti, et al., pp. 153-164

ISBN 978-1-60021-044-0
© 2007 Nova Science Publishers, Inc.

Chapter 10

The Psychophysiological Evaluation of Chronic Pain

Elon Eisenberg and Rafael L. Carrasso

It is well documented that patients who suffer from chronic pain often present with an overlay of psychological distress. A review of the literature clearly supports the notion that psychosocial traits often precede the onset of a chronic pain. Conversely, the chronic pain experience itself often contributes to the development of psychological disorders. Not uncommonly, acute onset of pain is associated with anxiety. In the case of persistent pain, the anxiety level is likely to decline whereas feelings of hopelessness and helplessness may evolve and lead to depression. Attention should therefore be paid to the psychological condition of every patient with pain, acute or chronic.

This chapter will provide an overview of the psychological diagnoses most commonly correlated with chronic painful conditions. It will examine the signs and symptoms that should alert the evaluating physician to the possible existence of psychological variables that often accompany ongoing physiological distress.

PSYCHOLOGICAL ILLNESS IN CHRONIC PAIN PATIENTS

The identification of psychological illness in chronic pain patients is not a new concept (see chapter 8). Throughout the years, researchers and clinicians have attempted to understand those chronic pain sufferers who fail to respond to conventional treatment alone.

I. Affective Disorders

Prevailing research identifies "Affective Disorders" categorized under the Axis I diagnosis in the DSM IV (American Psychiatric Association, 1994), as the most prevalent among the chronic pain population (Clauw 1995; Luscombe et al. 1995). Depression is considered by many clinicians to be natural consequence of chronic pain. Anger, frustration, anxiety and feelings of hopelessness due to persistent painful conditions, can result in an inability to cope effectively and increased maladaptive cognitions and behavior patterns in an otherwise healthy individual (Hitchcock et al. 1994; Fernandez and Turk, 1995; Reinking et al. 1995). This is demonstrated in studies of patients with a variety of chronic pain complaints such as back pain, who are unable to work or resume the leisure activities they once enjoyed (Weiser and Cedraschi, 1992; Gamsa, 1994). A subset of these patients may be predisposed to develop a chronic pain syndrome due to poor premorbid coping styles or perhaps an already existing psychological condition that may be the result of early parental or environmental influences (Elton et al. 1994). Studies on Reflex Sympathetic Dystrophy and abdominal painful conditions support this theory (Van Houdenhove et al. 1992; Kachwaha et al. 1994). In addition to depression, anxiety and "Adjustment Disorders" are most evident among chronic pain patients (Weiser and Cedraschi, 1992). Questionnaires such as the Coping Strategy Questionnaire (Rosenstiel and Keefe 1983), Beck Depression Inventory (Beck, 1961) and any general anxiety scale can be helpful during the assessment process (see chapter 13). .

II. "Somatoform Disorders"

The common feature of "Somatoform Disorders" is the presence of physical symptoms suggesting a medical condition without being fully explained by this condition (Smith, 1992; Eisendrath, 1995), or example, Somatization, Somatoform Pain Disorder, Conversion Disorder and Hypochondrosis. Psychological variables are judged to have an important role in the onset, severity, exacerbation or maintenance of these symptoms (Dworkin, 1994). These types of conditions are generally very recognizable by dramatic and persistent illness behavior and exaggerated symptomatology. The etiology of the Somatoform Disorders may be pre-existing emotional distress such as a neurosis, major depression or a history of trauma. The onset may also be the result of months or even years or growing disruption in a person's life that has rendered him or her emotionally, physically and spiritually disabled. These individuals continue to spend considerable time and money seeking out the "cure" for their pain. They develop a preoccupation with their painful condition and run the risk of additional problems such as family discord, social isolation and narcotic overuse. Somatoform Disorders are commonly evident in patients whose pain complaints are more diffuse and non-specific as well as in patients who carry a primary DSM IV diagnoses in the Affective Disorder category.

III. "Psychological Factors Affecting Medical Conditions", "Factitious Disorder" and "Malingering"

Often Somatoform Disorders are confused with the DSM IV diagnosis of "Psychological Factors Affecting Medical Conditions" (Schoen, 1993). In the former, there is no medical condition to account fully for the symptoms. In the latter diagnosis, psychological and behavioral factors are adversely effecting an existing medical condition. These factors are evident in the chronic pain population and include stress, depression, excessive use of substances and general problematic personality traits. Often patients with persistent pain may be intentionally inflicting physical harm to maintain or exacerbate symptoms. This type of behavior is diagnosed as "Factitious Disorder" and can have a psychological (sometimes psychotic) etiology. These individuals may have secondary gains in maintaining the sick role and therefore intentionally cause physical symptoms to exacerbate a medical condition. "Munchausen Syndrome" is defined as an individual's intent to spend an inordinate amount of time in the hospital and resume the sick role, for secondary and other gain purposes. The Factitious Disorders differ from "Malingering", where the secondary gain from elaborate symptomatology allows an individual to consciously avoid activities such as work or other responsibilities (Chibnall and Tait, 1994; Dush et al. 1994; Harness and Chase, 1994).

IV. "Post-Traumatic Stress Disorder"

Complains of persistent pain can sometimes exist in the absence of objective findings or no identifiable etiology. This can be very frustrating for both the physician and the patient. The diagnosis of "Post-traumatic Stress Disorder" (PTSD) common to victims of early abuse, is found to correlate with pain syndromes such as facial pain, and chronic pelvic and abdominal pain (Walker et al. 1995; Mathias et al. 1996). A recent study showed that Holocaust survivors who were referred to a Pain Clinic experienced higher pain and depression levels compared to age matched subjects, fifty years after World War II. The authors concluded "that experiencing the Holocaust atrocities at early life is likely to have an effect on its survivors' current pain" (Yaari et al. 1999). Individuals diagnosed with PTSD often carry the diagnosis of Somatoform Pain Disorder as well because their pain complaints are sometimes non-specific and their illness behavior appears very dramatic (Walling et al. 1994b). Not surprisingly with the PTSD population, the emotional sequelae often result in physiological deterioration and physical breakdown that may be difficult to understand and treat by the patient's physicians. Although symptoms are exacerbated by pre-existing physiological trauma, these individuals may have an initial physiological basis for their pain.

V. "Conversion Disorder"

The diagnosis of a "Conversion Disorder" indicates a psychological cause of physiological dysfunction, i.e. voluntary motor or sensory deficits suggestive of a neurological or medical condition. Symptoms may be inconsistent and therefore confusing to the caregiver. Conversion Disorder should not be diagnosed for unexplained pain alone, or during a course of Somatization Disorder. Even when following careful guidelines, patients can easily be misdiagnosed due to lack of knowledge of more appropriate diagnostic categories and limitations of objective assessments.

VI. "Personality Disorders"

The review thus far indicates that the majority of the physiological conditions related to chronic pain are within the Axis I diagnostic category. "Personality Disorders" (coded on Axis II), are also evident in this population (Fishbain et al. 1992; Mongini et al. 1992; Ham et al. 1994; Wade et al. 1994). The "Dependent Personality" is characterized as an excessive need to be taken care of. These individuals believe that they are unable to care for themselves. Their behaviors are designed to elicit caregiving, constant reassurance and nurturance from others. These individuals may have a history of rejection, criticism and pessimism about their own capabilities resulting in poor self-esteem and self-doubt. The features of the "Histrionic Personality" include excessive and pervasive attention seeking behavior. These individuals are dramatic in their presentation and often carry the diagnosis of Somatization Disorder as well. The "Borderline Personality" is marked by unstable, interpersonal relationships and impulsivity. These patients may seemingly have an inappropriate and uncontrollable affect, and may exhibit reckless behavior. In extreme cases, these individuals may demonstrate recurrent suicidal gestures or self-mutilating behavior. Familial patterns are evident in some Personality Disorders. They are associated with a variety of painful conditions and are generally marked by pathological communication patterns, dramatic and exaggerated responses to pain and self-destructive behavior. Personality Disorders may be less obvious until the occurrence of a traumatic event such as the development of a chronic pain problem. Personality inventories such as The Minnesota Multiphasic Personality Inventory (MMPI) as well as input of family members can be helpful in deciphering to what degree a patient's pain behavior and complaints are attributed to ongoing psychological distress or static personality traits (Deardorff et al. 1993; Parker et al. 1993; Gatchel et al. 1995).

VII "Substance Related Disorders"

Individuals who suffer from chronic pain sometimes have "Substance Related Disorders" such as the dependence or addiction to alcohol, recreational or prescribed drugs. A great deal of controversy continues to exist regarding to the use of opioids with the chronic pain population (Goldman 1993; Sees and Clark, 1993). Recommendations are made to use caution when prescribing narcotics to patients who may have a prior history of psychological illness or substance abuse (Schofferman, 1993). These individuals may use substances excessively or inappropriately to relieve both their physical and physiological pain. Iatrogenic effects from years of polypharmacy and misuse of certain substances is highly likely with a subset of these patients, since pain symptoms may persist or exacerbate overtime. Early detection of the potential misuse of substances is crucial. Many theorists believe that opioid use is safe for most individuals who have a chronic painful condition (Fishbain, 1992). Physicians should be encouraged to assess patients on an individual basis and consider pain medications when it is helpful for increasing functional activity such as resuming work.

Although patients with chronic pain are often psychologically distressed, it is sometimes difficult to determine whether this distress is antecedent to the onset of pain or caused by living with a chronic painful condition. The severity and nature of the psychosocial component is varied among this population. Many theorists would conclude that these emotional changes are likely to occur in individuals who are otherwise psychologically healthy. The prolonged pain experience can result in a person becoming worn down over time and thus present with emotional symptomatology such as anxiety, depression, increased hostility and hysterical behavior patterns. Regardless of whether the emotional distress preceded or followed the onset of pain, including a psychosocial assessment during a pain evaluation may be helpful for appropriate and successful intervention.

In the acute care setting, patients may exhibit early signs of poor coping ability, affective illness or excessive drug and alcohol use. Recent findings suggest that these variables are the *most consistent* predictions of the potential to develop maladaptive life patterns resulting from persistent pain (Stenger, 1992; Sullivan et al. 1994; Dworkin et al. 1992). Perhaps early detection and treatment could result in the prevention of a disabling pain cycle that may serve to unnecessary and unintentionally cripple a patient for many years following the pain onset.

THE PSYCHOPYSIOLOGICAL EVALUATION

In the remainder of the chapter an attempt will be made to understand how the psychological factors discussed above as contributors or as consequences of pain might be reflected in the physical evaluation of the pain patient. In other words, what should alert the clinician during an examination that significant psychological components are likely to be present. The acknowledgment of such factors is crucial for making the correct diagnosis, and for referring the patient to the appropriate care facility which in many cases is a multidisciplinary pain center. It may also save the patient multiple unnecessary and sometimes potentially harmful diagnostic and therapeutic procedures. Nonetheless, making an incorrect diagnosis of "psychological pain" may cause delay in the diagnosis and treatment of serious medical conditions. Therefore a careful (and thoughtful!) psycho-physical evaluation of the patient with chronic pain is almost always necessary.

Since chronic pain is a multidimensional experience which includes sensory, affective, cognitive and behavioral components, it is widely accepted that evaluation of a single dimension, such as pain intensity for example, will inevitably fail to capture the many qualities of pain and the pain experience (Melzack, 1975). Likewise, a limited physical examination which is restricted only to the painful site may often be misleading and result in inadequate diagnosis. The first rule then is to listen to the patient carefully and to examine the patient in a comprehensive manner. Special attention should be paid to the following points:

I. Anxiety and Depression

As mentioned above, pain is often associated with anxiety and depression. It is traditionally believed that anxiety accompanies acute pain and depression is found in chronic pain (Sternbach, 1977). However, Signs and symptoms of those two common conditions should always be looked for in any patient with chronic pain. It is usually relatively easy to determine the presence of anxiety. The patient may report of a wide variety of somatic complaints such as dizziness, diffuse paresthesias, tachycardia and tachypnea, increased muscle tension, headache and chest or abdominal pain. The physical examination can reveal restlessness, disorganized thoughts and speech, hyperhydrosis, elevated pulse and blood pressure, and increased muscle tone. Depression is not always as obvious, and can therefore be more difficult to detect. In order to make the correct diagnosis the clinician should look for the existence of affective (depressed mood, anhedonia, apathy or feelings of guilt, hopelessness, and helplessness), cognitive (loss of concentration and of general interest in the different aspects of life), and somatic (sleeplessness, loss of appetite, weigh loss, dry mouth and constipation) components of depression. In addition, the depressed patient may move and speak slowly, have a shallow or depressed facial expression and may have an overall neglected general appearance. Notably, a special sub-group of patients with 'masked depression' may present with a variety of symptoms, including pain, but without the typical symptom of depression (McCullough 1991). Once the presence of either anxiety or depression is suspected in a patient, their diagnosis can be further supported by the use of the appropriate psychological questionnaire, such as the Beck Depression Inventory (Beck et al. 1961) Symptom Check List-90 (Derogatis, 1977), or others. The diagnosis of depression and anxiety is important because they are often treatable, and without their resolution it may be difficult to successfully treat the pain problem per-se (Carrasso et al. 1979).

II. Non-Anatomical or Diffuse Pain Patterns

Since our knowledge of pain is still limited, the fact that a pain complaint does not fit a well-defined clinical diagnosis does not indicate that the pain is psychological. However, when the reported symptoms are in no way related to, or even contradict any reasonable anatomical or pathological mechanism, the presence of psychological factors should be suspected. A perfect example for such condition is a patient with a bulged or herniated lumbar disc (e.g. L4-5), who complains of pain, numbness, or pins and needles sensation in the entire lower extremity, from the groin down. The patient's examination reveals complete loss of sensation to all modalities and diffuse weakness (usually of the "give way" type) that involves again, the entire extremity. These signs and symptoms fail to fit, and even contradict, the anatomical mechanism expected in the case of nerve root irritation. This patient may or may not suffer real nerve root irritation, but is likely to have psychological components that alter the reasonable clinical picture.

Patients evaluated at pain centers frequently complain of diffuse pain that involves large body surfaces. Such pain patterns are nicely demonstrated by asking the patient to shade in the areas in pain on a pre-prepared human body drawing (Ransford et al. 1976). Diffuse pain patterns generally imply that psychological involvement is present, as no underlying known physiological mechanism can be detected. Only in a small number of specific medical conditions (e.g. polymayalgia rheumatica, metastatic cancer) can cause of diffuse pain. Most of these conditions are associated with abnormal physical, radiological or laboratory findings and their physiological pain mechanisms are known. It is true that in many of the patients with physically unexplained chronic pain, a precise psychological mechanism, which can by itself explain the entire pain picture, can not be found. However, psychological mechanisms often help in the understanding of the overall clinical picture in those patients. We recently completed a study in which chronic pain characteristics of Holocaust survivors were compared to those of age matched European-born chronic pain-sufferers who left Europe before World War II started (Yaari et al. 1999). The study showed significantly larger number of pain sites and significantly higher pain levels in Holocaust survivors. At the same time no differences between the groups were found in the degree of the physical illness. Part of the study conclusions were that the extreme psychological distress of experiencing the Holocaust atrocities at early life is likely to have an effect on its survivors' pain 50 years later.

III. Discrepancy Between Subjective Complaints and Objective Physical Findings

Objective physical findings to support their complaints of pain are absent in many patients with chronic pain (Turk and Melzach, 1992). Patients with trigeminal neuralgia for example typically lack neurological findings on examination (Farbell, 1984). Not uncommonly, tension type headache, atypical facial pain and other types of localized or diffuse pain syndromes are unaccompanied by any physical findings. In the majority of patients with trigeminal neuralgia or migraine headache ,the pain description is likely to be sufficient for making the correct diagnosis regardless of the normal examination. However, when the pain syndrome is not so well defined (such as in the case of atypical facial pain or chronic pelvic pain), and no objective findings are found to support the patient's complaints, psychological components are suspected. In those cases a more careful psychological evaluation is necessary. As mentioned earlier in this chapter psychological conditions such as anxiety, depression, somatoform disorder and others have all been suggested to have an association to pain. A major focus of recent research has been the possible connection between chronic painful conditions to early life trauma and abuse. Emerging evidence is now available to support a possible association of chronic back pain (Karol et al. 1992), pelvic (Toomey et al. 1992) pain, fibromyalgia (Taylor et al. 1995), and headache (Walling et al. 1994a), to early physical, sexual, or psychological abuse. At present, we do not have a clear understanding of the mechanisms relating psychological conditions to pain. But if such connections exist and play an important role in "creating" a chronic pain syndrome, a physiologically unexplained mismatch between subjective complaints and objective findings is much easier to understand.

A discrepancy between subjective complaints and objective findings may have the opposite clinical picture in which physicals findings such as paralysis are present but are not accompanied by an appropriate patient's response. This can sometimes be seen in patients with a conversion disorder. The patient appears unbothered or even comfortable with his paralyzed extremity (La Belle Indifference). Occasionally such a patient can present at a pain clinic with pain in the paralyzed organ (Miller, 1988). A most detailed neurological and psychiatric work up is usually required for making the correct diagnosis. Even then, the prognosis is often grave. We recently saw a young woman who underwent a below knee amputation of her lower limb for painful paralysis related to a conversion disorder, even though the correct diagnosis of conversion was made ahead of time.

Reflex Sympathetic Dystrophy (RSD; now also termed Complex Regional Pain Syndrome) and fibromyalgia are exceptions in this regard, in that defined physical findings, correlated with the subjective symptoms, are essential for the diagnosis (Wolfe et al. 1990; Boas, 1996). Despite that, many researches and clinicians believe that RSD and firbromyalgia are at least in part psychologically mediated (Taylor et al. 1995; Covington, 1996 for review). In sum, discrepancy between subjective symptoms and objective signs indicates strongly, but not exclusively, the involvement of psychological factors. Yet, a reasonable "match" between complaints and findings which usually suggests a physiological mechanism, not always precludes psychological involvement.

IV. Lack of Findings on Laboratory Tests

Not uncommonly, no abnormalities can be detected in a wide variety of laboratory and radiological studies in patients with chronic pain. Therefore, once the appropriate workup has been completed, one can relatively safely focus on the treatment or management of the pain rather than on repeatedly testing the patient over and over again. Over-testing can result in subjecting the patient to unnecessary risks (e.g. radiation), and reinforcing of pain behavior and over utilization of medical services. Interpretation of laboratory tests should always be done in relation to the clinical problem. It is well known now that bulged disc per CT or MRI can be found in a high percentage of the healthy population with no history of back pain (Jensen et al. 1994). Unfortunately, this fact is not well known by many clinicians. Patients, on the other hand, are often eager to discover what causes their pain and to treat it. Thus, an accidental radiological finding of bulged disc in a patient with chronic back pain may easily lead to unnecessary multiple procedures, such as epidural steroid injections or even surgery.

Lack of findings in tests should not automatically indicate a psychological problem. Most radiological studies demonstrate only static anatomical (in contrast to dynamic) changes which are sometimes irrelevant to the patient pain problem. Subsequent to whiplash injury for example, patients may suffer severe pain and impaired mobility that originates from ligaments, capsules or facet joints in the cervical spine. Sophisticated radiological studies like CT scan and MRI are almost automatically ordered for those patients and are often normal. However, simple flexion-extension lateral radiographs that can demonstrate a clear biomechanical problem such as instability of the cervical spine are not being performed. The right diagnosis is not being made and the patient is regarded as having "psychological pain". EMG and nerve conduction tests are often misinterpreted as well. A negative study in a patient with radicular pain does not indicate that the patient does not have "real pain". It only indicates that the large caliber afferents (which generally are unrelated to pain) are unaffected! At the same time, the small caliber fibers (Aδ and C) which are responsible for the conduction of painful stimuli have not been tested at all.

Lastly, our novel understanding of pain mechanisms such as primary afferent and dorsal horn neuron sensitization certainly raise the possibility that a short, transient tissue insult may result in persistent pain. Such pain may last far beyond the cessation of the insult itself (Dubner and Ruda, 1992). Those mechanisms may explain some forms of chronic pain in the absence of visible radiological or other laboratory abnormalities

V. "Pain Behavior"

"Pain behavior" is a term used by many pain clinicians to describe behaviors exaggerated, given the patient's medical history and physical examination. In other words "Pain behavior" usually implies psychological overlay. Practically it means that the patient's 'body language' expresses an unexpectedly severe pain. The patient may move slowly in a guarded fashion, maintain an abnormal body posture and have pain related facial expression, or may present with limited motion of different body parts. He may also verbally express being in severe pain. It may require a longitudinal observation at different situation, sometimes by more than one observer before those behaviors are validated, and "pain behavior" is determined with reasonable degree of certainty. Observation of "pain behavior" is only one part of the overall assessment of the pain experience and should be regarded this way. The term "pain behavior" should always be used with cautious, especially with patients from different cultures or ethnic backgrounds who may express their pain in ways which can be misinterpreted.

VI. Additional Factors

It has been others (Waddell et al. 1984) as well as our experience that several symptoms are likely to be related to psychological distress rather than physical illness: (a) Pain is always at the maximal level possible (or "pain is always 10/10" on a 0-10 scale), regardless of the patients activities; (b) Pain has been persistent over a long period of time, sometimes for years, without any periods of remission; (c) Lack of response to any of multiple previous interventions. In some cases, pain is aggravated by treatments that have to be stopped; (d)

Over-utilization of emergency medical services; (e) Presence of substance related disorders.

Again, these symptoms should be evaluated as part of the overall assessment, since it is impossible to make an appropriate diagnosis based on one symptom or sign in isolation.

In conclusion, it is important to acknowledge that for patients with chronic pain, physical evaluation by itself is insufficient. The presence of psychological and behavioral factors should always be considered during the assessment of these patients. More often than not the assessment of the chronic pain patient is a difficult and complex task, as there is no clear relationship between physical pathology, pain, and psychological distress. Moreover, not only anxiety and depression accompany chronic pain; many psychological conditions such as post traumatic stress disorder, conversion and somatoform disorders, substance abuse, personality disorders, and others can be detected among those who suffer chronic pain.

REFERENCES

American Psychiatric Association. *Diagnostic and statistical manual of mental disorders* (4th edition), Washington DC, 1994.

Beck, A.T., Ward, C.H., Mendelson, M,M,, Mock, J. and Erbaugh, J., An inventory for measuring depression, *Arch. General. Psych.*, 4 (1961) 561-571.

Boas, R.A., Complex regional pain syndromes: symptoms, signs, and differential diagnosis. In: W. Janig and M. Stanton-Hicks (Eds.), *Reflex Sympathetic Dystrophy: A Reappraisal.* IASP Press, Seattle, 1996, pp. 79-92.

Carrasso, R.L., Yehuda, S. and Streifler, M., Clomipramine and amitriptyline in the treatment of severe pain. *Intr J Neurosci* 9 (1979) 191-194.

Chibnall, J.T. and Tait, R.C., The pain disability index: factor structure and normative data, Arch. Physical. *Med. Rehabil.*, 75 (1994) 1082-1086.

Clauw, D.J., the pathogenesis of chronic pain and fatigue syndromes, with special reference to fibromyalgia, *Med. Hypothesis*, 44 (1995) 369-378.

Covington, E. C., Psychological issues in reflex sympathetic dystrophy. In: W. Janig and M. Stanton-Hicks (Eds.), *Reflex Sympathetic Dystrophy: A Reappraisal.* IASP Press, Seattle, 1996, pp. 191-215.

Deardorff, W.W., Chino, A.F., and Scott, D.W., Characteristics of chronic pain patients: factor analysis of the MMPI-2, *Pain*, 54 (1993) 153-158.

Derogatis, L.R., *SCL-90 administration, scoring and procedure manual.* Baltimore, MD: Johns Hopkins University Press 1977.

Dubner, R. and Ruda, M.A., Activity dependent neural plasticity following tissue injury and inflammation, *Trends Neurosci.*, 14 (1992) 96-103.

Dush, D.M., Simons, L.E., Platt, M., Nation, P.C. and Ayres, S.Y., Psychological profiles distinguishing litigation and nonlitigating pain patients: subtle, and not so subtle, *J. Personality Assess.*, 62 (1994) 299-313.

Dworkin, S.F., Somatization, distress and chronic pain, *Quality Life Res.*, 1 (1994) S77-83.

Eisendrath, S.J., Psychiatric aspects of chronic pain, *Neurol.*, 45 (1995) S35-36.

Elton, N.H., Hanna, M.M. and Treasure, J., Coping with chronic pain. Some patients suffer more, *Br. J. Psychiatry* 165 (1994) 802-807.

Farbell, D.F., Cranial neuralgias and other face pain. In P.D. Swanson (ed.), *Signs and symptoms in neurology*, J.P. Lippincott Company Philadelphia, 1984, pp. 230-236.

Fernandez, E. and Turk, D.C., the scope and significance of anger in the experience of chronic pain, *Pain* 61 (1995) 165-175.

Fishbain, D.A., Rosomoff, H.L. and R.S., Drug abuse, dependence, and addiction in chronic pain patients, *Clin. J. Pain*, 8 (1992) 77-85.

Gatchel, R.J., Polatin, P.B. and Kinney, R.K., Predicting outcome of chronic back pain using clinical predictors of psychopathology; a prospective analysis, *Health Psychol.*, 14 (1995) 415-420.

Gamsa, A., The role of psychological factors in chronic pain. I. A half century of study., *Pain*, 57 (1994) 5-15.

Ham, L.P., Andrasic, F., Packard, R.C. and Burdrick, F.L., Psychopathology in individuals with post-traumaticheadaches and other pain types, *Cephalalgia*, 14 (1994) 118-126.

Harness, D.M. and Chase, P.F., Litigation and chronic facial pain, *J Orofacial Pain*, 8 (1994) 289-292.

Hitchcock, L.S., Ferrell, B.R. and McCaffery, M., The experience of chronic nonmalignant pain. *J. Pain Symptom Manage.*, 9 (1994) 312-318.

Jensen, M.C., Brant-Zawadzki, M.N., Obuchowski, N., Modic, M.T., Malkasian, D. and Ross, J.S.,Magnetic resonance imaging of the lumbar spine in people without back pain, N. Engl. *J. Med.*, 331 (1994) 69-73.

Kachwaha, S.S., Chadda, V.S. and Bhardwaj, P., Value of clinico-psychiatric assessment in the diagnosis of chronic intractable pain in abdomen, *Indian J Gastroenterol.*, 13 (1994) 56-57.

Karol, R.L., Micka, R.G. and Kuskowski, M., Physical, emotional and sexual abuse among pain patients and health care providers; Implications for psychologists in multidisciplinary pain treatment centers, Proff. Psychol. *Res. Prac.*, 23 (1992) 480-485.

Luscombe, F.E., Wallace, L., Williams, J. and Griffiths, D.P., A district general hospital pain management program. First year experience and outcomes, *Anesthesia*, 50 (1995) 114-117.

Mathias, S.D., Kuppermann, M., Liberman, R.F., Lipschutz, R.C. and Steege, J.F., Chronic pelvic pain: prevalence, health-related quality of life, and economic correlates, *Obstetrics Gynecol.*, 87 (1996) 321-327.

McCullough PK., Geriatric depression: atypical presentations, hidden meanings. *Geriatrics.* 46 (1991) :72-76.

Melzack, R., The McGill Pain Questionnaire: Major properties and scoring methods, *Pain, 1* (1975) 277-299.

Miller, E., Defining hysterical symptoms, *Psychol. Med.*, 18 (1988) 275-277.

Mongini, F., Ferla, F. and Maccagnani C., MMPI profiles in patients with headache or craniofacial pain: a comparative study, *Cephalalgia*, 12 (1992) 91-98.

Parker, M.W., Holmes, E.K. and Terezhalmy, G.T., Personality characteristics of patients with temporomandibular disorders: diagnostic and therapeutic implications, *J. Orofacial Pain*, 7 (1993) 337-344.

Ransford, A.O., Cairns, D. and Mooney, V., The pain drawing as an aid to the psychological evaluation of patients with-low back pain, *Spine*, 1 (1976) 127-134.

Reinking, J., Tempkin, A. and Tempkin, T., Rehabilitation management of chronic pain syndrome, *Nur. Pract. forum*, 6 (1995) 139-144.

Rosenstiel, A.K. and Keefe, F.J., The use of coping strategies in low-back pain patients: Relatioship to patient characteristics and current judgement, *Pain*, 17 (1983) 33-40.

Schoen, M., Resistance to health: when the mind interferes with the desire to become well, Am. J. Clin. *Hypnosis*, 36 (1993) 47-54.

Schofferman, J., Long term use of opioid analgesics for the treatment of chronic pain of nonmalignant origin, *J pain symptom manage.*, 8 (1993) 279-288.

Sees, K.L. and Clark, H.W., Opioid use in the treatment of chronic pain: assessment of addiction, *J Pain Symptom Manage.*, 8 (1993) 179-188.

Smith, G.R., The epidemiology and treatment of depression when it coexists with somatoform disorders, somatization, or pain, Gen. Hosp. *Psychiatry*, 14 (1992) 265-272.

Stenger, E.M., Chronic back pain: view from a psychiatrist's office, *Clin. J. Pain*, 8 (1992) 242-246.

Sternbach, R.A., Psychological aspects of chronic pain, *Clin. Orthopedics*, 129 (1977) 150-155.

Sullivan, M., Katon, W., Russo, J., Dobie, R. and Sakai, C., Coping with marital support as correlates of tinnitus disability, Gen. Hosp. *Psychiatry*, 16 (1994) 259-266.

Swimmer, G.I., Robinson, M.F. and Geisser, M.E., Relationship of MMPI cluster type, pain coping strategy, and treatment outcome, *Clin. J. Pain*, 8 (1992) 131-137.

Toomey, T.C., Hernandez, J.T., Gittleman, D.F. and Hulka, J.F., Relationship of sexual and physical abuse to pain and psychological assessment variables in chronic pain patients, *Pain*, 53 (1993) 105-109.

Taylor, M.L., Trotter, D.R. and Csuka, M.E., The prevalence of sexual abuse in women with fibromyalgia, Arthr. *Rheumat.*, 2 (1995) 229-234.

Turk, C.T. and Melzack, R., The measurement of pain and assessment of people experiencing pain. In D.C. Turk and R. Melzack (eds.), *Handbook of Pain Assessment*, The Guilford Press, New York, 1992, pp. 3-12.

Van Houdenhove, B., Vasquez, G., Onghena, P., Stans, L., Vandeput, C., Vermaut, G., Vervaeke, G., Igodt, R. and Vertommen, H., Etiopathogenesis of reflex sympathetic dystrophy: a review and biopsychological hypothesis, *Clin. J. Pain*, 8 (1992) 300-306.

Wade, J.B., Dougherty, L.M., Hart, R.P., Rafii, A. and Price, D.D., A cononical correlation analysis of the influence of neuroticism and extroversion of chronic pain, suffering, and pain behavior, *Pain*, 51 (1992) 67-73.

Waddell, G., Main, C.J., Morris, E.W., DiPaola, M., and Gray, I.C., Chronic low-back pain psychologic distress, and illness behavior, *Spine*, 9 (1984) 209-213.

Walker, E.A., Katon, W.J., Hanson, J., Harrop-Griffins, J., Holm, L., Jones, M.L., Hichok, L.R. and Russo, J., Psychiatric diagnosis and sexual victimization in women with chronic pelvic pain, *Psychosomatics*, 36 (1995) 531-540.

Walker, E.A., Katon, W.J., Neraas, K., Jemelka, R.P. and Massoth, D., Dissociation in women with chronic pelvic pain, *J. Psychiatry*, 149 (1994) 534-537.

Walling, M.K., Reiter, M.A., O'hara, M.W., Milburn, A.K., Lilly, G. and Vincent, S.D., Abuse history and chronic pain in women: I prevalence of sexual abuse and physical abuse, *Obstet. Gyn.*, 84 (1994a) 193-199.

Walling, M.K., O'hara, M.W., Reiter, M.A., Milburn, A.K., Lilly, G. and Vincent, S.D., Abuse history and chronic pain in women: II A multivariaic analysis of abuse and psychological morbidity, *Obstet. Gyn.*, 84 (1994b) 200-206.

Weiser, S. and Cerdraschi, C., Psychosocial issues in the prevention of chronic low back pain - a literature review, Baillieres Clin. *Rheumatol.*, 6 (1992) 657-684.

Wolfe, F., Smythe, H.A., Yunus MB et. al., The American College of Rheumatology 1990 criteria for the classification of fibromyalgia. report of the Multicenter Criteria Committee,. Arthr. *Rheumat.*, 33 (1990) 160-172.

Yaari A, Eisenberg E, Adler R, Birkhan J., Chroinc pain in Holocaust survivors. *J Pain Symptom Manage* 17 (1999) 181-187.

In: The Handbook of Chronic Pain
Editors: S. Kreitler, D. Beltrutti, et al., pp. 165-181

ISBN 978-1-60021-044-0
© 2007 Nova Science Publishers, Inc.

Chapter 11

Psychological Evaluation of the Chronic Pain Patient

Shimon Shiri and Shulamith Kreitler

COMPREHENSIVE PATIENT EVALUATION

There is a growing awareness among pain theoreticians and practitioners of the vital importance of assessment for pain management. The goals of pain treatment are defined by and in term of the results of pain assessment. Accordingly, the last decades have witnessed a gradual change in the approach to pain assessment. The change consists mainly in the attempt to match pain assessment with the updated conception of pain itself. Since pain conception expanded from tissue damage to a multi-component phenomenon including emotional, cognitive and behavioral aspects, pain assessment too expanded beyond medical and psychophysiological measures (see chapters 11-12, this book) to include psychosocial aspects of pain. These developments in pain assessment conform to the guidelines of international organizations such as the WHO (1996) and the AHCPR (1994) for pain assessment. Thus, pain assessment turns into a comprehensive evaluation of the patient as a whole person, in which diverse teams of health professionals are expected to be involved.

In each of the following sections we will describe different assessment tools. The presented tools have been chosen because they are common and widely used, concern aspects that are of interest to many pain investigators and practitioners and meet the standard psychometric criteria. In view of the large number of tools, clinicians may be guided in their choice of tool by prior information they may have about the psychosocial environment of their patients, their special focused interest in a particular aspect, and by the psychometric qualities of the tools.

ASSESSMENT OF FUNCTIONING AND PSYCHOSOCIAL ASPECTS

Taking a broad biopsycosocial perspective requires assessing the patient's quality of life, daily functioning, the responses of significant others to the patients' pain and various other psychosocial aspects. (In addition, please see the tools presented in Chapter 6 of this book).

West Haven-Yale Multidimensional Pain Inventory (WHYMPI) – (Kerns, Turk and Rudy, 1985). This multifactor widely-used instrument is designed to assess a broad domain of psychosocial variables related to chronic pain. Theoretically it is based on the cognitive-behavioral perspective and therefore assesses patient's beliefs about their pain and the impact of pain on their lives and their social environment.

The WHYMPI has 52 items with scores ranging from 0 (= "never") to 6 (= "very frequently"). Items are divided into three parts, each containing several scales. Part I assesses perceived interference of pain in vocational, social/recreational and family/marital functioning. The scales of this part are: 1. pain sensitivity, 2. interference, 3. support, 4. life-control, and 5. affective distress. Part II assesses patients' perceptions of the responses of others to their demonstrations and complaints of pain. Three scales assess patients' perceptions of frequencies of 1. solicitous, 2. negative and 3. distracting responses. Part III contains four scales assessing frequency of participation in daily activities: 1. Household chores, 2. social activities, 3. outdoor work, and 4. activities away from home. The internal coefficients of reliability for these scales range from .72 to .90. Test-retest reliability coefficients range from .62 to .91 (Kerns et al., 1985; Kerns and Jacob, 1992). A recent study (Stroud et al, 2000) showed that the reliability values of the WHYYMP subscales were satisfactory, ranging from .69 to .90.

The WHYMP has been demonstrated as an effective measure in predicting psychosocial functioning, affective distress and reported pain after treatment (Kerns et al, 1986; Kerns and Haythornthwaite, 1988). The instrument was also shown to have prognostic value, predicting whether patients with a neck injury would develop chronic pain (Ingemar et al., 2002).

The McGill Pain Questionnaire (MPQ) - (Melzack, 1975). This questionnaire was designed to provide a quantitative measure of pain. In its construction process, participants were asked to classify words, obtained from clinical literature, relating to pain. On this basis, words were categorized into three classes: 1. Sensory – temporal, spatial, pressure, thermal and other sensory properties. 2. Affective qualities – fear, tension and other emotional aspects of pain experience, and 3. Evaluative – description of the overall intensity of the total pain experience. In the second part of the preliminary study, intensity values were attached to the verbal descriptors by groups of doctors, patients and students, so that each descriptor provides information also about pain intensity.

A short form of the MPQ was developed by Melzack (SF-MPQ) (Melzack, 1987) to allow a more rapid administration than the original MPQ. The SF-MPQ has 15 adjectives describing sensory and affective dimensions of pain, a visual analogue scale (VAS), and present pain index (PPI). Adjectives that were endorsed by 33% or more of patients experiencing different types of pain were chosen. Internal consistency estimates in the preliminary study for the sensory and the affective factors were .76 and .78, respectively. Recently the factorial validity of the SF-MPQ was supported by a study with chronic back pain patients (Wright et al., 2001). Confirmatory factor analysis yielded a two-factor solution, consistent with Melzack's (1987) original suggestion. Internal consistency estimates for these factors were .77 for both the sensory and the affective dimensions.

The SF-MPQ was translated into many languages and has been widely used with different chronic pain populations, in experimental settings, and for assessing pain treatment programs.

The Pain Experience Profile (PEP) - (Kreitler and Kreitler, 2004a). The PEP is specifically designed to assess the particular qualities of the pain experience. It is grounded in the theory of meaning (Kreitler and Kreitler, 1990) which provides for a comprehensive assessment of all the dimensions of pain's meaning, such as the affective, evaluative, locational, temporal, developmental, functional, quantitative, causal, sensory (thermal, pressure, etc.), etc. Each of the 30 meaning dimensions is represented by four phrases, and the respondent's task is to check whether the phrase fits his/her pain very much, somewhat, or not at all. The scores provide information about the components of pain that reflect the patient's experience, and about the complexity of the experience. Test-retest reliability over 4 weeks was .90. Validity is demonstrated in preliminary findings indicating the responsiveness of the patient to different pain therapies addressing differential aspects of pain experiencing.

The Illness Behavior Questionnaire (IBQ) – (Pilowsky and Spence, 1994). This inventory assesses an individual's ideas, affects and attribution of clinical symptoms. It has 62 items with a dichotomous yes/no response scale. Seven scales were obtained in a factor analysis: 1. General Hypochondriasis, 2. Disease Conviction, 3. Psychological versus Somatic Focusing, 4. Affective Disturbance, 5. Affective Inhibition, 6. Denial, and 7. Irritability. The IBQ is often used for detecting patterns and illness behaviors of psychosomatic disorders.

The IBQ has been shown to be sensitive to treatment effects among back pain patients (Waddle et al., 1989). Factor analysis provided support for the construct validity of its seven subscales. Further support for its discriminative validity was obtained in a study that showed the IBQ's efficacy to distinguish between clinical and non-clinical samples (Boyle, 2000).

Sickness Impact Profile (SIP) (Bergner Et Al., 1981) - This comprehensively tested and revised instrument was developed in an extensive process during multiple trials (Bergner et al., 1981). It contains 136 items assessing 12 categories: 1. sleep and rest, 2. eating, 3. work, 4. home management, 5. recreation and pastimes, 6. ambulation, 7. mobility, 8. body care and movement, 9. social interaction, 10. alertness behavior, 11. emotional behavior, and 12. communication. The first 5 scales are considered "independent", next 3 are "physical" and last 4 are "psychosocial".

In the preliminary study, overall reliability was high (Cronbach's alpha=.94). It was shown to be sensitive to changes achieved by psychological treatment for chronic pain patients (Turner and Clancy, 1988). Recently, in a one year long prospective study with critically ill patients (Lipsett et al., 2000), the SIP was demonstrated as a comprehensive, valid over time and sensitive tool, reflecting changes in patients status in overall score, physical health sub-scores, ambulation, social interaction, alertness and behavior, eating, and recreation. Its internal consistency was consistently high (Cronbach's alpha coefficients higher than .85).

Rolland and Morris Disability Questionnaire (RMDQ) (Roland and Morris, 1983). This widely applied and translated inventory is used particularly as a measure of disability with low-back pain patients. The original form contains 24 items with a dichotomous (yes/no) response scale. Items were chosen from the Sickness Impact Profile (Bergner et al., 1976), to cover a wide range of aspects of daily living, including walking, doing jobs around the house, resting, and dressing. Psychosocial contents are hardly addressed in this inventory. Scores range from 0 to 24, with higher scores representing greater disability.

The questionnaire is simple and can be completed in about 5 minutes. Short-term repeatability in the preliminary study yielded a reliability coefficient of .83. It compared well with a self-rated measure of pain, suggesting satisfactory validity.

In a modified version RM-18 (Stratford and Binkley, 1997), 6 items were deleted and dichotomous (yes/no) responses were replaced with a 7-point Likert scale ranging from 0 (= "disagree totally") to 6 (= "agree totally"). The modified version is highly correlated with the original RMDQ (Walsh and Radcliffe, 2002) and is sensitive to changes following participation in a multidisciplinary pain management program, based on a cognitive-behavioral intervention. The RM-18 discriminated effectively between low back pain patients with different levels of clinical and electromyographic severity (Leclaire et al., 1997).

Short Form 36 of Medical Outcome Study (SF-36) - (Ware and Sherbourne, 1992) – This widely used and translated questionnaire contains 36 items and assesses eight domains: 1. physical function, 2. role limitations due to physical problems, 3. bodily pain, 4. general health perception, 5. energy and vitality, 6. social function, 7. role limitations due to emotional problems, and 8. mental health. There is another unscaled single item measuring patients' assessment evaluation of their health change over the past year. These domains represent concepts that are most affected by disease and function and most frequently occur in widely used health surveys (Ware and Sherbourne, 1992). Item scores are coded, summed and transformed for each dimension, yielding a scale from 0 (= "worst possible health state") to 100 (= "best possible health state"). Two additional standardized scores can be calculated: the physical component summary and the mental health component summary.

The reliability of the questionnaires' eight scales has been assessed in many studies. A review of the first 15 published studies indicated that the median reliability coefficients was equal to or higher than .80, except for the social functioning scale, which had a median reliability of .76 across studies (Ware et al., 1993). The SF-36's validity has been demonstrated in many patient groups and languages (Ware, 2000). It is a generic measure and is therefore effective in estimating burden caused by various diseases. It has been studied frequently in patients with arthritis, back pain, depression, hypertension and diabetes (Shiley et al., 1996).

Improvements in a modified version, the SF-36 Version 2 (SF-36-II) (Ware and Kosinski, 1996) include simpler instructions and questionnaire items, five-level response choices instead of the dichotomous response choices for seven items in the two role functioning scales, greater comparability with widely used translations and cultural adaptations, and improved layout for questions and answers. Recently, the SF-36-II was demonstrated as an internally consistent instrument, with satisfactory construct validity (Jenkinson et al., 1999).

The Oswestry Low Back Pain Disability Questionnaire (Oswesrty) (Fairbank et al., 1980). This is a widely used measure of functional disability for low back pain patients. It is divided into 10 sections selected from experimental questionnaires, assessing limitations in various activities of daily living. The sections are: 1. pain intensity, 2. personal care 3. lifting, 4. walking, 5. sitting, 6. standing, 7. sleeping, 8. sex life, 9. social life, and 10. traveling. These sections were found to be most relevant to the problems suffered by low back pain patients. Each section contains six statements, describing a greater degree of difficulty in performing an activity. Statements are simply worded, containing usually one idea. Completing the questionnaire takes about 5 minutes and scoring takes about one minute.

In the preliminary study, the questionnaire was shown to be a valid indicator of observed disability and symptoms. Test-retest reliability was as high as .99 and internal consistency was shown to be satisfactory. Similarly to the Roland-Morris, the Oswestry was also found to be effective in discriminating between low back pain populations with different levels of clinical and electromyographic severity (Leclaire et al., 1997).

MEASURES OF PSYCHOLOGICAL AND EMOTIONAL STATUS

Numerous studies indicate that various types of chronic pain are associated with psychological distress. Hence, assessing the patients' psychological and emotional status is a necessary stage in the overall evaluation process. The use of self-report questionnaires may serve as an initial tool in a thorough evaluation of patients.

Beck Depression Inventory (BDI) (Beck et al., 1961). This inventory is designed to provide a quantitative assessment of the intensity of depression. The BDI includes 21 clinically derived categories, reflecting observed behavioral attitudes and symptoms of depressed patients. Categories refer to mood, guilt feelings, crying spells, irritability, social withdrawal and other behavioral manifestations of depression. Each category consists of 4 to 5 graded self-evaluative statements. Numerical values ranging from 0 to 3 are assigned to each statement, indicating the degree of severity.

In the preliminary study, all categories showed a significant relationship to the total score and the split-half reliability value was .86, reflecting high internal consistency. Validity, assessed by comparing the inventory scores to clinical judgments, was shown to be high as well. This inventory enabled discriminating between groups of patients with various degrees of depression (Beck et al., 1961).

The BDI-II was presented by Beck et al. (1996) as an upgraded tool, to address all nine of the symptoms for the diagnosis of a major depressive episode in accordance with the criteria of the American Psychiatric Association (4th ed.; DSM-IV). The psychometric properties of the BDI-II were assessed in a number of studies (Steer and Beck, 2000). It was shown to have a high internal consistency and moderate to high convergent validities.

Minnesota Multiphasic Personality Inventory (MMPI) – (Hathaway and McKinley, 1943). Historically, this inventory has been the most popular one for assessing the psychological status of pain patients. In its original form, it contained 566 items that formed 13 scales: three validity scales and 10 scales designed to assesses psychological disturbances. The MMPI was developed within a psychiatric orientation so as to enable assessing psychopathology, personality characteristics, stress and coping styles. A revised version, known as MMPI-2, was introduced in 1989 (Hathaway et al, 1989). It includes 90 fewer items and 68 modified items. It has an equal validity and includes the same clinical scales as the original version. In both versions, raw scores are converted into T-scores, to allow comparison with normative populations. Normative samples used for the MMPI-2 are more representative for the U.S. population in terms of education, religion and ethnic variability.

The MMPI has been criticized for its length, contamination of items with somatic preoccupation rather than psychopathology (e.g., Graham, 1993) and uncertainty of predictive validity of the profile patterns of chronic pain patients (Smythe, 1984).

Hospital Anxiety and Depression Scale (HADS) (Zigmond and Snaith, 1983). This widely used and studied inventory is designed to assess anxiety and depression among medical inpatients or outpatients. Items were selected on a theoretical basis, stressing distinctions between anxiety and depression. In order to prevent "noise" from the physical illness of patients, somatic symptoms, such as headaches, dizziness and fatigue were excluded. The questionnaire contains eight items for detecting anxiety and eight for detecting depression. In the preliminary study, reliability values for both samples were found to be satisfactory. Validity was demonstrated since scores on the two sub-scales correlated highly with psychiatric ratings.

In a review of about 200 studies on HADS in various patient populations, Herrman (1996) concluded that the HADS is an efficient, reliable and valid tool for assessing anxiety and depression among medical patients. In a more recent review (Bjelland et al., 2000) of 747 identified papers, the HADS was found as an internally consistent, concurrently valid, and efficient tool in assessing severity of anxiety and depression symptoms among psychiatric, somatic and primary care patients as well as in the general population.

Pain Anxiety Symptoms Scale (PASS) (McCracken et al., 1992). This inventory is designed to assess the role of fear of pain in exaggerated or persistent pain behaviors and to classify patients on the basis of the level of their pain-related anxiety. In its original form, the questionnaire contains 53 rationally derived items, consistent with the three-system model of fear (Lang, 1968). Pain behaviors are assessed in three response modalities: cognitive, physiologic and motoric. Patients respond to items describing the four following categories: 1. Fear of pain - fearful thoughts related to the experience of pain or anticipated negative consequences of pain, 2. Cognitive anxiety – cognitive symptoms related to the experience of pain, such as impaired concentration, 3. Somatic anxiety - physiological arousal related to the experience of pain, and 4. escape and avoidance – overt behavioral responses to pain. Respondents are asked to rate the frequency of occurrence of each of the behaviors on a 6-point scale, ranging from 0 (= "never") to 5 (="always"). Cronbach's alpha coefficients for these subscales ranged from .81 to .89 in the preliminary study. The questionnaire's construct validity has been moderate, as reflected in its correlations with other measures of anxiety. Concurrent validity was demonstrated as well, in relation to measures of disability, depression and medication use. Several studies provided further support for the PASS's construct validity, concurrent validity, and utility (e.g. McCracken and Gross, 1993; Burns et al., 2000).

General Health Questionnaire (GHQ) (Goldberg, 1978). This is a commonly used, extensively studied, and widely translated questionnaire for screening of psychiatric problems in medical settings. It attempts mainly to detect two classes of indications: Inability to carry out one's normal functions and the appearance of new symptoms, with distressing nature. In its original form, the questionnaire consisted of 60 items. Later, a shorter version with 28 items was developed (Goldberg and Hillier, 1979) which consists of four factor-analytically derived scales: "somatic complaints", "social dysfunction", "anxiety" and "depression", with demonstrated reliability and concurrent validity. At present different shortened versions of the questionnaire exist, including the GHQ-30, the GHQ-28, the GHQ-20, and the GHQ-12. The 12-item and the 28-item versions are the most extensively used. The 12-item version has been demonstrated to be as efficient as the 28-item version in screening of psychiatric morbidity (Goldberg et al, 1997). The GHQ asks whether the respondent has experienced a particular symptom or behavior recently. Items have four answers (less than usual, no more than usual, rather more than usual, or much more than usual), while different scoring procedures have been applied including the Likert procedure and verbal scores.

Center for Epidemiologic Studies Depression Scale (SES-D) (Radloff, 1977). This inventory was originally developed for use in large epidemiologic studies involving the general public. It contains 20 items, each corresponding to a specific symptom of depression, such as depressed mood, worthlessness, guilt, helplessness, loss of appetite, and sleep disturbances. Items were derived from several previously validated depression scales (i.e. Beck et al., 1961). The frequency with which each symptom has been experienced in the preceding week is assessed, using a 4-point Likert scale, ranging from 0 (= "rarely or none of the time") to 3 (= "most or all of the time"). Total scores range from 0 to 60, with higher scores indicating greater distress.

The instrument was shown to be reliable, with Cronbach's alpha coefficients ranging from .84 to .90 (Radloff, 1977) and from .90 to .93 in a recent study (Verdier-Taillefer et al, 2001). The CES-D also has satisfactory construct and predictive validity (Clark et al., 2002)

APPRAISAL OF BELIEFS, PERCEIVED SELF-EFFICACY AND COPING STYLES

Chronic pain patients may believe that pain necessarily causes disability, that it represents harm, that it can hardly be controlled and that it may last for ever. Beliefs of this kind may significantly affect various aspects of pain experience and coping. For example, low back pain patients who believe that organic factors are associated with their pain and treatment report higher levels of physical disability than those who believe that their pain is associated with psychological factors (Walsh and Radcliffe, 2002). Patients with internal locus of control may benefit more from rehabilitation programs than those with external locus of control (Harkapaa et al., 1991). Patients with greater sense of functional self-efficacy may achieve higher levels of function than those with a lower sense (Lackner and Carosella, 1999).

Beliefs are essentially cognitions of different kinds that are personally shaped or culturally shared. There are various categories of beliefs relevant for pain. Some are highly general philosophical assumptions about oneself, reality, life and ethics; some are beliefs that reflect attitudes and coping styles, such as locus of control or self-efficacy; some are beliefs that contribute to strengthening or weakening the tendency to maintain chronic pain; and finally, some are specific beliefs about pain, such as its duration and causes.

Many pain beliefs assessment instruments have been developed in the last two decades, some of which similar in coverage and even positively intercorrelated. Three major considerations have dictated the choice of instruments for presentation in this review: a validating process that consisted in comparing the questionnaire scores with external independent criteria such as observed behavior during rehabilitation programs; satisfactory concurrent validity; and theoretical and clinical significance of the tool and its scores (see also Chapter 17 section 'Cognitive Attitude-Based Therapy').

Pain Beliefs and Perceptions Inventory (PBAPI) (Williams and Thorn, 1989). The original form of the questionnaire assesses three factorially-derived belief dimensions: 1. Self-blame for the occurrence and maintenance of the pain; Perception of pain as mysterious and hardly comprehensible; and 3. Perceptions of the stability of pain and its enduring nature. The questionnaire includes 16 items to which the respondents are requested to respond expressing their agreement on a 4-point Likert type scale. Estimated reliability coefficients within each subscale ranged from .65 to .80 (Williams and Thorn, 1989), suggesting satisfactory internal consistencies. Its predictive validity was supported by findings indicating that the assessed beliefs were predictive of subjective pain intensity, multidisciplinary chronic pain treatment compliance, poor self-esteem, somatization and psychological distress, and were associated with attributions about health locus of control.

Williams et al. (1994) suggested a new scoring system referring to four factorially identified scales: Mystery, Self-blame, Pain Permanence, and Pain Constancy. These scales correlated with important pain indices, including pain quality and coping strategies. Each scale had unique associations, such as pain constancy with greater pain self-report, and self-blame with depression. Scores range between –10 to +10 for the pain permanence, -8 to +8 for pain constancy and mystery, and -6 to +6 for self blame. The new scoring system has been implemented in several studies since then (Ashgari and Nicholas, 2001; Turner et al., 2000).

Pain Self-Efficacy Questionnaire (PSEQ) (Nicholas et al., 1992). This questionnaire measures pain self-efficacy. It contains 10 items that measure strength and generality of the patient's self-efficacy regarding different 10 activities. Patients rate their abilities on a scale ranging from 0 (= "not at all confident") to 6 (="completely confident"). The total score ranges between 0-60. Test-retest reliability in the preliminary study (Nicholas et al., 1992) was .79. A higher reliability score, .94, was obtained in a study with low-back pain patients (Gibson and Strong, 1996).

The instrument effectively predicts functional impairment, use of active coping strategies, and medication use. Its validity was demonstrated in studies which showed that it predicted dropout from treatment in pain management programs (Coughlan et al., 1995) and correlated (.78) with perceived capacity for work related tasks (Gibson et al., 1996).

Survey of Pain Attitudes (SOPA) (Jensen et al., 1987). This is a well-researched instrument, with several versions. Its original version (Jensen et al., 1987) contained 24 items and was designed to assess five attitude scales: 1. Pain control, 2. Effectiveness of medications, 3. Pain-related disability, 4. Solicitous responses from others, and 5. Medical cure for pain. Reliability measures for these scales ranged between .56 to .73, with test-retest measures ranging from .80 to .91, reflecting a high degree of attitude consistency. The revised version (Jensen and Caroly, 1989) included 35 items and an additional scale of emotionality assessing pain-emotions interactions. A further scale assessing pain as evidence of physical harm was added later (Jensen et al. 1994). The version with 57 items seemed to possess high internal consistency within each of its subscales, and satisfactory test-retest reliability and convergent/discriminant validity (Jensen et al., 1994). It was shown to have predictive value in regard to patients' activity level, professional services utilization and psychological functioning. SOPA-B, a brief 30-item version of the SOPA, was designed by Tait and Chibnall (1997). Reliability values for its seven subscales are comparable to those of earlier versions of the SOPA, the only exception being 'medication', for which Cronbach's alpha reliability is .56. It is a brief questionnaire, clearly reflecting the seven dimensions of the original SOPA, and therefore possesses a practical value.

The Coping Strategies Questionnaire (CSQ) (Rosenstiel and Keefe, 1983). - This is a widely used and researched 50-item self-report questionnaire. In a preliminary study with low-back patients, 6 cognitive and 2 behavioral coping strategies were assessed. One subscale was dropped, as it failed to show satisfactory internal consistency. Participants indicated how often they have used each strategy on a 7-point scale ranging from 0 (=never) to 6 (=always). Patients also rated their control over pain and ability to decrease pain.

Internal reliability values for these subscales range from .71 to .85. Principal components analysis yielded three factors that accounted for 68% of the response variance. The preliminary study reported significant predictive value of the CSQ for several measures of adjustment including average pain, depression, state anxiety and functional capacity.

Several studies have confirmed the CSQ's internal consistency and predictive validity (Keefe et al., 1989; Martin et al., 1996). The CSQ was adapted for different languages populations, including children and adolescents (Reid et al., 1994).

The present version of the CSQ includes eight strategies grouped into four clusters: *I. Cognitive coping and suppression*: 1. Reinterpreting pain sensations (imagining something that is inconsistent with the pain); 2. Coping self statements (telling oneself that one can cope with the pain); 3. Ignoring pain sensations (denying the pain or its effects); *II. Helplessness*: 4. Catastrophizing (negative self-statements); 5. Control over pain; *III. Diverting attention and praying*: 6. Diverting attention (thinking of things that serve to distract one from the pain); 7. Praying or hoping (telling oneself to hope and pray for the pain to get better); *IV. Behavioral coping strategies*: 8. Increasing activity level (engaging in active behaviors that divert attention from the pain).

Pain Locus of Control (PLC) (Main and Waddell, 1991). This 20-item questionnaire measures two dimensions: 1. Pain control - beliefs about how well one can control one's pain and 2. Pain responsibility - beliefs about the degree of responsibility one holds for managing one's pain. Scores are on a four-point Likert scale ranging from "very true" to "very untrue". In the preliminary study (Main et al., 1991) reliability coefficients were satisfactory, and in a more recent study (Ashgari and Nicholas, 2001) they were .72 for pain control and .83 for the pain responsibility scale. Both dimensions have been shown to be sensitive to changes in pain management programs (Maine and Parker, 1989) and to predict future consulting behavior (Main and Wood, 1990).

The Arthritis Self-Efficacy Questionnaire (ASE). (Lorig Et Al., 1989) - This is a well studied 20-item questionnaire developed through consultation with patients and physicians and through study of four groups of chronic arthritis patients who took an arthritis self-management course. It refers to three factors: 1. self-efficacy for physical function, 2. self-efficacy for pain, and 3. self-efficacy for controlling other arthritis symptoms. Patients indicate their level of certainty for performing specific behaviors in each of these factors, on a scale ranging from 10 (= "very uncertain") to 100 (= "very certain"). The total score represents the sums of the scores across the three scales. Higher scores reflect greater self-efficacy. One month test/retest reliabilities for its subscales ranged from .85 to .90 in a preliminary study. Construct and concurrent validity have been satisfactory as well. The questionnaire has been found to be sensitive to changes occurring in the course of a rehabilitation program. In a recent study (Gaines et al., 2002) the ASE predicted successfully self reported functional performance among older women, but not among older men. A study with fibromyalgia female patients showed the ASE (Swedish version) to be sensitive to changes in health status following a self-management education and physical training program, whereby its correlations with pre and post health status measures were consistent with the questionnaire's theoretical assumptions (Lomi and Burckhardt, 1995).

Fear-Avoidance Belief Questionnaire (FABQ) (Waddel et al., 1993) - This 16-item questionnaire measures fear avoidance beliefs about work and physical activity. Scores are on a seven-point Likert scale, ranging from "strongly disagree" to "strongly agree". The questionnaire is based on theoretical assumptions on fear and avoidance behavior and is focused on patients' beliefs about the effects of physical activity and work on their low back pain. Principal-components analysis revealed two factors: fear avoidance beliefs about work and fear avoidance beliefs about physical activity, with internal consistency values of .88 and .77, respectively. Fear avoidance beliefs correlated highly with self-reported disability in activities of daily living and with work loss (Waddel et al., 1993).

Crombez et al. (1999) found the FABQ to be efficient in predicting self reported disability and poor behavioral performance. Also the German version was shown to be reliable and valid although it had a different factor structure from the original English version (Pfingsten et al., 2000).

Tampa Scale for Kinesiophobia (TSK) (Vlaeyen et al., 1996). This 17-item questionnaire measures the degree of fear of movement/(re)injury. Scoring is on a four-point Likert scale, ranging from "strongly disagree" to "strongly agree". A total score is calculated after inverting the scores of four items (nos. 4, 8, 12, 16). The TSK was shown to have fair internal consistency (Cronbach's alpha = .77). The preliminary study showed the TSK to be related to gender, compensation status, psychological measures (catastrophizing and depression), and to fear measures (social phobia, agoraphobia and fear of body injury, illness and death). Other studies showed that the TSK was efficient in predicting self reported disability and poor behavioral performance (Crombez et al., 1999) as well as avoidance behavior in chronic fatigue syndrome patients (Silver et al., 2002).

The Pain Beliefs Questionnaire (PBQ) (Edwards, 1992). This 20-item questionnaire assesses beliefs about the cause and treatment of pain. It includes two scales: "organic beliefs" (8 items) and "psychological beliefs" (4 items). Responses range from 1 (= "never") to 6 (= "always"). Internal reliability values in the preliminary study were .73 for the organic beliefs scale and .70 for the psychological beliefs.

The preliminary study reported that chronic pain patients emphasized the importance of organic aspects of pain while pain-free participants tended to stress the significance of psychological factors in pain.

The construct validity of the PBQ was supported by its association with the Multidimensional Health Locus of Control questionnaire (MHLC) (Wallstone and Wallstone, 1978). Chronic pain patients who scored high on the PBQ organic scale also scored high on the MHLC beliefs that powerful others, usually doctors or chance, control their pain. On the other hand, stressing the significance of psychological factor regarding pain was associated with beliefs that individuals have control over their health and well-being. The predictive validity of the PBQ was also demonstrated in a study with low back pain patients in whom reductions in "organic" pain beliefs were associated with improvements in reported disability (Walsh and Radcliff, 2002).

The Pain Cognitions Questionnaire - (PCQ) (Boston et al., 1990). This 30-item questionnaire was developed through a study with mixed chronic pain patients. An exploratory factor analysis revealed two positive factors (active positive coping strategies and passive optimism) and two negative factors (hopelessness and helplessness), with internal consistencies ranging between .66 and .80. Responses are on a four-point scale, ranging from "not at all" to "most of the time". It has good face validity and can be easily administered. Scores on the negative factors correlated with pain intensity, distress and behavior disruption, whereas scores on the positive factors did not correlate with patient functioning, which is consistent with other findings about successful coping.

The Cognitive Orientation of Pain Inventory (COPI) (Kreitler and Kreitler, 2004b). COPI resembles the other questionnaires in this section insofar as it assesses beliefs, but differs from them in the target of the assessment which is the motivational disposition for pain. The COPI has been developed in the framework of the cognitive orientation theory of physical wellness and disease which assumes that specific clusters of cognitions act as risk factors contributing to the formation and maintenance of physical disorders (Figer et al., 2002; Kreitler and Kreitler, 1991).

The cognitions predisposing toward a specific disorder are beliefs of four types reflecting contents relevant for that disorder. The four types of beliefs are: (a) *Beliefs about goals*, which express actions or states desired or not by the individual (e.g., 'I want to be respected by others'); (b) *Beliefs about rules and norms*, which express ethical, esthetic, social and other rules and standards (e.g., 'One should be assertive'); (c) *Beliefs about self*, which express information about oneself, such as one's habits, actions or feelings (e.g., 'I often get angry', 'I was born in Canada'); and (d) *General beliefs*, which express information about others and the environment (e.g., 'The world is a dangerous place'). Formally, the beliefs differ in the subject (in a and c it is the self, in b and d it is non-self) and in the relation between subject and predicate (in c and d it is factual, in b the desirable, in a the desired). Contents relevant for a particular disorder are identified by pretests conducted in accordance with a standard procedure based on a sequential testing of meanings. A motivational disposition is diagnosed when the individual has endorsed a high (above the mean) number of beliefs orienting toward the disorder in at least three of the belief types. The motivational disposition is assumed to be unconscious, nonvoluntary and not the function of rational decision-making.

The purpose of the COPI is to identify the individuals who have a motivational disposition for pain, to chart out the procedure of treatment for chronic pain patients by detecting the specific motivational elements that characterize them and to follow-up progress in their treatment, and to characterize different types of pains in terms of their correlates in terms of the motivational disposition.

The COPI has four parts, each refers to one of the belief types and contains statements referring to themes identified as relevant for pain, such as the expression of emotions, denial of negative emotions, guilt about getting help and attention from others, leaving problems unsolved, and compulsion for cleanliness and order. The participant is requested to check one of four response alternatives for each statement ("very true", "true", "not true", "not at all true"). There are four scores, one for each belief type, and scores for each theme. The reliability of the COPI is satisfactory (Cronbach's alpha in the range of .88 to .95). Its validity was demonstrated in studies that showed its ability to discriminate between chronic pain patients and controls (other types of chronic patients or healthy) as well as to predict who will respond positively to pain treatment.

CONCLUDING REMARKS

The variety of available assessment tools should not produce in the practitioner a sense of confusion but rather evoke confidence that we may be reaching the point where it will be possible to find the right kind of tool for each assessment need. Assessment gradually takes on the form of a two-component procedure: a core component that includes standard tools, and a peripheral or additional component that includes circumstantially selected tools, according to the specific needs of the particular patient in a particular therapeutic context. The striving should be to make the core component as rigidly standard as possible, across patients in diverse pain centers and countries, using the same tools and scores to improve communication within the broad pain experts' community. At the same time, the peripheral component should be rendered as flexible as possible to reflect the individual needs of the individual patient.

REFERENCES

Agency for Health Care Policy and Research (1994). *Clinical Practice Guideline No. 9: Management of cancer pain*. Rockville, MD, US Department of Health and Human Services [AHCPR Publication No. 94-0592]. HAmerican Psychological Association (1994*). Diagnostic and Statistical Manual of Mental Disorders* (4th ed.). Washington, DC: Author

Ashgari, A., and Nicholas, M. K. (2001). Pain self-efficacy beliefs and pain behavior. A prospective study. *Pain, 94*, 85-100

Beck, A. T., Steer, R. A., and Brown, G. K. (1996*). Manual for the Beck Depression Inventory*. San Antonio, TX: Psychological Corporation.

Beck, A., Ward, C.H., and Mendelson, M. (1961). Cognition, affect and psychopathology. *Archives of General Psychiatry, 24*, 495-500.

Bergner, M., Bobbitt, R.A., Pollard, W.E., et al. (1976). The sickness impact profile: development and final revision of a health status measure. *Medical Care, 19*, 787-805

Bergner, M., Bobbit, R.A., Carter, W.B., et al. (1981). The sickness impact profile. Validation of a health status measure. *Medical Care, 14,* 57-67.

Bjelland, I., Dahl, A.A., Haug, T.T., et al. (2002). The validity of Hospital Anxiety and Depression Scale. An update literature review. *Journal of Psychosomatic Research, 52,*69-77.

Boston, K., Pearce, S.A., and Richardson, P.H. (1990). The Pain Cognitions Questionnaire. *Journal of Psychosomatic Research, 34,*103-109.

Boyle, G.J. (2000). Discriminant validity of the illness behavior questionnaire and Millon Clinical Multiaxial Inventory-III in a heterogeneous sample of psychiatric outpatients. *Journal of Clinical Psychology, 56,* 779-791.

Burns, J.W., Mullen, J.T., Higdon, L.J., et al. (2000). Validity of the Pain Anxiety Symptom Scale (PASS): prediction of physical capacity variables. *Pain, 84,* 247-252

Clark, C.H., Mahoney, J.S., Clark, D., et al. (2002). Screening for depression in hepatitis C population: the reliability and validity of the Center for Epidemiologic Studies Depression Scale (CDS-D). *Journal of Advanced Nursing, 40,* 361-369.

Coughlan, G.M., Ridout, K.L., Williams, A.C., and Richardson, P.H.(1995). Attrition from a pain management programme. *British Journal of Clinical Psychology, 34* (Pt 3), 471-479.

Crombez, G., Vlaeyen, J.W, Heuts, P.H., et al. (1999). Pain-related fear is more disabling than pain itself: evidence on the role of pain-related fear in chronic back pain disability. *Pain, 80,* 329-339

Edwards, L.C., Pearce, S.A., Turner-Stokes, L., et al. (1992). The Pain Beliefs Questionnaire: an investigation of beliefs on the causes and consequences of pain. *Pain, 51,* 267-272

Fairbank, J.C.T., Couper, J., Davies, J.B., and O'Brien, J.P. (1980). The Oswestry Low Back Pain Disability Questionnaire. *Physiotherapy, 66,* 271-273.

Figer, A., Kreitler, S., Kreitler, M., and Inbar, M. (2002). Personality dispositions of colon cancer patients. *Gastrointestinal Oncology, 4,* 81-92.

Gaines, J.M., Talbot, L.A., and Metter, E.J. (2002).The relationship of arthritis self-efficacy to functional performance in older men and women with osteoarthritis of the knee. *Geriatric Nursing, 23,* 167-170.

Gibson, L., and Strong, J. (1996). The reliability and validity of a measure of perceived functional capacity for work in chronic back pain. *Journal of Occupational Rehabilitation, 6,* 159-175

Goldberg, D.P. (1978). *Manual for the General Health Questionnaire.* Sussex: DJS Spools.

Goldberg, D.P., Gater, R., Sartorius, N., et al. (1997). The validity of two versions of the GHQ in the WHO study of mental illness in the general health care. *Psychological Medicine, 27,* 191-197.

Goldberg, D.P., and Hillier, V.F. (1979). A scaled version of the General Health Questionnaire. *Psychological Medicine, 9,* 139-145.

Graham, J.R. (1993). *MMPI-2, assessing personality and psychopathology.* New ork: Oxford University Press.

Harkapaa, K., Jarvikoski, A., Mellin, G., et al. (1991). Health locus of control beliefs and psychological distress as predictors for treatment outcome in low-back pain patients: results of a 3-month follow-up of a controlled intervention study. *Pain, 46,* 35-41.

Hathaway, S.R., and McKinley, J.C. (1943). *The Minnesota Multiphasic Personality Inventory*. Minneapolis, MN: University of Minnesota Press.

Hathaway, S.R., McKinley, J.C., Butcher, J.N., et al. (1989). *Minnesota Multiphasic Personality Inventory-2: Manual for administration*. Minneapolis, MN: University of Minnesota Press.

Herrmann, C. (1997). International experiences with the Hospital Anxiety and Depression Scale – a review of validation data and clinical results. *Journal of Psychosomatic Research, 42,* 17-41.

Ingemar, O., Bunketorp, O., Sven, C., et al. (2002). Prediction of outcome in whiplash-associated disorders using West Haven-Yale multidimensional pain inventory. *Clinical Journal of Pain, 18,* 238-244.

Jenkinson, C., Brown, S.S., Petersen, S., et al. (1999). Assessment of the SF-36 in the United Kingdom. *Journal of Epidemiology and Community Health, 53,* 46-50.

Jensen, M.P., and Karoly, P. (1992). Pain-specific beliefs, perceived symptom severity, and adjustment to chronic pain. *Clinical Journal of Pain, 8,* 123-130.

Jensen, M. P., Karoly, P., and Huger, R. (1987). The development and preliminary validation of an instrument to assess patients' attitudes toward pain. *Journal of Psychosomatic Research, 31,* 393-400.

Jensen, M.P., and Caroly, P. (1989). *Revision and cross-validation of the Survey of Pain Attitudes*. Paper presented at the 10th Annual Scientific Sessions of the Society of Behavioral Medicine, San Francisco, CA

Jensen, M.P., Turner, J.A., and Romano, J.M. (1994). Relationship of pain specific beliefs to chronic pain adjustment. *Pain, 57,* 301-309.

Keefe, F.J., Brown, G.K., Wallstone, K.A., and Caldwell, D. S. (1989). Coping with rheumatoid arthritis: catastrophizing as a maladaptive strategy. *Pain, 37,* 51-56.

Kerns, R.D., and Haythornthwaite, J.A. (1988). Depression among chronic pain patients: Cognitive behavioral analysis and effect on rehabilitation. *Journal of Consulting and Clinical Psychology, 56,* 70-76.

Kerns, R.D., and Jacob, M.C. (1992). Assessment of the psychosocial context in the experience of pain (pp. 235-256). In D. C. Turk, and R. Melzack (Eds.), *Handbook of pain assessment*. New York: Guilford.

Kerns, R.D., Turk, D.C., Holzman, A.D., and Rudy, T.E. (1986). Comparison of cognitive-behavioral and behavioral approaches to outpatients treatment of chronic pain. *Clinical Journal of Pain, 1,* 195-203.

Kreitler, S., and Kreitler, H. (1990). *The cognitive foundations of personality traits*. New York: Plenum.

Kreitler, S., and Kreitler, H. (1991). Cognitive orientation and physical disease or health. *European Journal of Personality, 5,* 109-129.

Kreitler, S., and Kreitler, M. (2004a). Assessing the experiencing of pain. [in press]

Kreitler, S., and Kreitler, M. (2004b). The Cognitive Orientation of Pain Inventory: Who will be a pain patient? {in press]

Lackner, J.M., and Carosella, A.M. (1999). The relative influence of perceived pain control, anxiety, and functional self efficacy on spinal function among patients with chronic low back pain. *Spine, 1, 24,* 2254-2260; discussion 2260-2261.

Lang, P.J. (1968). Fear reduction and fear behavior: problems in treating a construct. In J. M Shilen (Ed.), *Research in Psychotherapy, Vol. 3* (pp. 90-103). Washington, DC: American Psychological Association.

Leclaire, R., Blier, F., Fortin, L., et al. (1997). A cross-sectional study comparing the Ostwestry and the Roland-Morris functional disability scales in two populations of patients with low back pain of different levels of severity. *Spine, 22*, 68-71.

Lipsett, P.A., Swoboda, S.M., Campbell, K.A. et al. (2000). Sickness Impact Profile Score versus a Modified Short-Form survey for functional outcome assessment: acceptability, reliability, and validity in critically ill patients with prolonged intensive care unit stays. *Journal of Trauma, 49*, 737-743.

Lomi, C., Burckhardt, C., and Nordholm, L. (1995). Evaluation of a Swedish version of the arthritis self-efficacy scale in people with fibromyalgia. *Scandinavian Journal of Rheumatology, 24*, 282-287.

Lorig, K., Chastain, R.L., Ung, E., Shoor, S., and Holman, H.R. (1989). Development and evaluation of a scale to measure perceived self-efficacy in people with arthritis. *Arthritis and Rheumatology, 32*, 37-44

Main, C.J., and Parker, H. (1989). Pain management programmes. In M. Roland and J. Jenner (Eds.), *Back pain: New approaches to rehabilitation and education.* Manchester, UK:Manchester University Press.

Main, C.J., and Waddell, G. (1991). A comparison of cognitive measures in low back pain: statistical structure and clinical validity at initial assessment. *Pain, 46*, 287-298.

Main, C. J., and Wood, P.L.R. (1990). The prediction of treatment outcome in patients with low back pain. Paper presented to the 3rd European Congress on Back Pain, Current Concepts and Recent Advances, Glasgow.

Matrin, M., Bradley, L.A., Alexander, R.W., et al. (1996). Coping strategies predict disability in patients with primary fibromyalgia. *Pain, 68*, 45-53.

McCracken, L.M., Zayfert, C., and Gross, R.T. (1992). The Pain Anxiety Symptoms Scale: development and validation of a scale to measure fear of pain. *Pain, 50*, 67-73.

McCracken, L.M., and Gross, R.T..(1993). Does anxiety affect coping with chronic pain? *Clinical Journal of Pain, 9*, 253-259.

Melzack, R. (1975). The McGill Pain Questionnaire: Major properties and scoring methods. *Pain, 1*, 277-299.

Melzack, R. (1987). The short-form McGill pain questionnaire. *Pain, 30*,191-197

Meyer-Rosberg, K., Burckhardt, C.S., Huizar, K., et al. (2000). A comparison of the SF-36 and Nottingham Health Profile in patients with chronic neuropathic pain. *European Journal of Pain, 5*, 391-403.

Nicholas, M.K., Wilson, P.H., and Goyen, J. (1992). Comparison of cognitive-behavioral group treatment and an alternative non-psychological treatment for chronic low back pain. *Pain, 48*, 339-347.

Pfingsten, M., Kroner-Herwig, B., Leibing, E., et al. (2000). Validation of the German version of the Fear-Avoidance Beliefs Questionnaire (FABQ). *European Journal of Pain, 4*, 259-266.

Pilowsky, I., and Spence, N.D. (1994). *Manual for the illness behavior questionnaire* (3rd Edition.). Adelaide, Australia: University of Adelaide, Department of Psychiatry.

Radloff, L. (1977). The CES-D scale: a self report depression scale for research in the general population. *Applied Psycological Measurement,1,* 386-401

Reid, G.J., Gilbert, C.A., McGrath, P.J., et al. (1994). Development of the pediatric pain coping checklist [abstract]. Paper presented at Third International Symposium on Pediatric Pain, Philadelphia, PA.

Roland, M, and Morris, R. (1983). A study of the natural history of back pain. *Spine, 8,* 141-144.

Rosentiel, A.K., and Keefe, F.J. (1983). The use of the coping strategies in chronic low back pain patients: Relationship to patient characteristics and current adjustment. *Pain,17,* 33-44

Shiley, J.C., Bayliss, M.S., Keller, S.D. et al. (1996). SF-36 health survey annotated bibliography: The first edition (1988-1995). Boston, MA: The Health Institute, New England Medical Center.

Silver, A., Haeney, M., Vijayadurai, P., et al. (2002). The role of fear of physical movement and activity in chronic fatigue syndrome. *Journal of Psychosomatic Research, 52,* 485-493.

Smythe, H.A. (1984). Problems with the MMPI (editorial). *Journal of Rheumatology, 11,* 417-418.

Steer, R.A., and Beck, A.T. (2000). The Beck Depression Inventory-II. In W.E Craighead and C.B. Nemeroff (Eds.), *The Corsini encyclopedia of psychology and behavioral science* (3rd ed.), Vol. 1 (pp. 178-9). New York: Wiley.

Tait, R.C., and Chibnall, J.T. (1997). Development of a brief version of the Survey of Pain Attitudes. Pain, 70, 229-35

Turner, J.A., and Clancy, S. (1988). Comparison of operant behavioral and cognitive-behavioral group treatment for chronic low back pain. *Journal of Consulting and Clinical Psychology, 56,* 261-266.

Turner, J., Jensen, M.P., and Romano, J. (2000). Do beliefs, coping and catastrophizing independently predict functioning in patients with chronic pain. *Pain, 85,* 115-125.

Verdier-Taillefer, M., Gourlet, V., Fuhrer, R., et al. (2001). Psychometric properties of the Center for Epidemiologic Studies Depression Scale in multiple sclerosis. *Neuroepidemiology, 20,* 262-267.

Vlaeyen, J.W., Kole-Snijders, A.M., Boeren, R.G., et al. (1995). Fear of movement/(re)injury in chronic low back pain and its relation to behavioral performance. *Pain, 62,* 363-372.

Waddell, G., Newton, M., Henderson, J., Somerville, D., and Main, C.J. (1993). A Fear-Avoidance Beliefs Questionnaire (FABQ) and the role of fear-avoidance beliefs in chronic low back pain and disability. *Pain, 52,* 157-168.

Waddell, G., Pilowsky, I., and Bond, M.R. (1989). Clinical assessment and interpretation of abnormal illness behaviour in low back pain. *Pain, 39,* 41-53.

Wallstone, K.A., and Wallstone, B.S. (1978). Development of the multidimensional health locus of control (MHLC) scale. *Health Education Monographs, 6,* 160-170.

Walsh, D.A., and Radcliffe, J.C. (2002). Pain beliefs and perceived physical disability of patients with chronic low back pain. *Pain, 97,* 23-31.

Ware, J.E. Jr. (2000). SF-36 health survey update. *Spine, 25,* 3130-3139.

Ware, J.E., and Kosinski, M. (1996). The SF-36 health survey (version 2) technical note. Boston MA: Health Assessment Laboratory. (Sept. 20, 1996; updates Sept. 27, 1997).

Ware, J.E., and Sherbourne, C.D. (1992). The MOS 36-item short form health survey (SF-36): I. Conceptual framework and item selection. *Medical Care, 30,* 473-483.

Ware, J.E., Snow, K.K., Kosinski M, and Gandek, B.(1993). *SF-36 health survey manual and interpretation guide.* Boston, MA: New England Medical Center, The Health Institute.

Williams, D.A., Robinson, M.E., and Geisser, M.E. (1994). Pain beliefs: assessment and utility. *Pain, 59,* 71-78.

Williams, D.A., and Thorn, B.E. (1989). An empirical assessment of pain beliefs. *Pain, 36,* 351-358.

World Health Organization (1996). *Cancer pain relief: With a guide to opioid availability* (2nd ed.). Geneva, Switzerland: Author.

Wright, K.D., Asmundson, G.J.G., and McCreary, D.R. (2001). Factorial validity of the short-form McGill pain questionnaire (SF-MPQ). *European Journal of Pain, 5,* 279-284.

Zigmond, A.S., and Snaith, R.P. (1983). The Hospital Anxiety and Depression Scale. *Acta Psychiatrica Scandinavica, 67,* 361-37

Part IV:
Medical Therapeutic Approaches

In: The Handbook of Chronic Pain
Editors: S. Kreitler, D. Beltrutti, et al., pp. 185-206

ISBN 978-1-60021-044-0
© 2007 Nova Science Publishers, Inc.

Chapter 12

Pharmacological Therapy of Pain: Connection Between Theory and Practice

David Niv , Alexander Maltsman-Tseikhin and Eric Lang

Despite the recent advances in information and technologies of treating pain, a lot remains to be discovered and invented. In this chapter an attempt will be made to review major developments concerning some of the physiological changes that occur in the nociceptive pathway after injury. Whenever possible, specific drugs or techniques will be described, with the caveat that in many cases the "magic bullet" has not yet been developed or not yet made the difficult path from compound to clinical drug. In addition, a connection between theoretical scientific background and practical use of some medications will be demonstrated that may be really helpful for practitioners to attain pain alleviation if not full pain control in their patients.

MODULATION OF PAINFUL STIMULI

Two kinds of modification in the nervous system occur following tissue injury: (a) *peripheral sensitization*, i.e., reduced threshold of nociceptor afferent peripheral terminals, and (b) *central sensitization,* i.e., an increased excitability of spinal neurons. Further, inflammatory pain can be produced by peripheral tissue damage, and neuropathic pain by damage to the nervous system.

There are two mechanisms contributing to changes in sensitivity in inflammatory pain. The first is increased sensitivity of high-threshold nociceptive primary sensory neurons when exposed to inflammatory mediators and other chemicals involved in tissue damage. The mediators are different inflammatory acute-phase reactants, which sensitize peripheral nociceptors and augment spinal input during inflammation (Figure 1). Peripheral sensitization mediates changes in thermal sensitivity in the immediate vicinity of tissue injury, with changes in the mechanical sensitivity of high threshold cutaneous mechanonociceptors in the joints.

The second mechanism is a change in the excitability of the neurons in the spinal cord, which lasts longer than nociceptive afferent inputs (viz. central sensitization) (Woolf, 1993).

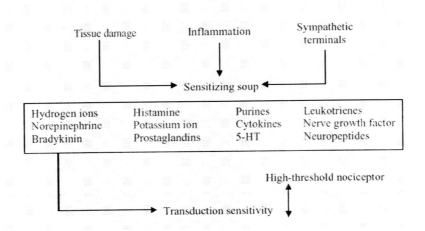

Figure 1. The transduction sensitivity of high-threshold nociceptors can be modified in the periphery by a combination of chemicals that act synergistically as a "sensitizing soup". These chemicals are produced by damaged tissue as part of the inflammatory reaction and by sympathetic terminals. 5-HT, 5-hydroxytryptamine. (Redrawn from Woolf, C.J. (1993). Preemptive analgesia – treating postoperative pain by preventing the establishment of central sensitization. *Anesthesia and Analgesia, 77,* 362-379).

PERIPHERAL MODULATION

Research targets the development of means for reducing peripheral sensitization by interfering with the inflammatory reactants that mediate the sensitivity of high-threshold nociceptor primary sensory neurons (Table 1). Let us focus first on **bradykinin**. It is formed through tissue damage and inflammation. *Antagonists of bradykinin B_2 receptor* are potent analgesic and anti-inflammatory agents in acute inflammatory pain, for example, the peptide HOE140 was tested successfully in mice (Heapy, Shaw and Farmer, 1993) and the bovine-derived polypeptide aprotinin in humans for reducing pain and swelling in third molar surgery (Brennan, Gardiner and McHugh, 1991). In cases of prolonged inflammation bradykinin B_1 receptors may also contribute to the maintenance of hyperalgesia. For example, the specific B_1 antagonist des-Arg9, (Leu8)-BK was effective in reversing or preventing hyperalgesia whereas the B_1 agonist des-Arg9-BK produced a small exacerbation of hyperalgesia (Perkins, Campbell and Dray, 1993).

Histamine mediates C fiber sensitivity in neuromas in animal models. It is produced, stored and released by mast cells in the neuroma, whose number increase after transection of the peripheral nerve and the formation of nerve end neuromas. In an animal model, a peripheral H_1 blocker relieved the pain resulting from neuroma formation (Seltzer, Paran, Eisen, and Ginzburg, 1991). This indicates that *histamine H_1 receptor antagonists* may be useful for treating pain in humans with painful neuromas.

Prostaglandins such as PGE_2 and PGI_2 are produced in inflamed tissue and mediate painful stimuli. Arachidonic acid production and the cyclooxygenase (COX) pathway produce prostaglandins. One of the two types of COX, specifically COX-2, is induced in response to inflammation. It was hypothesized that a specific **COX-2 inhibitor** would have a better side effect profile than other available *nonsteroidal anti-inflammatory drugs (NSAID's)* (Vane, Mitchell, Appleton et al., 1994).

Cyclo-oxygenase-2 inhibitors (COXIB's) - rofecoxib, celecoxib - offer some advantages over conventional non-steroidal anti-inflammatory drugs in their effects on the gastrointestinal tract and platelet function. However, significant adverse effects are still possible with COXIB's, including serious cardiovascular and renal complications that are especially relevant in the elderly (Mamdani, Juurlink, Lee et al., 2004).

Several *NSAID's* deserve special mention. *Nimesulide* possesses COX-2 specificity, has low toxicity and many analgesic effects with a rapid onset of action but may cause gastointestinal ulcers. *Nabumetone* is devoid of direct toxic effects on the gastric mucosa, and is well tolerated although it is not COX-2 specific. It has a slow onset of action and requires 3-6 days to achieve steady state plasma concentrations. *Etodolac* is also COX-2 specific and although it causes gastrointestinal effects, gastro-duodenal ulcers occur only rarely. Different clinical trials are in progress for testing new drugs with high COX-2 specificity, high potency and no gastrointestinal toxicity.

Norepinephrine released from peripheral nerve terminals may sensitize peripheral nociceptors and augment spinal nociceptive input. *Clonidine*, an *α_2-adrenergic agonist*, was shown to decrease hyperalgesia and pain in patients with sympathetically mediated pain syndromes (Davis, Treede, Raja, et al., 1991). Future research may lead to the discovery of further specific *peripheral adrenergic agonists,* which have fewer side effects than α_2-adrenergic agonists that can traverse the blood-brain barrier.

Cytokines, such as interleukin 1 and tumor necrosis factor, are released during inflammation and are potent hyperalgesic factors in animal models. *Cytokine-suppressive anti-inflammatory drugs (CSAID's)* are now being developed. For example, SKF 86002 inhibits lipopolysaccharide-induced interleukin productin and shows analgesic effects in acute and chronic pain models (Rang and Urban, 1995).

Sodium channel function is vital for normal function of excitable membranes. Abnormal sodium channel activity may play a role in the formation of neuropathic pain, which is often resistant to regular analgesic drugs. It was shown that spontaneous ectopic activity develops in damaged sensory neurons, which possibly results from abnormal accumulation of sodium channels in the cell membranes (Devor, 1994). The effectiveness of anticonvulsants, local anesthetics and anti-arrhythmic drugs in the treatment of neuropathic pain may be due to the fact that they are all sodium channel blockers (Butterworth and Stricharz, 1990; Devor, Wall and Catalan, 1992). Yet their effectiveness is limited by their multiple side effects (Virani, Mailis, Shapiro, 1997).

Table 1. Peripheral and Central Modulation of Nociceptive Stimuli

Mechanism of Action	Drug Therapy
Inhibits bradykinin B_2	HOE140 and other peptide and nonpeptide agents
Inhibits bradykinin and histamine	Aprotinin
Inhibits bradykinin B_1	Des-Arg9, (Leu8)-BK
Peripheral antihistamine H_1	Astemizole
NSAIDs: COX-2 antagonists	Nimesulide, etodolac, celecoxib, rofecoxib, and others
Peripheral or central α_2-adrenergic agonist	Clonidine patch, systemic and intrathecal clonidine, tizanidine
Interleukin production inhibitor	SKF 86002, other cytokine-suppressive anti-inflammatory drugs being developed
Sodium channel blockers	Anticonvulsants, local anesthetics, antiarrhythmic drugs
Gabapentinoids	Gabapentin, pregabalin
NK-1 receptor antagonist	CP96345 and other agents
Substance P depletion	Capsaicin and other vanilloids such as resiniferatoxin
Somatostatin analogues	Peptide analogues exist
CGRP antagonist	CGRP8-37
CCK antagonists	Devazepide, lorgumide
NMDA antagonists	AP-5, dizocilpine, dextromethotphan, phencyclidine, ketamine
Adenosine modulation	Al receptor agonists may prove useful
Potentiation of GABA	Midazolam
Antidepressant medications	Amitriptyline, SSRIs, and venlafaxine
Acetylcholine release	Neostigmine
Calcium channel blockade – N-type channels	SNX-111, SNX-159, SNX-239
Calcium channel blockade – L-type channels	Diltiazem, verapamil, nimodipine
Tissue transplantation	Adrenal medullary chromaffin cell transplant

SSRI, selective serotonin reuptake inhibitor; COX, cyclooxygenase; NSAID, nonsteroidal anti-inflammatory drug; GABA, γ-amniobutyric acid; NMDA, N-methyl-$_D$-aspartate; CCK, cholecystokinin; CGRP, calcitonin gene-related peptide.

Accordingly, there is a lot of interest in developing for pain treatment an anticonvulsant with fewer side effects or no capability of crossing the blood-brain barrier and of entering the central nervous system. Indeed, several anticonvulsant drugs have been released for clinical usage. Anticonvulsants without blocking sodium channels, include **gabapentin** and **pregabalin**, are a highly effective analgesic agents. Despite intensive study, the basis for gabapentin analgesia remains uncertain. Proposed mechanisms of analgesic actions for **non-sodium channel blocking** drugs revolve around effects on sensitized central neurons, such as direct or indirect inhibition of the release of excitatory amino acids, blockade of neuronal calcium channels, and augmentation of CNS inhibitory pathways via increasing GABA-ergic transmission. The best example of an effective non-sodium channel blocking anticonvulsant is *gabapentin*, a lipophilic GABA analog. Gabapentin was shown to be useful in treating humans with complex regional pain syndrome (reflex sympathetic dystrophy), neuropathic pain, postherpetic neuralgia and in migraine prophylaxis (Mellick and Mellick, 1997; Wetzel and Connelly, 1997; Backonja, Beydoun, et al., 1998; Rowbotham, Harden, Stacey, et al., 1998; Rowbotham and Petersen, 2001; Bennett and Simpson, 2004). In some pain centers, gabapentin is being used as first-line therapy for all types of chronic pain. Gabapentin does not reduce acute nociceptive pain (Hunter, Gogas, Hedley, et al., 1997; Jun and Yaksh, 1998). *Pregabalin* was shown to be useful in neuropathic pain associated with diabetic peripheral neuropathy and postherpetic neuralgia. Significant reduction of neuropathic pain occurs, on average, within 3 days of initiating pregabalin treatment (Rowbotham, Young, Sharma, 2004). Drugs of this kind have fewer side effects and a better toxicity-to-efficacy ratio than older generation anticonvulsants. The success of drugs acting by mechanisms other than sodium channel blockade indicates much future potential for analgesic/anticonvulsant drugs.

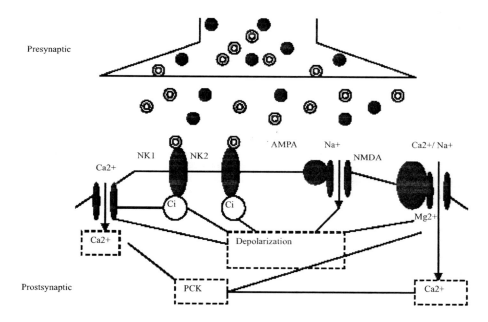

Figure 2. A model of the transmitter and cellular mechanisms that produce central sensitization. C fiber terminals release both the excitatory amino acid glutamate and neuropeptides, such as the tachykinins in the dorsal horn of the spinal cord. Glutamate can act on both α-amino-3-hydroxy-5-methyl-4-isoxazolepropionic and acid (AMPA) and *N*-methyl-ᴅ-aspartic acid (NMDA) receptors on postsynaptic membranes on dorsal horn neurons. Normally, the ion channels linked to the NMDA receptor is blocked by magnesium ion, but the block can be removed by a depolarization of the cell leading to an influx of calcium and sodium ions, which leads to a further depolarization. The tachykinins bind to neurokinin receptors NK-1 and NK-2, leading, via guanosine triphosphate (GTP) protein activation, to depolarization and to changes in second messangers. (Redrawn from Woolf, C.J. (1993). Preemptive analgesia – treating postoperative pain by preventing the establishment of central sensitization. *Anesthesia and Analgesia, 77,* 362-379).

CENTRAL MODULATION

Central sensitization includes changes in the receptive fields of spinal neurons that follow an increase in excitability produced by peripheral nociceptor inputs, leading to hypersensitivity to subsequent stimuli (Woolf, 1993). In recent years interest has focused on the central modulation of nociceptive signals. An understanding of the mediators that centrally modulate nociceptive pathways may reveal new methods and drugs for pain management. (see Figure 2 for the cellular mechanisms and transmitters producing central sensitization, and Table 1 for the therapeutic modalities).

Glutamate and substance P mediate facilitation of C fiber input in the dorsal horn (McMahon, Lewin and Wall, 1993). **Glutamate** acts on both **α-amino-3-hydroxy-5-methylisoxazole (AMPA)** and **N-methyl-D-aspartate (NMDA).** Many other mediators are assumed to modulate nociceptive transmission, including alterations in opioid peptide-mediated synaptic inhibition related to increased cholecystokinin elease, CGRP, somatostatin and various amino transmitters.

Neuropeptides. Substance P is the most intensively studied sensory neuropeptide. It is an important mediator in the nociceptive pathway, which acts on neurokinin-1 (NK-1) receptors that are up-regulated during hyperalgesic conditions (McCarson and Krause, 1994; Schafer, Nohr, Krause and Weihe, 1993). Through sustained depolarization of dorsal horn neurons, substance P contributes to "wind-up" pain (Randic and Urban, 1987).

Several *peptide* and *nonpeptide antagonists* specific for NK-1 receptors are available, as for example **CP96345** which showed good oral activity in a number of animal models but had cardiovascular side effects, which interfered with its analgesic properties (Snider, Constantine, Lowe, et al., 1991). *NK-1 antagonists* show promise as clinically viable analgesic drugs because they hardly affect the CNS – apart from their analgesic action and antiemetic effect - and appear to be relatively free of unwanted side effects (Gardner, Bountra, Bunce and Dale, 1994).

Capsaicin, a vanilloid that functions by depletion of substance P or by counterirritation, was originally extracted from hot peppers. As cream it is indicated for treating rheumatic pain and pain due to peripheral neuropathies, and in the form of intravesicular instillation it is beneficial for alleviating severe bladder pain and detrusor hyperreflexia related to spinal cord injury (Ishizuka, Igawa, Mattiasson and Andersson, 1994; Chandiramani, Peterson, Duthie and Fowler, 1996). Further development of capsaicin and similar materials of the same family, as resiniferatoxin and even alterations in the capsaicin molecule itself, will provide greater control over the medication, preventing the local irritation that often occurs at the beginning of treatment with capsaicin, and will explore the possibilities of intraneural and direct spinal or epidural administration of the drugs.

Somatostatin and its analogues octreotide and vapreotide produce analgesia in various animal models and in humans after intravenous, epidural or intrathecal administration in postoperative pain after upper abdominal surgery, articular pain, chronic pancreatitis and neoplastic pain (e.g. Betoin, Ardid, Herbet. et al., 1994). To date, only peptide analogues of somatostatin, which do not reach spinal sites unless administered intrathecally or epidurally, were described. Further, it is unclear whether somatostatin analogues cause analgesia by acting specifically on somatostatin receptors or surrogate opioids. Further research will clarify these and related issues concerning the action mechanisms of these agents.

Calcitonin gene-related peptide (CGRP) is another neuropeptide that hold promise for pain management. It is released by nociceptive afferent fibers in the dorsal horn in response to noxious stimuli. It potentiates the effect of substance P and produce slow depolarization in dorsal horn neurons (Morton and Hutchison, 1989).

Cholecystokinin (CCK) differs from other neuropeptides in that it appears to act indirectly by interaction with the opioid system. Intrathecally it antagonizes the analgesic effect of *opiates* acting on the mu receptor, but by itself under normal conditions it does not produce hyperalgesia. However, during stress, when the endogenous opioid systems are activted, CCK produces hyperalgesia like naloxone. *CCK antagonists* enhance the effects of morphine in animal models of neuropathic hyperalgesia (Xu, Hao, Seiger, et al., 1994). CCK receptor antagonists prevented morphine tolerance and enhanced morphine analgesia in animal models (Dourish, O'Neill, Coughian, et al., 1990). In humans similar drugs may be useful in order to enhance the analgesic potency of opiates while avoiding unwanted side effects.

Amino-acid antagonists. The NMDA receptor for **glutamate** is implicated in the generation the maintenance of central (spinal) state of hypersensitivity. Hence, *NMDA antagonists* may be useful in the treatment of hyperalgesia, indeed not for total abolishment of the pain but in order to prevent or block hyperalgesic states due to tissue or nerve damage, inflammation or ischemia. There is increasing preclinical and clinical evidence that *NR2B selective antagonists* of the NMDA receptors have analgesic effect in neuropathic pain. However, few studies examined the therapeutic potential of this class of drugs in chronic inflammatory pain states, where spinal NMDA receptors may also play a key role (Horvath, Felmerai, et al., 2004).

NMDA antagonists in combination with opioids may also help in the treatment of difficult clinical pain. The beneficial effects are due to the fact that opioids can act presynaptically on C fiber terminals to reduce transmitter release and thus produce synergistic inhibition with postsynaptically acting NMDA receptor antagonists (Dickenson, 1997). In addition, NMDA receptor antagonists seem to prevent the development of opioid tolerance (Elliot, Kest, Man, et al., 1995) and can thus be used for limiting the dose requirements for the individual drugs. However, the efficacy of NMDA receptor antagonists may be limited by side effects, such as anxiety and hyperacusis in the case of *ketamine* and other NMDA antagonists (Kristensen, Karlsten, Gordh and Berge, 1994). *Dextromethorphan* is also NMDA Glutamate receptor antagonist, widely available as an over-the-counter cough remedy. Two randomized clinical trials (Nelson, Park, Robinovitz, et al., 1997; McQuay, Carroll, Jadad, et al., 1994; Bostwick, 1996) showed that chronic treatment with dextromethorphan at an average dose of 400 mg per day reduced pain in patients with diabetic neuropathy to about 80% of the intensity reported by placebo-treated patients, a degree of pain relief approximating that shown in other studies of tricyclic antidepressants, mexiletine, and gabapentin. Side effects at this dose, especially confusion, were prominent during upward dose titration but mild after a maintenance dose was found. Patients with postherpetic neuralgia did not report pain relief in either study. Other NMDA receptor antagonists include *amantadine* and *memantine*. A single paper reports that a single intravenous infusion of amantadine temporarily reduced chronic postsurgical neuropathic pain (Pud, Eisenberg, Spitzer, et al., 1998). There are no chronic treatment studies with the commonly available oral form of this medication. Memantine, commonly used for the treatment of Parkinson's disease and Alzheimer's disease, is under study in AIDS-related neuropathy, diabetic neuropathy, and postherpetic neuralgia (Sang, et al., 1997).

In conclusion, blocking NMDA receptor function has been disappointing up to now because the selectivity of the available drugs for the nociceptive pathway is insufficient to produce analgesia without major negative effects.

Adenosine modulates nociceptive transmission in the periphery and in the CNS (in the superficial region of the dorsal horn): A_1 receptors mediate mainly inhibitory effects and are responsible for the antinociceptive action, and A_2 mediates mainly excitatory effects. The analgesic effects would have been useful if it were not for intolerable side effects: intrathecal administration is attended by motor impairment, while systemic administration results in cardiac depression and hypotension (Karlsten, Gordh and Post, 1992; Galer, 1995).

$α_2$Adrenergic agonists. The mechanism of action of $α_2$-adrenergic agonists seems to involve both inhibition of substance P release from primary afferent neurons and a postsynaptic inhibitory effect on dorsal horn neurons. Their analgesic effect has been recognized for some time, but their use is limited by unwanted side effects: *clonidine* causes hypotension and sedation, and *dexmedetomidine* produces motor disturbances in veterinary use. Also in selected patients with severe refractory complex regional pain syndrome (CRPS) the epidural application of clonidine showed a significant pain reduction   (Baron, 2004).

Benzodiazepines and potentiation of **Gamma-Aminobutiryc Acid (GABA)** neurotransmission. The dorsal horn neurons of the spinal cord or medulla receive information about noxious stimuli from primary afferent fibersin peripheral nerves and modulate this afferent information before it is transmitted to higher centers for pain perception. The modulating circuitry of the dorsal horn includes input from dorsal roots and trigeminal fibers as well as descending projections from higher centers, such as the nucleus raphe magnus of the rostral ventral medulla. The modulation makes use of both *excitatory and inhibitory neurotransmitters*. The main neurotransmitter used by the rostral ventral medulla is **serotonin (5-HT)** (Fields, Heinricher and Mason, 1991), but also the inhibitory neurotransmitters **GABA** and **glycine** are also involved to some extent (Antal, Petko, Polgar, et al., 1996).

The presented description of these pathways is supported by experimental evidence. Studies in animals using an axonal tracer and calcium-binding proteins for labelling descending neurons showed that *benzodiazepines* probably elicit their action by acting as agonists at GABA receptors (Antal, Petko, Polgar, et al., 1996). In dogs and rats lumbar intrathecal administration of *midazolam* (a benzodiazepine agonist) resulted in antinociceptive effect, whereas intraperitoneal administration of midazolam resulted in hyperalgesia (Niv, Whitwam and Loh, 1983; Niv, Davidovich, Geller and Urca, 1988).

There is experimental evidence that benzodiazepines have a similar activity in human pain models. The demonstrated ability of the opioid antagonist naloxone to antagonize flumazenil-induced analgesia (Gear, Miaskowski, Heller, et al., 1997) suggests that this agent activates endogenous opioid analgesic systems. *Midazolam* also produces antinociceptive effects and is useful in treating acute postoperative somatic pain, probably due to its interaction with the GABA-A receptor in the spinal cord. In patients with chronic mechanical low-back pain intrathecal midazolam was as effective in reducing pain as epidural methylprednisolone and required less medication in one half to one third of the patients during the 2-months follow-up period (Serrao, Marks, Morley and Goodchild, 1992).

Some studies with healthy volunteers showed that benzodiazepines reduce the affective-emotional aspect of pain (Chapman and Feather, 1973) but not the sensory-discriminative component (Serrao, Stubbs, Goodchild and Gent, 1989), and sometimes neither of the two components (Zacny, Coalson, Young, et al., 1995). In conditions where anxiety and muscle spasm potentiate each other, benzodiazepines may improve these two symptoms and interrupt this vicious cycle. Although controlled trials support the efficacy of benzodiazepines in certain disorders, such as chronic tension headache (Lance and Curran, 1964; Hackett, Boddie and Harrison, 1987) and temporomandibular joint dysfunction (Harkins, Linford, Cohen, et al., 1991), benzodiazepines have been ineffective in controlled trials of postherpetic neuralgia (Max, Schafer, Culnane, et al., 1988) and other chronic nonmalignant pain syndromes (Wilson, 1990). The most prominent and clinically relevant adverse effects of benzodiazepines are those related to dose-dependent, reversible CNS depression. The abuse potential of these drugs is a relative contraindication to use for periods longer than several weeks. Other than for short-term use in the treatment of acute muscle spasm, there is little evidence of a favorable risk-benefit profile to support the general use of benzodiazepines as adjuvant analgesics in chronic pain management.

One of the most useful categories of drugs for modifying pain perception is the **indolamines** (Hendler, 1981). A majority of the indolamines in the body are **serotonin (5-HT)** and related compounds. When serotonin is added to the CNS directly via the ventricle, it accumulates in the periventricular area. This increases the effectiveness of morphine analgesia (Sewell, Spencer, 1974). Other researchers have found that augmenting serotonin by giving precursors that cross the blood-brain barrier or inhibiting the presynaptic reuptake with a variety of antidepressant drugs (e.g., doxepin, amitriptyline, nortriptyline) enhances serotonin-mediated activities such as sleep, raised threshold to pain, antidepressant and antianxiety activities. Conversely, depletion of serotonin increases the perception of pain by lowering the pain threshold (Hendler, Cimini, Ma, et al., 1980).

Apart from the opioids and NSAID group of analgesics, *antidepressant* medications are probably the most commonly prescribed class of drugs for the treatment of chronic pain. *Tricyclic antidepressants (TCA's),* including *amitriptyline, imipramine, nortriptyline, desipramine, clomipramine,* and *doxepin*, are thought to provide increased inhibition of pain through block the reuptake of **serotonin (5-HT), noradrenaline,** or both at spinal dorsal horn synapses. This assumption is however contested by some (Lang, Hord and Denson, 1996). Tricyclic antidepressants (TCA's) have classically been used for pain control, notably in lower doses than for depression treatment (Lang, Hord and Denson, 1996). Their major disadvantages are a relatively narrow therapeutic-toxic ratio and frequent side effects: anticholinergic (e.g., tachycardia, urinary retention, visual problems), antihistamine-mediated (e.g., sedation, decreased gastric acid secretion), and orthostatic hypotension (Watson and Evans, 1985; Watson, Chipman, Reed, et al., 1992).

A review of 17 studies of the effectiveness and safety of various antidepressants in the treatment of neuropathic pain showed that antidepressants resulted in a decrease of more than 50% of the pain for about 30% of the patients who did not have serious side effects, had mostly better effects than placebo, and were more effective than benzodiazepines (Max, Schafer, Culnane, et al., 1988). No differences were found between the various TCA's (McQuay, Tramer, Nye, et al., 1996). Many of these neuropathic pain studies showed that a significant analgesic effect remained even when depressed patients were excluded from the analysis (Max, Culnane, Schafer, et al., 1987; Magni, 1991). The antidepressants in these studies relieved brief, lancinating pains as well as constant pains (Watson, Evans, Reed, et al., 1982; Kishore-Kumar, Max, Schafer, et al., 1990) and allodynia as well as spontaneous pain (Max, Kishore-Kumar, Schafer, et al., 1991; Max, Lynch, Muir, et al., 1992). Although the large majority of neuropathic pain trials were carried out in patients with either diabetic neuropathy or postherpetic neuralgia, single reports suggest that amitriptyline is superior to placebo in a poststroke central neuropathic pain (Leijon and Boivie, 1989) and a mixed group of nondiabetic peripheral neuropathies.

There is also relatively convincing evidence for the efficacy of tricyclic antidepressants in preventing tension and migraine headaches (McQuay, Moore, 1997). Three studies suggested benefit of tricyclics in atypical facial pain.

The *selective serotoninergic reuptake inhibitors (SSRI's)* have fewer side effects than the TCAs. Some studies showed their effectiveness for pain control (Sindrup, Gram, Brosen, et al., 1990). *Fluoxetine* and *amitriptyline*, mainly together, were useful in treating fybromyalgia, and fluoxetine was effective for rheumatic pain, headache and migraine, phantom limb pain and diabetic neuropathy (Rani, Naidu, Prasad, et al., 1996; Saper, Silberstein, Lake and Winters, 1994; Power Smith and Turkington, 1993; Theesen and Marsh, 1989).

Several other antidepressants were shown to have analgesic effects in animal models. Thus, *venlaflaxine hydrochloride* – a structurally novel antidepressant inhibiting the reuptake of serotonin and noradrenaline - was useful for thermal hyperalgesia and for producing a mild nonspecific analgesic effect (Lang, Hord and Denson, 1996), and *nefazodone* potentiated the analgesic effect of morphine with no effect on lethality and the gastrointestinal tract (Pick, Paul, Eison and Pasternak, 1992).

In neuropathic pain, there is strong evidence for the efficacy of tricyclic antidepressants, but other drugs including *gabapentin, opioids*, and *carbamazepine* may provide similar degrees of relief (Max and Gilron, 2001; Niv, Maltsman-Tseikhin, Lang, 2004; Niv, Maltsman-Tseikhin, 2005). Choice of drug will depend on the ability of the patient to tolerate side effects of the various drugs and the urgency of the need for pain relief (McQuay, Carroll, Jadad, et al., 1995). For example, in a patient with severe cancer-related neuropathic pain *opioids* may be the drug of first choice. In patients with ischemic heart disease or orthostatic hypotension, *gabapentin* or *pregabalin* would be preferable, as they are free of cardiovascular side effects. In the patient with insomnia or depression, the sedative and antidepressant effects of *tricyclics* would provide additional value. In headache, fibromyalgia, and atypical facial pain, tricyclics are considered first-line treatments.

Neostigmine. In dogs, sheep and rats spinal neostigmine produced analgesia alone or enhanced analgesia associated with α_2-adrenergic agonists (Hood, Eisenach and Tuttle, 1995). These effects are probably mediated by spinal M_1 and M_2 receptor subtypes. Intrathecal administration of neostigmine in humans has an analgesic effect. It produces increases in acetylcholine concentrations in cerebrospinal fluid without increases in norepinephrine concentrations or nitric oxide (Eisenach, Hood and Curry, 1997).

Intrathecal neostigmine in humans produced a dose-independent reduction in postoperative rescue analgesic consumption but higher doses were associated with increased postoperative nausea and vomiting (Lauretti, Mattos, Reis and Prado, 1997). In general, neostigmine may be more effective for somatic pain than for visceral pain (Lauretti and Lima, 1996).

Neostigmine acts synergistically with morphine for postoperative analgesia (Klamt, Slullitel, Garcia and Prado, 1997). It interacts well also with other drugs, enhancing their analgesia but not the side effects, for example, with clonidine or alfentanil.

Opioids. For many decades, these drugs, given alone or as part of a multimodal program, have been the most frequently used method of pain control. The reason for their popularity and widespread use is that in most countries of the world they are readily available and inexpensive, and when properly administered, provide effective pain relief.

Opioid agonists include *morphine, codeine, meperidine, dihydromorphinone,* and *methadone*, among others. *Morphine* is the reference standard for all the potent opioid analgesics. Among clinically used opioids, morphine gives the clinician the most options for effective routes of administration. It can be instilled directly via intrathecal and epidural routes. It has also been used for cancer pain using the intracerebroventricular route. There are also a number of protocols for using morphine either IV or subcutaneously for both continuous infusion and patient-controlled analgesia (PCA). There are myriad oral preparations, from oral solution and immediate-release tablets to the multiple sustained-release preparations that allow dosing once to three times daily rather than every 3 to 5 hours. The controlled-release preparations of morphine offer great advantages for long-term therapy in patients with terminal cancer pain and noncancer pain because they provide constant plasma level for long periods of time (Arner, Bolund, Rane, et al., 1982; Twycross, 1982; Gourlay, 1998). Side effects associated with the use of morphine are those common to all the opioids. Tolerance and physical dependence develop when morphine is given for a period of several weeks to months (Twycross and Ventafredda, 1980).

Meperidine (Pethidine) is a synthetic phenylpiperidine opioid analgesic often used interchangeably with morphine. Chronic dosing of meperidine can lead to accumulation of its active metabolite (normeperidine), which can result in CNS irritability (mood changes, anxiety, tremor, multifocal myoclonus, and occasionally seizures). This is the reason why meperidine is relatively contraindicated for the management of chronic cancer pain because of these potential complications (Miyoshi and Leckband, 2001).

Methadone is a synthetic opioid that is slightly more potent but less dependence-producing than morphine. Methadone produces less euphoria and less sedation than many other opioids. The long-term use of methadone seems to provide efficient analgesia in non-cancer parients and is well supported in patients with previous opioid related neurological side effects (Brabant, Nagels, Dobbels, 2004).

Agonist-Antagonist Derivatives include *buprenorphine, butorphanol, pentazocine* and others. Buprenorphine is a potent partial Mu receptor agonist and appears to be a Kappa receptor antagonist. It is approximately 30 times more potent than morphine when given IM.

The side effects are similar to those of morphine, but euphoria seems to be less frequent, whereas sedation is more evident.

The gastrointestinal effects of opioids are mediated by activation of Mu opioid receptors (MOR) located in the central and peripheral (gut) nervous systems. All MOR agonists used in clinical practice induce nausea, vomiting and bowel dysfunction with a poor correlation with the dose. There are no definite predictive factors, although they may be drug, route, dose, and patient related. Inter-individual difference is mainly associated with co-morbidity and genetic variations in pharmacokinetics/dynamics. The incidence and severity of GI adverse events may oblige to discontinue treatment. Nausea and vomiting are common after acute administration, but unpredictable after chronic use due to tolerance development. Bowel dysfunction occurs in all patients receiving opioids but tolerance develops very slowly, and constipation persists throughout treatment. The peripherally acting *opioid antagonist methylnaltrexone* could be beneficial in the management of nausea, vomiting and bowel dysfunction caused by opioid therapy (Puig, 2004).

In considering the side effects of opioids, special attention has been placed on sedation and cognitive deficits. In most patients, the sedative effects tend to diminish spontaneously after a few days as tolerance develops. However, in cases of persistent sedation, a reduction in total daily opioid dose can reduce the side effects providing adequate analgesia is maintained. The concomitant use of some NSAID's may also be of value, since these agents have a documented "opioid-sparing effect", and their analgesic synergism with opioids allows a reduction in the opioid dose. The potential interaction with other drugs that also induce sedation should be avoided such as the benzodiazepines, neuroleptics, and barbiturates, and alternative opioids to morphine should be considered (Foley, 1979; Daut and Cleeland, 1982; Ripamonti and Bruera, 1991).

Several trials seem to confirm that equi-analgesic dosages of either *tramadol* – a *nonopioid centrally acting synthetic analgesic* or *transdermal fentanil* may reduce the incidence of sedation compared with oral morphine even at low dosages (Beltrutti, Conte, Marcellino and Russo, 2004).

Multimodal therapeutic pain management plan prioritize the treatment of acute and chronic cancer pain. Standard pain management protocol in cancer population represented a fixed schedule opioid regiment with breakthrough pain control. This approach is usually effective but rarely completely eliminates the pain. All classes of opioids-naturally occurring, synthetic and semi synthetic for continuity of care and for breakthrough pain control use as a first line of treatment. Second line treatment – invasive strategies in order to improve balance between analgesia and side effects such neural blockade and neuroablative techniques. If balance between pain relief and side effects is suboptimal, consider the third line of treatment – regional analgesic technique-spinal route of delivery of opioid medication by intrathecal pump (Krakovsky, 2004) (see below).

Calcium channel blockers. **Calcium** flux is essential for normal sensory processing. Disrupting calcium ion movement may result in interference of normal sensory processing and thus contribute to antinociception. Thus, calcium administered intracerebroventricularly can produce hyperalgesia in rodents (Chapman and Way, 1982) and intracerebroventricular calcium chelators EGTA and EDTA and the inorganic inhibitor of calcium cellular influx lanthanum produce antinociceptive effects that are reversed by intracerebroventricular calcium (Schmidt and Way, 1980). However, intrathecally administered calcium may produce antinociception (Lux, Welch, Brase and Dewey, 1988).

Opioids and calcium transport are closely interrelated in the CNS. Morphine inhibits calcium ion influx through the receptor operated calcium channel in neuronal cells (Halpern and Bonica, 1984). L-type calcium channel blockers ***verapamil*** and ***diltiazem*** potentiate the antinociceptive effects of morphine and other opiate receptor agonists (Benedek and Szikszay, 1984). Further, calcium antagonizes the analgesic effects of opioids (Chapman and Way, 1982).

Since the side effects of perispinal opioids are dose-dependent, it is of importance to determine if intrathecal calcium channel blockers potentiate the analgesic effect of intrathecal opioids at doses that produce tolerable side effects. Different studies focused on investigating the antinociceptive usefulness of calcium channel blockers. In experimental animals it was found that intrathecal administration of morphine produced dose-dependent antinociception, whereas intrathecal administration of calcium channel blockers did not. But the combination of intrathecally administered calcium channel blockers with doses of intrathecal morphine of low or moderate effectiveness produced synergistic antinociception, with no changes in arterial pressure or heart rate (Omote, Sonoda, Kawamata, et al., 1993). In another study, animals were pretreated with L-type, N-type or P-type calcium channel blockers none of which affected normal sensory or motor responses but all three prevented the development of sensory mechanical hyperalgesia and allodynia (Sluka, 1997). Research of this kind has led to the hope that similar agents, such as SNX-111, an N-type voltage sensitive calcium channel blocker, may prove to be an efficacious antinociceptive agent in humans.

ADRENAL MEDULLARY CELLS

Transplantation of ***adrenal medullary tissue*** or isolated ***chromaffin*** cells into the spinal subarachnoid space was shown to significantly reduce pain in rodents without the development of tolerance (Sagen, 1992). These cells were selected because high levels of both opioid peptides and catecholamines that reduce pain independently and possibly synergistically when injected locally into the spinal subarachnoid space. The adrenal medullary transplants survive for prolonged periods and continue to produce high levels of both catecholamines and Met-enkephalin. Preliminary results with humans suffering from intractable malignant pain were encouraging and enabled reduction of complementary intrathecal and oral morphine. To achieve analgesia with high levels of Met-enkephalin in the CSF it seemed essential to have a large volume of grafted tissue. A progressive decrease in Met-enkephalin release was noted 2-4 months after the transplantation (Lazorthes, Bes, Sagen, et al., 1995).

The modality through which adrenal medullary transplants provide pain relief is still unclear. Some of the possibilities are intervention in the spinal NMDA-nitric oxide cascade or constant provision of opioid peptides augmented by intermittent nicotinic stimulation (Wang and Sagen, 1994). However, the studies with adrenal medullary cells indicate the potential use of this means for controlling pain without the disadvantages of treatment with narcotics, such as tolerance, systemic complications, potential infections caused by implantable pumps and need for repeated administration of the drugs.

DRUG DELIVERY SYSTEMS

Since the 1970s there has been a steady increase in the use of sustained release of pain control medications, such as *slow release forms* of *morphine* (MS-Contin, MCR), *oxycodone* (Oxycontin), and slow-release forms of *calcium channel blockers* and *β-adrenergic blockers*. In general, these medications work by controlling drug diffusion through polymeric matrices or the degradation of these polymers (Kurisawa and Yui, 1996).

Ongoing experiments focus on designing drug release systems that are activated by internal or external stimuli, for example, stimulus-responsive polymeric materials designed to release the drug in response to changes in temperature, pH, glucose concentration or release of ribosomal enzymes. Materials of this kind hold promise for drug delivery systems adapted to respond to the needs of patients with acute pain. In regard to chronic pain it is possible to consider methods for prolonging the duration of action of *local anesthetics* through the use of a slow-release system, for example, through an epidural injection, a facet block or very prolonged sympathetic blocks. Ongoing research is being performed for testing the efficacy and safety of different types and sizes of microspheres.

Patient-controlled analgesia (PCA) is a system of self-titration of a pain medication, which prevents sedation as well as breakthrough pain. In practice, keeping the drug levels in a narrow range enables to avoid both suboptimal and toxic doses.

Computer-assisted controlled infusions (CACI's) constitute a further development of great promise. The underlying concept is that the distribution of a drug, say opioid medication in the body resembles a pharmacokinetic three-compartment model: a central volume and two peripheral volumes – a "rapid" one and a "slow" one. Accordingly, when a medication is administered, it is initially present only in the central volume, and is then distributed into the peripheral volumes, first the rapid one and then the slow one, while at the same time the drug is also being eliminated from the body. Simulating by computer these changes in individual patients makes it possible to use the computer for controlling an infusion pump for maintaining at all times a constant level of the drug in the body. Current research is encouraging in regard to the potential use of CACIs in the future for pain control in patients with severe chronic pain (Egan, Gavin, Sutcliffe and Crankshaw, 1997).

SPINAL CORD STIMULATION, LASER STIMULATION, AND PULSED-DOSE ELECTRICAL STIMULATION

Spinal Cord Stimulation (SCS). Electrical SCS for the relief of pain is a method with many advantages and some problems. One problem is that SCS helps only patients with pain related to specific syndromes, such as failed back syndrome, complex regional pain syndrome (CRPS), multiple sclerosis, peripheral vascular disease, intractable angina or diabetic neuropathy but not pain related to other syndromes, such as cauda equina injury, paraplegic pain, phantom pain, postherpetic pain or intercostal neuralgia (Sanderson, Ibrahim, Waterhouse and Palmer, 1994).

Another problem is the generally limited paresthesia coverage of the currently available SCS systems. However, paresthesia coverage may be improved through the use of dual leads to produce an intensified targeted stimulation field. A third problem is that current battery technology requires either an implantable battery that must be replaced every several years or an external power source to transmit energy to a subcutaneous receiver that powers the SCS. Current research addresses all three problems so that the range of application of SCS and the underlying technology will be greatly improved.

Laser stimulation. Preliminary findings showed that low-power laser stimulation could help in controlling pain at least in some cases, such as postherpetic neuralgia, even if not in others, such as chronic orofacial pain (Hansen and Thoroe, 1990). This modality too will have to be further investigated in the future.

Pulsed-dose electrical stimulation. Pulsed-dosed electrical stimulation is applied nocturnally through a stocking, glove or tubular bandage. Beneficial effects were reported after a month's treatment for subjective, burning, diabetic neuropathic pain when protective sensation is grossly intact (Armstrong, Lavery, Fleischli and Gilham, 1997). This method promises usefulness for patients with complex regional pain syndrome of an extremity or with peripheral neuropathies.

SOME GENERAL CONCLUSIONS

The review presented in this chapter has mentioned a great number of modalities, treatments and medications for pain control. This multiplicity of methods reflects primarily the fact that the route from damaged tissue to pain experience is long, multi-staged and complex. Furthermore, it varies in different pain syndromes and perhaps individuals too. This implies that pain cannot be eliminated by one stroke or one particular all-purpose treatment. Yet the good news is that there exist many particular junctures along the complex route at which pain can be attacked. The result may be at least pain alleviation if not full pain control. However, each step of attacking pain is attended by two drawbacks: side effects which may range all the way from weak and manageable to intolerable and insurmountable, and the need for recurrent use of the treatment modality, at least in protracted or chronic pain. In view of the potential varied possibilities for eliminating pain and the difficulties of side effects and continued use of treatments, the road to full pain control is indeed long. But there is also a lot of justification for optimism in that we may be closing-in on the major pain syndromes while exploiting a growing number of treatment potentialities.

REFERENCES

Andreotti, B., Pouliou, A Kolotoura A., et al. (2004). Gabapentin for the treatment of neuropathic pain after failed back surgery. *Pain Practice*. Book of abstracts 3rd World Congress WIP, 266.

Antal, M., Petko, M., Polgar, E., Heizmann, C.W. and Storm-Mathisen, J. (1996).Direct evidence of an extensive GABAergic innervation of the spinal dorsal horn by fibers descending from the rostral ventromedial medulla. *Neuroscience, 73,* 509-518.

Armstrong, D.G., Lavery, L.A., Fleischli, J.G. and Gilham, K.A. (1997). Is electrical stimulation effective in reducing neuropathic pain in patients with diabetes? *Journal of Foot and Ankle Surgery, 36,* 260-263.

Arner, S., Bolund,C., Rane, A., et al., eds. (1982). Narcotic analgesics in the treatment of cancer and postoperative pain. *Acta Anaesthesiol Scand,* 26 (Suppl 74),1-78.

Backonja, M., Beydoun, A., Edwards, K.R. (1998). Gabapentin for the symptomatic treatment of painful neuropathy in patients with diabetes mellitus: a randomized controlled trial. *JAMA, 280*(21), 1831-1836.

Benedek, G. and Szikszay, M. (1984). Potentiation of thermoregulatory and analgesic effects of morphine by calcium antagonists. *Pharmacological Research Communications, 16,* 1009-1018.

Bennett, M.I., Simpson, K.H. (2004). Gabapentin in the treatment of neuropathic pain. *Palliat Med,* 18,5-11.

Betoin, F., Ardid, D., Herbet, A., Aumaitre, O., Kemeny, J.L., Duchene-Marullaz, P., Lavarenne, J. and Eschalier, A. (1994). Evidence for a central long lasting antinociceptive effect of vapreotide, an analog of somatostatin, involving an opioidergic mechanism. *Journal of Pharmacology and Experimental Therapeutics, 269,* 7-14.

Bostwick, J.M. (1996). Dextromethorphan-induced manic symptoms in a bipolar patient on lithium. *Psychosomatics,* 37,571-572.

Brennan, P.A., Gardiner G.T., and McHugh, J. (1991). A double blind clinical trial to assess the value of aprotinin in third molar surgery. *British Journal of Oral and Maxillofacial Surgery, 29,* 176-179.

Butterworth, J.F and Strichartz, G.R. (1990). Molecular mechanisms of local anesthesia: A review. *Anesthesiology, 72,* 711-734.

Chandiramani, V.A., Peterson, T., Duthie, G.S. and Fowler, C.J. (1996). Urodynamic changes during therapeutic intravesical instillations of capsaicin. *British Journal of Urology,77,* 792-797.

Chapman, C.R. and Feather, B.W. (1973). Effects of diazepam on human pain tolerance and pain sensitivity. *Psychosomatic Medicine, 35,* 330-340.

Chapman, D.B. and Way, E.L. (1982). Modification of endorphin/enkephalin analgesia and stress-induced analgesia by divalent cations, a cation chelator and an ionophore. *British Journal of Pharmacology, 75, 389-396.*

Daut, R.L. and Cleeland, C.S. (1982). The prevalence and severity of pain in cancer. *Cancer,* 50, 1913-1918.

Davis, K.D., Treede, R.D., Raja, S.N., Meyer, R.A. and Campbell, J.N. (1991). Topical application of clonidine relieves hyperalgesia in patients with sympathetically maintained pain. *Pain, 47,* 309-317.

Devor, M. (1994). The pathophysiology of damaged peripheral nerves. In P. Wall and R. Melzack (Eds.), *Textbook of Pain* (pp. 79-100). Edinburgh: Churchill Livingstone.

Devor, M., Wall, P.D., Catalan, N. (1992). Systemic lidocaine silences ectopic neuroma and dorsal root ganglion discharge without blocking nerve conduction. *Pain,* 48, 261-268.

Dickenson, A.H. (1997). NMDA receptor antagonists: Interactions with opioids. *Acta Anaesthesiologica Scandinavica, 41,* 112-115.

Dourish, C.T., O'Neill, M.F., Coughlan, J., Kitchener, S.J., Hawley, D. and Iversen, S.D. (1990). The selective CCK-B receptor antagonist L-365,260 enhances morphine analgesia and prevents morphine tolerance in the rat. *European Journal of Pharmacology, 176,* 35-44.

Dukes, E., Dworkin, R., Stacey, B., et al. (2004). The effect of pregabalin on health-related quality of life in patients with neuropathic pain: findings from ten randomized clinical trials. *Pain Practice.* Book of abstracts 3rd World Congress WIP, 270-271.

Egan, D., Gavin, N.C., Sutcliffe, N. and Crankshaw, D.P. (1997). Intravenous drug delivery devices and computer control. In P.F. White (Ed.), *Textbook of Intravenous Anesthesia* (pp. 517-544). Baltimore: Williams and Wilkins.

Eisenach, J.C., Hood, D.D. and Curry, R. (1997). Phase I human safety assessment of intrathecal neostigmine containing methyl- and propylparabens. *Anesthesia and Analgesia, 5,* 842-846.

Elliott, K., Kest, B., Man, A., Kao, B., Inturrisi, C.E. (1995). N-Methyl-D-aspartate (NMDA) receptors, mu and kappa opioid tolerance and perspective on new analgesic drug development. *Neuropsychopharmacology, 13,* 347-356.

Fields, H.L., Heinricher, M.M. and Mason, P. (1991). Neurotransmitters in nociceptive modulatory circuits. *Annual Review Neuroscience, 14,* 219-245.

Foley, K.M. (1979). The management of pain of malignant origin. In: Tyler, H.R., Dawson, D.M., eds. Current neurology, Vol 2. Boston: Houghton Mifflin, 279-302.

Freynhagen, R., Strojek, K., Rodriguez-Lopez, M., et al. (2004). Pregabalin in the management of chronic neuropathic pain syndromes: analysis of fixed- and flexible-dose regimens. *Pain Practice.* Book of abstracts 3rd World Congress WIP, 269.

Galer, B.S. (1995). Neuropathic pain of peripheral origin: Advances in pharmacologic treatment. *Neurology, 45,* S17-S25.

Gardner, C., Bountra, C., Bunce, K. and Dale, T. (1994). Anti-emetic activity of neurokinin NK-1 receptor antagonists is mediated centrally in the ferret. *British Journal of Pharmacology, 112,* 516.

Gear, R.W., Miaskowski, C., Heller, P.H., Paul, S.M., Gordon, N.C. and Levine, J.D. (1997). Benzodiazepine mediated antagonism of opioid analgesia. *Pain, 71,* 25-29.

Gourlay, G.K. (1998). Sustained relief of chronic pain: pharmacokinetics of sustained release morphine. *Clin Pharmacokinet, 35,* 173-190.

Hackett, G.I., Boddie, H.G., Harrison, P. (1987). Chronic muscle contraction headache: the importance of depression and anxiety. J Royal Soc Med, 80, 689- 91.

Halpern, L.M. and Bonica, J.J. (1984). Analgesics. In: Modell, W., ed. *Drugs of Choice.* St. Louis: Mosby, 207-247.

Hansen, H.J. and Thoroe, U. (1990). Low power laser biostimulation of chronic oro-facial pain: A double-blind placebo controlled cross-over study in 40 patients. *Pain, 43,* 169-179.

Harkins,S., Linford, J., Cohen, J., et al. (1991). Administration of clonazepam in the treatment of TMD and associated myofascial pain: a double blind pilot study. *J Craniomandib Disord*, 5, 179-186.

Heapy, C.G., Shaw, J.S., and Farmer, S.C. (1993). Differential sensitivity of antinociceptive assays to the bradykinin antagonist Hoe 140. *British Journal of Pharmacology, 108,* 209-213.

Hendler N., Cimini C., Ma T., et al. (1980). The comparison between cognitive impairment due to benzodiazepines and narcotics. *Am J Psychiatry,* 137, 828-830.

Hood, D.D., Eisenach, J.C. and Tuttle, R. (1995). Phase I safety assessment of intrathecal neostigmine methylsulfate in humans. *Anesthesiology, 82,* 331-343.

Hunter, J.C., Gogas, K.R., Hedley, L.R., et al. (1997). The effect of novel anti-epileptic drugs in rat experimental models of acute and chronic pain. *Euro J Pharmacol*, 324, 153-160.

Ishizuka, O., Igawa, Y., Mattiasson, A. and Andersson, K.E. (1994). Capsaicin-induced bladder hyperactivity in normal conscious rats. *Journal of Urology,* 152, 525-530.

Jun, J.H., Yaksh, T.L. (1998). The effect of intrathecal gabapentin and 3-isobutyl gamma-aminobutyric acid on the hyperalgesia observed after thermal injury in the rat. *Anesth Analg,* 86(2), 348-354.

Karlsten, R., Gordh, T. and Post, C. (1992). Local antinociceptive and hyperalgesic effects in the formalin test after peripheral administration of adenosine analogues in mice. *Pharmacology and Toxicology*, 70, 434-438.

Kishore-Kumar, R., Max, M.B., Schafer, S.C., et al. (1990). Desipramine relieves postherpetic neuralgia. Clin Pharmacol Ther, 47, 305-312.

Klamt, J.G., Slullitel, A., Garcia, I.V. and Prado, W.A. (1997). Postoperative analgesic effect of intrathecal neostigmine and its influence on spinal anaesthesia. *Anesthesia, 52,* 547-551.

Kristensen, J.D., Karlsten, R., Gordh, T. and Berge, O.G. (1994). The NMDA antagonist 3-(2- carboxypiperazin-4-yl)propyl-1-phosphonic acid (CPP) has antinociceptive effect after intrathecal injection in the rat. *Pain, 56,* 59-67.

Kurisawa, M. and Yui, N. (1996). [Recent trends in drug delivery systems using biomaterials]. *Nippon Rinsho, 54,* 2004-2011.

Lance, J.W. and Curran, D.A. (1964). Treatment of chronic tension headache. *Lancet,* 1, 1235-1238.

Lang, E., Hord, A.H. and Denson, D. (1996). Venlafaxine hydrochloride (Effexor) relieves thermal hyperalgesia in rats with an experimental mononeuropathy. *Pain, 68,* 151-155.

Lauretti, G.R. and Lima, I.C. (1996). The effects of intrathecal neostigmine on somatic and visceral pain: Improvement by association with a peripheral anticholinergic. *Anesthesia and Analgesia, 82,* 617-620.

Lauretti, G.R., Mattos, A.L., Reis, M.P. and Prado, W.A. (1997). Intrathecal neostigmine for postoperative analgesia after orthopedic surgery. *Journal of Clinical Anesthesia, 9,* 473-477.

Lazorthes, Y., Bes, J.C., Sagen, J., Tafani, M., Tkaczuk, J., Sallerin, B., Nahri, I., Verdie, J.C., Ohayon, E. and Caratero, C. (1995). Transplantation of human chromaffin cells for control of intractable cancer pain. *Acta Neurochirurgica Supplementum Wien, 64,* 97-100.

Leijon, G. and Boivie, J. (1989). Central post-stroke pain: a controlled trial of amitriptyline and carbamazepine. *Pain,* 36, 27-36.

Lux, F., Welch, S.P., Brase, D.A and Dewey, W.L. (1988). Interaction of morphine with intrathecally administered calcium and calcium antagonists: Evidence for supraspinal endogenous opioid mediation of intrathecal calcium-induced antiniciception in mice. *Journal of Pharmacology and Experimental Therapeutics, 246,* 500-507.

Magni, G. (1991). The use of antidepressants in the treatment of chronic pain: a review of the current evidence. *Drugs,* 42, 730-748.

Mamdani M., Juurlink D.N., Lee D.S. et al.(2004). Cyclo-oxygenase-2 inhibitors versus non-selective non-steroidal anti-inflammatory drugs and congestive heart failure outcomes in elderly patients: a population-based cohort study. *Lancet,* 363, 1751-1756.

McQuay, H.J., Carroll, D., Jadad, A., et al. (1994). Dextromethorphan for the treatment of neuropathic pain: a double-blind randomized controlled crossover trial with intrgral n-of-1design. Pain, 59, 127-133.

Max, M.B., Culnane, M., Schafer, S.C., et al. (1987). Amitriptyline relieves diabetic neuropathy pain in patients with normal or depressed mood. *Neurology,* 37, 589-596.

Max, M.B., Schafer, S.C., Culnane, M., et al. (1988). Amitriptyline, but not lorazepam, relieves postherpetic neuralgia. *Neurology,* 38, 1427-1432.

Max, M.B., Kishore-Kumar, R., Schafer, S.C., et al. (1991). Efficacy of desipramine in painful diabetic neuropathy: a placebo-controlled trial. *Pain,* 45, 3-9.

Max, M.B., Lynch, S.A., Muir, J., et al. (1992). Effects of desipramine, amitriptyline, and fluoxetine on pain in diabetic neuropathy. *N Engl J Med,* 326, 1250-1256.

Max, M.B.(1995). Thirteen consecutive well-designed randomized trials show that antidepressants reduce pain in diabetic neuropathy and postherpetic neuralgia. *Pain Forum,* 4, 348-353.

McCarson, K.E. and Krause, J.E. (1994). NK-1 and NK-3 type tachykinin receptor mRNA expression in the rat spinal cord dorsal horn is increased during adjuvant or formalin-induced nociception. *Journal of Neuroscience, 14,* 712-720.

McMahon, S.B., Lewin, G.R. and Wall, P.D. (1993). Central hyperexcitability triggered by noxious inputs. *Current Opinion in Neurobiology, 3,* 602-610.

McQuay, H.J., Carroll, D., Jadad, A.R., et al. (1995). Anticonvulsant drugs for management of pain: a systematic review. *BMJ,* 311, 1047-1052.

McQuay, H.J., Tramer, M., Nye, B.A., Carroll, D., Wiffen, P.J. and Moore, R.A. (1996). A systematic review of antidepressants in neuropathic pain. *Pain, 68,* 217-227.

McQuay, H.J., Moore R.A. (1997). Antidepressants and chronic pain. *BMJ,* 314, 763-764.

Mellick, G.A. and Mellick, L.B. (1997). Reflex sympathetic dystrophy treated with gabapentin. *Archives of Physical Medicine and Rehabilitation, 78,* 98-105.

Morton, C.R. and Hutchison, W.D. (1989). Release of sensory neuropeptides in the spinal cord: Studies with calcitonin gene-related peptide and galanin. *Neuroscience, 31*, 807-815.

Nelson, K.A., Park, K.M., Robinovitz, E., et al. (1997). High-dose oral dextromethorphan versus placebo in painful diabetic neuropathy and postherpetic neuralgia. *Neurology*, 48, 1212-1218.

Niv D., Maltsman-Tseikhin A. (2005). Postherpetic neuralgia: The Never-ending Challenge. *Pain Practice*, 5(4), 327-340.

Niv, D., Maltsman-Tseikhin, A., Lang, E. (2004). Postherpetic neuralgia: what do we know and where are we heading? *Pain Physician*, 7(2), 239-247.

Niv, D., Davidovich, S. Geller, E. and Urca, G. (1988). Analgesic and hyperalgesic effects of midazolam: Dependence on route of administration. *Anesthesia and Analgesia*, 67, 1169-1173.

Niv, D., Whitwam, J.G. and Loh, L. (1983). Depression of nociceptive sympathetic reflexes by the intrathecal administration of midazolam. *British Journal of Anaesthesia,* 55, 541-547.

Omote, K., Sonoda, H., Kawamata, M., Iwasaki, H. and Namiki, A. (1993). Potentiation of antinociceptive effects of morphine by calcium-channel blockers at the level of the spinal cord. *Anesthesiology*, 79, 746-752.

Perkins, M.N., Campbell E., and Dray, A. (1993). Antinociceptive activity of the bradykinin B1 and B2 receptor antagonists, des-Arg9, [Leu8]-BK and HOE 140, in two models of persistent hyperalgesia in the rat. *Pain, 53*, 191-197.

Pick, C.G., Paul, D., Eison, M.S. and Pasternak, G.W. (1992). Potentiation of opioid analgesia by the antidepressant nefazodone. *European journal of Pharmacology, 211*, 375-381.

Power Smith, P. and Turkington, D. (1993). Fluoxetine in phantom limb pain. *British Journal of Psychiatry, 163*, 105-106.

Pud, D., Eisenberg, E., Spitzer, A., et al. (1998). The NMDA receptor antagonist amantadine reduces surgical neuropathic pain in cancer patients: a double-blind, randomized, placebo-controlled trial. *Pain*, 75, 349-354.

Randic, M. and Urban, L. (1987). Slow excitatory transmission in rat spinal dorsal horn and the effects of capsaicin. *Acta Physiologica Hungarica, 69*, 375-392.

Rang, H.P. and Urban, L. (1995). New molecules in analgesia. *British Journal of Anaesthesia, 75*, 145-156.

Rani, P.U., Naidu, M.U., Prasad, V.B., Rao, T.R. and Shobha, J.C. (1996). An evaluation of antidepressants in rheumatic pain conditions. *Anesthesia and Analgesia, 83*, 371-375.

Ripamonti, C. and Bruera, E. (1991). Rectal, buccal, and sublingual narcotics for the management of cancer pain. *J Palliat Care*, 7, 30-35.

Rowbotham, M., Young, J.P., Sharma, U. (2004). Pregabalin reduces neuropathic pain associated with diabetic peripheral neuropathy or postherpetic neuralgia by 3rd day of treatment. *Pain Practice*. Book of abstracts 3rd World Congress WIP, 271.

Rowbotham, M.C., Harden, N., Stacey, B., et al. (1998). Gabapentin for the treatment of postherpetic neuralgia. *JAMA*, 280(21), 1837-1842.

Sagen, J. (1992). Chromaffin cell transplants for alleviation of chronic pain. *ASAIO Journal, 38*, 24-28.

Sanderson, J.E, Ibrahim, B, Waterhouse, D. and Palmer, R.B. (1994). Spinal electrical stimulation for intractable angina: Long-term clinical outcome and safety. *European Heart Journal, 15*, 810-814.

Sang, C.N., et al. (1997). A placebo-controlled trial of dextromethorphan and memantine in diabetic neuropathy and post herpetic neuralgia. American Pain Society abstracts.

Saper, J.R., Silberstein, S.D., Lake, A.E. and Winters, M.E. (1994). Double-blind trial of fluoxetine: Chronic daily headache and migraine. *Headache, 34*, 497-502.

Schafer, M.K., Nohr, D., Krause, J.E. and Weihe, E. (1993). Inflammation-induced upregulation of NK1 receptor mRNA in dorsal horn neurons. *Neuroreport, 4*, 1007-1010.

Schmidt, W.K. and Way, E.L. (1980). Hyperalgesia effects of divalent cations and antinociceptive effects of a calcium chelator in naïve and morphine-dependent mice. *Journal of Pharmacology and Experimental Therapeutics, 212*, 22-27.

Seltzer, Z., Paran, Y., Eisen, A., and Ginzburg, R. (1991). Neuropathic pain behavior in rats depends on the afferent input from nerve-end neuroma including histamine-sensitive C-fibers. *Neuroscience Letters, 128,* 203-206.

Serrao, J.M., Marks, R.L., Morley, S.J. and Goodchild, C.S. (1992). Intrathecal midazolam for the treatment of chronic mechanical low back pain: A controlled comparison with epidural steroid in a pilot study. *Pain, 48,* 5-12.

Serrao, J.M., Stubbs, S.C., Goodchild, C.S. and Gent, J.P. (1989). Intrathecal midazolam and fentanyl in the rat: Evidence for different spinal antinociceptive effects. *Anesthesiology, 70,* 780-786.

Sewell, R.D.E, Spencer, P.S.J.(1974). Modification of the antinociceptive activity of narcotic agonists and antagonists by intraventricular injection of biogenic amines in mice. *Br J Pharmacol, 51*, 140-141.

Sharma, U., Portenoy, R., Young, J., et al. Pregabalin in the treatment of painful diabetic neuropathy or postherpetic neuralgia: long-term effects. *Pain Practice*. Book of abstracts 3rd World Congress WIP, 269-270.

Sindrup, S.H., Gram, L.F., Brosen, K., et al. (1990). The selective serotonin reuptake inhibitor paroxetine is effective in the treatment of diabetic neuropathy symptoms. *Pain, 42*, 135-144.

Sluka, K.A. (1997). Blockade of calcium channels can prevent the onset of secondary hyperalgesia and allodynia induced by intradermal injection of capsaicin in rats. *Pain, 71*, 157-164.

Snider, R.M., Constantine, J.W., Lowe, J.A., Longo, K.P., Lebel, W.S., Woody, H.A., Drozda, S.E., Desai, M.C., Vinick, F.J. and Spencer, R.W. (1991). A potent nonpeptide antagonist of the substance P (NK1) receptor. *Science, 251*, 435-437.

Theesen, K.A. and Marsh, W.R. (1989). Relief of diabetic neuropathy with fluoxetine. *DICP, 23*, 572-574.

Twycross, R.G. (1982). Controlling pain in cancer patients. *Mod Med (Lond),* 8, 2.

Twycross, R.G. and Ventafridda, V. (1980). The continuing care of terminal cancer patients. New York: Pergamon Press.

Vane, J.R., Mitchell, J.A., Appleton, I., Tomlinson, A., Bishop-Baily, D., Croxtall, J. and Willoughby, D.A. (1994). Inducible isoforms of cyclooxigenase and nitric-oxide synthase in inflammation. *Proceedings of the National Academy of Science of the United States of America, 91*, 2046-2050.

Virani, A., Mailis, A., Shapiro L.E., et al. (1997). Drug interactions in human neuropathic pain pharmacotherapy. *Pain*, 73, 3-13.

Wang, H. and Sagen, J. (1994). Absence of appreciable tolerance and morphine cross-tolerance in rats with adrenal medullary transplants in the spinal cord. *Neuropharmacology, 33*, 681-692.

Watson, C.P.N., Chipman, M., Reed, K., et al. (1992). Amitriptyline versus maprotiline in postherpetic neuralgia: a randomized, double-blind, crossover trial. *Pain*, 48, 29-36.

Watson, C.P.N. and Evans, R.J. (1985). A comparative trial of amitriptyline and zimelidine in postherpetic neuralgia. *Pain*, 23, 387-394.

Watson, C.P., Evans, R.J., Reed, K., et al. (1982). Amitriptyline versus placebo in posherpetic neuralgia. *Neurology*, 32, 671-673.

Wetzel, C.H. and Connelly, J.F. (1997). Use of gabapentin in pain management. *Annals of Pharmacotherapy, 31*, 1082-1083.

Wilson, A. (1990). Comparison of flurbiprofen and alprazolam in the management of chronic pain syndrome. *Psychiat J Univ Ottawa*, 15, 144-149.

Woolf, C.I. and Chong, M.S. (1993). Preemptive analgesia: Treating postoperative pain by preventing the establishment of central sensitization. *Anesthesia and Analgesia, 77*, 362-379.

Xu, X.J., Hao, J.X., Seiger, A., Hughes, J., Hokfelt, T. and Wiesenfeld-Hallin, Z. (1994). Chronic pain-related behaviors in spinally injured rats: Evidence for functional alterations of the endogenous cholecystokinin and opioid systems. *Pain, 56*, 271-277.

Zacny, J.P., Coalson, D., Young, C., Klafta, J., Rupani, G., Thapar, P., Choi, M., and Apfelbaum, J.L. (1995). A dose-response study of the effects of intravenous midazolam on cold pressor-induced pain. *Anesthesia and Analgesia, 80*, 521- 525.

In: The Handbook of Chronic Pain
Editors: S. Kreitler, D. Beltrutti, et al., pp. 207-228
ISBN 978-1-60021-044-0
© 2007 Nova Science Publishers, Inc.

Chapter 13

Common Nerve Blocks Used in Pain Medicine

z

Richard L. Rauck

INTRODUCTION

The use of nerve blocks in regional anesthesia and pain medicine continues to evolve. Regional anesthesia in the operating room was prevalent when general anesthetic drugs or monitoring was considered unsafe or risky. As general anesthetics became safer, a swing occurred away from regional techniques. At present the use of regional anesthetic techniques in the operating room depends on the skill of the operator, the philosophy of the surgical and anesthesiologist practice, and other ethnic and socioeconomic factors.

Regional anesthesia has also evolved in acute pain medicine, following surgical and nonsurgical trauma. Emergency room physicians frequently perform a variety of minor nerve block procedures. Trauma surgeons often ask anesthesiologists to become involved with nonoperative trauma, particularly in patients with chest injuries whose respiratory function may be compromised.

Postoperatively, acute pain medicine has flourished. The initial impetus for acute pain management teams was given by the discovery of opiate receptors in the spinal cord [1]. Small amounts of opiates delivered into the epidural space provided excellent postoperative analgesia and decreased morbidity and mortality in subsets of patients.[2-3] As acute pain management teams developed into formal services, other regional techniques were reintroduced or gained favor because of their ability to extend into the postoperative setting. Techniques utilizing continuous catheters were favored by some as these avoided repeated injections.

As more nonanesthesiologists become involved in different aspects of nerve block techniques it becomes of paramount importance that they have complete knowledge of the potential risks and complications and how to manage them. This chapter will describe the more commonly used nerve blocks in acute pain and chronic pain medicine [see also 4-7]

EPIDURAL AND INTRATHECAL BLOCKS (CENTRAL NEURAXIAL ANESTHESIA)

Subarachnoid or intrathecal nerve blocks have been used to provide anesthesia since the report of Koller using cocaine in 1884 [8]. Epidural anesthesia has been around for much of this past century. Both techniques have provided excellent operative conditions for surgical and obstetrical procedures. The employed drugs were various local anesthetics. These were not popular sole agents during the postoperative setting because of their side effects. The discovery in 1977 of opiate receptors in the spinal cord led to a rapid expansion of this technique for postoperative pain management [1]. Small opiate doses delivered into the epidural space have proven very effective for controlling postoperative pain. They are often combined with low dose local anesthetics to take advantage of the synergism between these two classes of agents [9-10]. Although the doses need to be individualized, as a rule more drug is required for more painful procedures and younger (<40 years) patients.

Patients with either diagnosed or suspected obstructive sleep apnea should be carefully managed in the postoperative period. Opiates increase the risk of a respiratory event in these patients. If opiates are necessary they should be used judiciously and extra monitoring should be considered. Alternatively, we often avoid narcotic medications in these patients. If local anesthetics do not suffice one can add clonidine to the epidural infusion or provide alternative adjuvant analgesics such as ketorolac or other nonsteroidal antiinflammatory drugs.

The technique of epidural placement is not difficult yet requires practice and formal training. The epidural space extends from just inside the sacral hiatus to the top of the cervical spinal segments. Access to the epidural space is present throughout much of this distance. The spinal cord ends between the T12 and L2 vertebral bodies in the majority of patients. If the epidural space inferior to the L2 vertebral body is approached then any contact with the spinal cord should be avoided if the needle inadvertently punctures the dura. The L3 level can be accurately determined by physical palpation of the posterior, superior iliac spines.

Thorough prior eparation of the skin with a bacteriocidal/static solution is necessary. Sterile drapes should also be used to further decrease the risk of any life-threatening epidural or intrathecal infection. A midline approach to the epidural space is recommended, particularly in the lumber region and the lower thoracic spine. Once the epidural needle is seated in the ligamentum flavum a syringe should be attached and the loss of resistance technique employed.

At the most distal aspect of the spinal column the epidural space can be encountered via a caudal approach. In children the patient is often positioned lateral. Adults are more easily approached via a prone position. Great variability exists at the sacral hiatus where the epidural space is entered. Strict adherance to sterile technique is important when this block is performed. For single shot injections a 22 gauge, 3-5 cm needle can be used. The bevel is superior until the sacrococcygeal membrane is pierced, then rotated 180° to decrease the chance of the sharp bevel piercing the epidural plexus of veins which lies more prominantly on the anterior surface of the sacrum. If a catheter technique is intended then an epidural needle is most commonly used with a catheter subsequently passed 5-10 cm. Many newer chronic pain procedures utilize the caudal approach for passing sophisticated wires and catheters cephalad into the epidural space. Fluoroscopic guidance should be used when extensive manipulation is intended.

In the middle thoracic region the spinous processes are steeply angulated which makes a midline approach very difficult or impossible in many patients. Because of this angulation it is recommended by most practitioners that a paramedian approach be used when the epidural space is sought in the areas between T 4-8. In this area the tip of the spinous process lays across from the body of the next higher vertebral body. Restated, the tip of the T7 spinous process is felt where the lamina of T6 would be contacted. The epidural needle is inserted approximately 1 cm lateral to the spinous process. Local infiltration is initially injected prior to the epidural needle in the same area. The needle should contact the lamina where additional local infiltration can be injected. The epidural needle can be advanced to the lamina then walked off in a cephalad direction. Once the epidural space is entered a catheter should thread easily for 5-8 cm. The foramina are small in the thoracic space and the risk of the catheter exiting through an intervertebral foramina is much decreased compared to the lumbar region.

Cervical epidurals are also frequently performed for upper extremity surgery and in chronic pain for herniated cervical discs. The technique can be safely performed in either the lateral or sitting position. The most frequently entered spaces are C6-7 and C7-T1, because the spinous processes are easily palpated and flexion of the neck provides for excellent access to the epidural space in most patients. The width of epidural space is diminished in the cervical region so adherence to proper technique is essential.

Loss of resistance can be obtained with either a syringe, a hanging drop, or a running drop. Once the epidural needle is seated into the ligamentum flavum it is very helpful to remove one's hands from the needle and observe the direction of the needle. If the needle stays in the midline then ultimate successful placement is almost guaranteed. Most errors with cervical epidural placement occur when the needle tracks off midline. Catheter placement will almost always track to one side or the other within the epidural space. If it is important to have the catheter on a specific side, it is advisable to place the cervical epidural catheter under fluoroscopic guidance.

SUBARACHNOID BLOCK

Subarachnoid blocks are performed most frequently in patients undergoing surgical procedures. In these situations opiates are often added to the single shot injection to provide additional pain relief after the operation. Doses of morphine range from 0.2-0.5 mg in most cases. The first dose of systemic opiate following a subarachnoid dose should be given judiciously and with adequate monitoring.

Risks and Complications

Complications from epidural placement are few when good technique is utilized. Backache is possible from the minor trauma associated with needle placement. A risk of headache is present when an inadvertent dural puncture occurs. Experienced practitioners should have dural puncture rates of 1% or lower, whereas new practitioners would have rates >10%. The likelihood of a headache if a puncture occurs depends also on age, and is higher in the younger (< 40 years) patients [13-14].

If a headache occurs patients are encouraged to drink plenty of clear liquids, drink caffeine-containing products, and stay flat in bed until the headache resolves. If these measures are unsuccessful then an epidural blood patch is the recommended treatment. This procedure is performed with the epidural needle reintroduced in the same site and 15-20 ml of the patient's own blood injected into the epidural space. Success of blood patches is reported to exceed 90% but can be repeated if the initial attempt is unsuccessful. [15]

Infection is always a risk after any interventional technique. Fortunately, the epidural space has a rich blood supply and can fight infectious processes very well. However, epidural abscesses can occur and present very insidiously. A stiff neck and headache, the cardinal symptoms of an epidural abscess, are not always the presenting symptoms. If suspicions exist, a white blood count, sedimentation rate, and possibly an MRI are necessary.

Epidural hematomas represent another potentially catastophic complication of epidural blocks. Minimal bleeding in the epidural space occurs after many procedures. Fortunately, this is rarely significant nor does it cause any symptoms or complications. Most patients who develop clinically significant hematomas have bleeding dyscrasias prior to the procedure (16-17). Patients whose history suggests abnormal bleeding should have a PT/PTT and/or INR drawn. Patients who are receiving heparin, low molecular weight heparins (LMWH), coumadin, thrombolytic drugs such as streptokinase, or platelet inhibiting drugs should be considered at significantly increased risk, and epidural placement should be delayed until bleeding parameters are established and normalized. The delay is possible because most epidurals are placed electively. Full neurologic recovery after the timely diagnosis and effective treatment of an epidural hematoma is less than 40% [16-17].

It should be noted that a thoracic or cervical approach to the epidural space can be performed reliably and safely. However, the spinal cord exists in these regions, and precaution should be maintained to avoid trauma with the needle. Whenever possible, it is advisable to perform these procedures in awake patients to avoid needle trauma. If sedation is used judiciously patients can still adequately advise the practitioner if the needle has touched the spinal cord. If this occurs or is suspected, the practitioner should never inject saline or any other drug as the development of a syrinx can produce significantly more damage than what might occur with direct needle trauma. This author has reviewed several reports where significant trauma to the spinal cord has been alleged from repeated needle trauma to the spinal cord when patients in a state of sleep could not report important information about paresthesias. .

Finally, a posterior fusion to either the thoracic or cervical spine should be considered a relative contraindication to epidural placement through the surgical scar region. Epidural placement can be performed cephalad or caudal to the scar but the surgical procedure will often alter or obliterate the epidural space and make the loss of resistance technique unreliable. Cerebrospinal fluid may not flow freely and unrecognized needle trauma can occur to the spinal cord in these patients if the needle pierces the cord. If epidural placement must be done it should only be performed under fluoroscopic guidance with the patient awake and a skilled practitioner performing the procedure.

BLOCKS OF THE SYMPATHETIC NERVOUS SYSTEM

Stellate Ganglion Block

The stellate ganglion, named because of its anatomic, star-shaped appearance, lies on the anterior surface of the C7 anterior tubercle and the T1 transverse process. The C7 anterior tubercle is not easily palpated in many people and can be vestigial in others, therefore, many practitioners have opted to perform this procedure at the prominent C6 anterior tubercle, Chaussignac's tubercle. This bony landmark is easily palpated in most individuals but lies somewhat distant from the specific site of action. Thus, if the block is performed at C6 sufficient drug must be instilled to ensure block of the ganglion, and the patient's head should be raised after the procedure to aid diffusion of the drug caudad.

In two separate studies, Malmqvist et al., and Hogan et al., demonstrated the difficulty of reliably blocking this ganglion from the standard C6 approach [18-19]. In Malmqvist's study less than 20% of patients met 3 of 5 criteria for sympathetic denervation. In part, this may be related to the distant location of the ganglion from the block site. In Hogan's study, contrast was found to travel in varied places following the procedure, including the brachial plexus, cervical plexus, middle and superior cervical ganglion, and the contralateral prevertebral space. By comparing the high interpleural approach with the standard C6 approach [20], we found no difference in efficacy and, similar to Malmqvist, were unable to completely denervate the sympathetic chain with any regularity.

Anterior Approach at Chaussignac's Tubercle (C6)

To perform a stellate ganglion block at C6 the patient is positioned in the supine position, with a pillow under the shoulders. The C6 tubercle lies across from the cricothyroid cartilage which can be palpated to confirm correct location. The skin is aseptically cleansed and the nonoperative first or second finger locates the tubercle. Palpation should be done using firm, constant pressure of a single digit.

A 22 gauge, and a 3-4 cm needle suffice in >95% of patients. Sedation can be used in particularly anxious patients, yet is mostly unnecessary.

Once the tubercle is contacted it is important to maintain contact with the bone while the probing finger releases pressure and secures the hub of the needle. The needle is withdrawn minimally, less than 1 cm to make sure the needle is out of the periosteum. Aspiration is essential prior to injection since 0.5 ml injected into the vertebral artery has been reported to cause seizure activity. After negative aspiration 1 ml of local anesthetic is injected, aspiration performed again and signs of intrarterial injection are monitored, then additional local anesthetic injected. The total amount of solution can vary from 6-20 ml.

As stated above, the patient's head should be elevated approximately 30 degrees to facilitate caudal diffusion of the drug to the stellate ganglion. Confirmation of effective block extends beyond just a Horner's syndrome since this can be obtained by block of the cervical sympathetic chain without denervating the stellate ganglion.

Risks of this approach include intraarterial injection into either the vertebral or less likely the carotid artery. Seizures can occur with small amounts of local anesthetic (< 0.5 ml). Treatment of the seizure is symptomatic, usually requiring only oxygen. Pneumothorax is possible in patients who have a dome of pulmonary parenchyma in the area. This risk is more common with the C7 approach.

Subarachnoid and epidural diffusion of drug is possible. If sufficient drug passes into the aubarachnoid space a total spinal results necessitating artificial ventilation and frequent assurances to the patient. Muscle relaxation is not needed to intubate patients in this situation. Epidural diffusion rarely paralyzes the diaphragm but can cause breathing difficulties. Common side effects include brachial plexus diffusion of drug with resultant upper extremity paresis and block of the recurrent laryngeal nerve causing hoarseness and abduction of the ipsilateral vocal cord. If stridor occurs it does not require any treatment except reassurance.

APPROACH OF ANTERIOR TUBERCLE AT C7

The patient is positioned as in the C6 approach. The C7 tubercle is approximately 1-2 cm caudad from the C6 tubercle. Fluoroscopic guidance greatly aids in locating this landmark. If fluoroscopic guidance is available many practitioners currently block the stellate ganglion by this approach since C7 is closer to the site of action. The rest of the procedure is performed in the same manner as in the C6 approach. Contrast can be injected prior to local anesthetic to confirm location. This approach is also more commonly used for radiofrequency denervation or neurolytic administration. The risk of pneumothorax is enhanced with the C7 approach to the stellate ganglion. Piercing the lymphatic duct is possible when the procedure is performed on the right side; otherwise, the risks are the same as those associated with the C6 approach.

POSTERIOR APPROACH AT T1-2

The upper sympathetic chain and stellate ganglion can be reached via a posterior approach. The patient is positioned prone and the T2 vertebral spine is palpated. An 8-10 cm, 22 gauge needle is inserted 4-5 cm from the midline at the T2 vertebral body. This can be performed using fluoroscopic or CT guidance. The needle is positioned at the mid vertebral body level on a lateral view. While the sympathetic chain lies at the anterolateral border in the lumbar region, it is at the midvertebral body in the thoracic region.

Contrast should be injected prior to placing either local anesthetic or neurolytic solution. Because the needle is more posterior than in the lumbar sympathetic block one must check for medicine tracking back to the somatic nerve root or into the epidural space. The potential risk of pneumothorax must be considered in any patient who develops shortness of breath or chest pain. Treatment of pneumothorax can be conservative, a one-way valved catheter, or rarely a large-bore thoracostomy tube, depending on symptoms and the degree of pneumothorax.

CELIAC PLEXUS AND SPLANCHNIC NERVE BLOCKS

The greater, lesser, and least splanchnic nerves form from preganglionic sympathetic nerves of T5-9, T10-11, and T12 nerves, respectively, although individual variations occur. These nerves contain sympathetic efferent fibers and afferent visceral nociceptors. They travel together along the vertebral bodies and pierce the diaphragm at the T12-L1 level.

The celiac plexus is a diffuse network as it encircles the aorta at the origin of the celiac artery (L1). The plexus can extend for several vertebral segments and wraps the aorta with a greater percentage of fibers anterior to the aorta. Many different approaches have been described regarding block of the celiac plexus [21-26]. It is unclear if any of these variations is better than the more traditional approaches.

STANDARD POSTERIOR APPROACH

The most frequent approach to the celiac plexus is via a posterior insertion with a pillow positioned under the abdomen. Sterile prep and drape should always be employed. The patient is positioned prone with bilateral 12-18 cm 22 gauge needles inserted 7 cm from the midline. The needles are inserted opposite the L1-L2 vertebral body, beneath the 12th rib and directed cephalad to the anteror aspect of the L1 vertebral body. The diaphragm becomes an important landmark if the needles are placed posterior to the aorta and vena cava. The use of contrast and fluoroscopy can delineate the diaphragm in some cases. Otherwise, spread must be visualized in both the anteroposterior and lateral views to determine accurate needle placement.

An alternative to the above approach uses a single needle technique on the left side. Most practitioners who perform this technique will enter from the left side and position the needle anterior to the aorta at L1. Another modification has the needles pierce the skin 4-5 cm from the midline and advance off the transverse process rather than the vertebral body. This author has found this technique more difficult because of the difficulty of reliably positioning the needle inside the lateral border of the lamina as viewed on the anteroposterior radiograph.

SPLANCHNIC NERVE BLOCK

The splanchnic nerve block is performed with the patient in the prone position and a pillow under the stomach. Needles are inserted approximately 6-7 cm from the midline under the 12th rib. The needles are advanced toward T12 with the tips ultimately positioned near the anterolateral border of the T12 vertebral body. Contrast should be viewed to stay adjacent to the vertebral body in the anteroposterior plane and in the anterior one-third of the vertebral body on the lateral view. Needles can be positioned with fluoroscopic guidance using either a "tunnel" view or a standard anteroposterior view with lateral view confirmation.

ANTERIOR APPROACH

The anterior approach to the celiac plexus has been advocated for patients who cannot tolerate lying prone. The anterior approach uses a single 22 gauge entering the abdomen at the L1 interspace. The needle is guided posterior until it rests at the anterior border of the aorta. Contrast confirms placement and injection of local anesthetic or neuroloytic solution follows. An increased risk of infection has not been reported.

MEDICATIONS USED FOR CELIAC PLEXUS BLOCK

Diagnostic procedures are performed with local anesthetic. Commonly 15 ml of bupivicaine 0.25-0.5% with epinephrine 1:200,000 is injected through each needle (larger volumes if a single needle technique is used). Different volumes may also be used to mimic the volume anticipated for a neurolytic block. Corticosteroid, commonly celestone, is injected in patients with noncancer pain where a diagnostic block has already been performed, neurolytic solution is not presently indicated, and it is possible that adhesions or scarring are present around the celiac axis.

Neurolytic solutions commonly used today include phenol or alcohol. Phenol is injected in 6-12% solutions. Total phenol doses should not exceed 3 grams or 40 mg/kg (whichever is less). Volumes are commonly 15 ml per needle or 20-25 ml if only one needle is used. Alcohol has been recommended in concentrations from 50-100%. Pure alcohol is painful on injection and not frequently used at present. Lesser concentrations of alcohol can be diluted with bupivicaine to lessen the pain on injection. Phenol has a local anesthetic effect which can be seen early and help predict the ultimate efficacy of the block. While both solutions have their proponents, they have not tested in comparative trials. Alternatively, some practitioners prefer to neurolyse the splanchnic nerves using a radiofrequency technique at T11 and T12.

COMPLICATIONS

Complications of the celiac plexus block include intravascular, subarachnoid, or epidural injection. Pneumothorax has been reported when the needles are inadvertently positioned between T11-12 rather than beneath the 12th rib. Discitis is possible if needles inadvertently pass through an intervertebral disc. Nerve paresthesia and neuralgias can occur, predominantly L1.

More serious complications have occurred with the instillation of neurolytic solutions. Paralysis has occurred and attributed to either subarachnoid injection or vascular compromise of the tenuous spinal artery arising from the aorta, the artery of Adamkowitz. Injection of phenol into the aortic wall has resulted in subsequent aortic dissection and death. Somatic neuralgias, commonly of L1, often last 4-6 weeks, but can be permanent.

LUMBAR SYMPATHETIC NERVE BLOCK

The lumbar sympathetic chain migrates from the midvertebral region of the thoracic chain and lies at the anterolateral border of the vertebral bodies. Nerves in the lumbar sympathetic chain include sympathetic efferents and corresponding primary nociceptive afferents although the latter is debated.

Block of the sympathetic chain is performed for conditions involving sympathetically mediated pain (e.g. complex regional pain syndrome) or patients with vascular compromise, particularly small vessel disease. Block of the sympathetic chain will not affect blood flow if a fixed lesion is present in the more proximal, larger arteries of the lower extremity.

STANDARD APPROACH

The lumbar sympathetic chain is commonly blocked with the patient in the prone position and a pillow under the abdomen. Sterile prep and drape should be used. Needles are inserted at L2, L3, and L4. The modified Reid's approach uses one needle only at L2 with subsequent larger volumes of drug. No comparative studies have shown if either approach is more effective.

A 12-18 cm, 22 gauge needle is inserted through the skin 7 cm from midline. The needle is advanced to the vertebral body and then walked laterally to pass by the vertebral body. Unlike the celiac plexus approach the needle is advanced perpendicular to the vertebral axis. Fluoroscopic guidance shows a correctly placed needle to lie at the anterior border of the vertebral body on lateral projection and near the laminar plane on an anteroposterior view. Injecting contrast demonstrates good longitudinal spread without spill into the psoas muscle.

The block can be performed either unilaterally or bilaterally. While "crosstalk" has been reported between sides of the sympathetic chain, many practitioners perform unilateral block if the condition is one-sided. Bilateral block is reserved in those situations when unilateral block becomes ineffective over time.

MEDICATIONS

Local anesthetics are used for diagnostic and therapeutic considerations. Corticosteroids are not commonly indicated since inflammation of the chain itself is not common. Bupivicaine 0.25-0.50% solutions are commonly injected and epinephrine 1:200,000 is often added to prolong the effect. Volumes range from 3-5 ml, if 3 needles are used on each side of a bilateral block, to 15 ml when a single needle is used. Duration of the local anesthetic block is less than 24 hours but the analgesia is often prolonged for days to weeks. This author's clinical experience has been that patients who respond best to more permanent denervation techniques exhibit analgesia from the local anesthetics significantly beyond the expected duration of the local anesthetic.

Neurolytic solutions include phenol 6-10% and alcohol 50%. Comparative studies showed alcohol produces more frequent L1 neuralgias than phenol after lumbar sympathetic injection [27]. Otherwise, the 2 drugs do not differ in efficacy. Volumes up to 15 ml can be safely injected in a single needle technique. If multiple needles are used per side then the volume per needle is adjusted accordingly.

COMPLICATIONS

Intravascular injection of the aorta or inferior vena cava can occur. Somatic block of the L2-4 nerve roots results from posterior diffusion of drug or inaccuraate needle placement. Lumbar plexus block occurs if drug diffuses into the psoas muscle. Even though the psoas muscle is easily delineated on fluoroscopic images, drug diffusion to a respective nerve root can occur, but is uncommon and has little significance when local anesthetic is used. However, more permanent neuralgia can result if a neurolytic solution is used. Weakness of the lower extremity can occur following local anesthetic injection into the psoas muscle and can last for 24 hours or longer if an epinephrine containing solution of bupivicaine has been used.

Subarachnoid sleeves extend with the respective lumbar nerve roots beyond the intervertebral foramen in some patients. If the needle is placed in this location a total subarachnoid block can occur resulting in the need to control ventilation. If a neurolytic solution is injected the result can be disasterous. More commonly, the needle passes through one of these sleeves enroute to its final location at the anterolateral vertebral body. The result can be a low pressure, spinal headache. If this occurs, an epidural blood patch can be attempted but does not have the high success rate expected from spinal headaches after a traditional dural puncture.

Needles used for this block should not be inserted beyond 7 cm from the midline. The kidney lies nearby and CT images have demonstrated needles passing through renal parenchyma when inserted too laterally. Rarely, the needle can pass through a ureter or the lymphatic duct.

SUPERIOR HYPOGASTRIC BLOCK

The superior hypogastric plexus forms from the lumbar sympathetic chain. Sympathetic efferents and primary afferents are located within the plexus which is located at the anterior aspect of the L5-S1 vertebral body. The block is performed for patients with pain of pelvic origin. Particularly, patients with pelvic malignancies have been reported to experience good relief of pain from this procedure.[28]

APPROACH TO THE SUPERIOR HYPOGASTRIC PLEXUS

The patient is positioned prone with a pillow under the abdomen. Sterile prep and drape should be utilized. Bilateral 12-18 cm, 22 gauge needles are inserted approximately 7 cm from the midline across from the L4 vertebral body. The needles are directed caudally to the 5th lumbar vertebral body. Once contacted they are walked off the vertebral body to pass to the anterolateral surface.

Two structures, the iliac crest and the transverse process of L5, make this block technically difficult in some patients. Fluoroscopic guidance significantly aids in placement of needles for this procedure. Practitioners familiar with L5-S1 discography can utilize a similar "tunnel" approach to the superior hypogastric plexus. Alternatively, anterior and lateral projections demonstrate when the needle is in the correct position.

MEDICATIONS

Local anesthetics, commonly bupivicaine 0.25-0.50% with epinephrine 1:200,000, are injected for diagnostic purposes. Corticosteroids may be added for patients where the origin of pain from the plexus may be inflammatory in nature. However, injection of corticosteroids can alter the diagnostic information obtained from the block.

Patients with cancer pain and limited life expectancies who demonstrate good relief from local blocks should be considered for a neurolytic procedure. Phenol, commonly 10% solutions in renograffin, can be injected in volumes of 10-15 ml per side. Total doses should not exceed 3 grams or 40 mg/kg (whichever is less).

COMPLICATIONS

Complications include those listed above for other sympathetic blocks of the vertebral column. Additionally, the 5th lumbar nerve root is near the path of the needle and susceptible to injury. Paresthesias are usually transient and if neuralgias develop they commonly resolve in 4-6 weeks. To prevent a risk of discitis the needle should avoid the L5 disc. If the L5 disc is entered, passing through to the anterior surface where the plexus lies may be tried. If a transdiscal approach is intentionally used antibiotics is to be initiated to minimize the discitis risk.

Intravascular injection can occur through the common iliac arteries or veins. Negative aspiration and confirmation of contrast in the proper location should diminish this risk.

GANGLION OF IMPAR BLOCK

The most distal sympathetic structure, the ganglion of Impar, lies on the anterior surface of the sacrum at the sacrococcygeal junction. This structure is a single, midline structure and forms from the union of the sympathetic chains distal to the superior hypogastric plexus. The ganglion contains sympathetic efferents and possible primary afferents from structures of the perineum. This is a midline structure and can be blocked with a bent 22 gauge needle inserted distal to the tip of the coccyx, the anococcygeal ligament and directed along the anterior surface of the coccyx to the sacrococcygeal junction. Alternatively, the ganglion of Impar can be reached with a 22 gauge needle that pierces the sacrococcygeal ligament. Needle confirmation can be verified with fluoroscopy.

A diagnostic block is performed with bupivicaine 0.25-0.50%, 6-10 ml. Epinephrine, 1:200,000, is added to lengthen duration. If effective, neurolysis can be performed with phenol, 10%, 4-6 ml. Complications are uncommon but can occur if neurolytic solution is injected into the rectal wall or extends posteriorly into the epidural space.

PERIPHERAL NERVE BLOCKS

Most peripheral nerves are amenable to block for various conditions, for diagnostic or therapeutic purposes. Catheters can be employed to prolong the effect in the postoperative setting or to facilitate physical therapy maneuvers. Local anesthetic solutions are most commonly injected, and neurolytic solutions should be avoided in most situations secondary to the high risk of neuritis and neuralgia.

Intercostal Nerve Block

The intercostal nerves emerge from the intervertebral foramen of the T2-T12 interspaces. T1 forms the inferior aspect of the brachial plexus. T12 and sometimes T11 combine with L1 to form the iliohypogastric and ilioinguinal nerves. If one needs to block all divisions of the intercostal nerve, the procedure should be performed proximal to the posterior axillary line. The 2 most commonly selected sights for block are at the scapular line or via a paravertebral approach. Intercostal blocks cephalad to T7 are often performed via a paravertebral approach because of the location of the scapula. The rhomboid muscles protect the medial (posterior) aspects of the ribs and make palpation of the intercostal space difficult in many patients. Another approach to the intercostal nerves is through the interpleural space. Three approaches will be discussed here.

Standard Infrarib Approach

In the classic approach to the intercostal nerve the patient is positioned prone. The skin should be marked in the interspaces between the ribs intended for block. After prep and local infiltration of the skin, the skin is retracted cephalad to position the the skin marks over the ribs. A 23 gauge needle is inserted through the skin mark until the rib is contacted. The needle should still have a cephalad direction such that the tip can be advanced both under the rib and cephalad to where the neurovascular bundle lies.

After negative aspiration a total of 3-5 ml of local anesthetic, bupivicaine 0.5% with epinephrine 1:200,000, is injected. Volume of injectate per rib is based, in part, on the total number of ribs injected. Studies showed rapid and high absorption of local anesthetics from the intercostal space, thus total volumes should be calculated carefully [29-30]. Epinephrine prolongs the block and decreases the rate of vascular uptake.

Paravertebral Approach

The intercostal nerve can be blocked via a paravertebral approach with the patient in the prone position. Fluoroscopy greatly aids needle placement and diminishes the risk of pneumothorax. A 22 gauge, 7-10 cm, needle is inserted about 4-6 cm from the midline. A paresthesia confirms accurate positioning. A local anesthetic (2-3 ml) will block the nerve root.

It should be remembered that the intercostal nerve leaves the foramen and does not assume its infrarib location for several centimeters (near the neck of the rib), thus an infrarib approach at the paravertebral site is not reliable. Also, approximately 1/3 of patients will get epidural spread of local anesthetic following this block [31]. Limiting the volume per level diminishes the epidural effect in many patients.

Interpleural Approach

The interpleural approach to the intercostal nerves can be performed with the patient prone or in the lateral position. The most common entry site is beneath the scapula at approximately the T7 or T8 level. The midscapular line is often used although a slightly more proximal approach may facilitate ultimate spread of local anesthetic to the paravertebral site, a presumed site of action along with posterior diffusion to the intercostal nerve.

After prep, drape, and local infiltration a blunt, epidural-style needle is used. The needle is placed above the rib to avoid the neurovascular bundle. Saline or air can be used. Negative pressure in the interpleural space is pronounced, and the air in the syringe is completely sucked in when the interpleural space is encountered. This technique avoids the false loss of resistance found on entry into the intercostal space. Once the interpleural space is located the bevel is directed medially to facilitate catheter positioning in a medial direction. The syringe is removed and the catheter inserted quickly to avoid further air into the pleural cavity.

Complications

Common complications of intercostal block include pneumothorax and local anesthetic toxicity (CNS or cardiovascular). Infection, bleeding from transection of the intercostal artery, or nerve injury from needle trauma occur less commonly.

Pneumothorax occurs when the needle passes through the interpleural space and communicates with pulmonary parenchyma, allowing inspired air to pass into the interpleural space. If tension develops this can progress to a life-threatening situation. The intercostal block is one of the few procedures done in an outpatient setting that can cause mortality within 24-48 hours if not appropriately recognized by the patient or physician. It is imperative that patients be alerted to this complication. Some patients developing small pneumothoraces can be treated conservatively. Others can be managed with insertion of a one-way valve. Since blood is rarely involved, a patient with a pneumothorax from an intercostal block rarely requires a large bore thoracostomy tube. The intercostal space has the highest rate of vascular uptake following local anesthetic injection [30]. This demands consideration of total local anesthetic dose. Epinephrine is to be used in most patients unless a contraindication exists.

Upper Extremity Blocks

Many blocks and approaches to the nerves of the upper extremity have been reported in regional anesthesia textbooks. Only the more common ones will be discussed here. Notably, many of the approaches to the brachial plexus also produce effective denervation of the sympathetic fibers to the upper extremity since these sympathetic fibers travel together with the somatic nerves.

Interscalene Approach

The interscalene approach to the brachial plexus is utilized most often when surgery or analgesia of the upper arm or shoulder is needed. In a pain clinic this approach is excellent for frozen shoulders when one can combine physical therapy and active range of motion exercises.

The patient is positioned supine with a pillow under the shoulders. The interscalene groove is found posterior to the sternocleidomastoid (SCM) muscle. The entry point is at the C6 vertebral body in the interscalene groove.

After prep, drape, and local infiltration a 22 gauge, 4-6 cm needle is inserted at the C6 level. The needle is directly medially, slightly posteriorly, and caudally until a paresthesia or nerve stimulator identifies the nerve. After negative aspiration a test dose of local anesthetic with epinephrine is made. A total of 30-40 ml will anesthetize the entire brachial plexus although the lower levels (C8-T1) may be unreliably blocked. Dilute concentrations of local anesthetics can produce effective sensory block and sympathetic denervation without complete motor effects.

Supraclavicular Approach

The nerves of the brachial plexus are compactly arranged as superior, middle, and inferior trunks at the level of the supraclavicular space. Their close proximity to each other at this level allows for effective block with less local anesthetic. This makes the supraclavicular approach an excellent choice for intraoperative anesthesia. However, the risk of pneumothorax makes this approach less optimal in some outpatient settings. Also, it may less effective for shoulder block than the interscalene block.

Several approaches have been advocated for the supraclavicular block. Classically, the needle is inserted approximately 1 cm superior to the clavicle at the lateral border of the first rib. The practitioner can stand either at the head of the bed (Bonica's technique) or at the side of the patient (Moore's approach). The needle is directed inferiorly, laterally, and posteriorly. The goal is to reach the brachial plexus trunks as they pass over the first rib. To avoid a pneumothorax the needle should never be directed medially. If the plexus is not contacted initially, the needle is directed in an anterior or posterior gridlike fashion until a paresthesia or twitch is encountered. For a complete block at this level 30 ml suffice.

Infraclavicular Approach

The infraclavicular approach to the brachial plexus is an excellent method for insertion of a catheter for infusion of local anesthetics. This technique, described first by Raj (32), avoids the risk of pneumothorax. The insertion site is 1-2 cm inferior to the clavicle in the middle third of the clavicle. The clinician stands on the opposite side of the brachial plexus to be blocked. The nonoperative arm is placed over the previously prepped axillary artery. Using the axillary artery as a landmark the needle is directed toward the axilla until the brachial plexus is contacted. A nerve stimulator greatly aids in placement of this block.

Once the plexus is found, the needle can be directed alongside the plexus for 2-4 cm prior to threading the catheter. This allows the catheter to stay in contact with the plexus if later movement by the patient results in movement of the catheter. The infraclavicular approach works well for 2-7 day infusions of the brachial plexus because there is usually little movement of the upper chest where the catheter is anchored. Different catheter systems have been used.

Axillary Approach

The axillary block is the most common approach to the brachial plexus for many practitioners. A complete block at this level will denervate the medial, lateral, and posterior cords of the brachial plexus. The block is not adequate for anesthesia of the shoulder and can also miss the musculocutaneous nerve which often exits from the plexus above the level of the axilla. The block is preferred because of its ease to perform and the decreased risk of side effects such as pneumothorax. Like other approaches to the brachial plexus nerve injury, infection, intravascular injection, and hematomas can result with this approach. Catheters can be inserted via this approach and left for several days although movement of the axilla may increase the risk of catheter dislodgment compared to the infraclavicular approach. Theoretically, infection may be greater with prolonged infusions because of the nature of the axilla.

The axillary approach requires the patient to abduct the shoulder to approximately 90^0. In normal patients this is easily done but can be difficult in patients with disorders of the shoulder or upper extremity. The axilla is prepped and draped sterilely. The axillary artery is palpated and marked with an indelible pen to facilitate knowledge of its location. A 22-23 gauge, 3-6 cm needle is inserted near the apex of the axilla. A short bevel needle may avoid trauma to the nerve, although it may cause increased trauma if an intraneural injection occurs (33).

The axillary artery is the main anatomic landmark used in the axillary approach. If anesthesia/analgesia of the ulnar nerve is necessary the needle is inserted below the artery to block the medial cord. If the radial nerve is required then locating the posterior cord would be sought. A complete median nerve block would necessitate both the lateral and medial cords to be anesthetized. Location of the individual cords can be done by a paresthesia or nerve stimulator technique. Alternatively, a transarterial approach works because the brachial plexus at this level is encased in a sheath which greatly aids in dispersion of drug to all the cords. Some practitioners prefer injecting two cords or injecting both behind and in front of the axillary artery.

Complications of Brachial Plexus Injections

Each approach to the brachial plexus carries general risks and risks specific to the individual approach. General risks include infection, hematoma or bleeding, intravascular injection, and nerve injury. Patients should have these risks explained prior to the block. Debate exists concerning the paresthesia and nerve stimulator techniques. Selander et al argue that short beveled needles and nerve stimulation techniques decrease the risk of nerve injury (34). However, the paresthesia technique has been performed safely for many decades, and it is doubtful if it has greater risk of nerve injury than any other technique. Regarding nerve injury, the most important consideration centers on good technique. Practitioners have better results if they develop good skills with their hands, use needles prudently with no unnecessary movements, and understand the anatomy at the site of blockade.

Risks and complications of brachial plexus blockade exist which are specific to the approach used. The interscalene approach can produce either epidural or intrathecal injection if the needle is inserted too far. Epidural injections often do not produce a total block. Often respiratory embarassment or subjective complaints of respiratory insufficiency occur. Cerebrospinal fluid should be visible from the needle if it is intrathecal but would not be expected if the needle is in the epidural space. Injection of local anesthetic into the intrathecal space at this level will produce a total spinal block requiring ventilatory support until the block wears off. Intubation can be performed without the need for additional muscle relaxation. Since the patient is likely to feel anxious, assurance may help, and anxiolytics or amnestic agents should be considered.

Intravascular injection into the carotid or vertebral artery can occur with the interscalene approach. This risk is minimized with adequate and repeated aspiration during injection. Only a small amount of local anesthetic is required into these vessels to cause CNS symptoms. If a seizure occurs ventilation and oxygenation should be the primary concern. In most cases the amount of local anesthetic injected is small, the symptoms are noticed immediately, and the seizure is short-lived. Supportive measures usually suffice.

At the level of the supraclvicular space the brachial plexus trunks lie relatively close to the dome of the lung. The risk of pneumothorax has been reported to range from <1% to >10% in different reports.(35,36) These differences, in part, may result from the experience and skill of the practitioner. If performed properly the needle should not be directed medially toward the lung but laterally as it probes for the plexus. Nonetheless, all patients should be advised of this risk and the potential morbidity and mortality if it is not recognized and treated.

Outpatients should have discharge instructions which can be reviewed later if symptoms develop. It is optimal for the practitioner to oversee the management of this complication unless the patient is unable to return to the treating facility or the corresonding emergency department. Consultation with a pulmonologist is often prudent. Small pneumothoraces can be watched and almost all can be treated with one-way valve catheters.

The subclavian artery is located near the brachial plexus trunks at the supraclavicular space. There are usually no sequelae following puncture with a small needle. However, in patients with a bleeding disorder or if a large bore needle and catheter system is used significant bleeding may result. Unfortunately, it is difficult or impossible to place direct pressure over the subclavian artery at this location. Blood may pass into the thoracic cavity. In susceptible patients an alternative approach should be considered.

No specific risks exist for the infraclavicular or axillary approach. General risks noted above should be addressed during the informed consent process. Prolonged catheterization at these sites increases the risk of infection, and prophylactic antibiotics might be considered for some patients. Intravascular injection at the axillary level might not be as readily discernible as the interscalene approach allowing a much larger volume of injected local anesthetic prior to detection. Cardiovascular and CNS side effects may result.

Lower Extremity Blocks

In many pain centers lower extremity blocks are not utilized as frequently as upper extremity blocks. The nerves to the upper extremity are concisely arranged and travel together for a relatively long distance. Nerves of the lower extremity are somewhat together at the lumbar and lumbosacral plexuses, but complete denervation to the lower extremity is problematic via any single approach. Several of the more frequently blocked lower extremity nerves will be discussed here (for a more complete presentation see 4-7).

Lateral Femoral Cutaneous Nerve Block

The lateral femoral cutaneous nerve is composed of branches from the L2-3 nerves. Injury of this nerve can result in meralgia paresthetica. Chronic pain from the lateral femoral cutaneous nerve can arise from constricting clothing such as tight jeans. The nerve is occasionally injured during a protracted childbirth. Pain is observed down the lateral aspect of the thigh. The differential diagnosis includes stretch of the ilial tibial band or tensor fascia lata.

Block of the lateral femoral cutaneous nerve is readily performed as it comes around the anterior iliac spine. The patient is prepped, and a 22-23 gauge needle is inserted 2 cm medial and inferior to the superior aspect of the anterior iliac spine. A field block technique or a nerve stimulator can be used. A series of 4-6 blocks with local anesthetics, physical therapy, and a change to less tight fitting clothes cures the condition in many patients.

Femoral Nerve Block

The femoral nerve arises from posterior divisions of the anterior trunks of the L2-4 nerve roots. The femoral, lateral femoral cutaneous, and obturator nerves form the lumbar plexus within the psoas muscle. The obturator nerve forms from anterior divisions of the anterior trunks of L2-4 and the lateral femoral cutaneous nerve comes from L2-3.

The femoral nerve can be injured directly where it passes beneath the inguinal ligament at the groin. This can occur from constriction of the ligament, from a large femoral hernia, secondary to herniorraphy surgery, or through stab wounds to the back and during childbirth. The femoral nerve is also reponsible for much of the sensation within the knee joint, and pain from the knee is often transmitted through the femoral nerve. Block of the femoral nerve can be combined with physical therapy if adequate range of motion has not been regained after knee arthroplasty.

Block of the femoral nerve is most commonly performed at the inguinal ligament. The patient is sterilely prepped and a 22-23 gauge, 3-6 cm needle is inserted lateral to the palpable femoral artery and inferior to the inguinal ligament. The nerve lies outside the sheath cointaining the femoral artery such that a needle can be positioned within the sheath, outside the artery, and preclude effective distribution of drug to the nerve. The nerve has usually divided into numerous branches at this location which makes obtaining a paresthesia difficult. A nerve stimulator works well, and the twitch should be sought near the knee and not at the groin. Effective block is provided by 10-15 ml of solution. Outpatients should be instructed not to attempt walking after this block until full sensation and motor strength have returned.

Femoral Plexus Block

The femoral plexus is formed from the anterior divisions of the L2-4 nerve roots. The plexus is found in the psoas muscle. While the femoral plexus rarely is injured directly—

penetrating trauma or tumor—the nerves of the plexus often transmit chronic pain from a variety of origins.

The lumbar plexus is blocked via a posterior approach. The patient is positioned prone and prepped sterilely. An 8-12 cm, 22 gauge needle is inserted 4-6 cm lateral to the spinous process of the L2 or L3 vertebral body. The needle is inserted perpendicular to the skin. A loss of resistance technique has been used. Alternatively, the transverse process can be located and the needle directed laterally and slightly deeper than the transverse process. A total of 15-20 ml of local anesthetic is injected.

The 3-in-1 block has been described as an alternative method to block the 3 major nerves of the lumbar plexus.[37,38] The block is performed at the inguinal ligament similar to the femoral nerve block. Digital pressure is placed distal to the nerve, and 30-50 ml of local anesthetic are injected. In theory, retrograde flow of local anesthetic flows toward the lumbar plexus effecting a block of L2, L3, and L4. Debate exists about the accuracy of flow after large volume injection at the inguinal ligament.[41] In many patients local anesthetic diffuses easily between the femoral and lateral femoral cutaneous nerve at the inguinal ligament. Often denervation of the obturator nerve is not checked (nor required) with a 3-in-1 block and may be ineffectively blocked.

Sciatic Nerve Block

The sciatic nerve is the largest peripheral nerve in the human body and arises from the L4, L5, S1, and often S2 and S3 nerve roots. Innervation includes the posterior thigh and everything below the knee excepting the medial aspect of the leg (saphenous nerve). The sciatic nerve can be blocked at several sites including the buttock and posterior thigh [4-7].

The classic approach to the sciatic nerve is Reid's approach. The patient is positioned in a modified lateral position, and bony landmarks palpated and marked on the skin. The main ones are the greater trochanter, the posterior iliac spine and the sacral cornu. Midway between the posterior iliac spine and the greater trochanter a 2.5 cm line is drawn perpendicular to the original line. This represents the sciatic notch where the sciatic nerve emerges from the pelvis and passes posteriorly. Commonly the sciatic nerve has already split into its two components, the peroneal and tibial nerves.

Depending on the size of the patient a 22 gauge, 9-15 cm needle is inserted. When the nerve is contacted a paresthesia is encountered either in the distribution of the peroneal or tibial nerve. If a nerve stimulator is used a twitch should be seen below the knee. Ten to 15 ml of local anesthetic will denervate the sciatic nerve if the needle is sufficiently close to the nerve.

Other Peripheral Nerve Blocks

Neuromas are frequently encountered in chronic pain patients. These are often blocked for diagnostic and therapeutic reasons. Local anesthetics and corticosteroid preparations are initially employed. More permanent destruction of the neuromatous foci can be done although skin slough and other potential complications should be conveyed to the patient prior to proceeding.

Trigger point injections represent a common nerve block for patients with myofascial pain. They may help patients with acute muscle spasms such as torticollis. In chronic pain patients trigger point injections should be used as part of a multidisciplinary approach. Temporary relief of muscle spasm can enable introducing physical therapy, biofeedback or relaxation therapies.

There are many small peripheral nerves of the upper extremity, lower extremity, and trunk which are often blocked for diagnostic or therapeutic purposes in chronic pain clinics. Their description is beyond the scope of this chapter.

SUMMARY

Interruption of neural information via nerve blocking techniques has proved valuable to regional anesthesiologists during intraoperative and postoperative management of patients and for chronic pain practitioners. Perioperative management with nerve blocks and epidural catheters has gained wide acceptance and decreases the morbidity and mortality risks in subsets of surgical patients. The role of nerve blocks in chronic pain is both diagnostic and therapeutic.

REFERENCES

[1]   Yaksh TL, Rudy TA. Analgesia mediated by a direct spinal action of narcotics. *Science* 1976; 192: 1357-8.

[2]   Stenseth R, Sellevold O, Breivik H. Epidural morphine for postoperative pain: experience with 1085 patients. *Acta Anaesthesiol Scand* 1985; 29: 148-156.

[3]   Rawal N, Sjostrand, Christoffersson M, et al. Comparison of intramuscular and epidural morphine for postoperative analgesia in the grossly obese: Influence on postoperative ambulation and pulmonary function. *Anesth Analg* 63: 583-92, 1984.

[4]   Raj PP. Textbook of Regional Anesthesia, NY, Churchill Livingstone, 2002.

[5]   Jankovic D and Wells C. Regional Nerve Blocks, Edinburgh, Blackwell, 2001.

[6]   Cousins MJ and Bridenbaugh PO. Neural Blockade in Clinical Anesthesia and Management of Pain, 2nd edition, Philadelphia, J.B. Lippincott Co., 1988.

[7]   Chelly JE. Peripheral Nerve Blocks: A Color Atlas, Philadelphia, Lippincott Williams and Wilkins, 1999.

[8]   Gunther B. Karl Koller: Centennial of the discovery of local analgesia (1884). *Rev Med Chil.* 1984; 112: 1181-5.

[9]   Mourisse J, Hasenbos MAWM, Gielen MJM, Moll JE, Cromheecke GJE. Epidural bupivacaine, sufentanil or the combination for post-thoracotomy pain. *Acta Anesthesiol Scand* 1992; 36: 70-4.

[10]   Scheinen B, Asantila R, Orko R. The effect of bupivacaine and morphine on pain and bowel function after colonic surgery. *Acta Anaes Scand* 1987; 31: 161-4.

[11] Gastafsson LL, Schildt B, Jacobsen K. Adverse effects of extradural and intrathecal opiates: Report of a nationwide survey in Sweden. *Br J Anaesth* 1982; 54: 479-86

[12] Moore AK, Vilderman S, Lubenskyi W, McCans J, Fox GS. Differences in epidural morphine requirements between elderly and young patients after abdominal surgery. *Anesth Analg* 1990; 70: 316-20.

[13] Halpern S, Preston R. Postdural puncture headache and spinal needle design. *Anesthesiology.* 1994; 81: 1376-83.

[14] Lybecker H, Moller JT, May O, Nielsen HK. Incidence and prediction of postdural puncture headache: A prospective study of 1021 spinal anesthetics. *Anesth Analg* 1990; 70: 389-94.

[15] Brownridge P. The management of headache following accidental dural puncture in obstetric patients. *Anaesth Intensive Care* 1983; 11: 4-15.

[16] Kafiluddi R, Hahn MB. Epidural Neural Blockade, In *Practical Management of Pain*. Ed. Raj PP, 3rd edition, Mosby, St. Louis, 2000, 648-9.

[17] Vandermeulen EP, Van Aken H, Vermylen J. Anticoagulants and spinal-epidural anesthesia. *Anesth Analg* 1994; 79: 1165-77.

[18] Malmqvist ELA, Bengtsson M, Sorensen J. Efficacy of stellate ganglion block: A clinical study with bupivacaine. *Reg Anesth* 1992; 17: 340-7.

[19] Hogan QH, Erickson SJ, Haddox JD, Abram SE. The spread of solutions during stellate ganglion block. *Reg Anesth* 1992; 17: 78-83.

[20] Czop CL, Rauck RL, Koman LA, et al. Sympathetic denervation to the upper extremity in CRPS: Stellate ganglion block vs interpleural block. *Anesthesiology* 1997; 87: A754.

[21] Rykowski JJ, Hilgier M. Efficacy of neurolytic celiac plexus block in varying locations of pancreatic cancer: Influence on pain relief. Anesth 2000; 92: 347-54

[22] Brown DL, Bulley CK, Quiel EL. Neurolytic celiac plexus block for pancreatic cancer pain. *Anesth Analg* 1987; 66: 869-73.

[23] Ischia S, Ischia A, Polati E, Finco G. Three posterior percutaneous celiac plexus block techniques. *Anesthesiology* 1992; 76: 534-40.

[24] Bridenbaugh LD, Moore DC, Campbell DC. Management of upper abdominal cancer pain. Treatment with celiac plexus block with alcohol. *JAMA* 1964; 190: 877-80

[25] Moore DC. Celiac (splanchnic) plexus block with alcohol for cancer pain of the upper intra-abdominal viscera. *Adv Pain Res Ther* 1979; 2: 357-71.

[26] Yamamuro M, Kusaka K, Kato M, Takahashi M. Celiac plexus block in cancer pain management. *Tohoku J Exp Med* 2000; 192: 1-18.

[27] Cousins MJ, Reeve TS, Glynn CJ, Walsh JA, Cherry DA. Neurolytic lumbar sympathetic blockade: Duration of denervation and relief of rest pain. *Anaesth Intens Care* 1979; 7: 121-35.

[28] Plancarte R, Amescua C, Patt RB, Aldrete JA. Superior hypogastric plexus block for pelvic cancer pain. *Anesthesiology* 1990; 73: 236-9.

[29] Hecker BR, Fjurstrom R, Schoene RB. Effect of intercostals nerve blockade on respiratory mechanics and CO_2 chemosensitivity at rest and exercise. *Anesthesiology* 1989; 70: 13-20.

[30] Tucker GT, Moore DC, Bridenbaugh PO et al. Systemic absorption of mepivacaine in commonly used regional block procedures. *Anes* 1972; 37: 276-80.

[31] Purcell-Jones G, Pither CE, Justins DM. Paravertebral somatic nerve block: a clinical, radiographic, and computed tomographic study in chronic pain patients. *Anesth Analg* 1989; 68: 32-9.

[32] Raj PP, Montgomery SJ, Nettles D, et al. Infraclavicular brachial plexus block: A new approach. *Anesth Analg* 1973; 52: 887-904.

[33] Auroy Y, Narchi P, Messiah A, et al. Serious complications related to regional anesthesia: Results of a prospective survey in France. *Anesth* 1997; 87: 479-86.

[34] Selander D, Dhuner KG, Lundberg G. Peripheral nerve injury due to injection needles used for regional anesthesia. *Acta Anaesth Scand* 1977; 21: 182-5.

[35] Brown DL, Cahill DR, Bridenbaugh LD. Supraclavicular nerve block: Anatomic analysis of a method to prevent pneumothorax. *Anesth Analg* 1993;76:530-4.

[36] Weaver MA, Tandatnick CA, Hahn MB. Peripheral Nerve Blockade In *Textbook of Regional Anesthesia* Ed Raj PP, Churchill Livingstone, NY, 2002.

[37] Winnie AP, Ramamurthy S, Durrani Z. The inguinal paravascular technique of lumbar plexus anesthesia: The "3-in-1 block." *Anesth Analg* 1973; 52: 989-96.

[38] Tarkkila P, Tuominen M, Huhtala J, Lindgren L. Comparison of intrathecal morphine and continuous femoral 3-in-1 block for pain after major knee surgery under spinal anesthesia. *Eur J Anesthesiol* 1998; 15: 6-9.

In: The Handbook of Chronic Pain   ISBN 978-1-60021-044-0
Editors: S. Kreitler, D. Beltrutti, et al., pp. 229-246   © 2007 Nova Science Publishers, Inc.

Chapter 14

The Neurosurgical Approach to Chronic Pain

Zvi Harry Rappaport

INTRODUCTION

The neurosurgeon's involvement in the management of chronic pain patients, after a decade of decline, has shown a resurgence of interest. Pain specialists have developed a multidisciplinary approach including potent novel pharmacological agents that have significantly advanced the comfort of cancer patients in particular. There has been a shift away from destructive neural procedures with their replacement by intrathecal drug delivery systems and nervous system stimulation.

The past has seen a multitude of neurosurgical procedures the mechanism of which were often poorly understood and their long-term efficacy of dubious benefit. The pathophysiology of many chronic pain syndromes was poorly understood, creating difficulty in matching an appropriate surgical stratagem for treatment. The advances in recent years in our understanding of pain states have led to a more scientific approach to the surgical procedures available for treatment. Thus, the neurosurgeon is reassuming a more important role in the management of selected chronic pain syndromes. [14;15;79].

CLASSIFICATION OF CHRONIC PAIN FROM A SURGICAL PERSPECTIVE

Patients with chronic pain that are amenable to surgical therapy can be categorized into those with nociceptive pain such as cancer or spondylosis and those suffering from elements of deafferentation or central pain, such phantom pain or root avulsion injuries. The proper characterization of the pain entity, which is beyond the scope of this chapter, is critical in deciding upon the appropriate procedure.

A patient may be referred to a neurosurgeon with a so-called failed back syndrome. Is his pain related to a possibly occult segmental instability, discitis, continued neural compression or is he suffering from deafferentation pain secondary to chronic arachnoiditis? The type of pain pattern, the clinical examination, and a review of electromyographic and radiological studies will allow the neurosurgeon to choose the appropriate therapy. This may range from a reexploration of the operative site to a fusion procedure, or in cases of deafferentation, spinal cord stimulation.

Some pain syndromes contain both elements of nociception and deafferentation. A patient suffering from brachial plexus pain following radiation therapy for cancer involvement may describe sharp lancinating pains on top of a steady dull vice-like background pain. A dorsal root entry zone (DREZ) lesion would be expected to ameliorate the lancinating pain without affecting the background pain.

Trigeminal neuralgia is one of the chronic pain syndromes most amenable to therapy. On the other hand, atypical facial pain rarely responds to surgical intervention. The patient's description of his pain is crucial in making the diagnosis. If the pain is constant, crosses the midline, or is accompanied by significant numbness, partial trigeminal rhizolysis or microvascular decompression of the nerve root will probably be of no value.

This emphasis on the thorough evaluation of the painful phenomenology is the key to a successful neurosurgical approach to the patient. The neurosurgeon must remind himself of his limitations in the treatment of certain types of pain syndromes, especially those of central origin and when the etiology is obscure. Only by a meticulous patient selection process, can an appropriate risk/benefit ration of a specific neurosurgical procedure be established.

CLASSIFICATION OF NEUROSURGICAL PROCEDURES

Surgical stratagems may be divided into three classes (Table 1):

1. Structural surgery, such as debulking of a mass lesion, microvascular decompression of the trigeminal root, or decompressing an impinged spinal root.
2. Augmentative or neuro-modulation surgery: This includes electrical stimulation of brain, spinal cord, and peripheral nerves. Implantation of intrathecal drug delivery systems may also be included in this category.
3. Destructive or ablative surgery, in which neural tissue form the peripheral nerve through the spinal root, spinal cord, and the brain itself is damaged.

Wherever possible, structural surgery should be used to relieve chronic pain of nociceptive origin, such as in cancer [73]. It is contingent upon identifying the anatomical basis of the pain. By treating the cause of the pain process, especially if it is not of long-standing duration, pain may be relieved, without compromising neural function. If the disease process has, however, caused neural damage, the patient may be left with a deafferentation pain syndrome. Chronic radicular compression by a herniated disc may give rise to a dermatomal dysesthesia, which does not improve following decompressive surgery. In general the longer the duration of the nociceptive pain, the less likelihood for the patient to be pain-free following structural surgery.

The procedure of second choice is augmentative surgery, such as electrical neural stimulation and intrathecal drug delivery systems. It is used in both nociceptive and in deafferentation pain. Its advantage lies in it being a limited surgical procedure that can be performed under minor anesthesia. In addition, it is reversible. The disadvantage is in its high cost (now some 12,000$ for a fully implantable spinal cord stimulation kit) and rather burdensome follow-up requirements. Implanted neuro-augmentative systems require frequent fine-tuning, tend to break and loose their effectiveness with time. There is also a psychological cost for some patients, who have difficulty coping with the concept of being dependent on such a device for their well being.

Ablative procedures are among the oldest neurosurgical operations. They literally extend from toe to head. Proceeding up the neural axis, we start from neurectomy and sympathectomy to rhizotomy and DREZ. In the cephalic direction, there is cordotomy, mesencephalotomy, thalamotomy, and finally psychosurgery. These procedures have been most efficacious in intractable nociceptive pain, such as in metastatic cancer disease with limited life expectancy. While also widely utilized in the past for deafferentation pain, ablative procedures are not considered very effective in most of the latter pain syndromes. It is unreasonable to expect a pain condition arising from neural tissue damage to respond to additional neural tissue destruction. Furthermore by creating further deafferentation, painful dysthesthetic pain commonly developes after a latency period of several months to a year or two. This phenomenon certainly limits the applicability of ablative surgery in cases of benign chronic pain with a prolonged life expectancy. Exceptional responses of specific deafferentation pain syndromes to ablative procedures will be elaborated upon in the following sections [70].

CHRONIC PAIN SYNDROMES AMENABLE TO NEUROSURGICAL INTERVENTION

Patients with a wide spectrum of chronic pain syndromes are referred for neurosurgical evaluation. In only a minority of them is neurosurgical intervention appropriate. Patient selection depends on the diagnosis and the demonstration of pathology appropriate to the pain entity. Specific and appropriate drug therapy must have been shown inefficacious. Psychiatric or personality disorders as well as issues of permanent gain should be excluded. Finally, testing of the proposed procedure should be performed where possible. This may include bracing prior to a spinal fusion, anesthetic blocks of neural structures that are to be ablated, or a trial stimulation period prior to electrode implantation for electrical stimulation.

In the following section, we shall detail the approach to the more common chronic pain conditions that respond to neurosurgical intervention (Table 2).

CANCER PAIN

Intrathecal Morphine

Local tumor resection often provides significant pain relief for the patient, even if lacking oncologic value. This is especially true when there is spinal or brachial plexus metastatic involvement [73]. When oral and systemic narcotics are no longer effective, intrathecal spinal morphine can achieve pain relief without sedation [19;51]. An implantable pump system for continuous delivery may be considered if the patient is expected to survive more than 6 months [11;38]. For upper body, head and neck pain morphine may be administered by an intraventricular access system[33].

Ablative Procedures

Ablative neurosurgery in cancer pain has been largely replaced by intraspinal morphine. For those patients with segmental pain or who are unresponsive to intrathecal drug delivery, destructive operations are still useful. Sacral rhizotomy in the incontinent patient is a typical example. Rhizotomies may be performed percutaneously with radiofrequency (RF) heating electrodes under local anesthesia. Although easy to perform more than half the patients will develop anesthesia dolorosa in the affected area following several months. Rhizotomy should therefore be limited to patients with an estimated survival of three months or less [54]. For more diffuse unilateral pain, percutaneous RF cordotomy via a lateral C1-2 puncture provides pain relief [22;73]. The life expectancy of the patient should not exceed 9-12 months. After this time, the development of dysesthetic deafferentation pain becomes a problem. For bilateral diffuse pain, the high cervical cordotomy may be paired with an open contralateral open thoracic cordotomy. Bilateral high cervical cordotomy entails the unacceptable risk of sleep apnea, the so-called *Ondine's curse*. Bilateral cordotomy, even if performed at different spinal levels risks the loss of urinary continence by disturbing descending sphincter controlling sacral fibers [66].

For pelvic metastatic pain, thoracolumbar mid-line commissural myelotomy provides effective pain relief with a lesser risk to sphincter control. In this procedure, midline decussating pain fibers proceeding on to the anterolateral spinal tract are severed [15].

Specific ablative procedures have been found useful for certain pain pictures. In brachial plexus metastatic involvement or radiation induced brachial plexopathy DREZ RF spinal cord lesions have alleviated pain in a large percentage of cases [29;84]. More recently introduced techniques, CT guided percutaneous extralemniscal myelotomy and trigeminal tractotomy, have been successful for visceral pain and head and neck pain respectively [22].

CRANIOFACIAL PAIN

Trigeminal Neuralgia

Of all chronic pain syndromes trigeminal neuralgia is one of the most gratifying conditions to treat. Virtually all patients will respond at least initially to drug therapy (carbamazepine). Approximately half of the patients will eventually require neurosurgical intervention, being due to drug intolerance, side effects or drug failure. Three categories of interventional therapy are available: peripheral neurectomy, percutaneous rhizotomy, and open microvascular root decompression or rhizotomy. Stimulation of the trigeminal root is an investigational procedure and is rarely utilized in cases of refractory facial pain [82]. Gamma knife radiation therapy of the trigeminal neuralgia has recently been introduced. It suffers from a long latency period until pain relief sets in and its long-term follow-up is only presently being compiled [28;83].

A) Peripheral Neurectomy

In elderly fragile patients peripheral neurectomy especially of the suprorbital and infraorbital nerves provides effective pain relief within an approximately 12 month time frame [42;52]. Local dense anesthesia, the later development of dysesthesia, and the high long-term recurrence rate make this procedure unattractive for the patient with a longer life expectancy.

B) Percutaneous Trigeminal Rhizotomy

Three methods are commonly used: RF rhizolysis[40;77], retrogasserian glycerol injection[12;21;59], and trigeminal root balloon compression[5]. A percutaneous puncture of the foramen ovale is performed under fluoroscopic guidance (Fig. 1). Partial damage to the nerve root and ganglion is achieved by either heating (RF), chemically (glycerol), or by compression (balloon).

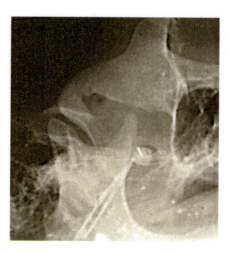

Figure 1. A fluoroscopic view of the foramen ovale with a spinal needle having been introduced percutaneously.

RF rhizolysis is the most senior of the three percutaneous procedures. The end-point of the procedure is obtaining an area of decreased sensation in the painful facial area. Patient cooperation during the stimulation testing procedure is important and is not readily obtained in some elderly patient. The recurrence rate is lower than the other two procedures; however the incidence of painful dysesthesia may be greater. For ophthalmic branch neuralgia, the risk of corneal hypesthesia is lower with the alternative procedures[15;74].

Glycerol rhizolysis does not require patient cooperation and has a lower incidence of facial dysesthesia. As it has a higher recurrence rate (70% of patients pain free at 1 year follow-up) than RF rhizolysis, repeat procedures may be necessary leading to the subsequent development of dysesthesia[58].

Balloon compression of the trigeminal root has a success rate intermediate between the previous two procedures. It entails a higher incidence of masticator dysfunction. As a large bore needle must be used for insertion, general anesthesia may be required making it less appealing in the authors eyes[10].

All three procedures are ablative in nature. As in any procedure that causes damage to the nervous system the danger of developing deafferentation pain exists. For the younger patient without significant medical risks a microvascular decompression procedure may be more appropriate for the long-term as it treats the structural cause of the pain producing pathology without damaging the nerve root.[57;76].

C) Microvascular Decompression

Most cases of trigeminal neuralgia are caused by vascular compression of the trigeminal root entry zone at the pons[20]. It is, however, important to exclude other causes of trigeminal neuralgia such as tumors compressing the trigeminal root (7% of cases) or multiple sclerosis (2% of cases) by performing an MRI scan prior to surgery.

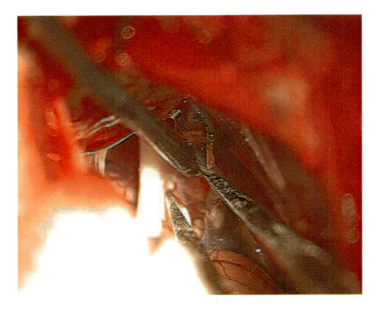

Figure 2. A view of the upper right cerebello-pontine angle. A compressing blood vessel (blue) is being separated from the trigeminal nerve root (white).

The advantage of this procedure lies in the resolution of the causative pathology and cessation of the pain without causing nerve root damage. Sensory deafferentation phenomena are thereby avoided. The initial success rate is in the order of 90% and the recurrence rate is of the order of 2% per year[2;36;71]. These outcome results are better than those obtained in percutaneous rhizotomies. The outcome is dependent on the zeal and the skill with which the surgeon can find the offending artery (Fig. 2). In cases where no definite arterial compression is visualized, a topographically appropriate partial sensory rhizotomy is performed[3;26]. The morbidity of the surgery should be within 4%. This low morbidity and virtually zero mortality are achieved by limiting the operation to patients less than 70 years of age and who do not suffer from major systemic diseases. In the older, high-risk patient, the percutaneous procedures would be more appropriate[57].

GLOSSOPHARYNGEAL NEURALGIA

Patients with glossopharyngeal neuralgia present with a frequency of less than 1% when compared to trigeminal neuralgia sufferers. Their clinical manifestations, moreover, are more variable. Generally pain is felt unilaterally in the throat region while swallowing or speaking. Autonomic manifestations such as syncope or bradycardia leading even to asystole are most dramatic manifestations of the syndrome. Surgical therapy in medically refractory patients can be expected to lead to good results in a high percentage of patients. Classically a glossopharyngeal open rhizotomy is performed with the addition of an upper third vagal rhizotomy. Complications include difficulty in swallowing with or without hoarseness [15]. In the seventies percutaneous RF rhizotomy via the pars nervosa of the jugular foramen gained popularity and became the procedure of choice. Bradycardia and vocal cord paralysis are the risks of this procedure [75]. As with trigeminal neuralgia, microvascular decompression has been successful in relieving glossopharyngeal neuralgia pain. Some authors routinely perform a rhizotomy following the vascular decompression [75]. Others have found that this is not necessary and have achieved long-term pain relief in over 75% of patients with minimal permanent side effects[27;62;71]. Percutaneous CT-guided RF trigeminal nucleotomy-tractotomy has recently been described as useful for complex cases [23]

Occipital Neuralgia

A common cause of medically intractable headache is occipital neuralgia. A diagnostic anesthetic block of the greater occipital nerve precedes referral for surgical intervention. The long-term results of classic occipital neurectomy have been unsatisfactory in general experience. Recurrent occipital neuralgia and deafferentation pain of the posterior scalp is frequently encountered. Modern surgical therapy has therefore switched to a more proximal target. The association with post-traumatic cervical spondylotic changes has led to decompression procedures of the C2-3 nerve roots in their foraminal course with some success[56]. More recently C1-3 intradural partial sensory rhizotomies [8;18] and C2 ganglionectomy[72] has been championed. While the reported results seem promising, the long-term results must still be evaluated before embracing these ablative procedures.

Cluster Headache

The medical treatment of cluster headaches has improved with the introduction of serotoninergic drugs. A substantial number of patients, however, continue to be intractable to therapy. RF ablation of the sphenopalatine ganglion has been useful in episodic cluster headaches, but unsuccessful in chronic patients[67]. Trigeminal rhizotomy may lead to corneal anesthesia and has an inconsistent beneficial effect[24;41]. It is doubtful whether section of the nervus intermedius improves outcome[41;64].

Percutaneous RF trigeminal rhizotomy is a less invasive procedure and has been successfully used for pain around the eye. Major pain in the malar and temporal area responded poorly[78]. Considering the disabling consequences of the accompanying corneal hypesthesia, glycerol trigeminal rhizolysis may be the initial invasive procedure of choice[17;68].

Atypical Facial Pain

Atypical facial pain is a poorly defined clinical entity that has a large variety of potential causes. It is one of the most difficult chronic pain entities to treat. Consequently, patients have been subjected to a large variety of surgical procedures ranging from local neurectomies to cerebral ablative procedures[15]. Success rates have varied greatly reflecting the lack of homogeneity of the patient population. Surgical procedures should not be performed if the pathophysiology of the pain syndrome remains obscure. In cases of trigeminal neuropathic pain, stimulation of the trigeminal root via a transoval percutaneously implanted electrode has shown some success, relieving pain in about half of the treated patients[82]. Movement of the electrode due to mastication limits the technical success rate of implantation. With technological improvements of the stimulation system, the utilization of this non-destructive procedure may entity [44]. Destructive lesions of the spinal trigeminal nucleus [6;13] should be viewed become more widespread. Motor cortex stimulation has recently shown some success in this as a therapy of last resort in non-malignant chronic facial pain.

FAILED BACK SYNDROME

Patients with chronic lower back and leg pain, following "failed" back surgery represent a significant proportion of the chronic pain clinic population. So-called failures include a variety of causes: Improper diagnosis with the in the a priori absence of a surgically correctable cause of the pain, psychological phenomena such as secondary gain, and bona fide pathophysiology such as instability, infection, persistent radicular compression and scarring. Traditionally reoperation has been met with a high failure rate that reaches up to two thirds of cases [45]. Accurate clinical correlation with ancillary diagnostic tests may improve the outcome of structural pain surgery in this syndrome. In cases, where root damage has already been established such as arachnoidal scarring, neuromodulation procedures are of value.

Spinal Cord Stimulation

Spinal cord stimulation has in the past been viewed as a "last resort" procedure for the failed back syndrome. However, with the introduction of programmable, multi-channel electrode arrays that can be inserted percutaneously, the efficacy of stimulation has improved considerably[7;30;35;46;50]. The procedure is mainly indicated for radiating leg pain, being rather ineffective for purely midline skeletal pain. Preoperative psychological screening has been found useful to increase the positive outcome rate[49]. The electrode is inserted percutaneously under local anesthesia. It is left in place if the paresthesia evoked by stimulation cover the area of radicular pain. Trial stimulation via an externalized lead wire is helpful in further selecting those patients most likely to benefit from the programmable internalized stimulator, which is rather expensive[49]. Two side by side electrodes may be implanted for bilateral radicular pain.

Ablative Surgery

As mentioned previously rhizotomy leads to very limited short-term pain relief as dysesthetic pain develops in a substantial number of patients following the procedure. A modification of this technique, dorsal root ganglionectomy has been tried to include afferent pain fibers that enter the spinal cord via the anterior roots. Here too results have been unrewarding[48].

Percutaneous RF facet denervation is used for the treatment of mechanical low-back pain. Following local anesthetic test blocks of the facet joint, which is a positive predictor of outcome, bilateral multilevel thermal lesions are made under fluoroscopic guidance at painful lumbar levels. The procedure's long-term efficacy rate is less than 50% both in virginal and in operated back patients. Being an essentially risk free outpatient procedure its selective use may still be warranted[47].

PAIN OF SPINAL CORD AND ROOT ORIGIN

Posttraumatic Pain

Following spinal cord injury, a variety of pain syndromes may coexist. Before considering specialized pain procedures, spinal osseous deformities and posttraumatic syringomyelia should be looked for and treated when appropriate. Therapeutic interventions may only target part of the pain symptomatology. In general segmental sharp, lancinating pain responds favorably to DREZ lesions of the cord [60;69], whereas chronic burning pain that is diffusely distributed responds poorly and inconsistently to surgery. Spinal cord stimulation has been notably unsuccessful in this type of pain. In paraplegic patients, cordectomy can relieve lancinating pains mainly in the lower cord. Again the steady, burning pain is unlikely to be affected [53;70;80].

Brachial Plexus Avulsion

Both the sharp lancinating aspect and the steady burning component of brachial plexus avulsion pain responds favorably to DREZ lesions[60;81]. Long-term satisfactory outcomes in over half the patients treated, makes this the procedure of choice in traumatic brachial plexus injury. The most extensive has been presented by Nashold's group[61]. Following laminectomy and opening of the dura mater, a RF electrode is inserted into the postero-lateral spinal sulcus in multiple adjacent sites and thermocoagulative lesions are created within the posterior spinal horn. An alternative surgical approach is utilized by Sindou [69]. Incisions are made into the posterior spinal horn at the dorsal root entry zone using a small blade with optical magnification. This procedure has also been successfully utilized in the spastic painful limb. Favorable results of this technique have been reported for lumbosacral plexus avulsions[39]. Pain producing plexus pathologies of other origins such as following radiation therapy or inflammation have poorer treatment outcomes[29;84].

Postherpetic Neuralgia

Surgical procedures for the relief of postherpetic neuralgia pain have generally been ineffective. Dorsal root rhizotomy and ganglionectomy have not resulted in consistent pain relief. Only a few authors have been satisfied with the results of spinal cord stimulation, and the procedure is not widely used for this condition[37]. DREZ lesions were performed for a number of years in treating postherpetic pain. The long-term efficacy does not justify its general recommendation in this entity. RF trigeminal nucleotomy has however shown long-term effectiveness in postherpetic facial pain and presents a viable option for refractory cases[4;9].

PERIPHERAL NERVOUS SYSTEM PAIN

Phantom Limb Pain

Chronic pain developing after limb amputation may be divided into stump related pathology and into a central pain phenomenon commonly called phantom limb pain. The former is generally dealt with by surgical reposition of the stump neuroma or local resection of the neuroma with fascicular ligation. Phantom pain is a more difficult problem to deal with. DREZ lesions have generally been unsuccessful for lower extremity phantom pain, but is useful in brachial plexus injuries[39;60]. Spinal cord stimulation has been most extensively applied. However, only some 50% will pass the trial stimulation period. Of those implanted, a long-term favorable outcome is obtained in another half of the patients[30;79]. When effective the stimulation system is used by the patient over years, and a dramatic improvement in his quality of life is obtained. Recently there have been reports to the effectiveness of motor cortex stimulation [65]. A wider experience is needed before this still experimental procedure can be recommended.

Post-Thoracotomy Pain

Chronic incisional pain following thoracotomy or mastectomy does not respond effectively to surgical treatment. Rhizotomy, RF intecostal neurectomy, ganglionectomy and DREZ lesions all have unsatisfactory records of accomplishment in this condition. Electrical stimulation of the affected nerves has shown some promise[55].

Pain After Peripheral Nerve Injury and Causalgia

Peripheral nerve injury especially in the upper extremity may give rise to chronic pain. Local exploration with untethering and external neurolysis is occasionally effective. Electrical nerve stimulation is initially effective in some two thirds of patients that have been screened by transcutaneous nerve stimulation. The long-term success rate of chronically implanted stimulation systems falls off to less than half in many clinical series[32;43]. The implantation is problematic in the lower extremity due to the involved movements. Technical improvements in electrode design and fixation may improve the success rate of this promising technique in the future[35].

Causalgia with accompanying reflex sympathetic dystrophy responds to sympathectomy[1]. The complex pathophysiology of this condition and the variability among the clinical syndromes treated creates difficulty in assessing the results of sympathectomy. The condition must be differentiated from chronic deafferentation pain, which can coexist.

PAIN AFTER BRAIN INJURY

The most common cause of chronic pain of cerebral origin is the so-called *thalamic syndrome* following a vascular injury (stroke) to the somatosensory tracts in the brain. The patient suffers from contralateral burning pain and hypersensitivity to touch. Stereotactic thalamic ablative procedures have largely been abandoned for in the treatment of chronic central pain. Deep brain stimulation in the postero-lateral nuclei of the thalamus when intact or in the posterior internal capsule also have disappointing long-term results[34] despite the occasional report to the contrary (Fig.3) [16;31;63]. It is here that the novel technique of motor cortex stimulation may have an impact, provided that the corticospinal tracts remain intact [24].

DISCUSSION

This survey of the surgical approaches to chronic pain illustrates the great efforts that neurosurgeons have undertaken to relieve patients from chronic pain and the difficulties in achieving this goal. With the exception of specific conditions such as cancer pain and trigeminal neuralgia, the record of accomplishment of surgical attempts is patchy at best. Yet faced with a patient whose quality of life is virtually non-existent and who may be suicidal, neurosurgeons have attempted pain-relieving procedures based on their anatomical understanding of the neural pathways involved. With the rapidly enlarging knowledge base in the field of pain, more tailored and less invasive forms of therapy have been found. Technological improvements have allowed the non-destructive techniques of intrathecal drug delivery and electrical stimulation to be applied successfully, replacing traditional ablative surgery. A multidisciplinary team approach to the chronic pain patient allows for appropriate screening of the patient.

Psychological evaluation, diagnostic blocks, drug therapy, and minimally invasive procedures should be included in more difficult cases prior to embarking on major surgery, especially if it is ablative. On the other hand, when a well-established surgical procedure is available, it should not be withheld for a lengthy period, turning the patient into a chronic pain invalid. The neurosurgeon must carefully evaluate the risk-benefit ratio of the available surgical options and bear in mind the principle of *primum non nocere*. The neurosurgical armamentarium has an ever evolving but well-defined role in the management of the chronic pain patient.

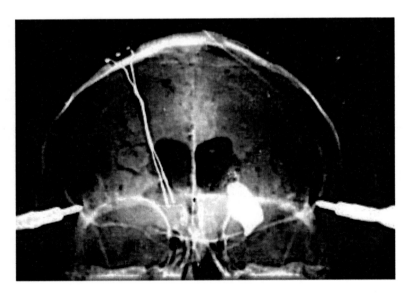

Figure 3. Two electrodes have been implanted in the right thalamus of a patient suffering from post-stroke deafferentation pain.

Table 1. Classification of surgical procedures for pain

Structural	Ablative	Augmentation
Decompressive surgery (spinal, nerve entrapment, microvascular decompression)	Sympathectomy, neurectomy	Electrical stimulation: deep brain, motor cortex, spinal cord, trigeminal root, peripheral nerve
Stabilization	Rhizotomy, rhizolysis ganglionectomy	Intraspinal and intraventricular drugs
Nerve repair and repositioning	DREZ, cordotomy, myelotomy, tractotomy	
	Mesencephalotomy	
	Thalamotomy	
	Cerebral leukotomy/cingulotomy	

Table 2. Chronic pain entities and their surgical therapy

Chronic Pain entity	Indications	Surgical Procedure
Cancer pain	Lower body pain Upper body pain	Spinal intrathecal morphine Intraventricular morphine
	Segmental pain or who are unresponsive to intrathecal drug delivery	Rhizotomy, cordotomy, DREZ lesion
	Visceral pain and head and neck pain	CT guided percutaneous extralemniscal myelotomy and trigeminal tractotomy
Trigeminal neuralgia	Elderly patients and those with high surgical risk	Percutaneous trigeminal rhizotomy (glycerol, RF, balloon compression)
	Patients with low surgical risk	Microvascular decompression
Glossopharyngeal neuralgia	Most patients	Microvascular decompression with or without partial rhizotomy
Occipital neuralgia	Patients that respond to appropriate anesthetic block	C2 ganglionectomy
Cluster headaches	Chronic cases uncontrolled by medication	Trigeminal glycerol rhizolysis
Atypical facial pain	Trigeminal neuropathy Only rarely indicated-	Trigeminal root, motor cortex stimulation Trigeminal tractotomy/nucleotomy
Failed-back syndrome	Preferable to ablative surgery	Spinal cord stimulation
Spinal-cord post-injury pain	Effective for lancinating but not chronic pain.	DREZ lesions
Brachial-plexus avulsion	Procedure of choice	DREZ lesions
Postherpetic neuralgia	May be effective in facial pain	RF trigeminal nucleotomy
Phantom limb pain	For lower limb pain For brachial plexus injuries	Spinal cord, motor cortex stimulation DREZ lesions
Post-thoracotomy pain	Following successful trial of TENS	Electrical stimulation of affected nerves
Peripheral nerve injury		Electrical stimulation of affected nerve
Causalgia	Following sympathetic block	Sympathectomy
Thalamic syndrome	Unreliable efficacy but preferable to ablative procedures	Deep brain and motor cortex stimulation

REFERENCES

[1]   AbuRahma A.F., Robinson P.A., Powell M., Bastug D. and Boland J.P.: Sympathectomy for reflex sympathetic dystrophy: factors affecting outcome. *Ann.Vasc.Surg.*, 8 (1994) 372-379.

[2]   Barker F.G., Jannetta P.J., Bissonette D.J., Larkins M.V. and Jho H.D.: The long-term outcome of microvascular decompression for trigeminal neuralgia. *N.Engl.J.Med.*, 334 (25-4-1996) 1077-1083.

[3]   Bederson J.B., Wilson C.B.: Evaluation of microvascular decompression and partial sensory rhizotomy in 252 cases of trigeminal neuralgia. *J.Neurosurg.*, 71 (1989) 359-367.

[4]   Bernard E.J., Jr., Nashold B.S., Jr., Caputi F. and Moossy J.J.: Nucleus caudalis DREZ lesions for facial pain. *Br.J.Neurosurg.*, 1 (1987) 81-91.

[5]   Brown J.A., Gouda J.J.: Percutaneous balloon compression of the trigeminal nerve. Neurosurg.*Clin.N.Am.*, 8 (1997) 53-62.

[6]   Bullard D.E., Nashold B.S., Jr.: The caudalis DREZ for facial pain. Stereotact.Funct.*Neurosurg.*, 68 (1997) 168-174.

[7]   Burchiel K.J., Anderson V.C., Brown F.D., Fessler R.G., Friedman W.A., Pelofsky S. et al.: Prospective, multicenter study of spinal cord stimulation for relief of chronic back and extremity pain. *Spine.*, 21 (1996) 2786-2794.

[8]   Dubuisson D.: Treatment of occipital neuralgia by partial posterior rhizotomy at C1-3. *J.Neurosurg.*, 82 (1995) 581-586.

[9]   Fox J.L.: Intractable facial pain relieved by percutaneous trigeminal tractotomy. *JAMA*, 218 (1971) 1940-1941.

[10] Fraioli B., Esposito V., Guidetti B., Cruccu G. and Manfredi M.: Treatment of trigeminal neuralgia by thermocoagulation, glycerolization, and percutaneous compression of the gasserian ganglion and/or retrogasserian rootlets: long-term results and therapeutic protocol. *Neurosurgery*, 24 (1989) 239-245.

[11] Gilmer-Hill H.S., Boggan J.E., Smith K.A. and Wagner F.C.J.: Intrathecal morphine delivered via subcutaneous pump for intractable cancer pain: a review of the literature. *Surg.Neurol.*, 51 (1999) 12-15.

[12] Gomori J.M., Rappaport Z.H.: Transovale trigeminal cistern puncture: modified fluoroscopically guided technique. *Am.J.Neuroradiol.*, 6 (1985) 93-94.

[13] Gorecki J.P., Nashold B.S.: The Duke experience with the nucleus caudalis DREZ operation. *Acta Neurochir.Suppl.*(Wien.), 64 (1995) 128-131.

[14] Gybels J.M.: Indications for neurosurgical treatment of chronic pain. *Acta Neurochir.*(Wien.), 116 (1992) 171-175.

[15] Gybels J.M. and Sweet W.H.: Neurosurgical treatment of persistent pain. *Karger*, *Basel*, 1989, 441 pp.

[16] Hariz M.I., Bergenheim A.T.: Thalamic stereotaxis for chronic pain: ablative lesion or stimulation? Stereotact.*Funct.Neurosurg.*, 64 (1995) 47-55.

[17] Hassenbusch S.J., Kunkel R.S., Kosmorsky G.S., Covington E.C. and Pillay P.K.: Trigeminal cisternal injection of glycerol for treatment of chronic intractable cluster headaches. *Neurosurgery*, 29 (1991) 504-508.

[18] Horowitz M.B., Yonas H.: Occipital neuralgia treated by intradural dorsal nerve root sectioning. *Cephalalgia*, 13 (1993) 354-360.

[19] Iacono R.P., Linford J., Sandyk R., Consroe P., Ryan M.R. and Bamford C.R.: Intraspinal opiates for treatment of intractable pain in the terminally ill cancer patient. Int.J.Neurosci., 38 (1988) 111-119.

[20] Jannetta P.J.: Microsurgical approach to the trigeminal nerve for tic doloreux. *Progr.Neurol.Surg.*, 7 (1976) 180-200.

[21] Jho H.D., Lunsford L.D.: Percutaneous retrogasserian glycerol rhizotomy. Current technique and results. *Neurosurg.Clin.N.Am.*, 8 (1997) 63-74.

[22] Kanpolat Y., Caglar S., Akyar S. and Temiz C.: CT-guided pain procedures for intractable pain in malignancy. *Acta Neurochir.Suppl.*(Wien.), 64 (1995) 88-91.

[23] Kanpolat Y., Savas A., Batay F. and Sinav A.: Computed tomography-guided trigeminal tractotomy-nucleotomy in the management of vagoglossopharyngeal and geniculate neuralgias. *Neurosurgery*, 43 (1998) 484-489.

[24] Katayama Y., Fukaya C. and Yamamoto T.: Poststroke pain control by chronic motor cortex stimulation: neurological characteristics predicting a favorable response. *J. Neurosurg.*, 89 (1998) 585-591.

[25] Kirkpatrick P.J., O'Brien M.D. and MacCabe J.J.: Trigeminal nerve section for chronic migrainous neuralgia. *Br.J.Neurosurg.*, 7 (1993) 483-490.

[26] Klun B.: Microvascular decompression and partial sensory rhizotomy in the treatment of trigeminal neuralgia: personal experience with 220 patients. *Neurosurgery*, 30 (1992) 49-52.

[27] Kondo A.: Follow-up results of using microvascular decompression for treatment of glossopharyngeal neuralgia. *J.Neurosurg.*, 88 (1998) 221-225.

[28] Kondziolka D., Lunsford L.D., Habeck M. and Flickinger J.C.: Gamma knife radiosurgery for trigeminal neuralgia. *Neurosurg.Clin.N.Am.*, 8 (1997) 79-85.

[29] Kori S.H.: Diagnosis and management of brachial plexus lesions in cancer patients. *Oncology*, 9 (1995) 756-760.

[30] Kumar K., Toth C., Nath R.K. and Laing P.: Epidural spinal cord stimulation for treatment of chronic pain--some predictors of success. A 15-year experience. *Surg.Neurol.*, 50 (1998) 110-120.

[31] Kumar K., Wyant G.M. and Nath R.: Deep brain stimulation for control of intractable pain in humans, present and future: a ten-year follow-up. *Neurosurgery*, 26 (1990) 774-781.

[32] Law J.D., Swett J. and Kirsch W.M.: Retrospective analysis of 22 patients with chronic pain treated by peripheral nerve stimulation. *J.Neurosurg.*, 52 (1980) 482-485.

[33] Lazorthes Y.R., Sallerin B.A. and Verdie J.C.: Intracerebroventricular administration of morphine for control of irreducible cancer pain. Neurosurgery, 37 (1995) 422-428.

[34] Levy R.M., Lamb S. and Adams J.E.: Treatment of chronic pain by deep brain stimulation: long term follow-up and review of the literature. *Neurosurgery*, 21 (1987) 885-893.

[35] Long D.M.: The current status of electrical stimulation of the nervous system for the relief of chronic pain. *Surg.Neurol.*, 49 (1998) 142-144.

[36] Lovely T.J., Jannetta P.J.: Microvascular decompression for trigeminal neuralgia. Surgical technique and long-term results. *Neurosurg.Clin.N.Am.*, 8 (1997) 11-29.

[37] Meglio M., Cioni B. and Rossi G.F.: Spinal cord stimulation in management of chronic pain. A 9-year experience. *J.Neurosurg.*, 70 (1989) 519-524.

[38] Mercadante S.: Problems of long-term spinal opioid treatment in advanced cancer patients. *Pain*, 79 (1999) 1-13.

[39] Moossy J.J., Nashold B.S., Jr., Osborne D. and Friedman A.H.: Conus medullaris nerve root avulsions. *J.Neurosurg.*, 66 (1987) 835-841.

[40] Moraci A., Buonaiuto C., Punzo A., Parlato C. and Amalfi R.: Trigeminal neuralgia treated by percutaneous thermocoagulation. Comparative analysis of percutaneous thermocoagulation and other surgical procedures. *Neurochirurgia.*(Stuttg.), 35 (1992) 48-53.

[41] Morgenlander J.C., Wilkins R.H.: Surgical treatment of cluster headache. *J.Neurosurg.*, 72 (1990) 866-871.

[42] Murali R., Rovit R.L.: Are peripheral neurectomies of value in the treatment of trigeminal neuralgia? An analysis of new cases and cases involving previous radiofrequency gasserian thermocoagulation. *J.Neurosurg.*, 85 (1996) 435-437.

[43] Nashold B.S., Jr., Goldner J.L., Mullen J.B. and Bright D.S.: Long-term pain control by direct peripheral-nerve stimulation. *J.Bone Joint Surg.*[Am.], 64 (1982) 1-10.

[44] Nguyen J.P., Lefaucheur J.P., Decq P., Uchiyama T., Carpentier A., Fontaine D. et al.: Chronic motor cortex stimulation in the treatment of central and neuropathic pain. Correlations between clinical, electrophysiological and anatomical data. *Pain*, 82 (1999) 245-251.

[45] North R.B., Campbell J.N., James C.S., Conover-Walker M.K., Wang H., Piantadosi S. et al.: Failed back surgery syndrome: 5-year follow-up in 102 patients undergoing repeated operation. *Neurosurgery*, 28 (1991) 685-690.

[46] North R.B., Ewend M.G., Lawton M.T., Kidd D.H. and Piantadosi S.: Failed back surgery syndrome: 5-year follow-up after spinal cord stimulator implantation. *Neurosurgery*, 28 (1991) 692-699.

[47] North R.B., Han M., Zahurak M. and Kidd D.H.: Radiofrequency lumbar facet denervation: analysis of prognostic factors. *Pain*, 57 (1994) 77-83.

[48] North R.B., Kidd D.H., Campbell J.N. and Long D.M.: Dorsal root ganglionectomy for failed back surgery syndrome: a 5-year follow-up study. *J.Neurosurg.*, 74 (1991) 236-242.

[49] North R.B., Kidd D.H., Wimberly R.L. and Edwin D.: Prognostic value of psychological testing in patients undergoing spinal cord stimulation: a prospective study. *Neurosurgery*, 39 (1996) 301-310.

[50] North R.B., Kidd D.H., Zahurak M., James C.S. and Long D.M.: Spinal cord stimulation for chronic, intractable pain: experience over two decades. *Neurosurgery*, 32 (1993) 384-394.

[51] Onofrio B.M., Yaksh T.L.: Long-term pain relief produced by intrathecal morphine infusion in 53 patients. *J.Neurosurg.*, 72 (1990) 200-209.

[52] Oturai A.B., Jensen K., Eriksen J. and Madsen F.: Neurosurgery for trigeminal neuralgia: comparison of alcohol block, neurectomy, and radiofrequency coagulation. *Clin.J.Pain*, 12 (1996) 311-315.

[53] Pagni C.A., Canavero S.: Cordomyelotomy in the treatment of paraplegia pain. Experience in two cases with long-term results. *Acta Neurol.Belg.*, 95 (1995) 33-36.

[54] Pagni C.A., Lanotte M. and Canavero S.: How frequent is anesthesia dolorosa following spinal posterior rhizotomy? A retrospective analysis of fifteen patients. *Pain*, 54 (1993)323-327.

[55] Picaza J.A., Hunter S.E. and Cannon B.W.: Pain suppression by peripheral nerve stimulation. Chronic effects of implanted devices. *Appl.Neurophysiol.*, 40 (1977) 223-234.

[56] Poletti C.E. : Proposed operation for occipital neuralgia: C-2 and C-3 root decompression. Case report. Neurosurgery, 12 (1983) 221-224.

[57] Rappaport Z.H.: The choice of therapy in medically intractable trigeminal neuralgia. *Isr.J.Med.Sci.*, 32 (1996) 1232-1234.

[58] Rappaport Z.H., Gomori J.M.: Recurrent trigeminal cistern glycerol injections for tic douloureux. *Acta Neurochir.*(Wien.), 90 (1988) 31-34.

[59] Rappaport Z.H., Magora F.: Trigeminal glycerol rhizolysis in the treatment of tic douloureux. *Eur.J.Anaesthesiol.*, 2 (1985) 53-57.

[60] Rath S.A., Seitz K., Soliman N., Kahamba J.F., Antoniadis G. and Richter H.P.: DREZ coagulations for deafferentation pain related to spinal and peripheral nerve lesions: indication and results of 79 consecutive procedures. Stereotact.*Funct.Neurosurg.*, 68 (1997) 161-167.

[61] Rawlings C.E., el-Naggar A.O. and Nashold B.S.J.: The DREZ procedure: an update on technique. *Br.J.Neurosurg.*, 3 (1989) 633-642.

[62] Resnick D.K., Jannetta P.J., Bissonnette D., Jho H.D. and Lanzino G.: Microvascular decompression for glossopharyngeal neuralgia. Neurosurgery, 36 (1995) 64-68.

[63] Richardson D.E.: Deep brain stimulation for the relief of chronic pain. Neurosurg.*Clin.N.Am.*, 6 (1995) 135-144.

[64] Rowed D.W.: Chronic cluster headache managed by nervus intermedius section. *Headache*, 30 (1990) 401-406.

[65] Saitoh Y., Shibata M., Hirano S., Hirata M., Mashimo T., and Yoshimine T. Motor cortex stimulation for central and peripheral deafferentation pain. Report of eight cases. *J. Neurosurg.*, 92 (2000) 150-155.

[66] Sanders M., Zuurmond W.: Safety of unilateral and bilateral percutaneous cervical cordotomy in 80 terminally ill cancer patients. J.Clin.Oncol., 13 (1995) 1509-1512.

[67] Sanders M., Zuurmond W.W.: Efficacy of sphenopalatine ganglion blockade in 66 patients suffering from cluster headache: a 12- to 70-month follow-up evaluation. *J.Neurosurg.*, 87 (1997) 876-880.

[68] Shetter A.G.: Pain surgery techniques for specialty neurosurgical practice. *Clin.Neurosurg.*, 40 (1993) 197-209.

[69] Sindou M.: Microsurgical DREZotomy (MDT) for pain, spasticity, and hyperactive bladder: a 20-year experience. *Acta Neurochir.*(Wien.), 137 (1995) 1-5.

[70] Sindou M., Jeanmonod D. and Mertens P.: Ablative neurosurgical procedures for the treatment of chronic pain. *Neurophysiol.Clin.*, 20 (1990) 399-423.

[71] Sindou M., Mertens P.: Microsurgical vascular decompression (MVD) in trigeminal and glosso-vago-pharyngeal neuralgias. A twenty year experience. *Acta Neurochir.Suppl.*(Wien.), 58 (1993) 168-170.

[72] Stechison M.T., Mullin B.B.: Surgical treatment of greater occipital neuralgia: an appraisal of strategies. *Acta Neurochir.*(Wien.), 131 (1994) 236-240.

[73] Sundaresan N., Di Giacinto G.V. and Hughes J.E.: Neurosurgery in the treatment of cancer pain. *Cancer*, 63 (1-6-1989) 2365-2377.

[74] Sweet W.H.: Percutaneous methods for the treatment of trigeminal neuralgia and other faciocephalic pain; comparison with microvascular decompression. *Semin.Neurol.*, 8 (1988) 272-279.

[75] Taha J.M., Tew J.M.J.: Long-term results of surgical treatment of idiopathic neuralgias of the glossopharyngeal and vagal nerves. *Neurosurgery*, 36 (1995) 926-930.

[76] Taha J.M., Tew J.M.J.: Comparison of surgical treatments for trigeminal neuralgia: reevaluation of radiofrequency rhizotomy. *Neurosurgery*, 38 (1996) 865-871.

[77] Taha J.M., Tew J.M.J.: Treatment of trigeminal neuralgia by percutaneous radiofrequency rhizotomy. *Neurosurg.Clin.N.Am.*, 8 (1997) 31-39.

[78] Taha J.M., Tew J.M., Jr.: Long-term results of radiofrequency rhizotomy in the treatment of cluster headache. Heiadache, 35 (1995) 193-196.

[79] Tasker R.R.: Management of nociceptive deafferantation and central pain by surgical intervention. In: H.L.Fields, (Ed.). *Pain syndromes in neurology.* [7] Butterworths , London, 1990., pp.143-200

[80] Tasker R.R., De Carvalho G.T. and Dolan E.J.: Intractable pain of spinal cord origin: clinical features and implications for surgery. *J.Neurosurg.*, 77 (1992) 373-378.

[81] Thomas D.G.: Brachial plexus injury: deafferentation pain and dorsal root entry zone (DREZ) coagulation. Clin.Neurol.Neurosurg., 95 *Suppl* (1993) S48-S49.

[82] Young R.F.: Electrical stimulation of the trigeminal nerve root for the treatment of chronic facial pain. *J.Neurosurg.*, 83 (1995) 72-78.

[83] Young R.F., Vermeulen S.S., Grimm P., Blasko J. and Posewitz A.: Gamma Knife radiosurgery for treatment of trigeminal neuralgia: idiopathic and tumor related. *Neurology*, 48 (1997) 608-614.

[84] Zeidman SM, Rossitch EJ and Nashold B.S.J.: Dorsal root entry zone lesions in the treatment of pain related to radiation-induced brachial plexopathy. *J.Spinal.Dis.*6(1993) 44-47.

In: The Handbook of Chronic Pain   ISBN 978-1-60021-044-0
Editors: S. Kreitler, D. Beltrutti, et al., pp. 247-272   © 2007 Nova Science Publishers, Inc.

Chapter 15

Implantable Devices and Drug Delivery Systems

Giancarlo Barolat and Ashwini D. Sharan

A – ELECTRICAL STIMULATION

A.1 – Spinal Cord Stimulation

A.1.a – History

The first experiments in the Western world on the use of electricity for pain control were conducted in 1840 by Moritz-Heinstrich Romber with galvano-puncture [1]. The gate control theory has focused interest in dorsal column stimulation. In 1967 Shealy inserted the first dorsal column stimulator in a human suffering from terminal metastatic cancer[3]. Shortly afterwards, the first two solid state transcutaneous electrical nerve stimulators (TENS)[3] were produced. Subsequently, electrodes have been implanted utilizing a variety of techniques: via a laminectomy in the subarachnoid space, between the two layers of the dura or in the epidural space[4] . The percutaneous technique was introduced later [5].

In spinal cord stimulation (SCS) the initial stimulating systems were only radio-frequency (RF) driven passive receivers. In the mid-seventies the first implantable pulse generators powered by a lithium battery were introduced. At first stimulation was delivered through a unipolar electrode, and only later bipolar arrays were introduced. In all the different types of percutaneous and plate-type arrays up to that time the contact combinations were hardwired and could not be reprogrammed after the pulse generator was implanted. This changed in 1980 with the introduction of the percutaneous quadripolar electrode with contact combinations that could be reprogrammed noninvasively through an external transmitter.

In the late seventies there was a surge of enthusiasm for SCS with thousands of patients undergoing implantation. Poor patient selection, technical problems with the equipment and implantation by inexperienced physicians led to a large number of poor results. In the early eighties the procedure fell into disrepute. Gradually, over the last 10 years SCS has regained acceptance in the management of chronic non-malignant pain. At present its role in the treatment of pain is well established. Moreover, it is being used also by other specialities, primarily anesthesiology[7], rehabilitation medicine, and orthopedic surgery, with newer applications in conditions, such as refractory angina pectoris, intestitial cystitis and occipital neuralgia. The success of this modality has further increased following the codification of the standards for electrode placement[8].

A.1.B- Equipment: Electrodes and Pulse Generators

There are several major implantable technologies:

(1) – Percutaneous electrodes (Table 1, Figure 1, Figure 2)

Percutaneous electrodes are particularly appealing. They can be inserted without any incision, which is advantageous for a trial stimulation to assess candidacy for a permanent implant. Further, the electrodes can be advanced over several segments in the epidural space, thus enabling the testing of several spinal cord levels in order to determine optimal electrode position, as well as the relative adequacy of an implantable pulse generator versus a radiofrequency device. With the insertion of multiple parallel electrodes different configuration matrices can be constructed, so as to create highly focused electrical fields. A major disadvantage of percutaneous electrodes is their tendency to migrate.

Table 1. Percutaneous Electrodes

Percutaneous Electrodes				
Company	Name	Contacts	Contact Length (mm)	Contact Spacing (mm)
Medtronic[1]	Pisces Quad	4	3	6
	Quad	4	3	4
	Compact	4	6	12
	Quad Plus	8	3	6
	Octad[x]			
	Verify[y]	4	3	6
ANS[2]	Octrode	8	3	4
	Cervitrode	7	3	4/28[z]
	Quattrode – 7mm	4	3	4
	Quattrode – 10mm	4	4	6

[1] – Medtronic Inc., Minneapolis, MN
[2] – Advanced Neuromodulation Systems, Allen TX
[x] – only for use with Mattrix system
[y] – temporary screening lead
[z] – 4 contacts at 4mm and 4 at 28mm

In percutaneous implantation the electrodes must be placed under fluoroscopic guidance. Temporary percutaneous electrodes can be easily removed in the implanting physician's office. In implanting permanenet percutaneous electrodes a surgical incision is required for anchoring the electrode in place, extension wires must be tunnelled a few inches away from the insertion site, and a return trip to the operating room is necessary for removing or internalizing the electrode.

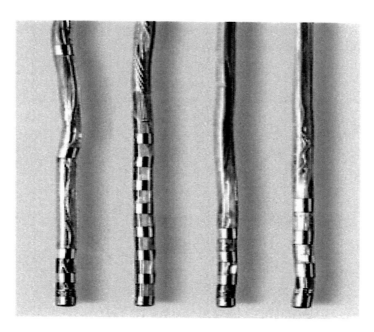

Figure 1. Percutaneous electrodes by Advanced Neuromodulation Systems. Quattrode 10mm, Quattrode 7mm, Octrode, Cervitrode (left to right).

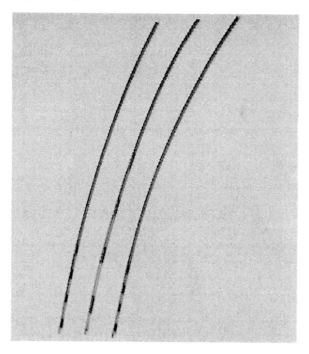

Figure 2. Percutaneous electrodes by Metronic Inc. Pisces Compact, Pisces Quad Plus, and Pisces Quad electrode (left to right).

(2) – Plate electrodes (Table 2, Figure 3, Figure 4)

Plate-type electrodes – also called ribbon electrodes, paddle electrodes, or laminotomy electrodes – require implantation under direct vision [10]. Most implants can be made through a skin incision 2.5-4 cm long. The amount of bony removal is usually minimal. The implanting physician can usually explore 4 to 5 levels in the thoracic spine and 5 to 6 levels in the cervical spine by advancing the electrode in either a cephald or a caudal direction. Implantation under direct vision may be safer in the upper thoracic and cervical areas. Multiple arrays or different electrode configurations can be constructed also with plate electrodes. The main advantage of plate electrodes consists in their higher stability in the dorsal epidural space and lesser propensity to migrate. Plate electrodes seem to have a broader stimulation pattern and lower stimulation requirements [11]. Plate electrodes are recommended as the single option in cases of previous spine surgery at the implant levels.

Table 2. Plate Electrodes

Plate Electrodes					
Company	Name	Contacts (#)	Contact Length (mm)	Contact Spacing (mm)[a]	Paddle Dimension (mm)
Medtronic[1]	Resume II	4	4[b]	6	44 x 8 x 1.8
	Resumt TL[x]	4	4[b]	6	44 x 6.6 x 1.37
	Specify	8	3 x 2	6 [2]	44.5 x 8 x 1.7
	Symmix	4	2 x 6	diamond[c]	44.2 x 10 x 1.7
	On-Point PNS	4	4	6	44 x 6.6 x 1.4[d]
ANS[2]	Lamitrode 88	16	4.1[e]	7	74 x 10 x 1.6
	Lamitrode 8	8	4[b]	7.1	70 x 7.5 x 1.6
	Lamitrode 44	8	4.1[e]	7	45 x 10 x 1.6
	Lamitrode 4	4	4.1[b]	10	43 x 7.9 x 2.0
	Lamitrode 22	4	4.1[b]	7.6	20 x 7.9 x 2.0

[1] – Medtronic Inc., Minneapolis, MN
[2] – Advanced Neuromodulation Systems, Allen TX
[a] – spacing between array
[b] – round
[c] – diamond configuration
[d] – with a mesh skirt that extends 5mm beyond paddle
[e] – rectangle
[x] – thinner and smaller than Resume II1

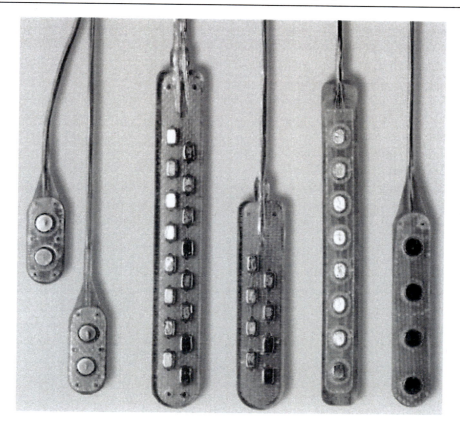

Figure 3. Plate electrodes by Advanced Neuromodulation Systems. Lamitrode 4, Lamitrode 8, Lamitrode 44, Lamitrode 88, and Peritrode (also called Lamitrode 22) electrodes (left to right).

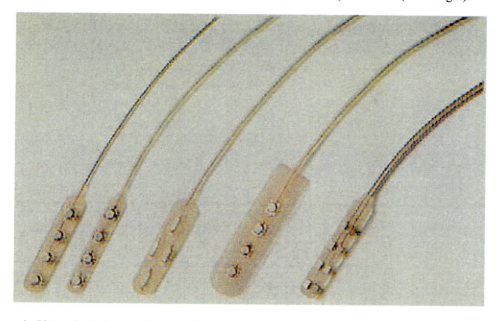

Figure 4. Plate electrodes by Metronic Inc. Specity, On Point, Symmix, Resume TL, and Resume electrodes (left to right).

(3) - Pulse generators and radio frequency (RF) receivers (Table 3, Figures 5, 6, 7)

Electrical stimulation consists of rectangular pulses delivered to the epidural space through implanted electrodes. Two types of systems are currently available: a completely implantable pulse generator (IPG) and a RF coupled pulse generator with an implantable receiver. The IPG contains a lithium battery. Activation and control occur through an external transcutaneous telemetry device. Once activated, it can be turned on and off through a small magnet that the patient is advised to carry at all times. The magnet also allows some minimal control over stimulation parameters. More extensive control of the unit can be attained through a small portable unit. The electrical combinations can be modified only by a console kept by the implanting physician. Life span of the battery is about 2.5-4.5 years, varying with usage and with the utilized parameters. Available lithium powered pulse generators allow stimulation with fine resolution increments of 0.05 V and with rates up to 130 Hz. Replacing the battery requires a surgical procedure in an outpatient clinic. IPG's with rechargeable batteries are currently available from all 3 major manufacturers (Advanced Bionics, Advanced Neuromodulation Systems and Medtronic). The devices can be recharged transcutaneously by applying a charger to the skin over the implanted IPG. At the battery end of life, the IPG still will need to be replaced surgically, but their duration should surpass the one of the non-rechargeable units.

RF driven systems consist of a passive receiver, implanted subcutaneously, and a transmitter, which is worn externally. An antenna applied to the skin in correpondence with the receiver is connected to the transmitter which sends the stimulation signals transcutaneously. In order for the system to function, the transmitter has to contain charged alkaline batteries, and the antenna must make adequate contact with the receiver. This requires the patient to wear the external system in order to receive the stimulation. RF driven systems can deliver stimulation with rates up to 1,400 Hz, and can be customized to deliver more power than the corresponding lithium-powered systems..

Both systems present advantages and disadvantages. The main disadvantage of the RF systems is the inconvenience of having to wear the antenna and the radio-receiver. The main disadvantage of the rechargeable IPG is the fact that the patient has to remember to recharge periodically. This could constitute a significant obstacle in older people or in relatively non-compliant individuals. Contact between the IPG and the external charging unit might also be problematic.

Table 3. Pulse Generators

Pulse Generators/ Receivers							
Company	Name	Power Source	Number of Independent Channels	Contacts Powered	Rate	Amplitude	Pulse Width
						(maximum)	
				(#)	(PPS)	(V)	(ms)
Medtronic[1]	Itrel 3	Internal lithium Battery	1	4	130	10.5	450
	Xtrel	RF[z]	1	4	1400	10	200
	Mattrix	RF[z]	2	8	240	12	500
ANS[2]	MNR-98[a]	RF[z]	1	8	1500	12	500
	MNR-904[b]	RF[z]	1	4	1500	12	500
	MNR-916[c]	RF[z]	2	8	1500	12	500
	MNR-940[d]	RF[z]	3	12	1500	12	500
	MNR-944[e]	RF[z]	2	16	1500	12	500
	MNR-988[f]	RF[z]	4	16	1500	12	500

[1] – Medtronic Inc., Minneapolis, MN
[2] – Advanced Neuromodulation Systems, Allen TX
[z] – Radiofrequency
[a] – Leads: Cervitrode[2], Octrode[2]
[b] – Leads: Quattrode[2], Peritrode[2], Lamitrode[2]
[c] – Leads: 2 Octrode[2]
[d] – Magnatrode[2]
[e] – Leads: 2 Quattrodes[2]
[f] – Omnitrode[2]

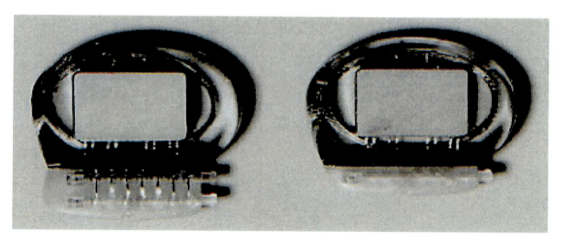

Figure 5. Radiofrequency coupled Pulse generators by Advanced Neuromodulation MNR (98 or 904) and MNR (914 or 944) (left to right).

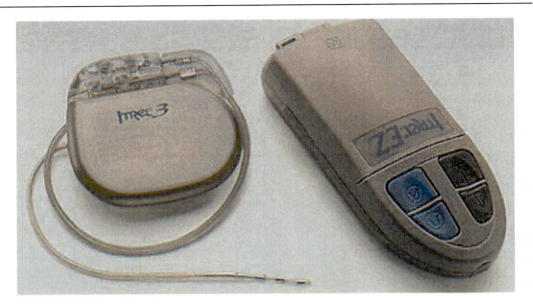

Figure 6. Battery powered Pulse generators by Metronic Inc. Itrel 3 fully implantable pulse generator (left) and the EZ Patient Programmer (right).

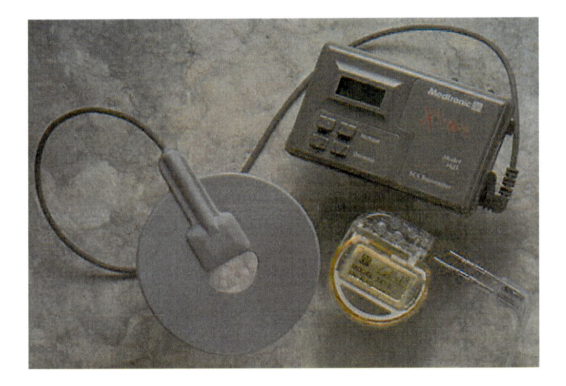

Figure 7. Radiofrequency coupled Pulse generators by Metronic Inc. Radiofrequency antenna (left) attached to the Xtrel programmer (top right) and the implantable receiver (bottom right)ublication Cooperation.

(4) - Conclusions

With modern technology both percutaneous and plate batteries are safe and effective ways of delivering electrical stimulation to the spinal cord. In some cases there are clear indications for applying one of the two methods (i.e., a percutaneous system in the case of an outpatient percutaneous trial, or a "laminotomy" system in the case of prior spine surgery). In all other cases both techniques can be used interchangeably, in with the preferences of the implanting physician. The authors prefer to use the"laminotomy system" because of its greater stability and predictability in positioning in patients with previous surgery and scarring.

The decision of using an IPG versus a RF should be tailored to the individual patient. An RF allows for a wider range of usage but is inconvenient because it has an external attachment. An IPG may be cosmetically more appealing but would require another surgical procedure to replace the battery, and does not give the patient full control over all the parameters of stimulation.

A.1.C – Implantation Techniques

Various surgical techniques have been developed for implanting the different devices. All depend to some extent on anesthesia. The distribution of the stimulation-induced paresthesia is vital to the efficacy of the modality for pain control. Electrode implantation can be performed either under monitored (local anesthetic and intravenous sedation) or under general anesthesia. With modern anesthetic techniques, testing an awake patient yields superior results and allows for immediate feedback regarding the stimulation-induced paresthesia. Under general anesthesia, it is difficult to assess the presence of undesired concomitant motor stimulation and one can rely only on the radiolographical position and on evoked motor or sensory responses to assure proper electrode positioning.

The anesthetic management is of crucial importance for the success of the procedure. The patient must be fully awake and cooperative during the testing phase and the degree of intravenous sedation should be carefully titrated. One should try to avoid any discomfort to the patient and to strive to obtain complete amnesia of the pain that may be perceived during the implant. Generous anesthetic infiltration with a long acting agent minimizes the requirements for intravenous sedation. Most patients are put in a lateral decubitus position and the anesthesiologist places a laryngeal mass airway (LMA). As the patient emerges from anesthesia, the LMA is removed and conversation may be held with the patient.

A.1.D - Indications

SCS has been used for a variety of pain conditions and is particularly indicated for neuropathic pain, including reflex sympathetic dystrophy, failed low back syndrome, nerve injury, phantom limb pain, spinal cord injury and interstitial cystitits. Recently the senior author has extended the indications to include intractable pain due to neurogenic thoracic outlet syndrome, and temporo-mandibular joint syndrome refractory to other surgical interventions. SCS has been used successfully for treating severe pain due to ischemic disease of the lower extremities and intractable angina pain. In selected patients SCS can produce at least 50% pain relief in 50-60% of the implanted patients. With proper follow-up care, these results can be maintained even up to twenty years.

(1) – Complex Regional Pain Syndrome

Currently the senior author has implanted over 350 patients for managing CRPS type 1 pain. SCS does not appear to change the disease course but should be considered after the patient has been through a variety of treatments. In these patients implantation is more difficult than in any other patient group, and there is a serious risk of aggravating the original pain or causing a new pain/allodynia at the implanted site. The pain often spreads to other body parts and it is challenging to be able to cover all the affected areas with stimulation.

Four studies reported on the clinical efficacy of SCS for CRPS type 1. In 1989, Barolat et al.[10] reported pain reduction in 10 out of 13 implanted patients. No patient was made completely pain free but all 10 reported a definitive difference when stimulation was stopped. In 1997 Kumar et al.[12] presented a median follow-up of 41 months on 12 patients with permanently implanted leads, 8 of whom reported near complete resolution of their symptoms and 4 maintained good relief. Kemlar et al.[13] reported 23 cases with improvement in 78%. Oakley and Weiner did a prospective study of 19 patients with CRSP implanted with spinal cord stimulation systems [14]. Of the 10 patients for whom detailed long-term efficacy data was collected, 3 reported full relief and 7 partial. In all studies permanent morbidity for the procedure has remained extrememly low. The authors have used SCS with good results for pain relief in patients in whom the symptomatology has spread to multiple body parts.

(2) – Brachial Plexitis/Neuroactic Thoractic Outlet Syndrome

This can be a highly successful application of spinal cord stimulation, which however present distinct challenges. Most of these patients complain of pain in the upper extremity, the shoulder, the trapezius, the axilla, and the anterior upper chest area. With the available systems, stimulation of all areas with one electrode is often not feasible. Pain control would require mostly the use of two electrodes or of the Cervitrode (ANS) percutaneous electrode for complex upper body pain syndromes because it has seven irregularly spaced contacts. Further, a two-channel stimulating device may be indicated, since the setting for the upper cervical region can differ from the one required to optimally stimulate the axilla and anterior chest area. Another difficulty is the extreme hyperesthesia present in the brachial plexus region as well as in the trapezius, often extending larger areas of the posterior thorax. Any surgical manipulation in these hypersensitive areas must be avoided. Tunnelling the implanted wires must be planned carefully and at a distance from the hypersensitive areas in order to prevent excruciating pain and intolerance to the implanted system.

(3) - Failed Back Surgery Syndrome (FBSS)

FBSS is vaguely defined and includes pain localized in the center of the lower lumbar area, in the buttocks, persistent reticular pain, or diffuse lower extremity(s) pain. Most published series distinguish between back and leg pain, but the details of the pain syndromes are rarely defined. SCS is accepted in the treatment of leg pain, but its widespread use for pain in the lower lumbar area still remains to be defined. Obtaining stimulation in the low back with the currently available electrodes is extremely difficult. Even with direct stimulation to the low back, the pattern of paresthesis is often replaced in time by an unpleasant segrmentary band of stimulation which negates the benefits of the procedure. Jay Law's[15] pioneering work showed that stimulation in the low back can be obtained only if one uses multiple arrays of closely spaced bipols at T9-T10. The best configuration is one where two octopolar electrodes are placed parallel on each side of the physiological line. North et al. recently challenged this concept by advocating the use of a single quadripolar electrode in midline [16]. So far no data exist as to the long-term behavior of single versus dual electrodes. The longitudinal studies by North [17] showed that in patients with post-surgical lumbar arachnoid or epidural fibrosis without surgically remediable lesions, SCS is superior to repeated surgical interventions on the lumbar spine (for back and leg pain) and to dorsal ganglionectomy (for leg pain). In his study there were 50 patients with FBSS who averaged 3.1 operations prior to SCS implantation. Successful outcome (at least 50% pain relief and patient satisfaction with the result) was obtained in 53% of patients at 2.2 years. Turner et al.'s [18] systematic review, based on 41 studies from 1966 to 1994, showed that 50-60% of the patients with FBSS reported > 50% pain relief from the use of SCS. Burchiel et al. [19] conducted a prospective multi-center study with one year follow up and also reported 55% success. Medication usage and work status were not significantly changed. None of the studies differentiated between axial back and leg pain. Nor did their data differentiate. Most implanting physicians share the experience that SCS is far more effective for reticular pain than for axial low back pain.

(4) - Phantom Limb

The largest published study was made by Krainic with 6 amputees implanted between 1972 and 1974[20]. The patients suffered from a combination of pains: phantom pain, localized stump pain, and a painful throbbing stump. Initially good pain relief (over 50%) was obtained in 45% of the patients. Yet with long-term follow-up of 2-5 years, there was a significant decline in the level of pain relief. Only one of the 13 patients who initially had over 75% pain relief was still enjoying these results. Overall 23% of the patients still had good pain relief, 20% had fair and 57% had none. Pain relief was clearly correlated with the ability to cover the painful area with stimulation-induced paresthesia. Both phantom pain and stump pain were affected by SCS while painful throbbing of the stump was not affected if associated with attacks of severe phantom or stump pain. All patients reported that stimulation was more effective on background pain than on attacks of severe pain.

(5) - Post-Herpetic Neuralgia

The effectiveness of SCS in post-herpetic neuralgia seems controversial. Meglio reported good success in 6 of 10 implanted patients [21]. Others have been unable to reproduce this success rate. None of the published series contain more than a handful of patients. In the senior author's experience this pain is not very responsive to stimulation. The stimulation-induced paresthesia is often felt as sharp and annoying and is not tolerated by the patients.

(6) - Spinal Cord Injury

The results of SCS on spinal cord injury pain have been disappointing. Tasker identified three main types of pain in the spinal cord injury patient: steady burning or dysesthetic pain, intermittent lancinating pain, and evoked pain [22]. Only the first type was relieved to some extent by SCS (36% of the patients in contrast to 0% and 16% in the other two types).

Further, there were no good results in patients with steady pain and complete spinal cord injury.

(7) – Angina

The role of SCS in managing refractory angina pectoris seems to be very promising. The few well-documented studies have uniformly shown good results in relieving anginal pain[24,25,27]. The results have been maintained in long-term follow-up and have been sustantiated by a reduction in the intake of nitrates. There is evidence that SCS has effects beyond pain relief, such as reduction in ST segment depression and improvement in exercise capacity, time to angina and recovery time, all of which suggest a reduction in ischemia. Yet since this has not been demonstrated by a myocardial perfusion study, it is likely that any perfusion changes are small, occur mainly in the ischemic area and are difficult to demonstrate. This may not be unlike the results of SCS in peripheral vascular disease, where microcirculatory tests were unable to detect the minute yet significant changes in microcirculatory parameters.

Vulink et al.[28] conducted a prospective study on quality of life changes in patients with refractory angina pectoris implanted with SCS. Both the pain and the health aspects of quality of life improved significantly after 3 months of SCS. Social, mental, and physical aspects of quality of life were improved after one year of SCS. It is unlikely that SCS for anginal pain would conceal an acute MI because patients treated with SCS who underwent an MI noted the difference in pain[29].

Since the mechanism of action of SCS as well as the relation between pain and myocardial ischemia are unclear, we do not know whether the pain relief is due to direct depression of the nociceptive signals in the spinal cord or represent a secondary gain from reduction in ischemia [30-31]. Foreman has shown that dorsal column stimulation inhibits the activity of spinothalamic tract cells evoked by activation of the cardiac sympathetic afferents or by intracardiac bradykinin. On the other hand, the effects of stimulation may be equivalent to those of sympathectomy and may be due to producing a prolonged inhibition of the hyperactive sympathetic system, as was shown experimentally in the rat [32].

(8) - Chronic Critical Limb Ischemia (CCLI)

Cook et al.[33] were the first to suggest in 1973 that the indications for SCS may extend beyond intractable pain control. A group of patients with multiple sclerosis who underwent SCS experienced not only pain relief but also an improvement in mobility as well as in sensory and bladder function. Cook et al. noted apparent improvement in lower limb blood flow and subsequently used SCS in patients whose primary problem was peripheral vascular disease (PVD)[34]. In 1981 Meglio and Cioni[35] reported pain relief and ulcer healing in a patient with advanced peripheral arterial insufficiency. In 1988 Jacobs[36] published clinical evidence that SCS improved the microcirculation as measured by capillary microscopy. Since then several large studies [38-39] reported by cardiologists, vascular surgeons and neurosurgeons provided evidence that the long term results of SCS include significant pain relief and ulcer healing. SCS for CCLI is widely practiced in Europe, with over 7000 patients having been implanted, while the US the medical establishment has remained more skeptical[46].

While SCS may not be considered an alternative to revascularization procedures, it should become an option when the latter are no longer deemed feasible. Pathological conditions that constitute appropriate indications for implantation include arteriosclerosis, arteriosclerosis with diabetes, Buerger's disease, Raynaud's disease, and embolic occlusive disease. Most of the published experience is with lower extremity problems, but results for upper extremity ischemic pain have been encouraging [40]. Currently the main goal of the procedure is to relieve pain, and the best results are obtained in ischemic pain. Other types of pain (e.g., epicritic ulcer pain, osteomyelitis pain) do not respond nearly as well.

There is some evidence that SCS facilitates healing of ulcers less than 3 sq. cm. but not gangrene. Hence it seems likely that SCS produces an increase in microcirculation in the affected area. The mechanism responsible for increased blood flow in individuals with peripheral vascular disease is probably inhibition of the sympathetic system. This phenomenon occurs within the spinal cord at the local level and is not related to antidromic activation of afferent fibers. The possible role of locally released vasoactive peptides is still unclear. Whether the effects on pain and blood flow are due to the same mechanisms is unknown, although some evidence suggests that pain relief is secondary to the microciculatory changes. Multiple mechanisms may be assumed to be operating simultaneously [43-45].

The patient must understand the treatment modality and be compliant. These requirements are not insignificant as the majority of patients are old (which may decrease their ability to master new technology) and ill with many ailments (which renders follow-up care difficult and unreliable). The best candidates seem to be individuals who have ischemic pain (rest or alaudication), no ulcers or gangrene, and are sufficiently motivated and intelligent to understand the treatment modality and the rigorous follow-ups.

A.1.E – Complications

With the proper expertise, complications are rare. The most serious one, which is shared with any type of spine surgery, is paralysis. The authors are aware of instances of severe neurological deficits that have occurred during SCS procedures. Other complications include infection of the implanted hardware (in about 3-5%), though it did not spread to the nervous system or caused any neurological impairment; persistent but not permanent pain at the implant site (in about 5%); reclacitrant cerebrospianl fluid leakage, that required surgical revisions (in a few patients); and breakage of the implanted hardware (in about 10%).

A.1.F Programming (Figure 10)

Implanting a SCS system is only one of the factors involved in the successful implementation of the modality. Titration of the electrical parameters and careful follow-up of the patients are just as important. After implantation two factors must be carefully evaluated. One is the distribution of paresthesis based on the contact polarities attempting to have the best electrical characteristics providing the broadest coverage of the painful area. Given the complexity of the available systems, the process should be performed by a dedicated trained health professional, preferably with computer-assisted patient interactive programming[48]. The ability to download into the pulse generator/receiver several programs which can be later recalled by the patient at the push of a button has greatly facilitated the management of the implanted systems. The second factor is the assessment of three electrical parameters which are important for programming SCS for the individual: the perception threshold (i.e., the voltage at which the patient begins to perceive paresthesia) [49] , the discomfort threshold (i.e., the voltage at which the patient perceives the stimulation a uncomfortable), and the usage range (i.e., the difference between the discomfort and the perception thresholds, which reflects the therapeutically useful stimulation range).

Once the optimal combination and stimulation voltage have been established, other electrical parameters must be assessed in order to optimize the stimulation. A most important one is the rate of stimulation.. Even though most patients will choose rates in the range of 20 to 100 Hz, there is a high individual variability (e.g., patients with specific neuropathic pain syndromes may respond better to higher stimulation rates over 250 Hz)[47]. It is not unusual for optimal stimulation parameters to be fully established only several weeks after implantation.

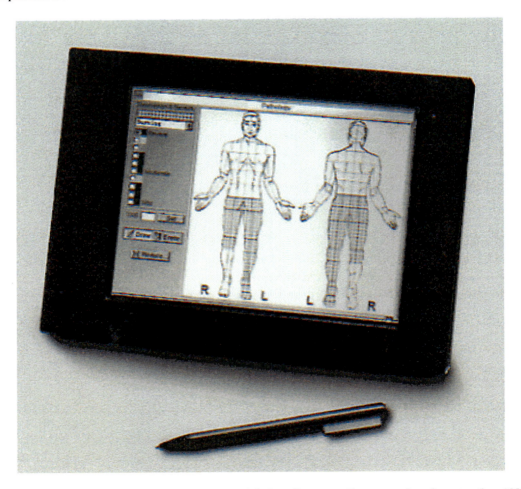

Figure 10. PainDoc by Advanced Neuromodulation Systems. Computer Interface to the ANS radiofrequency coupled pulse generators.

A.1.G – Conclusions

SCS has been performed for about 25 years, in the course of which it has become a more reliable and safe procedure, though its results are not perfect. Careful follow-up of the patients is necessary for successful long-term success because equipment related problems can arise at any time. Yet, as compared with the other modalities, the magnitude of its long-term results with 50% success rate over a few years follow-up, is not easily matched.

A.2 – Peripheral Nerve Stimulation (Pns)

A.2.A – History and Evolution

In order to test the predictions of the gate control theory, Wall and Sweet , in 1967 stimulated on themselves the infraorbital nerve, producing brief hypoalgesia[50]. The technique was gradually refined specifically designed plate electrodes were developed that could be laid on the nerve and sewn to the epineurum [54-55].

A.2.B - Indications and Related Issues

PNS is predominantly indicated if a patient's pain maps out to one or two specific nerve distributions. Racz has advocated the simultaneous utilization of SCS and PNS in patients with widespread pain affecting one extremity due to nerve injury. Alternatively, PNS could be indicated in more widespread pain syndromes where the inciting cause was clearly a traumatic lesion to a major peripheral nerve (i.e., a CRPS type 1 affecting the upper extremity in case of median nerve damage during a carpal tunnel procedure). The anatomical arrangement of peripheral nerves creates some difficulties and some opportunities as compared to the brain or the spinal cord. The opportunity rests on a better codified and predictable distribution and pattern of paresthesia than in the central nervous system. Nevertheless, within the peripheral nerve, motor and sensory fibers are in close proximity and often intermingled. Sunderland noted that the orientation and position of nerve fascicles vary constantly within the nerve trunk and a predetermined map for motor and sensory distributions cannot be obtained [56]. Since the motor fibers have a threshold equal to or lower than the sensory ones, selective creation of paresthesia without undesirable motor contractions is often difficult to achieve. This is different from the spinal cord where the motor and sensory tracts have separate and well-defined locations.

Peripheral nerves which have commonly been used for stimulation include the ulnar, median, tibial, common peroneal and sciatic. Implantation of pripheral nerve stimulators has been made predominantly in patients with pain related to direct or indirect trauma, causalgia, brachial plexopathy, or post-herpetic neuritis.

A.2.C – Complications

The most significant complications of PNS have been related to ischemic damage of the nerve. This may have been related to nerve compression due to inappropriately tight cuff electrodes and have since been reduced with the use of in-line electrodes. Electrode breakage has been observed particularly when the system crossed more than one joint.

A.2.D – Results

The results of PNS have been better in the upper extremity than in the lower extremity. Nashold reported a 52.6% success rate in the upper extremity in 19 patients and a 31% success rate in the lower extremity in 16 patients. He defined a success as a subjective estimate of more than 90% relief, increased physical activity, abstinence from analgesic, and continued use of the stimulator[52]. Schon et al. reported on a series of 19 patients with intractable lower extremity pain managed with PNS. A total of 22 limbs were implanted. Follow-up averaged 14 months. Post-operatively pain and function improved an average of 4 and 3 points respectively on a scale of 0-10 [57].

Sweet in 1976 reported on 69 implanted patients, most of them with traumatic neuropathy. He reported an initial success rate of 43%, which, at a longer follow-up, decreased to 25% [58]. Similar results were reported by Campbell and Long [59]. Some of the failures were certainly attributable to equipment failure or electrode breakage, which during the first two decades, plagued implantable neurostimulation systems.

Hassenbush and Racz have championed the use of PNS in patients with CRPS type 1 [54,55,60]. Hoyen reported on 76 patients with Complex Regional Pain Syndrome type 1 implanted with peripheral nerve stimulators. Most patients had symptoms predominantly in one nerve distribution in the upper extremity. The author concluded that PNS has a definite role in the management of these conditions [61].

No study to date has provided a definitive answer to the efficacy of this technique. Gybels and Sweet [62] presented a summary of outcome in 1219 patients treated from 1972 to 1986. They reported short-term success rates of 66% and long-term success rates of 50%. With patient selection criteria, these results may be increased up to 83% and 65%, but there is a tendency towards lessening pain relief with time [63-64]. Other factors that have influenced results have included patient selection, techniques of localization, electrode type and application, and anatomical variation of motor and sensory nerve fascicles.

A.2.E – New Applications

A new concept was introduced by Weiner with the implantation of percutaneous electrodes subcutaneously in the occipital region to stimulate the occipital nerve [65]. This technique has been utilized to treat refractory occipital neuralgia which has failed to respond to other medical and surgical measures. In 1998 Weiner et al.[65] reported that out of 28 patients pain relief was excellent in 61%, good in 32%, and poor in 7%.

Alo et al. reported on a novel technique to cannulate the nerve roots with percutaneous electrodes and used it on selective lumbar and sacral nerve root stimulation for the treatment of chronic pain [66-67]. Five patients who have been unresponsive to conservative treatment and to spinal cord stimulation underwent a percutaneous trial with lumbo-sacral nerve root stimulation. Paresthesia coverage was above 75% in all patients, with a mean paresthesia coverage of 82%. VAS scores declined from a mean of 9.8 to 3, and four patients requested permanent implantation.

A.3 - Deep Brain Stimulation

A.3.A – History

The work of Heath and Mickle in 1954 set up the framework for the modern concepts of DBS [68-69]. Reynold described "stimulation-produced analgesia"[70-72] and demonstrated that electrical stimulation of the periaqueductal gray (PAG) in rats could produce analgesia, while further studies demonstrated elevation of opioid neurotransmitters after DBS [71-75]. Reynolds and others showed that activating the periaqueductal gray matter by electrical stimulation mobilized the brain's own peptides to activate descending serotonergic pathways that blocked nociceptive impulses [70,76].

A.3.B – Targets

PAG and periventricular gray matter (PVG) stimulation have been shown to be beneficial for relief of nociceptive pain, including chronic back pain, neck pain, and cancer pain. Paresthesia producing stimulation has been possible with stimulation of the ventrocaudal nucleus, medial lemniscus, or thalamic radiations. Thalamic stimulation, including the ventralis posterolateralis and posteromedialis nuclei, has been utilized only for the treatment of neuropathic pain. This has included peripheral neuropathy, radiculopathy, thalamic syndrome, trigeminal neuropathy, traumatic spinal cord lesions, causalgic pain, phantom limb pain, post-herpetic neuralgia, anesthesia dolorosa [69,71,72]. Even though this distinction applies to most patients, individual patients may actually respond to the stimulation of one or another site regardless of their predicted pain syndrome. Some authors routinely place an electrode in the sensory thalamus and one in the PAG/PVG and decide during the trial which will be the most effective target[72]. The exact mechanism for such relief is still unclear but probably depends on complex central pathways. Additional target sites for stimulation have been proposed including the internal capsule, and the motor cortex[77].

A.3.C – Equipment

The most commonly utilized electrode for DBS is a coaxial lead composed of platinum-iridium powered by either the Medtronic radiofrequency-coupled device by a lithium powered pulse generator.

A.3.D - Implantation Technique and Indication

DBS is a stereotactic procedure whereby one or more electrodes are implanted in the depths of the brain matter. Following placement of the stereotactic frame, the targets are localized with imaging devices - computerized tomography (CT) or magnetic resonance imaging (MRI). The surgical implantation of the lead is performed according to the usual stereotactic implantation techniques. Electrical stimulation of the sensory nuclei of the thalamus results in contralateral tingling paresthesia that exhibit a somatotopic arrangement linked to the stimulated area. As with other neurostimulation procedures, pain relief occurs only in the areas where the paresthesia is felt. Stimulation of the PAG/PVG gives rise to a pleasant sensation of warmth and general well being. Higher voltage stimulation, however, may elicit feelings of fear and anxiety accompanied by tachycardia and blood pressure elevation.

A.3.E – Results

A few retrospective studies have shown positive effects of DBS on chronic pain. A review [72] of DBS found that 572 of 964 patients (59%) experienced satisfactory pain relief, and a large group of patients, including patients with back and leg pain, experienced a long lasting pain reduction of at least 50%. Levy reported 31% relief in 141 patients with average follow-up of 80 months [78].

Significant improvement for neuropathic pain ranges between 30 –78% and for nociceptive pain between 25–81% [76]. Cancer related pain and chronic low back pain seem to have greater success although there may be a tolerance effect with time. It has also been suggested that unilateral PVG stimulation can be effective for bilateral pain. The published results are often difficult to interpret since the methodologies are far from being uniform and the classification of the effectiveness are highly variable.

A.3.F – Complications

Complications are fortunately rare, but can be disastrous. They include intracranial bleeding (subdural hematoma or intracerebral hemorrhage), permanent neurological deficits including hemiplegia and paresis, sensory loss, diploplia, lead breakage, and malfunction of the pulse generator. Young has reported a 3.7% permanent and 26% temporary complication rate [72].

A.3.G – Conclusions

Even though DBS has been performed for almost three decades, there are no large prospective studies on its efficacy. The FDA has classified it as an investigational procedure that needs approval as a new application. The current role of DBS in chronic pain management is unclear and limited. Very few neurosurgical centers have the expertise to successfully implement the modality. At present DBS should be viewed as the last resort, to be implemented permanently only after successful trial stimulation.

B – INTRASPINAL DRUG DELIVERY

Intrathecal pump delivery systems provide a further alternative for the treatment of chronic pain syndromes, whose feasibility and usefulness have been empirically established [82-83].

B.1 – Equipment (Table 4, Figures 8, 9)

The majority of the implantable pumps are made of titanium, and have a thickness of 2-3 cm and weigh between 110-200 gm. They generally come with their own refill kits and catheter attachments, and can be punctured between 500-2000 times through a self sealing silicone septum; they have bacterial retentive filters, and most models are available with a direct access port which allows one to inject and withdraw directly from the CSF, bypassing the drug delivery chamber.

Table 4: Specifications for Implantable Pump

Company	Name	Type	Power	Reservoir capacity (ml)	Weight (g)	Flow rate range (ml/24hr)	Side port	Bacterial filter
Medtronic[1]	Synchromed 8610h	Motor/Variable Flow Rate	Battery	18	185	0.6-21	no	no
	" 8611h	Motor/Variable Flow Rate	Battery	18	185	0.6-21	no	yes
	" 8615s	Motor/Variable Flow Rate	Battery	18	205	0.1-21	yes	yes
	" 8615Ls[b]	Motor/Variable Flow Rate	Battery	18	205	0.1-21	yes	yes
	" 8616-10	Motor/Variable Flow Rate	Battery	10	190	0.1-23	no	yes
	" 8617-10	Motor/Variable Flow Rate	Battery	10	190	0.1-23	yes	yes
	IsoMed 8472-20-xx	Passive/Fixed Flow Rate	Propellant	20	113	0.5-1.5	yes	yes
	" 8472-35-xx	Passive/Fixed Flow Rate	Propellant	35	116	0.5-1.5	yes	yes
	" 8472-60-xx	Passive/Fixed Flow Rate	Propellant	60	120	0.5-1.5	yes	yes
Arrow[2]	3000	Passive/Fixed Flow Rate	Propellant	30	137	0.5-2	yes[a]	no
INFUSAI	100	Passive/Fixed Flow Rate	Propellant	47	187	1-6	no	yes
D[3]	400	Passive/Fixed Flow Rate	Propellant	47	208	1-6	yes	yes

xx – identifies flow rate

[1] – Medtronic Inc., Minneapolis, MN

[2] – Arrow International, Inc., Walpole, MA

[3] – Intermedics INFUSAID, Inc., Norwood, MA

[a] – in line bolus port

[b] – has 3 pre-attached surgical fixation loops

Pumps can be divided in two groups, depending on whether their mechanism of delivery is a propellant or battery operated. Propellant pumps do not contain a motor and utilize the body temperature to provide expansion of an inert substance which, via expansion, results in the delivery of medication through the intrathecal catheter. Their drawback is that in order to modify the delivery rate of the medication, the pump must first be completely emptied.

The lithium battery powered model utilizes a microprocessor which regulates a peristaltic pump. This system enables modifying the dosage of the medication non-invasively and delivery of the drug with different programmable modes. But it requires more frequent refills and skin punctures, and surgical replacement of the batteries at the end of their battery life.

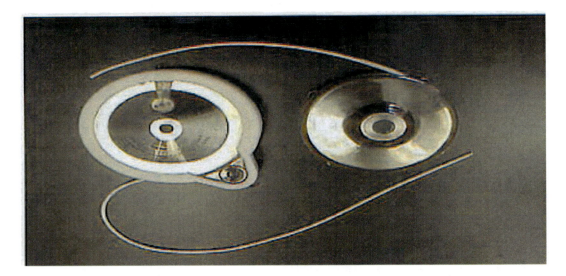

Figure 8. Implantable Pumps by Metronic. Synchronized and IsoMed (left to right).

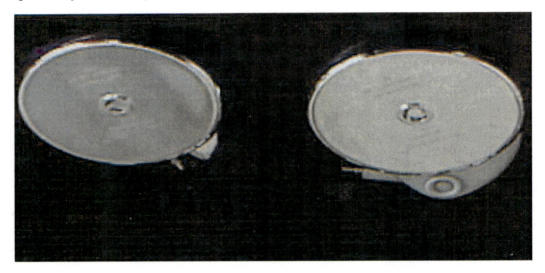

Figure 9. Implantable Pumps. Arrow Intenational Model 3000 and Intermedics INFUSAID Model 400 (left to right)

B.2 - Implantation Indications And Techniques

Intraspinal drug delivery devices have been implanted for both malignant pain and chronic benign pain. Successful implantation of a pump requires a significant commitment and an infrastructure. It is highly advisable that all patients undergo a screening trial and that they have greater than 50% subjective pain relief, have no undesirable side effects, and be infection free. The criteria for implantation in patients with malignant pain [84] include life expectancy greater than three months without tumor encroachment on the thecal sac, intolerable side effects from systemic opioids, or strong opioid use without adequate relief.

The procedure can be performed under general or monitored anesthesia. The pump is usually placed in the lower quadrant of the abdomen. The catheter is inserted in the subarachnoid space with a puncture at the lowest lumbar spine level available. The size of the patient and the configuration of the abdomen dictate the exact position of the device. The chest wall may constitute an alternative implant site.

B.3 – Complications

There are a number of complications, each of which can be treated in line with the severity of the phenomena and the state of the patient. The major complications are: (a) Leakage of CSF along the catheter track and into the pump pocket; (b) Infections of different kinds: superficial, of the subcutaneous tissues, hardware infection, local epidural and subdural abscesses, and CNS infections; (c) Catheter migration; (d) Radicular irritation; (e) Catheter occlusion; (f) Granuloma at the catheter tip; (g) Overdose as a result of pump malfunction or improper injection of the refill directly through the direct access port.

B.4 –Conclusions

Intraspinal drug delivery systems have a definite role in the management of chronic pain. Their utilization in the management of malignant pain could greatly reduce the need for ablative procedures, such as cordotomy or rhizotomy or high doses of oral or intravenous narcotics.

The exact relative role of intraspinal drug delivery versus neurostimulation is not yet clear. To our mind, implanting an intrathecal pump carries a higher degree of commitment and a greater risk of complications than an electrical stimulator. Patients with implanted pumps experience systemic and hormonal changes that are not observed with electrical stimulation. The side effects might be subtle and hard to recognize, especially in a patient with a CRPS type 1.

The possible complications are serious, some even potentially lethal. The implanting physician must be prepared to care for most of the patient's medical problems, regardless of whether they are related to the implanted pump, since other health professionals might decline caring for patients with implanted devices with which they are not familiar. In most centers in the US, pump implantation is usually considered only after the patient has failed a neurostimulation procedure. Exceptions occur and each case must be assessed individually.

The availability of new medications which might be more effective and specific for the various pain syndromes makes the use of drug delivery systems very appealing and assures a further growth of this modality.

REFERENCES

[1]   Schiller F. (1990). The history of algology, algotherapy, and the role of inhibition. *Hist. Phil.* Life Sci. 12; 27-50.

[2]   And 3. Shealy C.N. and Cady R.K. Historical perspective of pain management. In: R.S. Weiner (Eds.). Pain Management: A Practical Guide for Clinicians. 5th ed. St. Lucie Press, Florida, 1998, 7-15.

[3]   Hoppenstein R. : Electrical stimulation of the ventral and dorsal columns of the spinal cord for relief of chronic intractable pain. *Surg. Neurol.* 4 (1975) 187-194.

[4]   Dooley D.M. : Percutaneous electrical stimulation of the spinal cord. *Assoc. Neurol.* Surg. Bal Harbour, Fla, April 1975

[5]   Racz G.B., McCarron R.F., and Talboys P : Percutaneous dorsal column stimulator for chronic pain control. *Spine* 14(1) (1989) 1-4.

[6]   Barolat G. : Epidural spinal cord stimulation. Anatomical and electrical properties of the intraspinal structures and clinical correlations. Neuromodulation 2 (1998) 63-71.

[7]   Barolat ·G., Schwartzman R., and Woo R. : Epidural spinal cord stimulation in the management of reflex sympathetic dystrophy. Stereo. *Funct. Neurosurg.* 53 (1989) 29-39.

[8]   North R., Kidd D.H., Olin J., and Sieracki J.M. : Spinal cord stimulation electrode design: a prospective randomized comparison of percutaneous and insulated paddle electrodes. Abstracts of the 4th International Congress of the INS (1998) 211.

[9]   Kumar K., Nath R.K., and Toth C. : Spinal cord stimulation is effective in the management of reflex sympathetic dystrophy. *Neurosurg.* 40 (1997) 503-509.

[10]   Kemler M.A., Barendse G.A.M., Van Kleefe M., Van Den Wildenberg F.A.J.M., Weber W.E. : Electrical stimulation in of reflex sympathetic dystrophy: retrospective analysis of 23 patients. *J. Neurosurg* (Spine). 1 (1999) 79-83.

[11]   Oakley, J.C. and Weiner, R.L. : Spinal cord stimulation for complex regional pain syndrome: a prospective study of 19 patients at two centers. *Neuromodul 2* (1999) 47-50.

[12]   Law J.D. : Spinal stimulation in the "failed back surgery syndrome": Comparison of technical criteria for palliating pain in the leg vs. in the low back. *Acta Neurochir.* 117 (1992) 95.

[13]   North R., Kidd D.H., Olin J., Sieracki J.M., and Cutchis P.N. : Spinal cord stimulation for axial low back pain: single versus dual percutaneous electrodes. Abstracts of the 4th International Congress of the INS (1998) 212

[14] North R.B., Ewend M.G., Lawton M.T., Kidd D.H., and Piantadosi S. : Failed back surgery syndrome: Five-year follow-up after spinal cord stimulator implantation. *Neurosurg.* 28 (1991) 692-699.

[15] Turner J.A., Loeser J.D., and Bell K.G.. : Spinal cord stimulation for chronic low back pain: a systematic literature synthesis. *Neurosurg* 37(6) (1995) 1088-1096.

[16] Burchiel K.J., Anderson V.C., Brown F.D., Fessler R.G., Friedman W.A., Pelofsky S., Weiner R.L., et al. : Prospective, multicenter study of spinal cord stimulation for relief of chronic back and extremity pain. *Spine* 21(23) (1996) 2786-2794.

[17] Krainick J.U., Thoden U., and Riechert T. : Pain reduction in amputees by long-term spinal cord stimulation: Long-term follow-up study over 5 years. *J. Neurosurg.* 52 (1980) 346-350.

[18] Meglio M., Cioni B., Prezioso A., and Talamonti G. : Spinal cord stimulation in the treatment of postherpetic pain. *Acta Neurochir.* 46S (1989) 65-66.

[19] Tasker R.R., DeCarvalho G.T., and Dolan E. : Intractable pain of spinal cord origin: clinical features and implications for surgery. *J. Neurosurg.* 77 (1992) 373-378.

[20] DeJongste M.J.L., Haaksma J., Hautvast R.W.M., Hillege H.L., and Meyler J.W. : Effects of spinal cord stimulation on daily life myocardial ischemia in patients with severe coronary artery disease. A prospective ambulatory ECG study. *Br. Heart J.* 71 (1994) 413-418.

[21] DeJongste M.J.L., Hautvast R.W.M., Hillege H.L., and Lie K.L. : Efficacy of spinal cord stimulation as an adjuvant therapy of angina pectoris, A prospective randomized study. *J. Am. Coll. Cardiol.* 23 (1994) 1592-1597.

[22] Sanderson J.E., Brooksby P., Waterhouse D., Palmer RB., and Neubauer K. : Epidural spinal electrical stimulation for severe angina: a study of its effects on symptoms, exercise tolerance and degree of ischaemia. *Eur. Heart J.* 13 (1992) 628-33.

[23] Vulink N., Overgaauw D., Jesserun G., TenVaarwerk I., Kropmans T., ven der Shans C., Middel B., Staal M., and DeJongste M : The effects of spinal cord stimulation on quality of life in patients with therapeutically chronic refractory angina pectoris. *Neuromodulation* 2 (1999) 33-40

[24] Andersen C., Hole P., and Oxhoj H. : Will SCS treatment for angina pectoris pain conceal myocardial infarction? Abstracts of the First Meeting of the International Neuromodulation Society, Rome (1992) 39

[25] Thamer V., Deussen A., Schipke J.D., Tolle T., and Heush G. : Pain and myocardial ischemia: the role of the sympathetic system. *Bas. Res. Card.* 85s1 (1990) 253-266.

[26] Meller S.T. and Gebhart G.F. : A critical review of the afferent pathways and the potential chemical mediators involved in cardiac pain. *Neurosc.* 48 (1992) 501-24.

[27] Linderoth B., Gazelius B., Franck J., and Brodin E. : Dorsal column stimulation induces release of serotonin and substance P in the cat dorsal horn. *Neurosurg.* 31 (1992) 289-297.

[28] Cook A.W. and Weinstein S.P. : Chronic dorsal column stimulation in multiple sclerosis. N.Y. *St. J. Med.* 73 (1973) 2868-2872.

[29] Cook A.W., Oygar A., Baggenstos P., Pacheto S., and Keriga E : Vascular disease of the extremities: electrical stimulation of the spinal cord and posterior roots. N.Y. State *J. Med.* 76 (1976) 36-38.

[30] Meglio M., Cioni B., Dal Lago A., DeSantis M., Pola P., and Serricchio M. : Pain control and improvement of peripheral blood flow following epidural spinal cord stimulation. case report. *J. Neurosurg.* 54 (1981) 821-823.

[31] Jacobs M.J., Jorning P.J., Joshi S.R., Kitslaar P., Slaaf D.W., and Reneman R.S. : Epidural spinal cord electrical stimulation improves microvascular blood flow in severe limb ischemia. *Ann. Surg.* 207 (1988) 179-183.

[32] Horsh S. and Claeys L. : Epidural spinal cord stimulation in the treatment of severe peripheral arterial occlusive disease. *Ann. Vasc. Surg.* 8 (1994) 468-474.

[33] Sampere C.T., Guasch J.A., and Paladino C.M. : Spinal cord stimulation for severely ischemic limbs. *Pace* 12 (1989) 273-279.

[34] Robaina F., Dominguez M., Diaz M., Rodriguez J., and deVera J. : Spinal cord stimulation for relief of chronic pain in vasospastic disorders of the upper limbs. *Neurosurg.* 24 (1989) 63-67.

[35] Linderoth B., Fedorcsak I., and Meyerson B. : Peripheral vasodilatation after spinal cord stimulation: animal studies of putative effector mechanisms. *Neurosurg* 28 (1991)187-195.

[36] Linderoth B., Gunasekera L., and Meyerson B. : Effects of sympathectomy on skin and muscle microcirculation during dorsal column stimulation: animal studies. *Neurosurg.* 29 (1991) 874-879.

[37] Sanchez-Ledesma M.J., Garcia-March G., and Silva I. : Role of vasoactive neuropeptides in the segmentary vasomotor response following spinal cord stimulation. an experimental study. Stereo. Funct. *Neurosurg.* 54-55 (1990) 224-231.

[38] LoGerfo F. : Epidural spinal cord electrical stimulation: an unproven methodology for management of lower extremity ischemia. *J. Vasc. Surg.* 13 (1991) 518-519.

[39] North R., Sieracki J., Fowler K., Alvarez B., and Cutchis P. : Patient-interactive microprocessor-controlled neurological stimulation system. *Neuromodul 1* (1998) 185-193

[40] He J., Barolat G., Holsheimer J., and Struijk .JJ. : Perception threshold and electrode position for spinal cord stimulation. *Pain* 59 (1994) 55-63.

[41] Wall P.D. and Sweet W. : Temporary abolition of pain in man. *Science* 155 (1967) 108-109.

[42] Racz G.B., Browne T., and Lewis R. : Peripheral stimulator implant for treatment of causalgia caused by electrical burns. *Text Med.* 84 (1988) 45-50.

[43] Racz G.B., Lewis R., Heavner J.E., et al. : Peripheral nerve stimulator implant for treatment of causalgia. In: Stanton-Hicks M, (Ed.) Pain and the sympathetic nervous system. Kluwer Academic Publishers, Norwell, MA, 1990 225-239.

[44] Sunderland S. : The intraneural topography of the radial, median, and ulnar nerve. *Brain* 68 (1945) 243-200.

[45] Schon L.C., Lam P.W.-C., Anderson C.D., Easley M.E., and Timka H.J. : Preliminary results of peripheral nerve stimulation for intractable lower extrremity nerve pain. *Abstracts of the 4th International Congress of the INS*, Lucerne (1998) 173.

[46] Sweet W.H. : Control of pain by direct stimulation of peripheral nerves. *Clin. Neurosurg.* 23 (1976) 103-111.

[47] Campbell J.N. and Long D.M. : Peripheral nerve stimulation in the treatment of intractable pain. J. *Neurosurg.* 45 (1976) 692-699.

[48] Hassenbusch J., Stanton-Hicks M., Schoppa D., Walsh J.G., and Covington E.C. : Long-term results of peripheral nerve stimulation for reflex sympathetic dystrophy. *J. Neurosurg.* 84 (1996) 415-23.

[49] Hoyen H.A. : Peripheral nerve stimulation for chronic regional pain syndrome. *Abstracts of the 4th International Congress of the INS*, Lucerne (1998) 109.

[50] Gybel J.M. and Sweet W.H. : Neurosurgical management of persistent pain. In: KargerBasel (Ed.), New York, 1989.

[51] North R.B., Kidd D.H., Z.M., James C., and Long D.M. : Spinal cord stimulation for chronic intractable pain: experience over two decades. Neurosurg. 32 (1993) 384-395.

[52] Shetter A.G. : Spinal cord stimulation in the treament of chronic pain. *Curr. Rev.* Pain 1(3) (1997) 213-222.

[53] Weiner R.L., Alo K.M., Feler C., Oakley J, Naumann C., Stepniewski M., Keller H, Redko V., and Yland M.J. Nerve stimulation in the treatment of occipital neuralgia. *Abstracts of the 4th International Congress of the INS*, Lucerne (1998) 225.

[54] Alo K.M., Yland M.J., and Redko V. A novel technique to selective nerve root cannulation in the treatment of chronic pain. *Abstracts of the 4th International Congress of the INS*, Lucerne (1998) 283.

[55] Alo K.M., Yland M.J., Redko V, Feler C., and Naumann C. Lumbar and sacral nerve root stimulation (NRS) in the treatment of chronic pain: a novel anatomic approach and neuro stimulation technique. *Neuromodulation* 2 (1999) 23-31.

[56] Heath R.G. and Mickle W.A. : Evaluation of seven-years experience with depth electrode studies in human patients. In E.R. Ramey and D.S. O'Doherty DS (Eds.). Electrical studies on the unanesthetized brain. Paul B. Hoeber, New York 1960, 214-247.

[57] Kumar K., Toth C., and Nath R.K. : Deep brain stimulation for intractable pain: a 15 year experience. *Neurosurg* 40(4) (1997) 736-751.

[58] Reynold D.V. : Surgery in the rat during electrical analgesia induced by focal brain stimulation. *Science* 164 (1969) 444-445.

[59] Young R.F. : Periaqueductal and periventricular stimulation for pain. In J.R. Youmans (Ed.). Neurological surgery. W.B. Saunders Company, Philadelphia, 1996, 3528-3540.

[60] Young R.F. : Deep-brain stimulation for the treatment of chronic pain. Cur. Rev. Pain 1(3) (1997) 182-191.

[61] Adams J.E. : Naloxone reversal of analgesia produced by brain stimulation in the human. *Pain* 2 (1976) 161-166.

[62] Hosobuchi Y., Adams J.E., and Linchitz R. : Pain relief by electrical stimulation of the central gray matter in humans and its reversal by naloxone. *Science* 197 (1977) 183-186.

[63] Richardson DE and Akil H. : Pain reduction by electrical brain stimulation in man: part II. chronic self administration in the periventricular gray matter. *J Neurosurg* 47 (1977) 184-194.

[64] Tasker R.R. and Vilela Filho O. : Deep brain stimulation for the control of intractable pain. In J.R. Youmans (Ed.). Neurological surgery. W.B. Saunders, Philadelphia, 1996, 3512-3527.

[65] Hosobuchi Y. : Subcortical electrical stimulation for control of intractable pain in humans. Report of 122 cases (1970-1984). J. *Neurosurg.* 64 (1986) 543-553.

[66] Levy R.M., Lamb S., and Adams J.E Treatment of chronic pain by deep brain stimulation: long-term follow-up and review of the literature. *Neurosurg.* 21 (1987) 885-893.

[67] Sjoberg M., Nitescu P., Applegren L., and Curelaru L Long-term intrathecal morphine and bupivacaine in patients with refractory cancer pain. Results from a morphine: bupivacaine dose regimen of 0.5:4.75 mg/ml. *Anesth.* 80 (1994) 284-297.

[68] Winkelmuller M and Winkelmuller W : Long term effects of continuous intrathecal morphine opioid treatment in chronic pain of nonmalignant etiology. *J. Neurosurg.* 85 (1996) 458-467.

[69] Krames, E.S. : Intraspinal opioid therapy for nonmalignant pain. Curr. Rev. *Pain.* 1 (1997) 198-212.

In: The Handbook of Chronic Pain   ISBN 978-1-60021-044-0
Editors: S. Kreitler, D. Beltrutti, et al., pp. 273-296   © 2007 Nova Science Publishers, Inc.

Chapter 16

Radiation Therapy Pain of Malignant and Non-Malignant Origin

S Pergolizzi, E. G. Russi and G. Marchetti

INTRODUCTION

Radiation therapy is a discipline devoted to management of patients with cancer and other diseases using ionizing radiation. With the discoveries of W Roentgen in 1895 and M Curie in 1898 radiation therapy has became the most effective non-surgical tool for malignant disease treatment for much of the 20th century.

The aim of radiotherapy is to deliver an accurately measured dose of irradiation to a defined anatomic volume with low damage to healthy tissue [3]. Intrinsic to the understanding of radiation therapy is the concept of therapeutic ratio, which, as in pharmacology, is the ratio of benefits to side effects of a therapeutic tool. The radiation oncologist's primary concern is treatment of patients with malignant tumors. When choosing to treat pain from benign diseases that do not respond to other therapeutic modalities, the risks of delayed damage from ionizing radiation, such as carcinogenesis and genetic damage, should be kept in mind.

Patients with incurable neoplastic disease can have a long-term survival, in terms of months as well as years. In this clinical setting radiotherapy has an integrative role in the framework of the medical antalgic therapy. It is designed both to control chronic pain and symptoms linked to the neoplastic disease and to improve the quality of remaining life.

The palliative choice sometimes is more difficult with respect to definitive therapy and it depends on multiple variables present at the time of the therapeutic strategy (i.e. long history of disease, iatrogenic disease by previous treatments).

This chapter will focus on explaining the following:

a) Principles of radiological physics and radiation therapy treatment machines;
b) Fractionation schedules for palliative irradiation;

c)   Basic concepts of palliative radiotherapy;
d)   The role of clinical evaluations in decision making;
e)   Description of clinical pictures according to anatomical site of neoplastic disease;
f)   Radiation therapy of benign diseases.

PRINCIPLES OF RADIOLOGICAL PHYSICS AND RADIATION THERAPY TREATMENT MACHINES

The radiation oncologist employs a particular drug: the ionizing radiation. An electromagnetic radiation is called "ionizing" when its energy has the capability to ionize the atoms. It is generally believed that injury to nucleic acids is the most important mechanism by which radiation kills cells. The damage to DNA yields both a cellular transformation (genetic harm) and a cellular death.

Table 1a Acute and early or subacute side effects of radiation therapy

Confined to irradiation volume

	Erythema
Skin	Epilation
	Breakdown
Brain	Cerebral edema with headache
	Alopecia
Head	Otitis
	Conjunctivitis
	Mucositis
	Dry mouth
Head and Neck	Taste deficit
	Dysphagia
	Glottis edema
	Dysphagia (esophagitis)
Chest	Radiation Pneumonitis
	Temporary EKG changes
	Acute nephritis
Urinary tract	Frequency, Dysuria, Hematuria (cystitis)
Gastrointestinal Tract	
	Nausea, Vomiting
Stomach	Gastritis
	Acute enteritis with diarrhea
Small intestine	Nausea, Vomiting
	Infarction
	Tenesmus
Colon and Rectum	Rectal hemorrhage
	Systemic (out from irradiation volume)
Anorexia	
Fatigue	
Malaise	

Table 1b.Chronic or late side effects of radiation therapy

Skin	Telangectasia
	Fibrosis
	Necrosis
Brain	Severe gliosis and atrophy with Somnolence, intellectual deficit
	Necrosis
Head	Cataract
	Temporo-mandibular joint fibrosis
Head and Neck	Xerostomia
	Mandibular necrosis
	Pharyngeal-cervical esophageal stricture
	Esophageal stricture
	Lung fibrosis
Chest	Chronic cor pulmonale (secondary to interstitial fibrosis)
	Constrictive pericarditis
Urinary tract	Nephrosclerosis with benign or malignant hypertension
Gastrointestinal Tract	
Stomach	Gastric ulcer
Small intestine	Segmental enteritis
	Stenosis
Colon and Rectum	Segmental colitis
Rectal ulcer	
Strictures	
Fistula	

The effects of ionizing radiation, delivered by collimated beams directed to the tumor volume within the body, include neoplastic tissue and healthy structures. On normal tissues, this action can produce both acute and early or subacute (during treatment or 1-3 months after fractionated and single-dose therapy) as well as chronic or late (months or years after fractionated therapy) side effects, although every effort is made to reduce these in palliative treatment.

Irradiation gives rise to acute side effects during the therapy. These effects can be divided into two groups: those confined to the irradiated volume, and the systemic ones. These two groups of effects are summarized in Table 1 (Table 1a and Table 1b)

There are two different ways to deliver radiotherapy: by external beam and by isotopes. External radiation therapy is delivered using machines that generate different voltage; according to the energy the units are divided in:

Megavoltage (MV) unit (Linear Accelerator, Cobalt, Cyclotron); Kilovoltage (kV) or orthovoltage and superficial unit (X-ray machine). In the MV setting the nature of the beam is Photon, Electron and Particle (neutrons, pi-mesons, protons). At these levels of energies the beams penetrate without damaging the skin. The MV units are employed to irradiate deep lesions; up to date the particles have been used experimentally. The kV machines produce low energy photon beam that do not spare the skin. These kV energies are used to treat superficial lesions and skin tumors (see Appendix).

Isotopes can be divided into two groups:

1. "Sealed sources" for intracavitary applicators and interstitial implants (needles): cesium-137 and iridium-192. These sources are used mainly in gynecologic, head and neck, and skin tumors.
2. "Unsealed sources": Iodine-131 for thyroid cancer, Strontium-39 for pain from bone metastases.

PRINCIPLES OF FRACTIONATION SCHEDULES

Although some early radiation therapy was given as large single doses, fractionation was soon introduced because the output of machines was low and experiments on the response of testis to radiation showed that fractionation resulted in more inhibition of spermatogenesis than skin desquamation. Since skin was the dose-limiting normal tissue for low-energy X-rays and tumors proliferated like the seminiferous epithelium, it was deduced that dose fractionation would yield a favorable therapeutic advantage.

Biology of Dose Fractionation

The basic principles are:

*   Late responding tissues are more sensitive to changes in dose per fraction than are early responding tissues. As a result, increasing dose per fraction will increase the severity of late responses on healthy tissues. Spinal cord, optic nerve and perhaps peripheral nerves are intolerant of large dose fractions.
*   Late responding tissues are spared little or not at all by extending the overall treatment duration because their target cells turn over very slowly.
*   Acutely responding normal tissues can undergo extensive re-population during a protracted course of radiation therapy. There is a lag period between the initiation of radiation therapy and the onset of re-population.
*   Tumors, like acutely responding normal tissues, have the capacity to repopulate during an extended course of radiation therapy, but also only after a lag period.
*   The smaller the dose per fraction, the greater the self-sensitizing effect of cell cycle redistribution. This is presumed to occur in tumors and acutely responding normal tissues, but not in non-proliferating (late-responding) normal tissues [4].

Based on these basic principles, commonly used regimens involve doses per fraction of 1.8-2Gy, and treatment frequencies of 5 fractions per week. Using these doses, a total dose of 60-70Gy/6-7 weeks is delivered with safety.

In palliative radiation therapy, where the aim is to relieve symptoms, the dose per fraction is higher (3-10Gy) and the total dose is lower (10-45Gy).

BASIC CONCEPTS OF PALLIATIVE RADIOTHERAPY

The aim of radiation therapy should be defined "curative" or "palliative". In the curative setting the purpose is to "cure", so radiotherapy is delivered to patients in which there is a good probability of long-term survival; palliative irradiation is employed when there is no chance of the patient surviving for long period and thus, the aim of this treatment is the patient's comfort and quality of life.

Loco-regionally recurrent and metastatic cancer can cause strong symptoms such as pain due to nerve involvement with or without bone destruction. In this case prognosis is poor as well as quality of life [5,6].

The aims of palliative irradiation are:

1. Local control of neoplastic growth (i.e. control of fungation and ulceration);
2. Neoplastic cytoreduction (i.e. prevention of blockage of hollow viscera or veins).

The symptomatic irradiation is a unique form of palliation in which the aim is to control the pain caused by neoplastic disease. Symptomatic radiotherapy should be consistent with patient's tolerance, reducing number of hospital accesses and length of overall treatment, so that precious remaining time away from family is not excessive. Table 2 presents the clinical settings in which radiotherapy has a palliative objective.

Table 2.Indications for palliative radiation therapy

Pain	(bone metastases, carcinomatous neuropathy, involvement of the soft tissues)
Bleeding	(from exophytic bleeding tumors such as cervical and bladder cancer)
Fungation and ulceration	(skin metastases, head and neck cancer, locally recurrent breast carcinoma)
Oncologic emergencies Brain metastases	(superior vena cava syndrome, spinal cord compression)
Blockage of hollow viscera	(obstruction of the bronchi, esophagus, upper aerodigestive tract, bile ducts, ureteres)

ROLE OF CLINICAL EVALUATIONS IN DECISION MAKING

Clinical evaluation in palliative treatment choice is often difficult because of the necessity to consider many prognostic variables linked both to the patient and to the disease.

Hence we must reflect on the following three factors: (a) Overall survival; (b) Radiotherapy correlated side effects; and (c) Psychological impact on the patient

The first step in clinical decision-making should be the evaluation of the full extent of the tumor, node and metastases (TNM Staging) by whatever means available, including the surgical approach (biopsies) and imaging studies.

In the evaluation of treatment programs to be pursued, it is important to define whether the metastasis is a single or solitary lesion, or a metastasis as a part of more general systemic disease. In the former situation, aggressive programs of management should be pursued in order to maximize the potential for long-term control and disease-free interval. In the latter case, more conservative treatment techniques are appropriate in order to maintain local control but allow for continued long-term comfort.

It should be emphasized that in metastatic disease different tumors are characterized by different life expectancy. Thus, in patients with metastatic breast cancer we can identify three risk groups according to the sites of metastatic spread and "history" of disease: Low-, intermediate and high risk with a median survival times of 45.5, 24.6, and 10.6 months, respectively. For example, in the low-risk group patients without hepatic metastases and with a disease-free survival longer that 24 months are included [7].

The median survival of patients with bone metastases from lung cancer is 3.6 months [8].

The estimate life expectancy is inexact at best. Even experienced oncologists and hospice workers tend to overestimate the prognosis by an average of 3.4 weeks [9].

Unfavorable predictive prognostic factors about both the efficacy of the radiotherapy and survival can be considered:

(a) Metastatic disease in site/s prone to severe side effects linked to irradiation (liver, kidney) and/or presenting technical difficulty in treatment planning (pleura, peritoneum, pericardium).
(b) Bedridden patients. ECOG performance status >2
(c) Anemia.
(d) Hypercalcemia.
(e) Disease free survival (time from first neoplastic diagnosis to first progression disease in distant site/s) < 24 months
(f) Three or more sites of metastatic disease
(g) Presence of metastases without primitive tumor control
(h) Poor patient compliance to the treatment
(i) Karnofsky performance status < 50
(j) Physical complaints of dry mouth, shortness of breath, and difficulty swallowing

In palliative therapy a certain probability of significant side effects of therapy may not be acceptable and then no major iatrogenic conditions should be seen.

In a palliative setting it is highly important for the radiation oncologist to deliver a dose to the "metastatic volume" to ensure the maximum symptomatic control, while keeping at the lowest possible level any damage of radiation treatment in the surrounding normal tissues.

Last but not least, a cost-benefit evaluation will have an impact on the decision for radiotherapy in terminally ill patients. In the face of an ever tightening restriction of financial resources, this issue increasingly requires the attention of the medical profession. Analysis of the general health costs shows that the largest amount of money spent arises during the last year of his life. Guidelines for avoidance of futile medical procedures have been proposed but have proved to be almost not feasible as they are valid only if prognosis can be calculated with certainty [10]. However, rarely will a prognosis be definitely desperate, and in this era of ever rising legal fees for malpractice and omission of intervention, fewer radiation therapists will take the risk of deciding that a patient is lost and deserves no further treatment rather than the best supportive care [11].

The therapeutic decisions need often to be taken under pressure regarding time, the demands of the patient and relatives and on the part of referring colleagues. Moreover, in the case of failure or serious toxicity, the radiation oncologist alone has to take the responsibility.

DESCRIPTION OF CLINICAL PICTURES ACCORDING TO ANATOMICAL SITE OF NEOPLASTIC DISEASE

This section will describe both the clinical pictures and the role of radiotherapy in the palliative management of locally-advanced, recurrent and metastatic neoplastic disease causing painful symptoms. According to current radiotherapeutic principles the management of these diseases is based on site of anatomical localization rather than histology.

Cancer in the Brain, Spinal Cord and Nerves

Headache and impaired cognition are the most common symptoms in brain primary, recurrent, and metastatic tumors.

Palliation in Glioblastoma Multiforme

Older age and poor performance status at presentation are unfavorable prognostic factors for patients with glioblastoma (GB). Some studies suggest that in such patients a shorter, palliative course of radiotherapy may confer similar benefits compared to a radical course.

Bauman et al [12] reported the results of a prospective study of short-course radiotherapy in poor prognosis glioblastoma multiforme using a short-course whole brain radiotherapy (30 Gy/10 fractions/2 weeks). The authors demonstrated that elderly patients with a low pretreatment KPS (< or = 50) may be treated adequately with a short, palliative course of radiotherapy. Elderly patients with a higher pretreatment KPS (> 50), however, may benefit from a higher dose radiotherapy regimen. Another study [13] showed that patients treated with short course radiotherapy (37.5Gy in 15 daily fractions) in GB had comparable median survival to that of other series of radical radiotherapy.

Palliation in Brain Metastases

Brain metastases are the most common endocranial tumors among adults, occurring up to 10 times as frequently as primary tumors. Metastases to the brain are also the most frequent metastatic neurologic complication of systemic cancer [14].

Brain metastases develop when tumor cells that originate in tissues outside the central nervous system spread to directly involve the brain. Endocranial metastases may involve the brain parenchyma, the cranial nerves, the blood vessels (including the dural sinuses), the dura, the leptomeninges, and the inner cranial vault. Of the intracranial metastases, the most common are intraparenchymal metastases.

Headache from multiple brain metastases can be treated with radiation therapy and dexamethason. The most frequent primary tumor anatomic sites are lung, breast and unknown primaries [15]. Brain metastases due to cancers from the pelvic region or gastrointestinal tract are uncommon. Soft tissue sarcomas rarely metastasize to the brain, despite the presence of extensive metastases in other sites. Malignant melanoma has the highest percentage of brain metastases with respect to other primary sites.

The most important prognostic factors influencing treatment are the performance status, a disease-free survival interval longer than 1 year, the presence of multiple brain metastases and the presence of extracerebral metastases [16].

The following functional scale is valuable in predicting prognosis in patients with brain metastases [17].

Level I	Fully functional; no sign of disease
Level II	Fully functional; not able to work
Level III	Bedridden patients; needs help half of the time
Level IV	Requires help all of the time

For patients in whom survival is expected to be very short, for example a few weeks, and for those in whom symptoms from brain metastases are not the prominent problem, withholding radiation would be a reasonable option [18].

Borgelt et al [19], from the RTOG (Radiation therapy Oncology Group), conducted two randomized studies comparing fractionation schedules and total doses of irradiation for the palliative irradiation of brain metastases (from 20Gy in five fractions to 40Gy in 20 fractions/4 weeks). The results were the same in the different treatment groups.

The RTOG studies demonstrated that short treatment schedules provide as good a palliation as longer radiation schedules 1[9, 20].

In conclusion, the advantages of a short schedule are less time spent by the patients in the hospital, reduced costs, and maintenance of the same level of palliation.

Techniques for irradiation of patients with brain metastases are generally simple and can be carried out in all radiation oncology departments. Current treatment guidelines include use of opposed lateral whole brain fields and treating both fields daily to reduce dose inhomogeneity. Equipment for optimal beam energy range includes Cobalt 60 through 6MV accelerators.

Palliation in Metastatic Spinal Cord Compression

Compression of the spinal cord and nerve roots is second only to brain metastases as the most frequent neurologic complication of cancer[21]. About 5% of patients with systemic cancer have epidural metastases at autopsy [22], and nearly 20% of patients with neoplastic involvement of the vertebral column develop spinal cord compression [23].

Despite widespread bony deposits and even partial vertebral collapse, cord compression is rare, but when it occurs, it may become catastrophic [17].

The most important prognostic factor in patients with spinal cord compression is the degree of neurologic deficit before definitive therapy. Ambulation can be maintained for about 80% of patients who can walk at presentation [24]; in patients who are paraplegics the prognosis is poorer and they rarely recover walking capacity. Therefore, the results of treatment are good when the diagnosis is made early. Heightened awareness of signs and symptoms, wiith an emphasis on the significance of back pain, are the key to successful management.

The extradural space can be involved by paraspinal tumors (primary or metastatic), but the epidural compression is most commonly caused by a vertebral metastasis breaking through the posterior bony spinal canal and invading the epidural space.

A postmortem analysis [25] demonstrated that severe cord compression from vertebral metastases resulted from vertebral body collapse in 75% of cases and from epidural tumor extension in 25% of cases.

Changes in the spinal cord that arise from compression range in severity from reversible edema to irreversible necrosis. Some studies [26-28] emphasize that epidural compression of the cord impairs blood flow through perforating arteries and draining veins, whic leads to secondary changes including spinal cord edema, ischemia, and infarction.

Clinically, cord compression can be divided into two types: gradual and rapid. In the "gradual" type, sensory radiculopathy precedes weakness by months. In "rapid" type, sensory and motor dysfunction occur quickly, and the patient has paraparesis or paraplegia.

Pain is the initial symptom in 70% to 95% of patients [29-30]. The pain can be local or radicular. Local pain is present in almost all cases, and it is usually close to the site of compression [29]. Local pain is usually constant, dull, aching, and progressive. The level of involved vertebral body can usually be established by gentle spinal percussion [31].

Weakness, present in approximately 80% of patients, is the second most common symptom [29,30].

The most important diagnostic tool is the Magnetic resonance imaging (MRI). In addition to its diagnostic accuracy, MRI is extremely useful in planning radiotherapy or surgery. Identification of paravertebral tumors and outline of additional sites of vertebral involvement by MRI provide important information for designing radiotherapy portals.

Patients diagnosed with epidural cord compression should be treated immediately.

The primary aim of treatment is preservation or recovery of neurologic function and palliation of pain. Although untreated epidural cord compression is not fatal *per se*, the loss of ambulation is associated with shortened survival [32,33]. When the diagnosis of epidural compression has been made, high dose dexamethasone (10-90mg) should be started.

Over the last 15 years, treatment of metastatic spinal cord compression has been increasingly oriented to radiation therapy alone, reserving surgery for selected cases [34]. Studies [35, 36], comparing radiation therapy alone and irradiation plus surgery, showed the same results but a better quality of life for patients treated with radiation therapy alone.

Patients with no histologic diagnosis, with recurrent epidural compression in a previously radiated site, with worsening of neurologic signs during radiotherapy, with cord compression due to retropulsion of bone, with neoplastic diseases known to have limited radioresponsiveness (i.e. malignant melanoma), and fragments, should be considered for surgical resection. Other patients can be treated effectively with radiotherapy alone.

Techniques for irradiation of patients with metastatic spinal cord compression are generally simple and can be executed in all radiation oncology departments. Current treatment guidelines include use of anteroposterior or opposed lateral radiation fields. Equipment for optimal beam energy range include Cobalt 60 through 6-15 MV accelerators. On rare occasions the choice could be 20MeV electrons (for example, in a cervical epidural compression after laminectomy). Doses of 20Gy in four to five fractions are effective [37]. According to other authors [34], we prefer to deliver 30Gy over 2 weeks (3Gy per fraction).

During irradiation, patients are maintained on dexamethasone, and dose tapering occurs 3 weeks after the completion of radiation therapy.

Palliation in Nerve Infiltration

Tumor infiltration of nerve causes pain syndromes in patients with primary locally-advanced, recurrent and metastatic cancer. Clinically, it is possible to distinguish tumor infiltration of [38]:

Peripheral nerve->	Peripheral neuropathy
	Intercostal neuropathy
Plexus->	Cervical plexopathy
	Brachial plexopathy
	Lumbosacral plexopathy
	Celiac plexopathy
Root->	Radiculopathy
	Leptomeningeal metastases

Radiotherapy is often helpful in situations where tumor infiltrates directly into nerve and/or soft tissues, in which case it is usually administered in combination with steroids or non-steroidal anti-inflammatory drugs. Higher doses of radiation may be required in these instances than for treatment of bone pain.

Radiculopathy from metastatic disease should be treated in the same manner as epidural spinal cord compression. (for cervical plexopathy, see neoplastic disease in the head and neck; for intercostal neuropathy and brachial plexopathy, see chest neoplastic disease; for celiac and lumbosacral plexopathy, see neoplastic disease in the abdomen-pelvis).

Cancer in the Head And Neck

Palliative radiotherapy has a great role in the management of recurrent cancer causing pain and in metastatic disease affecting the head and neck.

Metastases of the Cranial Vault

Tumor infiltration of bone in the cranial vault needs a radiation treatment when there is a pain syndrome (rarely). In this rare occasion the choice could be 6-12MeV electrons to spare the brain.

Metastases of the Skull Base

Specific syndromes associated to metastatic spread at the base of the skull have been described and they are usually, but not always, a late finding in the course of a neoplastic disease [39, 40].

The success of radiotherapy in controlling pain from jugular foramen and middle fossa syndromes, clivus and parasellar metastases or sphenoid sinus metastases is well established. In these cases the irradiation should be directed to the base of the skull and it requires that the inferior edge of the portal be at the line drawn from the inferior orbital ridge to the mastoid tip. An orbital block should be used. Equipment for optimal beam energy range includes Cobalt 60 through 6 MV accelerators. Doses of 30Gy in ten fractions are effective.

Metastases of the Orbital Region

With the increasing efficacy of systemic chemotherapy used as an adjuvant to surgery and radiation therapy, metastatic disease to the choroid and/or orbital structures is increasing in frequency [41]. Orbital metastases are associated with retro-orbital or frontal headache, often with diplopia, visual loss, proptosis, and extraocular nerve palsies. In these instances, a lateral Co60 or 4-6MV field encompassing the orbit is employed. Doses of 20-30Gy (3-5Gy per fraction) are delivered.

Cervical Plexopathy

Cervical plexopathy may result from loco-regionally invasion by head and neck cancers or pressure from enlarged lymph nodes. Symptoms are primarily sensory in the distribution of the plexus, and are referred as aching preauricular, postauricular, or neck pain [42].

Because loco-regionally advanced head and neck cancer are sometimes suitable for radical irradiation, palliation is reserved to recurrent cancer previously irradiated and in metastatic disease in neck from distant tumors. In the former situation, aggressive management programs should be pursued. In the latter cases a short course therapy (10-30Gy in 1-10 fractions) can achieve some symptomatic responses.

Neoplastic Disease in the Chest

Brachial Plexopathy

Brachial plexopathy can be caused by tumor infiltration or radiation damage, if prior irradiation has been given to that area. Brachial plexopathy is associated most commonly with carcinoma of the lung (primary or metastatic) and breast (supraclavicular nodes metastases), as well as lymphoma [43].

Pain is an early symptom, and it often precedes other neurologic findings; therefore an early recognition with referral for treatment is essential to limit neurologic morbidity.

The lower cord of the plexus (C7-T1) is affected most frequently, and pain is characteristically experienced as diffuse aching in the shoulder with radiation down the arm (to the elbow and medial aspect of the hand) [44].

Early diagnosis of brachial plexopathy secondary to tumor and prompt administration of radiation therapy can alleviate neurologic symptoms in most patients. If symptoms are longstanding, the likelihood of alleviating them is considerably decreased.

Equipment for optimal beam energy range includes Cobalt 60 through 6 MV accelerators.

Doses of 30Gy in ten fractions are effective.

Chest Wall Pain

Chest wall pain is due to involvement of the parietal pleura from primitive or metastatic lung cancer. Tumor progression can result in the invasion of ribs and intercostal nerves.

When the treatment for rib metastases is necessary, either electron beam or tangential photon beams may be used, depending the patient's anatomy and compliance. We deliver a single dose of 10Gy using Cobalt 60 or 4-6MV linear accelerator. In this instance a careful delineation of the disease allows the best clinical results, both to limit the risk of acute-late pulmonary toxicity and to reduce the risk of "geographic miss".

Superior Vena Cava Syndrome

Superior vena cava syndrome (SVCS) is caused by tumor growth in the superior mediastinum and it is an acute or subacute oncologic emergency with typical clinical features that require prompt action. SVCS was first described as a clinical entity by Hunter W in 1757, in a patient with syphilis [45]. The most common presenting symptoms are shortness of breath, facial swelling, cough, headache, chest pain, and dysphagia.

The pathophysiology of the SVCS is related to obstruction of venous drainage in the upper part of the thorax, with increased venous pressure; a prolonged superior vena cava obstruction may lead to irreversible thrombosis, central nervous system damage, or pulmonary complication. Benign causes of SVCS include goiter, superior vena cava thrombosis, pericardial constriction.

Up to date cancer accounts for an estimated 97% of all cases of SVCS [46] and the syndrome is most common in patients with carcinoma of the lung and malignant lymphoma.

Radiotherapy has been advocated as standard treatment for most patients with SVCS [47,48]. It is used as the initial treatment if a histologic diagnosis cannot be established and the clinical status of the patient is deteriorating; however, recent reviews suggest that SVC obstruction alone rarely represents an absolute emergency that requires treatment without a specific diagnosis [49,50].

The fractionation schedule of radiation usually includes two to four large initial fractions of 300 to 400 cGy, followed by additional daily doses of 1.8 to 2Gy to complete the definite course of radiation therapy [51].

Cancer in the Abdomen-Pelvis

Celiac Plexopathy

Celiac plexus is located immediately inferior to the celiac artery; it lies on the anterolateral surface of the aorta from the T12 to L2 vertebral levels.

Abdominal pain is the most common symptom in patients with pancreatic carcinoma. In a study of patients with pancreas cancer, 45% had moderate or severe pain and 38% had no pain. Among the patients who had pain, 90% complained of abdominal pain in the chest, and 48% had lumbosacral pain [52].

Celiac nerve block has been performed for many years to treat intractable pain, usually secondary to pancreatic carcinoma; the efficacy of celiac plexus block approaches 90%, but the quality and duration of analgesia was rarely stated.

Symptom relief has been reported with radiation therapy [53-55], but the quality and duration of pain control has not been studied prospectively in a large group of patients with pancreas cancer.

To our knowledge there are no prospective studies comparing the effectiveness of radiation and nerve blocks in patients with pain refractory to medical management, nor is the optimal approach to treating the various types of pain experienced by patients well established.

Lumbosacral Plexopathy

Several distinct patterns of symptoms have been identified in lumbosacral plexopathy [56, 57]. The upper plexus syndrome may involve the ileoinguinal, iliohypogastric, and/or genitofemoral nerves, and is characterized by lower abdominal and groin pain, often accompanied by sensory loss but rarely motor loss. The lower plexus syndrome may involve sacral plexus, pudendal plexus, and pudendal, obturator nerves. It is associated with numbness of the foot, and flexor weakness of the ankle and knee.

Suspected plexopathy must be differentiated from invasion of the spinal cord or cauda equina. The patients have pelvic, perineal and leg pain; numbness or paresthesias along the distribution of involved nerves; muscular weakness and focal paralysis of muscle [5, 58]; and, less commonly, sphincter disturbance.

Lumbosacral neuropathy may be caused by infiltration or compression of the plexes and nerves from abdomen-pelvic malignancies or from lymphatic and osseous metastases of extraabdomen-pelvic tumors.

The surgical obliteration of the perivisceral fascial layers can explain the high frequency of pelvic neuropathy from postsurgical pelvic recurrences because recurrent tumor, without the fascial planes as barriers against endopelvic diffusion, can easily spread into the extraperitoneal pelvic space and involve the pelvic plexi and nerves [57].

The level of plexus involvement can be obtained by dermatomal somatosensory findings and must be confirmed by CT and/or MRI performed from L2 to perineum.

Most patients with lumbosacral plexopathy died within a year from the time of diagnosis [5,56,59]. Radiation therapy has role in the palliation of lumbosacral plexopathy. In this instance we strongly support [5,58,60] the use of megavoltage external beam irradiation (Cobalt 60, 6-15MV linear accelerator) with treatment fields encompassing only the site where the disease involves the lumbosacral plexus or its branches. He whole of the pelvis should be included in the radiation field only when a pan-sacralplexopathy is clinically diagnosed. The total dosage to deliver is 10-20Gy (1-5 fractions).

Metastatic Cancer in The Skeletal System

The most common cause of pain in cancer is bone infiltration. Malignant bone metastases occur in 30-70% of all patients with cancer (mainly for patients with lung, breast, and prostate primaries) [61]. Pain from bone metastases is usually constant, but may be greatest at night and it is often worse with movement or weight bearing.

Mechanisms of bone pain remain incompletely understood, but a biochemical explanation is attractive to explain how even small lesions can produce severe pain; probably there is stimulation of periosteal nociceptors *via* different mechanisms [62]. Four major mechanisms of pain from bone metastases have been described [93]:

(a) Stimulation of nerve endings in endosteum as result of release of hum from destroyed bone (PGE2, bradykinin, substance P, histamine);

(b) Stretching of periosteum by tumor enlargement;

(c) Fractures; and (d) Tumor growth into surrounding nerves and/or tissues.

Both treatment of metastases to bone and mechanisms of pain relief after radiation therapy are in general poorly defined. Further, the published guidelines for irradiation in cases with bone metastases are especially confusing because of the great variation in results of clinical trials and reports of treatment of a large variety of patients using different scoring methods and reporting techniques [63].

It is important to stress that patients with predominant bone metastases have longer duration of survival than patients with predominantly visceral metastases [64]. But, with long survival times, uncontrolled progression in the skeletal system may result in a lengthy period of severe disabling symptoms.

In general, an ambulatory patient who has localized pain, fewer than four sites of metastases without visceral sites (lung, liver, central nervous system), and no hypercalcemia is an excellent candidate for successful long-term palliation and survival [17].

Radiation therapy

Radiation therapy can be delivered using three forms of treatment: Local-field radiation therapy, Wide-field radiation therapy, and Radionuclide therapy.

(a) *Local-field radiation therapy* is the conventional treatment of bone metastases; it treats the involved bone and yields a pain relief rate of 80 to 90% [65]. Local-field irradiation is delivered using photon beam from megavoltage units (from Cobalt 60 to 6-15 MV linear accelerators).

Tong et al [66] reported the results of a RTOG randomized study on 756 patients with both solitary and multiple site of bone metastases using different total radiation doses and fractionations (20 *vs* 40.5Gy for solitary localization; 15 *vs* 20 *vs* 25 *vs* 30Gy for multiple site). All the schedules were effective and a median duration of pain relief of 12 weeks was observed.

Blitzer et al [67] reported a re-analysis of the study by Tong where they combined patients with solitary and multiple metastases, giving more power to the data, and included need for re-treatment. Blitzer observed that a more protracted course of irradiation (270cGyx15 fractions in solitary and 300cGyx10 fractions in multiple) was more effective in the pain control. There has been considerable interest in the administration of large, single fractions for bone metastases. A Royal Marsden Hospital randomized study [68] compared a single fraction of 8Gy *vs* 30Gy/10 fractions. No difference was found, in terms of speed of onset or duration of pain relief, between the two groups.

(b) is *Wide field (half-body, hemibody) radiation therapy* a form of "systemic" radiation therapy and can be used as primary palliative therapy for widespread symptomatic bone metastases [69,70], or as an adjuvant to local-field irradiation to reduce the later expression of occult metastases and the need for re-treatment [71].

Wide field irradiation provides pain relief ranging from 64% to 100%; approximately 50% to 66% of patients maintain pain relief for the remainder of their lives [63]. The fields must be shaped to reduce dose to sensitive structures such as lung, gut, kidney, and liver. Moreover, critical structures that have received previous irradiation up to tolerance must be blocked.

Wide field irradiation is delivered using MV units (from Co60 to 15MV linear accelerators) given through antero-posterior and postero-anterior portals.

It is possible to distinguish three types of treatments:

1. Upper wide-field treatments (from C1 to L2-3)
2. Lower wide-field treatments (from L3-4 to above the knees)
3. Mid-body wide-field treatments (from L1 to upper third of the femurs)

The optimal single-dose for upper wide field is 6Gy, and for lower or mid-body wide field it is 8Gy [69]. Zelefsky et al [70] used wide-field irradiation in a fractionated schedule to a higher total dose (25-30Gy in 8-10 fractions, three fractions per week).

(c) *Radionuclide therapy* is the systemic use of radioisotopes (unsealed sources) for bone pain. It is currently regarded as suitable for comparison with wide-field irradiation, but appears to have major disadvantages in terms of pain relief and toxicity. Using Strontium 89 in the treatment of bone metastases, response rate ranges from 37% to 91%; onset of pain relief occurs at 10 to 20 days, maximum relief requires up to 6 weeks, and median duration of pain relief is 12 weeks [63].

Skin Metastases

Superficial tumor fungation and ulceration is a disfiguring disorder that may be associated with pain. The most common of such tumors are locally recurrent and metastatic breast cancer on the chest wall, fungating head and neck cancer and malignant melanoma. The use of few large radiation fractions can be helpful for patients with a very poor prognosis. In these cases it is advisable to administer a superficial irradiation using electrons or low energy photons produced by x-ray machines.

CANCER CAUSING BLOCKAGE OF HOLLOW VISCERA

Any hollow organ may produce pain from obstruction by the presence of tumor into the lumen or by extrinsic compression. In these cases the role of radiation therapy (external MV or brachiterapy with "Sealed sources") may be helpful, although more data are needed.

Radiation Therapy of Benign Diseases

Radiation therapy is an accepted treatment for benign diseases that do not respond to other therapies. The report of the Committee on Radiation Treatment of Benign Disease of the Bureau of Radiological Health recommends the following [72]:

(a) Iinfants and children should be treated with irradiation only in very special cases; (b) direct irradiation of organs prone to late effects (thyroid, eye, gonads, breast) should be avoided; and (c) meticulous radiation protection techniques should be used at all times.

Kopicky and Order [73] analyzed the current use of radiation therapy for benign disease by radiation oncologists. The data showed that there is a very great difference in opinion about optimal dose and fractionation for treatment of most of the diseases.

Here we describe some examples of the use of irradiation for benign disease causing pain.

Orbital Pseudotumor

Lymphoid diseases of the orbit include three groups: pseudolymphoma (orbital pseudotumor and reactive hyperplasia); atypical lymphoid hyperplasia and malignant lymphoma [74]. Orbital pseudotumor is a benign idiopathic orbital unilateral or bilateral inflammation. Extensive lymphocytic infiltration produces inflammatory signs including pain. Patients are usually diagnosed with bioptic procedures. A 4-6 MV photon beam is used with unilateral or bilateral temporal fields posterior to the lens [75]. The radiation dose is 20-23.6 Gy with ultimate local control of 70-100% [76,77]. Patients must be followed closely, because subsequent systemic lymphoma is reported in 30% of patients [76,78].

Bursitis and Tendinitis

These disorders are caused by degenerative and inflammatory changes in tendons that could lead to calcium deposit, inflammation of the bursa, rupture and discharge of calcified material into the bursa. Bursitis and tendinitis principally affect the shoulder and calcification may occur both without and with pain, tenderness, and limitation of motion. Limited radiation fields encompassing only the disease are employed and the total dose delivered is of 6-10Gy. Therapy results are less satisfactory in chronic cases than in acute and subacute disease.

Peyronie's Disease

It is an idiopathic inflammatory lesion of the corpora cavernosa that could lead to the formation of localized or extensive plaques or nodules. In this case a painful angulation of the erect penis occurs. Some authors believe that irradiation is effective because pain is relieved in more than 70% of patients [79, 80]. The treatment requires a careful lead shielding of the gonads; doses range from 5Gy in one fraction to 24Gy (2-3Gy per fraction) [79-81].

Ameloblastoma

Ameloblastoma is a slow-growing neoplasm with few symptoms in the early stages. In advanced stages there may be facial deformity or loosening of the teeth or denture [82] and pain. The treatment of choice for ameloblastoma is surgery with adequate margins. Postoperative radiation therapy is rarely used as part of the initial therapy [83]. Irradiation has generally been applied to patients with advanced disease or after multiple surgical failures. Hence, the cure rate is unknown. The lesions respond well to radiotherapy and complete remission occurs delivering 50-60Gy (2Gy per fraction) [84].

Vertebral Hemangiomas

Most vertebral hemangiomas are asymptomatic and require no treatment, but there may be back pain. In this case a combined therapeutic approach of surgery and radiotherapy is usedd [85]. Radiation therapy alone has been used with the administration of 30-40Gy/3-4 weeks/2Gy per fraction; the results show a good symptomatic response rate [86, 87].

Ectopic Ossification

Experimental and clinical data support effectiveness of perioperative radiotherapy to prevent heterotopic ossification after hip surgery or trauma. This pathological entity occurs in 30% of patients undergoing hip arthroplasty [88]; the incidence is greater than 60% when risk factors are present: osteoarthritis, history of heterotopic bone formation, ankylosing spondylitis and diffuse idiopathic skeletal hyperostosis [89]. Postoperative ossification in the soft tissues can become symptomatic showing pain and impaired movement. Kolbl et al [90] performed a randomized trial comparing early postoperative irradiation (single 5Gy vs single 7Gy) vs. the use of nonsteroidal antiinflammatory drugs (indomethacin 2 x 50 mg/day for 1 week) for prevention of heterotopic ossification following prosthetic total hip replacement.

The authors report that a single fraction of 7Gy is more effective than irradiation with a single 5 Gy fraction or use of indomethacin. The efficacy of a single dose of 7Gy is confirmed by the data of another randomized study by Knelles et al [91]. Radiation treatment is given through anterior and posterior fields that encompass the soft tissues surrounding the hip joint.

Acute Postoperative Parotitis

This complication is now a rarity. It occurs 5 weeks after surgery in dehydrated patients, and radiation may avoid the necessity for incision and drainage. Pain decreases within a few hours and complete remission occurs after 4-5 days [92]. A total dose of 7.5-10Gy is given (daily dose of 2-2.5Gy) with orthovoltage x-rays, cobalt 60 or electrons through a lateral portal encompassing the parotid gland with 2-cm margins [75].

REFERENCES

[1]   Iaap. Subcommitte On Taxonomy: Pain Terms: A List With Definitions And Notes On Usage. *Pain*, 8(1980) 249-252.

[2]   Janjan N.: Pain Management. In: Perez C.A. And Brady L.W. (Eds.). Principles And Practice Of Radiation Oncology, 3rd Ed, Lippincott-Raven Publishers, Philadelphia, 1997, Pp. 2227-2241.

[3]   Perez C.A., Brady L.W., Roti Roti J.L.: Overview. In: Perez C.A. And Brady L.W. (Eds.). Principles And Practice Of Radiation Oncology, 3rd Ed., Lippincott-Raven Publishers, Philadelphia, 1997, Pp. 1-78.

[4]   Palcic B., Skarsgard L.D.: Reduced Oxygen Enhancement Ratio At Low Doses Of Ionizing Radiation. *Radiat. Res.*, 100 (1984) 328-339.

[5]   Russi E.G., Pergolizzi S., Gaeta M., Mesiti M., D'aquino A., Delia P.: Palliative-Radiotherapy In Lumbosacral Carcinomatous Neuropathy. Radiother. *Oncol.*, 26 (1993) 172-173.

[6]   Pergolizzi S., Settineri N., Santacaterina A., Maisano R., Frosina P., Loria F., Nardella G., Garufi G., Sansotta G., De Renzis C.: Prognostic Factors In Ambulatory Patients With Inoperable Locoregionally Recurrent Rectal Cancer Following Curative Surgery. *Anticancer Res.*, 19 (1999). In Press.

[7]   Yamamoto N., Watanabe T., Katsumata N., Omuro Y., Ando M., Fukuda H., Tokue Y., Narabayashi M., Adachi I., And Takashima S.: Construction And Validation Of A Practical Prognostic Index For Patients With Metastatic Breast Cancer. *J. Clin. Oncol.*, 16 (1998) 2401-2408.

[8]   Harrington K.D.: The Management Of Acetabular Insufficiency Secondary To Metastatic Malignant Disease. J. Bone Joint Surg. A., 53 (1981) 653-659.

[9]   Forster L.E., Lynn J.: Predicting Life Span For Applicants To Inpatient Hospice. Arch. *Intern. Med.*, 148 (1988) 2540-2543.

[10]   Emanuel E.J., Emanuel L.L.: The Economics Of Dying- The Illusions Of Cost Savings At The End Of Life. *N. Engl. J. Med.*, 330 (1994) 540-544.

[11]   Becker H.D., Di Rienzo G.: Interventional Bronchoscopy In Treatment Of Bronchial Carcinoma. In: Carpagnano F And De Lena M (Eds.). Recent Advances In Lung Cancer, Masson Spa, Milano, 1995, Pp. 221-234.

[12]   Bauman G.S., Gaspar L.E., Fisher B.J., Halperin E.C., Macdonald D.R., Cairncross J.G.A Prospective Study Of Short-Course Radiotherapy In Poor Prognosis Glioblastoma Multiforme.Int. J. Radiat. *Oncol. Biol. Phys.*, 29 (1994) 835-839.

[13]   Hoegler D.B., Davey P.: A Prospective Study Of Short Course Radiotherapy In Elderly Patients With Malignant Glioma. *J. Neurooncol.*, 33 (1997) 201-204.

[14]   Loeffler J.S., Patchell R.A., Sawaya R.: Section 1. Metastatic Brain Cancer. In: V. T. Devita, Jr., S. H., S. A. Rosenberg (Eds.). Cancer: Principles And Practice Of Oncology, Fifth Edition, Lippincott-Raven Publishers, Philadelphia, 1997, Pp 2523-2606.

[15]   Gelber R., Larson M., Borgelt B., Kramar S.: Equivalence Of Radiation Schedules For The Palliative Treatment Of Brain Metastases In Patients With Favourable Prognosis. *Cancer*, 48 (1981) 1749-1753.

[16]   Haie-Meder C., Pellae-Cosset A., Laplanche A., Lagrange J.L., Tuchais C., Nogues C., Arriagada R.: Results Of A Randomized Clinical Trial Comparing Two Radiation Schedules In The Palliative Treatment Of Brain Metastases. Radiother. *Oncol.*, 26 (1993) 111-116

[17]   Kagan A.R.: Radiation Therapy In Palliative Cancer Management. In: Perez C.A. And Brady L.W. (Eds.). Principles And Practice Of Radiation Oncology, 2nd Edition, J.B. Lippincott Co., Philadelphia, 1992, Pp. 1495-1507

[18]   Coia L.R., Aaronson N., Linggood R., Loeffler J., Priestman T.J.: A Report Of The Consensus Workshop Panel On The Treatment Of Brain Metastases. Int. J. Radiat. Oncol. *Biol. Phys.*, 23 (1992) 223-227.

[19]   Borgelt B., Gelber R., Kramer S., Brady L.W., Chang C.H., Davis L.W., Perez C.A., Hendrickson F.R.: The Palliation Of Brain Metastases: Final Results Of The First Two Studies Of The Radiation Oncology Therapy Group. Int. J. Radiat. *Oncol. Biol*. Phys., 6 (1980) 1-9, 1980

[20]   Kurtz J., Gelber R., Brady L., Carella R., Cooper J.: The Palliation Of Brain Metastases In A Favorable Patient Population: A Randomized Clinical Trial By The Radiation Therapy Oncology Group. Int. J. Radiat. Oncol. *Biol. Phys.*, 7 (1981) 891-895.

[21]   Posner J.B.: Management Of Central Nervous System Metastases. *Semin. Oncol.*, 4 (1977) 81-91.

[22]   Barron K.D., Hirano A., Araki S., Terry R.D.: Experiences With Metastatic Neoplasms Involving The Spinal Cord. *Neurology*, 9 (1959) 91-96.

[23]   Siegal T., Siegal T.: Current Considerations In The Management Of Neoplastic Spinal Cord Compression. *Spine*, 14 (1989) 223-228.

[24]   Harrington K.D.: New Information On Neuromuscolar Disorders. General Orthopaedics. *Spine.*Anterior Decompression And Stabilization Of The Spine As A Treatment For Vertebral Collapse And Spinal Cord Compression From Metastatic Malignancy. *Clin. Orthop.*, 233 (1988) 177-197.

[25] Kakulas B.A., Harper C.G., Shibasaki K., Bedbrook G.M.:Vertebral Metastases And Spinal Cord Compression. *Clin. Exper. Neurol.*, 15 (1978) 98-113.

[26] Doppman J.L., Girton M.: Angiographic Study Of The Effect Of Laminectomy In The Presence Of Acute Anterior Epidural Masses. *J. Neurosurg.*, 45 (1976) 195-202.

[27] Arguello F., Baggs R.B., Duerst R.E., Johnstone L., Mcqueen K., Frantz C.N.: Pathogenesis Of Vertebral Metastasis And Epidural Spinal Cord Compression. *Cancer*, 65 (1990) 98-106.

[28] Ushio Y., Posner R., Posner J.B., Shapiro W.R.: Experimental Spinal Cord Compression By Epidural Neoplasms. *Neurology*, 27 (1977) 422-429.

[29] Gilbert R.W., Kim J.H., Posner J.B.: Epidural Spinal Cord Compression From Metastatic Tumor: Diagnosis And Treatment. *Ann. Neurol.*, 3 (1978) 40-51.

[30] Stark R.J., Henson R.A., Evans S.J.W.: Spinal Metastases. A Retrospective Survey From A General Hospital. *Brain*, 105 (1982) 189-213.

[31] Fuller B.G., Heiss J., Oldfield E.H.: Section 2. Spinal Cord Compression .In: V. T. Devita, Jr., S. Hellman, S. A. Rosenberg (Eds.). Cancer: Principles And Practice Of Oncology, Fifth Edition, Lippincott-Raven Publishers, Philadelphia, 1997, Pp 2523-2606.

[32] Leviov M., Dale J., Stein M., Ben-Shahar M., Ben-Arush M., Milstein D., Goldsher D., Kuten A.: The Management Of Metastatic Spinal Cord Compression: A Radiotherapeutic Success Ceiling. Int. J. Radiat. Oncol. *Biol. Phys.*, 27 (1993) 231-234.

[33] Sioutos P.J., Arbit E., Meshulam C.F., Galicich J.H.: Spinal Metastases From Solid Tumors. Analysis Of Factors Affecting Survival. *Cancer*, 76 (1995) 1453-1459.

[34] Maranzano E., Latini P., Checcaglini F., Ricci S., Panizza B.M., Aristei C., Perrucci E., Benvenuti S., Corgna E., Tonato M.: Radiation Therapy In Metastatic Spinal Cord Compression.*Cancer*, 67 (1991) 1311-1317.

[35] Portenoy P., Limpton R.B., Foly K.M.: Back Pain In The Cancer Patients: An Algorithm For Evaluation And Management. *Neurology*, 37 (1989)134-138.

[36] Aabo K., Walbom-Jorgensen S.: Central Nervous System Complications By Malignant Lymphomas: Radiation Schedule And Treatment Results. Int. J. Radiat. Oncol. *Biol. Phys.*, 12 (1986) 197-202

[37] Rate W.R., Solin L.H., Turrisi A.T.: Palliative Radiotherapy For Metastatic Malignant Melanoma: Brain Metastases, Bone Metastases, And Spinal Cord Compression. Int. J. Radiat. Oncol. *Biol. Phys.*, 15 (1988) 859-864.

[38] Foley K.M.: Supportive Care And The Quality Of Life Of The Cancer Patient. Section 1: Management Of Cancer Pain. In: Devita V.T., Hellman S., Rosenberg S.A. (Eds.). Cancer, Principles And Practice Of Oncology, 4th Ed., Jb Lippincott Co, Philadelphia, 1993, Pp 2417-2448.

[39] Greenberg H.S., Deck M.D.F., Vikram B: Metastasis To The Base Of The Skull: Clinical Findings In 43 Patients. *Neurology*, 31 (1981) 530-537.

[40] Elliot K., Foley K.M.: Neurologic Pain Syndromes In Patients With Cancer. Crit. *Care Clin.* 6 (1990) 393-420.

[41] Brady L.W.: Radiotherapy For The Eye- Tolerance Issues And Therapeutic Strategies For Benign And Malignant Problems. In: Proceedings Of The American Society For Therapeutic Radiology And Oncology, 39th Annual Meeting Orlando, Florida, 1997.

[42] Patt R.B.: Classification Of Cancer Pain And Cancer Pain Syndromes. In: Patt Rb (Ed.). Cancer Pain, Jb Lippincott Co, Philadelphia, 1993, Pp. 3-22.

[43] Kori S.H., Foley K.M., Posner J.B.: Brachial Plexus Lesions In Patients With Cancer:100 Cases. *Neurology*, 31 (1981) 45-50.

[44] Batzdorf U., Brechner V.L.: Management Of Pain Associated With The Pancoast Syndrome. *Am. J. Surg.*, 137 (1979) 638-646.

[45] Hunter W.: History Of Aneurysm Of The Aorta With Some Remarks On Aneurysm In General.M. *Observ. Inq.* (London), 1 (1757) 323.

[46] Helms S.R., Carlson M.D.: Cardiovascular Emergencies. *Semin. Oncol.*, 16 (1989) 463-470.

[47] Goodman R.: Superior Vena Cava Syndrome. Clinical Management. *Jama*, 231 (1975) 58-61.

[48] Perez C.A., Presant C.A., Van Amburg A.L. Iii: Management Of Superior Vena Cava Syndrome. *Semin. Oncol.*, 5 (1978) 123-134.

[49] Yellin A., Rosen A., Reichert N., Lieberman Y.: Superior Vena Cava Syndrome: The Myth -- The Facts. Am. Rev. Respir. *Dis.*, 141 (1990) 1114-1118.

[50] Ahmann F.R.: A Reassessment Of The Clinical Implications Of The Superior Vena Caval Syndrome. *J. Clin. Oncol.*, 2 (1984) 961-969.

[51] Rubin P., Ciccio S.: High Daily Dose For Rapid Decompression. In: Deeley T. (Ed). Modern Radiotherapy: Carcinoma Of The Bronchus, Appleton-Century-Crofts, New York, 1971, Pp. 354-378.

[52] Greenwald H.P., Bonica J.J., Bergner M.: The Prevalence Of Pain In Four Cancers. *Cancer*, 60 (1987) 2563-2569.

[53] Haslam J.B., Cavanaugh P.J., Stroup S.L.: Radiation Therapy In The Treatment Of Irresectable Adenocarcinoma Of The Pancreas. *Cancer*, 32 (1973) 1341-1345.

[54] Gastrointestinal Tumor Study Group: Radiation Therapy Combined With Adriamycin Or 5-Fluorouracil For The Treatment Of Locally Unresectable Pancreatic Carcinoma. *Cancer*, 56 (1985) 2563-2568.

[55] Green N., Beron E., Melbye R.W., George F.W. 3d: Carcinoma Of Pancreas-Palliative Radiotherapy. Am. J. Roentgenol. Radium Ther. *Nucl. Med.*, 117 (1973) 620-622.

[56] Jaekle K.A., Young D.F., Foley K.M.: The Natural History Of Lumbosacral Plexopathy In Cancer. Neurology, 35 (1985) 8-15

[57] Gaeta M., Pandolfo I., Russi E., Blandino A., Volta S., Racchiusa S.: Pelvic Carcinomatous Neuropathy. Ct Findings And Implications For Radiation Treatment Planning. J. Comput. *Assist. Tomogr.*, 12 (1988) 811-816.

[58] Russi E.G., Gaeta M., Pergolizzi S., D'aquino A., Mesiti M., Raffaele M., Di Carlo M., Delia P., Romeo F.: Pelvic Carcinomatous Neuropathy: Clinical, Radiologic, Therapeutic Implications. G. Ital. *Oncol.*, 10 (1990) 77-84.

[59] Ampil F.L.: Palliative Irradiation Of Carcinomatous Lumbosacral Plexus Neuropathy. Int. J. Radiat. Oncol. *Biol. Phys.*, 12 (1986) 1681-1686.

[60] Russi E.G., Gaeta M., Pergolizzi S., Settineri N., Frosina P., De Renzis C.: Antalgic Radiotherapy In Lumbosacral Carcinomatous Neuropathies. *Radiol. Med.*, 87 (1994) 858-864.

[61] Russi E.G., Marchetti G., Pergolizzi S., D'aquino A.: Metastatic Bone Disease. Tipolito Saste, *Cuneo*, 1989, Pp 42.

[62] Healey J.: The Mechanism And Treatment Of Bone Pain. In: Arbit E. (Ed). Management Of Cancer-Related Pain, Futura, New York, 1993, Pp 515-526.

[63] Powers W.E., Ratanatharathorn V.: Palliation Of Bone Metastases. In: Perez C.A. And Brady L.W. (Eds.). Principles And Practice Of Radiation Oncology, 3rd Ed., Lippincott-Raven Publishers, Philadelphia, 1997, Pp 2199-2217

[64] Leone B.A., Romero A., Rabinovich M.G., Vallejo C.T., Bianco A., Perez J.E., Machiavelli M., Rodriguez R., Alvarez L.A.: Stage Iv Breast Cancer: Clinical Course And Survival Of Patients With Osseous Metastases At Initial Diagnosis. Am. *J. Clin. Oncol.*, 11 (1988) 618-622.

[65] Nielsen O.S., Munro A.J., Tannock I.F.: Bone Metastases: Pathophysiology And Management Policy. *J. Clin. Oncol.*, 9 (1991) 509-524.

[66] Tong C., Gillick L., Hendrickson F.R.: The Palliation Of Symptomatic Osseous Metastases: Final Results Of The Study By The Radiation Therapy Oncology Group. *Cancer*, 50 (1982) 893- 899.

[67] Blitzer P.H.: Reanalysis Of The Rtog Study Of The Palliation Of Symptomatic Osseous Metastasis. *Cancer*, 55 (1985) 1468-1472

[68] Price P., Hoskin P.J., Easton D., Austin D., Palmer S.G., Yarnold J.R.: Prospective Randomised Trial Of Single And Multifraction Radiotherapy Schedules In The Treatment Of Painful Bony Metastases. Radiother. *Oncol.*, 6 (1986) 247-255.

[69] Salazar O.M., Rubin P., Hendrickson F.R, Komaki R., Poulter C., Newall J., Asbell S.O.,Mohiuddin M., Van Ess J.: Single-Dose Half-Body Irradiation For Palliation Of Multiple Bone Metastases From Solid Tumors: Final Radiation Thrapy Oncology Group Report. *Cancer*, 58 (1986) 29-36.

[70] Zelefsky M.J., Scher H.I., Forman J.D., Linares L.A., Curley T., Fuks Z.: Palliative Hemiskeletal Irradiation For Widespread Metastatic Prostate Cancer: A Comparison Of Single Dose And Fractionated Regimens. Int. J. Radiat. Oncol. *Biol. Phys.*, 17 (1989) 1281-1285.

[71] Poulter C.A., Cosmatos D., Rubin P., Urtasun R., Cooper J.S., Kuske R.R., Hornback N.,Coughlin C., Weigensberg I., Rotman M.: A Report Of Rtog 8206: A Phase Iii Study Of Whether The Addition Of Single Dose Hemibody Irradiation To Standard Fractionated Local Field Irradiation Is More Effective Than Local Field Irradiation Alone In The Treatment Of Symptomatic Osseous Metastases. Int. J. Radiat. Oncol. *Biol. Phys.*, 23 (1992) 207- 214.

[72] Bureau Of Radiological Health: A Review Of The Use Of Ionizing Radiation For The Treatment Of Benign Disease, Vol 1, Rockville, Md, Us Department Of Health, Education And Welfare, 1977, Pp1-2.

[73] Kopicky J., Order S.E.: Survey And Analysis Of Radiation Therapy Of Benign Disease. In: National Research Council, Ed: A Review Of The Use Of Ionizing Radiation For The Treatment Of Benign Disease, Vol Ii, Rockville, Md, Us Department Of Health, Education And Welfare, 1977, P13.

[74] Knowles D. M. 2d, Jakobiec F. A.: Orbital Lympoid Neoplasms: A Clinicopathologic Study Of 60 Patients. Cancer, 46 (1980) 576-589.

[75] Serber W., Dzeda M., Hoppe R.: Radiation Treatment Of Benign Disease. In: Perez C.A. And Brady L.W. (Eds.) Principles And Practice Of Radiation Oncology, 3rd Ed., Lippincott-Raven Publishers, Philadelphia, 1997, Pp 2167-2185.

[76] Austin-Seymour M.M., Donaldson S.S., Egbert P.R., Mcdougall I.R., Kriss J.P.: Radiotherapy Of Lymphoid Diseases Of The Orbit. Int. J. Radiat. Oncol. *Biol. Phys.*, 11 (1985) 371-379.

[77] Lanciano R., Fowble B., Sergott R.C., Atlas S., Savino P.J., Bosley T.M., Rubenstein J.: The Results Of Radiotherapy For Orbital Pseudotumor. Int. J. Radiat. Oncol. *Biol. Phys.* 18 (1990) 407-411.

[78] Barthold H.J., Harvey A., Markoe A.M., Brady L.W., Augsburger J.J., Shields J.A.: Treatment Of Orbital Pseudotumors And Lymphoma. Am. *J. Clin. Oncol.*, 9 (1986) 527-532.

[79] Helvie W.W., Ochsner S.F.: Radiation Therapy In Peyronie's Disease. *South Med. J.*, 65 (1972) 1192-1196.

[80] Rodrigues C.I., Hian Njo K., Karim A.B.: Results Of Radiotherapy And Vitamin E In The Treatment Of Peyronie's Disease. Int. J. Radiat. Oncol. *Biol. Phys.* 31 (1995) 571-576.

[81] Mira J.G., Chahbazian C.M., Del Regato J.A.: The Value Of Radiotherapy For Peyronie's Disease: Presentation Of 56 New Case Studies And Review Of The Literature. Int. J. Radiat. Oncol. *Biol. Phys.* 6 (1980) 161-166.

[82] Goldberg S.J., Friedman J.M.: Ameloblastoma: Review Of The Literature And Report Of Case. *J. Am. Dent. Assoc.* 90 (1975) 432-438

[83] Million R.R., Cassisi N.J., Mancuso A.A.: Oral Cavity. In: Million R.R And Cassisi N.J. (Eds.). Management Of Head And Neck Cancer. A Multidisciplinary Approach. 2nd Ed., J.B. Lippincott Co, Philadelphia, 1994, Pp321-400.

[84] Atkinson C.H., Harwood A.R., Cummings B.J.: Ameloblastoma Of The Jaw: A Reappraisal Of The Role Of Megavoltage Irradiation. *Cancer*, 53 (1984) 869-873.

[85] Mcallister V.L., Kendall B.E., Bull J.W.D.: Symptomatic Vertebral Hemangiomas. *Brain*, 98 (1975) 71-80.

[86] Faria S.L., Schlupp W.R., Chiminazzo H.: Radiotherapy In The Treatment Of Vertebral Hemangiomas. Int. J. Radiat. Oncol. *Biol. Phys.*, 11 (1985) 387-390.

[87] Schild S.E., Buskirk S.J., Frick L.M., Cupps R.E: Radiotherapy For Large Symptomatic Hemangiomas. Int. J. Radiat. Oncol. *Biol. Phys.*, 21 (1991) 729-735.

[88] Ritter M.A., Vaughan R.B.: Ectopic Ossification After Total Hip Arthroplasty: Predisposing Factors, Frequency And Effect On Results. J. Bone Joint *Surg. Am.*, 59 (1977) 345-351.

[89] Gregoritch S.J., Chadha M., Pelligrini V.D., Rubin P., Kantorowitz D.A.: Randomized Trial Comparing Preoperative Versus Postoperative Irradiation For Prevention Of Heterotopic Ossification Following Prosthetic Total Hip Replacement: Preliminary Results. Int. J. Radiat. Oncol. *Biol. Phys.*, 30 (1994) 55-62.

[90] Kolbl O., Knelles D., Barthel T., Kraus U., Flentje M., Eulert J.: Randomized Trial Comparing Early Postoperative Irradiation Vs. The Use Of Nonsteroidal Antiinflammatory Drugs For Prevention Of Heterotopic Ossification Following Prosthetic Total Hip Replacement. Int. J. Radiat. Oncol. *Biol. Phys.*, 39 (1997) 961-966

[91] Knelles D., Barthel T., Karrer A., Kraus U., Eulert J., Kolbl O.: Prevention Of Heterotopic Ossification After Total Hip Replacement. A Prospective, Randomised Study Using Acetylsalicylic Acid, Indomethacin And Fractional Or Single-Dose Irradiation. *J. Bone Joint Surg. Br.*, 79 (1997) 596-602

[92] Gustafson J.R.: Acute Parotitis. *Surgery*, 29 (1951) 786-788

[93] Scarantino C.W., Konski A.A.: The Role Of Radiation Therapy In The Management Of Bone Metastases. In: Proceedings Of The American Society For Therapeutic Radiology And Oncology. 39th Annual Meeting Orlando, Florida, 1997.

APPENDIX

Absorbed Dose

In 1953, the International Committee on Radiological Units and Measurements introduced the concept of adsorbed dose and named this unit *rad*. Absorbed dose is defined in terms of the energy deposited by the radiation beam as it passes through the medium of interest. The *rad* represents the absorption of 0.01 joule per kilogram of the medium:

1 rad = 0.01 J/kg

The SI unit for absorbed dose is 1 J/kg and is called a *Gray (Gy)*.

Notice that 100 rad = 1 J/kg = 1 Gy. Therefore, 1 *rad* = 1 *centigray (cGy)*.

Part V:
Psychosocial Therapeutic Approaches

In: The Handbook of Chronic Pain
Editors: S. Kreitler, D. Beltrutti, et al., pp. 299-321

ISBN 978-1-60021-044-0
© 2007 Nova Science Publishers, Inc.

Chapter 17

Psychological Approaches to Treatment of Pain: Sensory, Affective, Cognitive and Behavioral

Shulamith Kreitler and Michal Kreitler

The psychological approaches to pain treatment denote a series of therapeutic techniques defined first, by being nonpharmacological and noninvasive, and second, by utilizing psychological processes for controlling pain. In the present context we will refer only to techniques whose efficacy has been examined in experimental studies conforming to accepted methodological criteria and with samples of adults. This chapter will provide first, a general overview of all techniques, second, a set of criteria for characterizing and evaluating them, third, a brief presentation of major techniques (not presented in other chapters), and fourth, a summary presenting main conclusions about applying the techniques.

OVERVIEW OF THE PSYCHOLOGICAL TECHNIQUES

Classification of the techniques. According to the widely accepted approach to pain, pain consists of nociception, based on the damaged tissue, and the following four components: (a) sensations, such as strong/intense, burning, penetrating, slashing, deep/superficial and localized/ irradiating; (b) emotions, such as anxiety, depression, fear, anger, irritability and despair; (c) cognitions, such as identifying the input or sensation as pain, attitudes about the pain and how it will be or should be handled, appraisal of the severity of the pain and the situation, and expectancies about the future; and (d) behaviors, such as external expressions of pain (e.g., sighing, crying, screaming, grimacing), complaining, holding or rubbing the painful area, motor pain behaviors (e.g., limping), isolating oneself or seeking out others, avoiding physical movements and moving cautiously, as well as consumption of medication.

The updated more comprehensive conception adds quality of life as a domain afflicted by pain and reflecting beneficial effects of pain treatments (see Chapter 5, this book).

The different psychological techniques focus on different components of pain as their sole or major target. Accordingly, it is possible to classify the techniques into the following four groups:

I.   Psychological techniques targeting the sensory component of pain: Guided imagery, hypnosis, auto-suggestion, relaxation, biofeedback, distraction/displacement of attention, music therapy; meditation;

II. Psychological techniques targeting the affective component of pain: Supportive therapies (social support, family support, supportive psychotherapy), meaning-based control of negative emotions, dynamic psychotherapy, and art therapy;

III. Psychological techniques targeting the cognitive component of pain: educational/didactic information-based techniques, cognitive attitude-based therapy, and cognitive coping therapy.

IV. Psychological techniques targeting the behavioral component of pain: operant conditioning, environmental therapy, coping by means of behavioral strategies (behavioral therapy), cognitive orientation therapy.

PRESENTING THE TECHNIQUES: SOME CAVEATS

The above classification is based on the target of each technique rather than on the means they use. The targeted pain component and the means used by the technique may differ or not. Thus, guided imagery may target the sensory component but is based on applying cognitive means. Further, the classification reflects the major target of each technique, although it is evident that some techniques target explicitly or implicitly more than one pain component.

Most psychological treatments of pain are in fact comprehensive programs for managing pain, consisting of a combination of different techniques, used sometimes in their original form, more often in a modified form. Even a title as "cognitive-behavioral therapy" that apparently denotes an original technique represents a combination of different techniques to which more techniques are often added freely. Another example is "meditation" which at least in its Western applications consists of an aggregate of different techniques. Since none of the combinations of techniques is consensually accepted or has been widely tested, in the present context we will deal with the basic techniques. However, we will keep as close as possible to the format of the techniques as they are commonly used rather than analyzing them artificially into their components.

Another difficulty in describing the techniques is that most can be applied for attaining different goals. Thus, guided imagery may be used for controlling pain directly or indirectly, by promoting relaxation, control of anxiety, rehearsing coping strategies, etc. Thus, it is necessary to distinguish between the means and the contents, or the technique and the goal. In describing the techniques we will stick to their major uses, emphasizing the elements common to their different variants.

CRITERIA FOR CHARACTERIZING THE PSYCHOLOGICAL APPROACHES TO PAIN TREATMENTS

The following criteria are proposed for the characterization as well as evaluation of the different techniques. Therefore they have both a theoretical-scientific value for promoting research and further development of psychological pain therapies as well as applied-clinical value for facilitating orientation and choice of technique by the practitioner.

1. *Mode of application:* refers to the means, procedures, methods and stages characterizing the application of the technique.
2. *Tools or instruments used in application:* refers to actual instruments that may be necessary for applying the technique, such as a biofeedback machine.
3. *Targeted pain component(s):* refers to the primary and secondary pain components targeted by the technique, as well as domains of quality of life likely to be affected by the technique directly or indirectly and hence may be used for assessing its effects.
4. *Breadth of effect(s):* refers to the range of effects expected to be attained through the application of the technique, expressed in terms of the scale from narrow to broad (e.g., more than one pain component, several domains of quality of life).
5. *Extent of investment required for preparing application:* refers to the amount of time, training, and other resources required before the technique can be applied, for example, training of patient, preparing informative booklets or video, etc.
6. *Qualifications in terms of pain characteristics:* refers to adequacy of technique for specific types of pain, characterized in terms of acute vs. chronic, pain intensity (e.g., low, medium, high), pain duration (i.e., of specific pain events and their frequency as well as overall period since pain onset), and pain related to specific kinds of underlying diseases (e.g., osteoporosis, rheumatism, fibromyalgia, back pain). Further pain characteristics may prove to be of importance, e.g., cyclic nature of pain, extent of painful area, pain location, etc.
7. *Duration of effect:* refers to the length of time during which the treatment is expected to have beneficial effects, namely, whether the effects are limited to the activation of the technique, whether they are essentially limited to the activation but can be extended beyond it (e.g., as in hypnosis through post-hypnotic instructions), or whether the effects are not limited by the actual activation of the technique.
8. *Conditions of operation:* refers to whether the technique may be applied on a one-to-one basis in individual sessions, in the form of groups, or larger audiences.
9. *Psychological processes involved in the technique:* refers to major psychological processes that characterize the operation of the technique, are activated or mobilized by it, and determine its efficacy, such as suggestion in the case of hypnosis, or conditioning in the case of operant learning.
10. *Dependence on the therapist:* refers to the extent to which the application of the technique depends on the health professional, namely, on his/her continued active involvement in the process, for example, complete dependence in the case of

dynamic psychotherapy, partial in the case of the guided imagery or relaxation (if the patients are taught to apply the methods on their own), and minimal in the case of the didactic technique (if previously prepared materials are used).

11. *Requirements from the patient:* refers to requirements that may range from passive understanding in the case of the didactic methods to more active and specific requirements, such as cooperation, adherence, persistence or homework in the case of other methods.

12. *Qualifications in regard to patients*: refers to limiting conditions that specify exclusion criteria and determine selection of patients for each technique, such as fantasy in the case of guided imagery, at least average intelligence in the case of the didactic methods.

13. *Risks and shortcomings*: refers to possible adverse effects of the technique insofar as the pain is concerned as well as in domains other than pain, such as paradoxical enhancement of pain, increased disability, or increased dependence and passivity.

14. *Evaluation of the technique's efficacy:* refers to the effects of the technique as manifested in the per cent of patients affected positively by its application and the extent to which it decreases pain.

PAIN TREATMENT APPROACHES FOCUSED ON THE SENSORY COMPONENT

The specific techniques include guided imagery, suggestion and auto-suggestion, biofeedback, relaxation, distraction/displacement of attention, music therapy and hypnosis. We will describe briefly each technique (except hypnosis which is dealt with separately in chapter19), focusing in the text on the mode of application, emphasizing the elements common to the different variants of the technique, and summarizing the information about the other 13 criteria in Table 1.

Guided Imagery

Pain control is attained by means of imagery produced by the patient and shaped to a certain extent by the therapist prior to treatment or in the course of it (Hammond, 1990). It may be used with prior preparations that are minimal (e.g., closing one's eyes, concentrating) or longer (e.g., relaxing, hypnotic induction). The following are most potent images for pain control: (a) Endowing the pain with some metaphoric form and then moving it in fantasy to some other bodily site where it disturbs less, removing it altogether from the body (by some tunnel, with a scoop etc.), or dissociating it from oneself (e.g., by inserting between it and oneself space, distance, an object, a natural obstacle, etc.); (b) Transforming the pain sensation, for example, in terms of the quality of the sensation (e.g., to itching, tingling, numbness, warmth, etc.), duration of the sensation (e.g., compressing time to very brief duration or very fast passage), or its intensity (e.g., imagining that the pain is a certain color or substance that gradually loses saturation, dissolves, evaporates, melts, decomposes and eventually even disappears); (c) Blocking pain through suggestions of anesthesia or analgesia, for example, by using numbness in the pain area or "flipping switches" in the brain to disconnect pain messages; (d) Destroying the pain by some external agent, such as, freezing wind, sealing off (so that supplies for the pain are cut off), a hammer, an absorbing sponge, a scraper, an anesthetic, a magical spell, etc.; and (e) Changing the pain's meaning, e.g., to beneficial, soothing, necessary for healing, protection, etc.

Suggestion and Auto-Suggestion

Pain control is attained by imposing on the pain sensations an interpretation with positive connotations, e.g., healing is proceeding as planned, all is well, tissue or organ are in good shape or will soon be, etc. (Barber, 1984; Kreitler and Kreitler, 1977). The suggestive interpretation is provided in soothing, repetitive, fixed phrases that are pronounced for extended periods of time (e.g., 10 to 20 minutes), repeatedly, by the therapist (viz. suggestion) or by the patient (viz. auto-suggestion) or by both at different times (e.g., by the therapist in the clinic, by the patient at home). The suggestions refer mostly to the beneficial outcomes (e.g., there is no pain, you feel no pain, the pain has disappeared) rather than to the means whereby these outcomes can supposedly be attained (e.g., disconnecting channels to the brain, moving the pain to another site). Suggestions constitute the core of another technique that is often called "coping self-statements" which is based on silent or spoken statements the patient says to himself/herself and which express managing, mastering or reinterpreting the painful sensations (Meichenbaum, 1985; Turk, Meichenbaum and Genest, 1983).

Biofeedback

Pain_control is attained by acquiring voluntary control over physiological responses related to the pain (Basmajian And Deluca, 1985; Schwartz and Associates, 1995). This is made possible by providing the patient systematic and relatively immediate information about these physiological responses that are normally subliminal. The common procedure consists in monitoring by the therapist of the patient's bodily responses (e.g., muscle tension, skin temperature, heart rate, blood flow) on a machine and feeding the information back to the patient through an auditory or visual stimulus (that decreases or increases in line with the physiological tension). The electrodes are attached to some organ, for example, to a tense muscle group in the case of headache. The patient is offered a number of strategies for controlling the tension, e.g., relaxing imagery, repetition of relaxing phrases, deep breathing, stopping thinking. During the training sessions (which may range from 12 to 36 or more), the patient learns to identify means that decrease the tension. At this point generalizing the learned skills from the office to real life takes place. In this stage the patient is encouraged to practice the successful means as often as possible (even 10-20 times a day) in daily life and regular surroundings, using different cues instead of the machine feedback.

Relaxation Therapy

Pain control is attained by learning to relax major muscles by specific acts (Lichstein, 1988). One well-known method consists in methodically tensing and then relaxing specific muscle groups in a given sequence, as specified by the progressive muscle relaxation procedure (Jacobson, 1929). Starting with, say, 14 muscle groups (e.g., lower arms and hands, upper arms, calves, lower legs) the relaxation becomes gradually deeper, and the muscle groups are clustered step-by-step into larger units (e.g., lips, eyes, jaw, lower forehead and upper forehead are grouped as 'face'). In addition to the training sessions themselves (often 9 or more), the patient is instructed to practice relaxation also on his/her own, as often as 10-20 times a day, applying tension-release exercises (as in the training sessions), or relaxation by recall (viz. thinking about one's muscles so as to prevent their contraction or increase of tension in them), or cue-controlled relaxation (viz., binding a relaxation strategy contingent for example on deep breathing to a self-produced cue, such as thinking to oneself the word 'relax'). After termination of training, applying the procedures should go on, even if at a reduced pace.

There exist also other methods for relaxation, e.g., by concentrating on one's body and "draining away" the tension by focusing attention on tension-laden problem areas; by using peaceful, comforting imagery; by lying down motionless or sitting still for extended periods of time, say, 20-30 minutes; by systematic physical movement, e.g., walking; by assuming specific bodily postures for extended periods of time, such as the yoga "asanas"; or by breathing exercises, sometimes coupled with suggestion focused on reducing autonomic arousal, as in autogenic training (Linden, 1993) (see also e.g., Kravette 1982; Monaghan and Diereck, 1999).

Distraction/Displacement of Attention

Control of pain is attained by removing attention from the pain itself or reducing awareness of it. There are two major procedures for attaining this. One consists in focusing attention on something other than pain, often an object, preferably a common object in one's immediate environment, or some idea, preferably a word or a phrase (e.g., "mantra"), or a simple activity, such as walking or breathing. The other procedure consists in emptying one's mind of all contents, that is, letting nothingness or emptiness control one's awareness. The success of these procedures depends on persistence in the act and practice over time (McCaul and Malott, 1984).

Table 1. Characterization of the pain treatment approaches focused on the sensory component in terms of 13 criteria

Criteria	Guided imagery	Suggestion and Auto-Suggestion	Biofeedback	Relaxation	Distraction/ Displacing Attention	Music therapy
Tools	None (audiotape)	None (audiotape)	Biofeedback machine	None (audiotape)	None (audiotape)	Recorded music, tapes
Pain components	Sensations (affects)	Sensations (affects)	Sensations	Sensations, affects	Sensations, affects	Sensations, affects
Breadth of effect	Medium	Medium	Medium	Medium	Medium	Medium
Investment prior to application	Medium	Small	Large	Large	Medium	None
Pain qualifications	Mainly acute pain: any intensity	Mainly acute pain; up to medium intensity	Mainly acute pain: up to medium intensity	Acute and chronic pain: any intensity	Mainly acute pain; up to medium intensity	Mainly acute pain: any intensity
Duration of effect	Limited to operation; extensible	Limited to operation	Limited to operation	Limited to operation	Limited to operation	Limited to operation
Conditions of operation	Individual, group	Individual, group	Individual	Individual, group	Individual, group	Individual, group
Psychological processes	Imagery, metaphorization, suggestion	Suggestion, self-regulation	Imagery, self-regulation	Self-regulation	Cognitive control, suggestion	Imagery, self-regulation
Dependence on therapist	Not obligatory, small	Not obligatory, small	Necessary, large	Necessary, large	Not obligatory, medium	None
Requirements from patients	Concentration, persistence, practice	Concentration	Concentration, persistence, compliance, practice	Concentration, persistence, compliance practice	Concentration, persistence, compliance	Listening
Patients' qualifications	Hypnotizability, fantasy, no introspection barriers	Suggestibility	Persistence, self-control, fantasy	Persistence, self-control, fantasy	Self-control	None
Risks, shortcomings	Absorp. in fantasies	None	Intruding thoughts, panic, difficulty of generalization	Intruding thoughts, panic, difficulty of generalization	None	None
Efficacy: Patients improved %	40-60%	~40%	15-25%	15-30%	~25%	75-80%
Pain reduction %	~50%	20-30%	50-60%	50-60%	60-70%	25-40%

Note. The characterizations are designed mainly to serve orientation purposes rather than as summaries of the empirical evidence. They are based on references mentioned in the text. The characterization in terms of the mode of application (criterion 1) is presented in the text. For explication of the the criteria see text.

Notably, some meditation practices seem to use the mentioned techniques, even though with a different emphasis. This applies in general to meditation that promotes concentration practices (e.g., transcendental meditation) and in particular to 'mindfulness meditation' which cultivates intentional, nonreactive, nonjudgmental awareness of the present moments. The claim is that by focusing completely on the present, for example, by attending to breathing, one's field of awareness becomes the present in its fullness, that is, the present exclusively without any accompanying connotations (Kabat-Zinn, Massion, Hebert and Rosenbaum, 1998). It will be noted that this procedure is based on distraction, culminating paradoxically in focusing on the sensation of pain, which however is reduced to its bare essentials and thus diminished.

Music Therapy

Pain control is attained by exposure to music while one experiences pain or is exposed to a painful procedure. Music therapy is discussed separately from art therapy because it differs from it in procedure (music therapy consists in passive exposure to music whereas art therapy may involve active expressive elements) and in the underlying beneficial processes (music therapy may affect pain through vibrations, evoked images, enhanced sense of control, and distraction, whereas art therapy relies more heavily on the expressive elements) (Campbell, 1997; Chesky and Michel, 1991; Krout, 2001; Lepage, Drolet, Girard, et al., 2001; Maslar, 1986; Rider, 1985).

Concluding Remarks about the Treatments Focused on the Sensory Component

Despite the different theoretical backgrounds and different modes of application, the six described approaches share several important elements. First, they all attempt to reduce pain by manipulating the meaning assigned to the messages from the damaged area or tissue. Thus, guided imagery does it by means of images, distraction by means of changes in focus of attention, and music therapy by reinterpreting them in terms of tones and vibrations. Second, all techniques are based on some cognitive change rather than, say, behavioral change. Third, though the major target of these techniques is sensations, they also attain change in affect that contributes to reduction in pain.

PAIN TREATMENT APPROACHES FOCUSED ON THE AFFECTIVE COMPONENT

The specific techniques include supportive therapies, meaning-based control of negative emotions, dynamic psychotherapy, and art therapy. We will describe briefly each technique, focusing in the text on the mode of application, emphasizing the elements common to the different variants of the technique, and summarizing the information about the other 13 criteria in Table 2.

Supportive Therapies

The different variants of this approach include social support, family support and supportive psychotherapy. The attempt to attain pain control is based on legitimizing pain, expressing empathy for the suffering pain patient, encouraging the pain patient to share his or her experiences and suffering, strengthening the pain patient by emphasizing that he/she is not alone and can rely on the sympathy, understanding and help of others. The main emphasis is placed on constructing a trusting relationship with the patient, expressing compassion and sympathy, and providing comfort and reassurance. By these means the loneliness and depression of the patient are alleviated, and the feelings of isolation, neglect and rejection by others may be greatly reduced. These effects may increase the likelihood of pain control first, because the patient may have greater motivation to undergo treatment for pain control; second, because the patient may devote more efforts to recovering rather than to convincing others of his/her suffering; and third, because the patient may feel strengthened through the support and hence better able to challenge the pain. Some studies demonstrate beneficial effects of social support on pain (Feldman, Downey and Schaffer, 1999; Klapow, Slater, Patterson et al., 1995). The support may be provided by the therapist or clinician, by family members or friends on their own or in line with guidance by the therapist, or by other pain patients in the framework of support groups, with or without participation of a therapist (viz. self-help groups) (Bradley et al., 1987; Tunks and Mersky, 1990).

Meaning-based Control of Negative Emotions

Pain control is attained by means of a systematic change in specific cognitive styles of information processing which promote negative emotions accompanying and maintaining pain. The cognitive styles consist in particular tendencies of meaning assignment to inputs that have been empirically identified and were shown to enhance negative emotions, in particular anxiety (Kreitler and Kreitler, 1985, 1987, 1990a). These cognitive styles relate to all kinds of inputs rather than to pain alone, and consist in assigning to inputs metaphoric or symbolic meanings (e.g., Life – is like a ship in a stormy ocean), expressing personal meanings more than interpersonally-shared meanings, and emphasizing feelings, evaluations and cognitive contents evoked by the input (e.g., Life - is depressing, difficult, and reminiscent of crises). The meaning-based procedure for weakening negative emotions consists in strengthening cognitive styles that are antithetic to those mentioned above, namely, assigning to inputs specific well-defined meanings attributively or comparatively (e.g., Life – is a biological event, different from non-organic phenomena), expressing interpersonally-shared meanings, and emphasizing actions and sensory-qualities of the inputs (e.g., Life – keeps the heart active, is manifested in the forms and colors of the living species). The training of the adequate cognitive styles is performed in 1-2 brief sessions, according to a structured protocol.

Table 2. Characterization of the pain treatment approaches focused on the affective component in terms of 13 criteria

Criteria	Supportive therapies	Meaning-based control of negative emotions	Dynamic psychotherapy	Art therapy
Tools	None	None	None	Art materials
Pain components	Affects	Affects, cognitions	Affects, cognitions	Affects, cognitions
Breadth of effect	Narrow	Medium	Medium	Medium
Investment prior to application	None	Medium	Large	Medium
Pain qualifications	Chronic (acute), up to medium intensity	Chronic or acute, any intensity	Chronic, any intensity	Chronic, up to medium intensity
Duration of effect	Brief	Long	Long	Medium
Conditions of operation	Individual or group	Individual or group	Individual or group	Individual or group
Psychological processes	Decrease of loneliness, strengthening self-confidence	Strengthening cognitive styles of meaning assignment to inputs	Acquiring insight, resolving conflicts	Catharsis, emotional expression, insight, creativity
Dependence on therapist	Necessary, large	Necessary, medium	Necessary, large	Necessary, medium
Requirements from patients	Sharing experiences, readiness to accept support	Cooperating in learning and applying the method	Motivation for change, introspection readiness, emotional life	Cooperating in art projects, emotional life, motivation for self-expression
Patients' qualifications	Ability to share experiences helps but is not obligatory	Understanding the instructions of the procedure	Readiness to invest time and money in treatment, at least mean IQ	Interest and minimum skills in the arts, persistence and motivation
Risks, shortcomings	Intensification or maintenance of pain, increase of secondary gain of pain	None	Centering one's life on pain	None
Efficacy: Patients improved % Pain reduction %	75% up to 10%	70-80% ~50% (dependence on neg. emotions)	10-25% up to 70%	10-20% up to 25%-30%

Note. The characterizations are designed mainly to serve orientation purposes rather than as summaries of the empirical evidence. They are based on references mentioned in the text. The characterization in terms of the mode of application (criterion 1) is presented in the text. For explication of the the criteria see text.

Dynamic Psychotherapy

Pain control is attained by a protracted process of dynamically-oriented psychotherapy designed to enable the patient develop insight into unconscious processes, gain psychodynamic understanding of one's motivations, resolve conflicts, overcome traumata from earlier life periods, get catharsis by expressing emotions (mainly anger, depression, helplessness, loss), weaken guilt and the associated tendencies of self-destruction and self-punishment, and learn to replace inefficient coping strategies with more efficient and healthy ones (Aronoff, 1999; Grzesiak, Ury, and Dworkin, 1996). There exist different therapeutic approaches – gestalt, Freudian, Adlerian, analytical, existentialist, psychodramatic, and others – that apply a wide array of different specific means for attaining understanding, conflict resolution, emotion expression and self-control to the point where the patient is emotionally free from the need to succumb to pain and suffering. The liberation from emotional conflict, burdens and barriers is assumed to be the key to liberation from pain, or at least from the element of intense suffering that forms one of its components. Most approaches emphasize psychological treatment of the person as a whole (Pinsky and Malyon, 1979; Sarno, 1976) and rely mainly on verbal communication. Since several major psychodynamic themes underlying pain may be assumed to be characteristic of many pain patients, the psychodynamic approach is often applied also in a group setting.

Art Therapy

Pain control is attained by means of expressing oneself through the media of the arts, including visual arts, dance or movement, writing or telling of stories, writing poetry, photographing, acting, film making, singing and playing of music (as distinguished from listening to music). It is generally assumed that no expertise or prior learning in the arts is necessary, although it is helpful. The major therapeutic processes of art therapy are the expressive-creative dimension, which is implemented by the production of the artistic output, the cognitive-symbolic dimension, which is promoted by the guidance of the therapist, and the interactive-analytic dimension, which consists in the direct and art-mediated communication between the patient and the therapist (Luzzatto and Gabriel, 1998). There are three major kinds of art therapy: (a) studio-based art therapy provides the patient different art materials in a safe and nonevaluative environment, encouraging him/her to experiment with them so as to express freely one's internal world, including positive and negative feelings; (b) group art therapy uses the group dynamics as a therapeutic means, e.g., all members express the same theme or use the same medium, or discuss their art after completion; (c) individual art therapy consists in using the different potentialities of art therapy, tailored by the therapist to the patient's needs. The major therapeutic components of art therapy are the production of an art object, and communicating about it with the therapist or the other group members or both. The expression of one's internal world through the medium of art provides catharsis, the possibility to communicate to others one's feelings and thus overcome the sense of loneliness and isolation, and the chance to gain insights into one's innermost self as well as discover new ways of coping. The artistic expression is deeper and more complete than the regular verbal one, not in the least because it includes also the symbolic-metaphoric level. It constitutes also an outlet for creativity, which is pleasurable and contributes to enhancing the patient's self-esteem. The process and products of art therapy may be used by the therapist to attain different goals, such as, relaxation, insight in line with different dynamic approaches, or pain alleviation by images which are objectified rather than merely fantasized (see "guided imagery") (e.g., Ferszt, Massotti, Williams et al., 2000; Vick and Sexton, 1999).

Concluding Remarks about the Treatments Focused on the Affective Component

The described treatments focus on affects as the key to pain alleviation. The impact of supportive therapies on affects is direct but limited to the positive affects evoked in response to comforting words, encouragement and sympathy expressed by others. The effect on pain is limited in extent and duration. None of the other three described techniques affects emotions directly. The meaning-based technique functions by transforming tendencies of meaning assignment, dynamic psychotherapy by promoting insight and resolution of emotional conflicts, and art therapy by facilitating emotional expression with the accompanying creative, metaphoric-symbolic and communicative elements. The impact of these three techniques on affects is deeper and longer lasting than the impact of the purely supportive therapies. The meaning-based technique targets pain-involved affects more specifically than dynamic psychotherapy and art therapy and hence its effect on pain is more focused and definite. In addition, it requires a much shorter training with the patient.

PAIN TREATMENT APPROACHES FOCUSED ON THE COGNITIVE COMPONENT

The specific techniques include educational/didactic information-based techniques, cognitive attitude-based therapy, and cognitive coping therapy. We will describe briefly each technique, focusing in the text on the mode of application, emphasizing the elements common to the different variants of the technique, and summarizing the information about the other 13 criteria in Table 3.

Educational/Didactic Information-Based Techniques

Pain control is attained by providing information to the patient about the pain – mainly, its source (the underlying physical problem or disease, physiological processes involved, details of the medical procedure that causes it), expected duration, nature (e.g., cycles, kind of sensations), its components, function, the effect of analgesics, the situation after pain control is attained, and other relevant matters. The underlying assumption is that information about the pain may contribute to pain control mainly by reducing the patient's anxiety, as well as by helping the patient prepare for the pain and its vicissitudes or enabling better coping with it. Information is often provided to patients in groups in the form of lectures or discussion meetings (see Table 3 for further media). Sometimes the information is provided not only to the patients but also to their spouses or caretakers, so that they could act on the information, or help the patients apply it. Patient education interventions are used with a wide range of patients, by different health professionals (Daltroy and Liang, 1988; Lorig, Lubeck, Kraines, et al., 1985; Melzack, Taenzer, Feldman, et al., 1981). In recent years the popularity of the educationl techniques has increased because getting information has come to be considered as one of the basic patients' rights and a step towards empowering patients in the medical setting. Failure to get adequate information and explanation of one's pain is the most frequently reported source of patient dissatisfaction and the attendant lower rates of compliance with treatment and improvement in pain control (Deyo and Diehl, 1986).

Cognitive Attitude-Based Therapy

Pain control is attained by changing attitudes of patients concerning pain and its management. The underlying assumption is that attitudes play a role in the matrix of factors determining pain, so that enhancing 'positive' or functional attitudes or weakening dysfunctional ones could promote pain control. Patients' beliefs concerning their pain are good predictors of the patients' long-term rehabilitation (Jensen, Turner and Romano, 1994; Lackner, Carosella and Feuerstein, 1996). Major topics of relevant beliefs are etiology of pain (e.g., somatic only or also psychological, one's blame vs. unfortunate accident), diagnostic expectations, treatment expectations, and outcome goals (e.g., complete cure vs. relief). The following are the most common inventories for assessing pain beliefs: (a) The Pain Beliefs Questionnaire (Gottlieb, 1984) measuring disability expectation, self-efficacy, depression, and pain as threat; (b) Survey of Pain Attitudes (Jensen and Karoly, 1989), measuring beliefs about pain control, solicitude, medical care, disability, medication and emotions; and (c) Pain Beliefs and Perception Inventory (Williams and Thorn, 1989), measuring beliefs about stability of pain, self-blame and mysteriousness of pain. Changing attitudes in the desired direction is done, for example, by group discussions, providing supportive information, and using illustrative models (Bradley, 1996; Feldman, Phillips and Aronoff, 1999; Keefe, Beaupré and Gil, 1996).

Table 3. Characterization of the pain treatment approaches focused on the sensory component in terms of 13 criteria

Criteria	Educational/didactic information-based technique	Cognitive attitude-based therapy	Cognitive coping therapy
Tools	Booklets, video, films, tapes	Booklets, video, films, tapes	None
Pain components	Cognitions	Cognitions, affects	Cognitions, affects
Breadth of effect	Narrow	Medium	Medium
Investment prior to application	Little	Medium	Medium
Pain qualifications	Acute or chronic, up to medium intensity	Mainly chronic, any intensity	Mainly chronic, any intensity
Duration of effect	Limited	Medium	Medium
Conditions of operation	Group, individual	Group, individual	Group, individual
Psychological processes	Comprehension	Comprehension, self-control	Self-regulation
Dependence on therapist	Minimal, not obligatory	Medium	Medium
Requirements from patients	Passive listening	Attitude formation	Learning and unlearning of strategies, motivation, generalization
Patients' qualifications	At least medium IQ, concentration	At least medium IQ, decision-making	Medium IQ, learning, generalization
Risks, shortcomings	Excessive focusing on pain, increase of anxiety	Excessive dealing with pain, increase of anxiety	Focusing on inadequate strategy
Efficacy: Patients improved% Pain reduction %	~30% 5%-10%	40%-50% 10%-20%	60%-70% ~50%

Note. The characterizations are designed mainly to serve orientation purposes rather than as summaries of the empirical evidence. They are based on references mentioned in the text. The characterization in terms of the mode of application (criterion 1) is presented in the text. For explication of the the criteria see text.

Cognitive Coping Therapy

Pain control is attained by promoting in the patients acquisition of adequate cognitive skills for managing the pain, such as active problem solving, use of coping self statements (e.g., I will overcome this pain) and humor, and avoiding inadequate cognitive skills, such as catastrophizing or overgeneralization (see Chapter on Quality of Life and Coping). The major means used for helping patients learn the adequate strategies and unlearn the inadequate ones are information, discussion, modeling, reinforcement (rewards and punishments), rehearsal, generalization of the strategies to everyday life settings and providing supports for maintenance of the learned strategies (Bradley, 1996). Often cognitive coping strategies constitute part of cognitive-behavioral therapy but this is neither always the case nor is it necessary on theoretical or clinical grounds. Cognitive therapy is commonly done in the setup of group therapy, and spouses may be involved in the treatment (Keefe, Beaupré and Gil, 1996).

Concluding Remarks about the Treatments Focused on the Cognitive Component

The three_described techniques form a kind of continuum with respect to the depth of cognitive processes they engage for pain control. The educational/didactic information-based techniques rely primarily on information. All they require from the patient is listening and comprehension. It is implicitly assumed or expected that the information would be used beneficially by the patient, but this is neither required nor explicitly indicated. Thus, these techniques may be described as "staying on the surface" of cognition. The cognitive attitude-based therapy probes deeper. It seeks to affect the attitudes of the patient, which are based on information but engage also more complex processes. Hence, the patient is not merely provided information which he or she may use as they think fit, but the patient is required explicitly to take a stand and espouse particular attitudes in regard to pain. These attitudes consist of beliefs about pain that are conducive to better pain control. Finally, cognitive coping therapy probes even deeper. It goes beyond attitudes into coping strategies, which are based on beliefs but engage even more complex processes. Thus, each of the three techniques is based partly on the other. Accordingly, each in turn is also more complex, requires more from the patient and from the therapist and is a more powerful tool for pain control.

PAIN TREATMENT APPROACHES FOCUSED ON THE BEHAVIORAL COMPONENT

The specific techniques include conditioning, environmental therapy, family therapy, behavioral therapy, and cognitive orientation therapy. We will describe briefly each technique, focusing in the text on the mode of application, emphasizing the elements common to the different variants of the technique, and summarizing the information about the other 13 criteria in Table 4.

Table 4. Characterization of the pain treatment approaches focused on the behavioral component in terms of 13 criteria

Criteria	Conditioning	Environmental therapy	Family therapy	Behavioral therapy	Cognitive orientation therapy
Tools	None	Alternate sites or objects	None	None	None
Pain components	Behaviors	Behaviors, affects	Behaviors, affects	Behaviors	Behaviors, cognitions, affects
Breadth of effect	Narrow	Narrow	Medium	Medium	Large
Investment prior to application	Large	Little	Medium	Large	Large
Pain qualifications	Chronic, up to medium	Chronic, up to medium	Chronic, weak	Chronic, any intensity	Acute or chronic, any intensity
Duration of effect	Medium	Short	Short	Medium	Long
Conditions of operation	Mostly individual	Individual	Individual or group	Group mostly	Group of individual
Psychological processes	Conditioning, learning, generalization	Conditioning, mostly respondent	Learning	Learning, coping	Changing unconsious cognitive motivations
Dependence on therapist	Large	Minimal	Small	Large	Medium
Requirements from patients	Motivation, cooperation, persistence	Readiness to change environment	Cooperation	Learning ability, motivation, active approach	Cooperation, compliance in applying method
Patients' qualifications	Motivation	None	None	At least average IQ	Ability to comprehend instructions
Risks, shortcomings	Encouraging passive approach	None	Encouraging passive approach	Focusing on inadequate strategy	None
Efficacy: Patients improved %	25%-35%	10%-15%	25%-35%	60%-75%	80%-90%
Pain reduction %	~40-50%	10%-15%	~15%	50%-65%	~85%

Note. The characterizations are designed mainly to serve orientation purposes rather than as summaries of the empirical evidence. They are based on references mentioned in the text. The characterization in terms of the mode of application (criterion 1) is presented in the text. For explication of the the criteria see text.

Conditioning

Pain control is attained by learning adaptive behaviors designed to replace maladaptive pain behaviors the patient had learned before. The major mechanisms used for learning are the same as those assumed to have been operative in acquiring the maladaptive behaviors, namely respondent and operant conditioning. The main difference between these two kinds of learning is that according to respondent conditioning the main factor in learning behavioral or emotional responses is the pairing of the original stimulus, say, pain, with another stimulus, say, the doctor's office, whereas according to operant conditioning, the main factor is the consequence of behavior, namely, the reward or punishment that followed it. Thus, in order to eliminate maladaptive behaviors, it is recommended to eliminate or reduce exposure to the external stimuli that have come to elicit these behaviors or apply consistently punishment if they occur (viz., 'extinction'). In order to let the patient acquire adaptive behaviors, it is recommended to evoke them often in the presence of previously neutral stimuli (viz., 'discriminative stimulus control'), reward their occurrence consistently (viz. 'reinforcement'), and approach gradually the level of the desired behavior (viz., 'shaping'). The treatment (often called 'operant conditioning') includes a stage of a preliminary functional behavior analysis, followed by the learning itself in a series of systematically structured sessions, and concludes with generalizing the learning to everyday life settings, coupled with a maintenance procedure over time designed to prevent relapse (Sanders, 1996).

Environmental Therapy

The attempt to attain pain control is based on removing the patient as much as possible from his or her regular environment, which includes many originally neutral stimuli that have come to be conditioned to the pain behaviors and evoke them. This therapy is based primarily on the principles of respondent conditioning (see 'Conditioning') (Fordyce, 1976). The removal from one's environment may take the form of actual physical removal to another geographic location, for shorter or longer periods of time (e.g., to a clinic or hotel for recovery, or another house). Sometimes the change of location may be secondary to a major goal, such as undergoing pain treatment in a pain center or an inpatient ward. Removal may also take the form of changing stimuli and objects in one's regular environment, e.g., changing placement of furniture, color of walls, replacing objects with which the patient has a lot of contact (e.g., bed, armchair, office chair), or adding new objects so that the overall atmosphere or shape of the regular environment is changed. If one opts for a loose meaning of the term environment, then change of wardrobe or hairdo may also be recommended.

Family Therapy

Pain control is attained by changing pain-relevant behaviors and beliefs of family members interacting closely with the patient (viz., 'significant others'). Family therapy is based on the assumption that family members are the providers of major types of rewards (e.g., love, support, encouragement, comforting), and punishment (e.g., expressions of anger, irritation, frustration, blame) to the patient. Hence, the behaviors of family members to the patient may have been a major factor in the emergence of pain and its maintenance. Accordingly, in line with operant conditioning principles, their behaviors may be used for changing the patients' pain behaviors, for example, by teaching them to identify the patient's adaptive and maladaptive behaviors and to provide systematic reward to adaptive behaviors and systematic punishments to maladaptive ones. Accordingly, family members may become therapists-by-proxy. Another variant of family therapy focuses on the pain-relevant beliefs and attitudes of family members, thus engaging their direct or indirect help in changing the patient's beliefs and attitudes (see "Cognitive attitude-based therapy') (Feldman et al., 1999; Kerns and Payne, 1996).

Behavioral Therapy or Coping by Means of Behavioral Strategies

Pain control is attained by promoting in the patients both acquisition of adaptive behavioral strategies for reducing and handling pain, such as active problem solving (e.g., exercising, returning gradually to work, engaging in social activities), or using the help of others in a constructive way, as well as avoiding nonadaptive behavioral strategies, such as complaining, excessive use of analgesics, or overcautious motor movements. The major goal is the enhancement of adequate coping. The main means applied in the process of learning are setting specific goals, reinforcement (rewards and punishments), rehearsal, generalization of the coping strategies to everyday life settings and providing supports for maintenance of the learned strategies (Bradley, 1996). Often behavioral coping strategies are integrated into cognitive-behavioral therapy but this is neither ubiquitous nor necessary. Behavioral therapy is often practiced in the context of groups (Keefe et al., 1996).

Cognitive Orientation Therapy

Pain control is attained by increasing the number of relevant beliefs that were identified by previous studies as promoting release from pain behaviors and mechanisms (Kreitler and Kreitler, 1990b). The underlying rationale is that behaviors as well as physiological responses are guided by cognitive contents and processes, specific for each type of behavior or response (Kreitler and Kreitler, 1991). Relevant beliefs are defined in terms of form and contents. In terms of form, there are four basic types of beliefs: beliefs about goals (e.g., "I want to do as much as possible for others"), beliefs about rules and norms (e.g., "One should do as much as possible for others"), beliefs about oneself (e.g., "I don't do too much for others"), and general beliefs, referring to others and reality (e.g., "Doing things for others often entails not doing things for oneself"). In terms of contents, there are particular themes that were found to characterize individuals who did not develop chronic pain or if they did overcame it. Themes of this kind include, for example, doing for others just enough so as not to encroach on satisfying one's own needs, comfort, etc; and being satisfied with doing one's best without striving for perfection. Mobilizing beliefs supporting themes of this kind is done by adding the adequate beliefs rather than by suppressing inadequate beliefs, and by evoking the adequate beliefs in the patient himself or herself (by evoking memories or generating meanings) rather than by implanting or suggesting the beliefs. Further, special care is taken to ensure that the adequate beliefs represent the four types of beliefs and not fewer types. Increasing the number of beliefs referring to the different themes across the four types of beliefs produces in the patient a cognitive-motivational orientation supporting release from pain. This orientation is neither conscious, nor voluntarily controlled. The therapy is carried out in a systematic manner, according to a structured sequence of themes, and is based on the use of processes, such as meaning generation, clustering of beliefs, and memory evocation.

Concluding Remarks about the Treatments Focused on the Behavioral Component

The described techniques are all designed to reduce pain by changing pain's behavioral component, but they differ in the means applied for attaining this goal: learning processes based on respondent and operant conditioning along the lines of early behaviorism, learning of behavioral coping strategies along the lines of higher-level cognitive learning theory, and formation of cognitive clusters orienting toward the adequate responses along the lines of meaning-anchored learning. Thus, these techniques represent the whole continuum of psychological theoretical approaches to the formation and change of behavior from behaviorism, through cognitive learning theory to meaning-anchored cognition. Despite their different theoretical backgrounds, these techniques may be applied conjointedly, mixing the specified means to different degrees.

THE ROLE OF PSYCHOLOGICAL THERAPIES IN THE CONTROL OF PAIN

In our description of the techniques an attempt was made to describe them in as pure a form as possible. However, in actual implementation they are often combined in different forms. Thus, cognitive-behavioral therapy often includes therapies based on operant and respondent conditioning, educational/didactic information-based therapy, cognitive attitude-based and cognitive coping therapies, relaxation, behavioral therapy and family therapy (Bradley, 1996). A program such as "psychological management of chronic pain" (Philips and Rachman, 1996) includes the educational/didactic techniques, distraction of attention, biofeedback, relaxation and behavioral therapy. Sometimes the different techniques are applied in consecutive sessions with the patient (Bradley, 1996); sometimes several are applied together in the same session (Creamer, Singh, Hochberg et al., 2000). Some techniques tend often to be applied together more than others, for example, guided imagery, suggestions, hypnosis and relaxation, or behavioral coping and cognitive coping. However, all types of combination may be attempted and often are. Thus, the presentation in this chapter of each technique separately has the advantage of providing the practitioner clear information that enables understanding the techniques, analyzing the components of each pain control program, or setting up a new program designed to express one's own approach to pain control, or tailored to the needs of a specific group of homogeneous or heterogeneous patients. Indeed, the multiple components of pain – sensations, affects, cognitions and behaviors – require the use of different techniques and facilitate their combined application.

However, the psychological approaches to pain control may not only be combined with each other but also with the medical approaches to pain control, pharmacological or surgical. It is of special importance to emphasize this possibility which is an integral component of the multidisciplinary approach to the treatment of pain. Combining the psychological approaches with the medical approaches is recommended on two grounds. First, the multi-component nature of pain not only enables combining the different approaches and facilitates the combinations, but actually requires them. Treating pain only by means of psychological or only by means of medical techniques is in danger of overlooking important components of pain so that the outcome is both incomplete and unstable. Second, the complex nature of pain as a physio-psycho-social phenomenon renders it likely that the physiological and psychological dimensions interact in the production and maintenance of pain. Hence, in order to obtain deep-reaching and durable effects of medical treatments it is advisable to apply psychological techniques conjointedly with the medical ones. Thus, a patient who has undergone cognitive orientation therapy which has produced a cognitive motivational orientation for overcoming pain, would be highly receptive to the effects of medical interventions and may accordingly react to them much faster, would need lower amounts of analgesics, and would be freed from the pain for long periods of time, perhaps permanently. Thus, one important role of psychological approaches to the treatment of pain is to obtain reduction or elimination of pain, to the maximum possible degree that the technique allows in a certain kind of patient. Yet another role, at least as important if not more, is to intensify, enhance, facilitate, extend and increase the effect of medical therapies in the context of treating pain as a whole in the person as a whole.

REFERENCES

Aronoff, G. M. (1999). Psychodynamics and psychotherapy of the chronic pain patient. In G. M. Aronoff (Ed.), *Evaluation and treatment of chronic pain* (3rd ed.) (pp. 283-289). Baltimore, MD: Williams and Wilkins.

Barber, T. X. (1984). Hypnosis, deep relaxation, and active relaxation: Data, theory, and clinical applications. In R. L. Woolfolk and P. M. Lehrer (Eds.), *Principles and practice of stress management* (pp. 164-166). New York: Guilford Press.

Basmajian, J. V., and DeLuca, C. J. (1985). *Muscles alive: Their functions revealed by electromyography*. Baltimore: Williams and Wilkins.

Bradley, L. A. (1996). Cognitive-behavioral therapy for chronic pain. In R. J. Gatchel and D. C. Turk (Eds.), *Psychological approaches to pain management* (pp. 131-147). New York: Guilford.

Bradley, L. A., Young, L. D., Anderson, J. O., Turner, R. A., Agudelo, C. A., McDaniel, L. K., Pisko, E. J., Semble, E. J., and Morgan, T. M. (1987). Effects of psychological therapy on pain behavior of rheumatoid arthritis patients: Tretment outcome and six-month follow-up. *Arthritis and Rheumatism, 30,* 1105-1114.

Campbell, D. (1997). *The Mozart effect.* London: Hodder and Straughton.

Chesky, K. S., and Michel, D. E. (1991). The Music Vibration Table (MVT): Developing a technology and conceptual model for pain relief. *Music Therapy Perspectives, 9,* 32-38.

Creamer, P., Singh, B. B., Hochberg, M. C., and Berman, B. M. (2000). Sustained improvement produced by nonpharmacologic intervention in fibromyalgia: Reslts of a pilot study. *Arthritis Care and Research, 13,* 198-204.

Daltroy, L. H., and Liang, M. H. (1988). Patient education in the rheumatic diseases: A research agenda. *Arthritis Care and Research, 1,* 161-169.

Deyo, R. A., and Diehl, A. K. (1986). Patient satisfaction with medical care for low-back pain. *Spine, 11,* 28-30.

Ferszt, G. G., Massotti, E., Williams, J., and Miller, J. R. (2000). The impact of an art program on an inpatient oncology unit. *Illness Crisis and Loss, 8,* 189-199.

Feldman, S. I., Downey, G., and Schaffer, N. R. (1999). Pain, negative mood, and perceived support in chronic pain patients: A daily diary study of people with reflex sympathetic dystrophy syndrome. *Journal of Consulting and Clinical Psychology, 67,* 776-785.

Feldman, J. B., Phillips, L. M., and Aronoff, G. M. (1999). A cognitive systems approach to treating chronic pain patients and their families. In G. M. Aronoff (Ed.), *Evaluation and treatment of chronic pain* (3rd ed.) (pp. 213-222).Baltimore, MD: Williams and Wilkins.

Fordyce, W. E. (1976). *Behavioral methods for chronic pain and illness.* St. Louis, MO: C. V. Mosby.

Goeppinger, J., Arthur, M. W., Baglioni, A. J., Jr., Brunk, S. E., and Brunner, C. M. (1989). A reexamination of the effectiveness of self-care education for persons with arthritis. *Arthritis and Rheumatism, 32,* 706-717.

Gottlieb, B. S. (1984). *Development of the Pain Beliefs Questionnaire: A preliminary report.* Paper presented at Association for the Advancement of Behavior Therapy, Philadelphia,PA.

Grzesiak, R. C., Ury, G. M., and Dworkin, R. H. (1996). Psychodynamic psychotherapy with chronic pain patients. In R. J. Gatchel and D. C. Turk (Eds.), *Psychological approaches to pain management* (pp. 148-178). New York: Guilford.

Hammond, D. C. (Ed.) (1990). *Handbook of hypnotic suggestions and metaphors.* New York: Norton (The American Society of Clinical Hypnosis).

Jacobson, E. (1929). *Progressive relaxation.* Chicago, IL: University of Chicago Press.

Jensen, M. P., and Karoly, P. (1989). *Revision and cross-validation of the Survey of Pain Attitudes (SOPA).* Presented at the 10th Annual Meeting of the Society of Behavioral Medicine, San Francisco, CA.

Jensen, M. P., Turner, J. A., and Romano, J. M. (1994). Correlates of improvement in multi-disciplinary treatment of chronic pain. *Journal of Consulting and Clinical Psychology, 62,* 172-179

Kabat-Zinn, J., Massion, A. O., Hebert, J. R., and Rosenbaum, E. (1998). Meditation. In J. Holland (Ed), *Psycho-oncology* (pp. 767-779). New York: Oxford University Press.

Keefe, F. J., Beaupré, P. M., and Gil, K. M. (1996). In R. J. Gatchel and D. C. Turk (Eds.), *Psychological approaches to pain management* (pp. 259-282). New York: Guilford.

Kerns, R. D. and Payne, A. (1996). Treating families of chronic pain patients. In R. J. Gatchel and D. C. Turk (Eds.), *Psychological approaches to pain management* (pp. 283-304). New York: Guilford.

Klapow, J. C., Slater, M. A., Patterson, T. L., Atkinson, J. H., et al. (1995). Psychosocial factors discriminate multidimensional clinical groups of chronic low back pain patients. *Pain, 62,* 349-355

Kravette, S. (1982). *Complete meditation.* Atglen, PA: Whitford Press.

Kreitler, H., and Kreitler, S. (1977). Introduction to the book "Autosuggestion in accordance with the method of Emile Coué" by Brooks. In S. H. Brooks, *Autosuggestion in accordance with the method of Emile Coué.* Tel Aviv: "A", Alef.

Kreitler, H., and Kreitler, S. (1978). Art therapy: Quo vadis? *Journal of Art Psychotherapy, 5,* 199-209.

Kreitler, S., and Kreitler, H. (1985).The psychosemantic determinants of anxiety: A cognitive proach. In H. van der Ploeg, R. Schwarzer and C. D. Spielberger (Eds.), *Advances in Test Anxiety Research, Vol. 4* (pp. 117-135). Lisse, The Netherlands and Hillsdale, NJ: Swets and Zeitlinger and Erlbaum.

Kreitler, S., and Kreitler, H. (1987). Modifying anxiety by cognitive means. In R. Schwarzer, H. M. van der Ploeg and C. D. Spielberger (Eds.), *Advances in Test Anxiety Research, Vol. 5* (195-206). Lisse, The Netherlands and Hillsdale, NJ: Swets and Zeitlinger and Erlbaum.

Kreitler, S., and Kreitler, H. (1990a). *The cognitive foundations of personality traits.* New York: Plenum.

Kreitler, H., and Kreitler, S. (1990b). Cognitive primacy, cognitive behavior guidance and their implications for cognitive therapy. *Journal of Cognitive Psychotherapy, 4,* 155-173.

Kreitler, S., and Kreitler, H. (1991). Cognitive orientation and physical disease or health. *European Journal of Personality, 5,* 109-129.

Krout, R. E. (2001). The effect of single-session music therapy on the observed and self-reported levels of pain control, physical comfort and relaxation of hospice patients. *American Journal of Hospice and Palliative Care, 18,* 383-390.

Lackner, J., Carosella, A., and Feuerstein, M. (1996). Pain expectancies, pain and functional self-efficacy expectancies as determinants of disability in patients with chronic low back disorders. *Journal of Consulting and Clinical Psychology, 64,* 212-220.

Lepage, C., Drolet, P., Girard, M., Grenier, Y., and DeGagne, R. (2001). Music decreases sedative requirements during spinal anesthesia. *Anesthesia and Analgesia, 93,* 912-916.

Lichstein, K. L. (1988). *Clinical relaxation strategies.* New York: Wiley.

Linden (1993). The autogenic training method of JH Schultz. In P. M. Lehrer and R. L. Woolfolk (Eds.), *Principles and practice of stress management* (pp. 205-230). New York: Guilford.

Maslar, P. M. (1986). The effect of music on the reduction of pain: A review of the literature. *Arts in Psychotherapy, 13,* 215-219.

McCaul, K. D., and Malott, J. M. (1984). Distraction and coping with pain. *Psychological Bulletin, 95,* 516-533.

Melzack, R., Taenzer, P., Feldman, P, and Kinch, R. A. (1981). Labour is still painful after prepared childbirth training. *Canadian Medical Association Journal, 125,* 357-363.

Monaghan, P., and Diereck, E. G. (1999). *Meditation: The complete guide*. Novato, CA: New World Library.

Philips, H. C., and Rachman, S. (1996*). The psychological management of chronic pain: A treatment manual* (2nd ed.). New York: Springer Publishing.

Pinsky, J. J., and Malyon, A. K. (1979). The eclectic nature of psychotherapy in the treatment of chronic pain syndromes. In B. L. Crue (Ed.), *Chronic pain: Further observations from City of Hope National Medical Center*. New York: SP Medical and Scientific Books.

Rider, M. S. (1985). Entertainment mechanisms are involved in pain reduction, muscle relaxation and music-mediated imagery. *Journal of Music Therapy, 22,* 183-192.

Sanders, S. H. (1996). Operant conditioning with chronic pain: Back to basics. In R. J. Gatchel and D. C. Turk (Eds.), *Psychological approaches to pain management* (pp. 112-130). New York: Guilford.

Sarno, J. (1976). Chronic back pain and psychic conflict. *Scandinavian Journal of Rehabilitation Medicine, 8,* 143-153.

Schwartz, M.S. and Associates (1985). *Biofeedback: A practitioner's guide* (2nd ed.). New York: Guilford Press.

Tunks, E. R., and Mersky, H. (1990). Psychotherapy in the management of chronic pain. In J. J. Bonica (Ed.), *The management of pain* (pp. 1753-1754). Philadelphia, PA: Lea and Febiger.

Turk, D. C., Meichenbaum, D., and Genest, M. (1983). *Pain and behavioral medicine: A cognitive-behavioral perspective*. New York: Guilford.

Vick, R. M., and Sexton, R. K. (1999). Interplay of art making practices and migraine headache pain experience. *Headache Quarterly, 10,* 287-291.

Williams, D. A., and Turner, B. E. (1989). An empirical assessment of pain beliefs. *Pain, 36,* 351-358.

In: The Handbook of Chronic Pain
Editors: S. Kreitler, D. Beltrutti, et al., pp. 323-334

ISBN 978-1-60021-044-0
© 2007 Nova Science Publishers, Inc.

Chapter 18

Psychological Approaches to Pain Management: Behavioral Modification

Janice M. Livengood

Behavioral intervention encompasses two broad categories of theory: the operant learning model and the respondent, or Pavlovian, conditioning model. Both of these theoretical positions have played a role in chronic pain management by systematically altering the consequences of pain behavior through non-reinforcement, while rewarding well behaviors so that healthy behavior is more satisfying to the patient (Grzesiak 1982, p.31).

OPERANT BEHAVIORAL MODEL

The role of operant learning in chronic pain was first proposed by Fordyce (1973; 1974; 1976; 1978; Fordyce, et al 1968a; 1968b; 1973) who suggested pain behaviors may be maintained by environmental contingencies once the acute pain phase ends. Grimacing, limping, and guarding as well as pain complaints, inactivity, and medication misuse are examples of pain behaviors. Visible indications of autonomic arousal include pallor, perspiration, and increased respiration.

The central premise of the operant behavioral model is that any behavior reinforced with a reward will have an increased probability of recurrence given the same or similar antecedent conditions. Proponents of this view suggest patients have learned rewarding consequences of pain expression; therefore, to alter or modify chronic pain behavior requires a reversal of contingencies so that pain behaviors are no longer rewarded while well behaviors receive increased attention and positive reinforcement (Kalsher et al., 1985). The individual is then more likely to engage in well behavior because of subsequent positive consequences.

Three general sets of conditions can lead to the development of an operant pain problem: (1) pain behavior receives direct and positive reinforcement such as increased attention or desired medication; (2) pain enables the individual to avoid unpleasant tasks; and (3) health or well behaviors are not rewarded and may even be punished through such admonitions as, "Take it easy" (Grzesiak, 1982). Thus, preoccupation with pain can lead to maladaptive behaviors such as prolonged inactivity, medication misuse and pain complaints. Unknowingly, family and friends may reward these behaviors by suggesting the patient rest, volunteering to perform his or her chores, and offering medications (Kientz, et al 1983).

The operant view is further expanded to the development of passive behaviors. Pain behaviors, subjective experiences of pain, and physiological correlates of pain are subject to operant learning mechanisms (Linton et al., 1984a, 1984b, 1985; Flor and Birbaumer, 1994). For example, patients with reinforcing, solicitous spouses reported significantly lower pain thresholds (i.e., indicated pain much sooner) when the spouses were present, compared to the group with non-reinforcing spouses (Flor and Birbaumer, 1994). Operant learning is thought to influence all levels of the pain experience and may establish powerful memories for pain-related responses (Flor and Birbaumer, 1994).

RESPONDENT BEHAVIORAL MODEL

The respondent, or Pavlovian, pain-conditioning model assumes pain is an unconditioned stimulus leading to numerous physiological reactions. These physiological reactions are conditioned by simultaneous presentation of stimuli with the pain experience. If these learned associations occur often and with great intensity, pain may develop and continue to be maintained by the respondent learning process. The learned pain response is no longer necessarily related to the initial cause of acute pain, although it may be localized at the same site and may have comparable qualities (Silver et al., 1975; Linton et al., 1984a, 1984b; Flor and Birbaumer, 1994; Waschulewski-Floruss et al., 1994). Stimuli once associated with pain, such as certain body positions, movements, emotions, or external situations, may acquire a pain-inducing function through respondent conditioning.

Fordyce (1976) distinguished between respondent and operant pain. Respondent pain is a response to a specific antecedent stimulation, i.e., is a signal of disease or biologic malfunction. Operant pain, however, is pain expression that has been shaped by its reinforcing consequences in the environment. Examples of reinforcing consequences include current or potential economic compensation; medications; nurturing and avoidance of undesired social, vocational or family responsibilities. When respondent pain lasts for a prolonged period of time it can, according to proponents of this theory, take on operant qualities, i.e., when respondent pain behavior is rewarded the pain behavior is likely to continue (Grzesiak 1982, p.31).

ASSESSMENT AND INTERVENTION

The scientific method is utilized in behavioral assessment and intervention (see Table 1). First, the patient's environment related to his/her pain problem is assessed, which is considered parallel to a literature review in scientific research. The patient's target behavior related to his/her pain problem is then identified, which is parallel to defining the research hypothesis and dependent variable. Treatment goals are defined, which is parallel to defining the independent variable. Next, treatment is applied with periodical re-administration of behavioral measures to assess treatment efficacy. If necessary, treatment methods are modified until treatment goals are achieved. This is considered parallel to applying the independent variable and measuring the dependent variable. Treatment methods and results are then discussed with the patient to help him/her apply the treatment to other aspects of his/her life, which is considered parallel to evaluating and discussing results in scientific research. As is outlined by this comparison, assessment is a continual and integral part of behavior therapy.

Table 1. Comparison Of Behavioral Assessment With The Scientific Method

Pre-treatment behavioral baseline related to the patient's pain problem is established	Literature review
Target behaviors are identified	Research hypothesis and dependent variable(s) are defined
Treatment goals are defined	Independent variables are defined
Treatment is applied with periodical re-administration of behavioral measures to assess treatment efficacy and, if necessary, treatment is modified to achieve treatment goals	Independent variables are applied and the dependent variable is measured
Treatment method and results are discussed with the patient to help him/her apply the treatment to other aspects of his/her life	Scientific research results are evaluated and suggestions for future research are discussed

Assessment

Behavioral therapists utilize a variety of assessment methods including self-monitoring by the patient, direct observation by the therapist and patient-completed questionnaires.

Self-Monitoring

Patients who are asked to self-monitor keep records that are then summarized and reviewed by the therapist. The goal is to establish a pre-treatment behavioral baseline in order to evaluate treatment efficacy and to establish whether treatment effects can be maintained after therapy is terminated (Keefe and Crisson 1988, p 61). Behaviors measured by self-monitoring include activity level and compliance with a scheduled exercise program. Patient-maintained diaries may determine activity level with hourly entries indicating amount of time spent reclining, sitting, standing, and walking (Fordyce 1976). Treatment is then designed to increase the patient's activity level. Social reinforcement and extinction of pain behavior are reportedly effective in increasing activity levels while simultaneously decreasing pain medication intake (Keefe and Crisson 1988; Fordyce 1976).

Physical therapists often have patients keep self-monitoring diaries to determine patient compliance with a scheduled exercise program. Advantages of self-monitoring methods include simplicity, low cost, and ease of administration over days and weeks of treatment. Limitations include lack of reliability due to possible under reporting or exaggeration of pain or activity level (Keefe and Crisson 1988, pp 62-3).

Direct Observation

Pain management professionals can observe and assess overt pain behaviors including pain complaints, painful facial expressions, guarded movements, grimacing, sighing, or rubbing the painful area. Reliability and validity of the observation method were supported by the finding that a sample of low-back-pain patients with positive physical findings displayed significantly higher rates of pain behavior than patients who did not have positive physical findings (Keefe and Crisson, 1988, pp. 63-65).

Electromechanical devices to monitor activity levels in chronic pain patients have been used to assess uptime and quantify gait abnormalities (Keefe and Crisson 1988). A pressure transducer placed in patients' shoes to examine gait patterns in chronic low back pain patients indicated that pain patients walked more slowly, took shorter steps, and did not demonstrate a normal symmetrical gait pattern (Keefe and Hill, 1985).

Self-report Questionnaires

Examples of self-report instruments for investigating physical symptoms include the Sickness Impact Profile, Chronic Illness Problem Inventory, Stanford Health Assessment Questionnaire, and the Oswestry Disability Index for Low Back Pain.

The Sickness Impact Profile (SIP), a behavior-based measure of health status, has demonstrated good reliability and validity as a measure of dysfunction among chronic pain patients. It is easily administered, has high reliability and validity and provides useful clinical information about disabilities in various areas including physical functioning, communication, and cognitive and social activity (Gilson, et al, 1985; Williams, 1988; Bergner, et al, 1981; Bergner, 1984; Gilson, et al, 1985),

The Chronic Illness Problem Inventory (CIPI) is shorter and more easily scored than the Sickness Impact Profile. Reliability and validity data demonstrate its ability to document patients' specific problems in areas of health care behaviors, physical limitations, psychosocial functioning, and marital adjustment (Kames, et al 1984; Romano et al., 1992).

The Stanford Health Assessment Questionnaire (HAQ), developed for use with arthritis patients, measures physical and functional disability. Disability, pain, economic, drug side effect and drug toxicity dimensions are measured by the HAQ (Fries, 1983; Fries, 1991; Ramey et al., 1992; Fries et al, 1994; Hubert et al., 1994; Leigh et al., 1994).

The Oswestry Disability Index for Low Back Pain is brief and easily scored. It includes measures of pain intensity and the patient's perceived need for pain medication, as well as limitations regarding personal care, lifting, walking, sitting, standing, sleeping, sexual activity, social activity and ability to travel (Soini et al., 1993; Osterbauer et al., 1993; Little et al., 1994; Hupli et al., 1996; Tiusanen et al., 1996a; Tiusanen et al., 1996b; Hurri et al., 1998; Kankaanpaa et al., 1998;).

Intervention

Behavior therapy is a diverse collection of therapies used to decrease maladaptive behaviors and increase more adaptive behaviors (Swanson et al, 1976; Swanson et al, 1979; Turner and Chapman 1982; Bakris and Zorumski, 1983; Kientz et al, 1983; White et al, 1986; Livengood 1994a, 1994b, 1995, 1996a, 1996b). These therapies emphasize current, versus previous, behaviors and utilize a scientific approach to the study and treatment of maladaptive behaviors.

The goal of operant behavior intervention is to decrease operant, or learned, pain behaviors and replace them with well behaviors. A change in environmental contingencies must occur so pain behaviors are not rewarded while desired behaviors are reinforced. Desirable behaviors to produce, decrease, maintain or eliminate are identified in contingency management intervention. Effective rewards are also identified. Treatment involves instructing medical staff and family members to ignore pain behaviors and reward activity (Turner and Chapman 1982; Swanson et al, 1976; Swanson et al, 1979; White et al, 1986). Verbal reinforcement is especially powerful for helping patients decrease medication, increase activity level, and comply with physical therapy regimens.

Medication reduction can be accomplished in inpatient treatment facilities with behavioral intervention (Bakris and Zorumski, 1983; Swanson, et al 1976). During the first week of inpatient care, the average daily dosage is determined. Medication is then changed to a fixed schedule with dosage based on the mean daily dose of the first week. Patients are informed the medication dosage will be tapered after which medication is withdrawn gradually by giving patients unmarked capsules so they have no knowledge of the tapered rate. Rationale for this approach is twofold: (1) a pharmacologically rational dosage regimen is provided and (2) availability of medicine is not contingent on patient request, which could reinforce pain behavior. A contract is negotiated with the patient for stepwise decreases of analgesic and sedative drugs while patients and their families are educated about drugs and their proper use (Kientz et al, 1983). Medications are administered on a regular time schedule and not on patient demand.

Operant conditioning approaches are concerned with chronicity defined in terms of patients' illness behavior. Outcome measures emphasize decreased utilization of medication and decreased use of the health care system as well as return to normal activity levels. A limitation of behavior modification is emphasis of a strict behavioral definition of chronic pain while ignoring mental processes associated with persistent pain. A behaviorist's goal is to change behaviors, whereas relieving the patient's subjective state of suffering is not formally acknowledged as a goal.

While this author advocates use of cognitive behavioral therapy over strict behavioral approaches, the following case demonstrates successful utilization of behavioral intervention to increase activity level, patient compliance with physical therapy and use of relaxation skills, while decreasing medication use.

CASE ILLUSTRATION

A 60-year-old, married, Caucasian, obese female presented with lower back pain of ten years duration following a work-related injury. The patient rated her pain as five on a 0-10 point scale with some numbness and tingling in the lower extremities. Treatment reportedly included surgery one year post injury, physical therapy, a TENS unit, relaxation training, biofeedback, and narcotic medication. According to the patient, none of these had helped for any length of time, although she acknowledged that she had not complied with her prescribed treatment other than taking narcotic medications.

The patient arrived at our pain center in a wheelchair and demonstrated difficulty standing which her physician attributed to disuse and inactivity versus organic pathology. Her medical evaluation revealed bilateral trigger points along the entire paraspinous musculature with no vertebral column abnormalities and no gross limb defects. She was given an Emory classification of one (Brena and Koch 1975) indicating low physical pathology and high pain behavior. She was wheel chair dependent for no diagnosed medical reason. Her physician concluded there were no identifiable objective findings underlying her reported pain and diminished sensation. The patient's medical plan of treatment included referral for psychological evaluation, aggressive physical therapy, a weight reduction program, discontinuation of narcotic medication and a prescription for anti-inflammatory medication.

The patient's psychological evaluation revealed a history of depression with previous anti-depressant medication treatment attempts reportedly resulting in patient non-compliance. A psychosocial history indicated the patient married at age 16 to her current husband. Two children and a number of grandchildren resulted from this union. With ten years of education, the patient began work at age 30 in a school cafeteria and reported a sporadic work history due to work-related injuries. She admitted she had no desire to return to work with little motivation to do "anything" stating her retired husband could manage the housework and cooking without her help. She described total reliance on her husband, stating she was ill and could not be expected to maintain the household or help with their elderly parents. Her apparent sick role had its roots in childhood, possibly modeled by an older sister and mother who were described as being "disabled". As a child she reportedly had to feign illness to get attention from her parents and family because her older sister, described as having chronic health problems, received most of the family's attention. The patient's sick role was maintained throughout adulthood and enabled her to obtain economic compensation for work-related injuries while avoiding undesirable social and family responsibilities. Nurturing support from her husband, adult children and friends, as well as reliance on narcotic medications, were additional rewards.

Psychological intervention included a review of pain management skills, relaxation training, and stress management skills with which the patient had reportedly not complied. Behavioral intervention included a patient-maintained diary of pain intensity including time patterns related to pain, along with behaviors or thoughts that accompanied pain. These were then examined for underlying patterns of behaviors accompanying her pain, with particular attention given to the role of others, interactive patterns between spouse or other family members and/or avoidance of responsibility. She was also asked to maintain a medication diary.

A behavioral modification program was found to be the most useful means of helping the patient comply with physical therapy, regular use of relaxation skills, and decreased medication usage. While the patient was not seemingly motivated to utilize skills to decrease her pain intensity, decrease medication or resume family or household responsibilities, she was motivated to shop for items to decorate her home; therefore, a token economy system was begun with the patient. With input from her physical therapist and nutritionist for weight reduction, a task list and frequency with which she was to perform each task per day was designed. She engaged in physical therapy for an agreed upon number of repetitions and times per day for which she received an agreed upon number of token points. Relaxation training, positive affirmations or any cognitive-behavioral homework assignments were completed an agreed upon number of times per day for which token points were earned. At the end of each day the patient totaled her number of earned points and then totaled the number of earned points at the end of the week. Points were converted into money with which she purchased items to decorate her home. With input from her pain physician, a token economy system was simultaneously utilized to wean her from narcotic medication.

In conjunction with the above token economy, the patient engaged in both individual therapy and couples therapy. The patient's husband learned to identify illness behaviors and reward only well behaviors. He initially reported difficulty complying with this plan because he was accustomed to responding automatically to his wife's requests. With the help of couples therapy, the patient and her husband identified and changed the system within which they had been living.

The result of behavioral intervention with this patient was increased activity and decreased focused on pain. Her pain intensity, depression and anxiety improved from regular use of pain management skills, physical therapy, increased activity, improved diet and compliance with taking anti-inflammatory and anti-depressant medication. She was successfully weaned from narcotic medication. Clearly, behavioral modification helped improve treatment compliance; although, the behavioral methods were used within a family systems framework which addressed underlying cognitive and interpersonal issues.

CONCLUSION

Behavioral modification has been successfully used with chronic pain patients to decrease medication use (Anderson, et al 1977; Sternbach, 1977; Cinciripini et al., 1982; Kientz, et al 1983; Klein, 1985; King, et al 1994); extinguish pain behaviors and reinforce well behaviors (Anderson, et al 1977; Klein, 1985; Rainville, et al 1997); increase activity level (Anderson, et al 1977; Sternbach, 1977); decrease pain (National Institute of Health Report, 1996; White et al, 1986) and decrease visits to health care professionals (Caudill et al., 1991). Behavioral modification has been successfully used in treating the following pain sites: headache (Hansotia, 1986); pelvic pain (Hahn, et al 1989); chronic back pain (Klein, et al 1985; Vlaeyen et al., 1989; Rainville, et al, 1997); abnormal gait (Klein, et al 1985); somatization disorders (Klein, et al 1985); irritable bowel syndrome (Drossman and

Thompson, (1992); temporomandibular disorders (Clark, et al 1990; Smith, 1985; Dworkin, 1997; Turk, 1997) and posttraumatic pain syndromes (Muse, 1986). Long-term follow-up studies ranging from one to eight years indicate continued efficacy with behavioral intervention (Roberts et al., 1980; Roberts et al., 1993). It is the opinion of this author that behavioral modification is best used in conjunction with cognitive-behavioral and family systems intervention.

REFERENCES

Anderson T.P., Cole T.M., Gullickson G., Hudgens A. and Roberts A.H.: Behavior modification of chronic pain: a treatment program by a multi disciplinary team. *Clin. Orth. and Rel. Res*, 129 (1977) 96-100.

Bakris G.L. and Zorumski C.F.: Chronic pain: A pharmacologic review and behavior modification approach. *Pain Management*, 73 (1983) 119-128.

Bergner M., Bobbit R.A., Carter W.B. and Gilson, B.S.: The sickness impact profile: development and final version of a health status measure. *Med. Care*, 19 (1981) 787-805.

Bergner M.: The sickness impact profile. In: N.K. Wenger, M.F. Mattson and C.D. Furberg (Eds.). *Assessment of Quality of Life in Clinical Trials of Cardiovascular Therapies*, LeJacq, New York, 1984, pp. 152-159.

Brena S.F. and Koch D.L.: A pain estimate model for qualification and classification of chronic pain states. *Anesthesiol. Rev.*, (1975) 8-13.

Caudill M., Schnable R., Zuttermeister P., Benson H. and Friedman R.: Decreased clinic use by chronic pain patients: response to behavioral medicine intervention. *Clinical J. of Pain*, 7 (1991) 305-310.

Cinciripini P.M. and Floreen A.: An evaluation of a behavioral program for chronic pain. *J. of Beh. Med.*, 5 (1982) 375-389.

Clark G.T., Seligman D.A., Solberg W.K. and Pullinger, A.G.: Guidelines for the treatment of temporomandibular disorders. *J. of Craniomandibular Dis.: Facial and Oral Pain*, (1990) 80-87.

Drossman D.A. and Thompson W.G.: The irritable bowel syndrome: review and a graduated multi component treatment approach. *Annals. of Internal. Medicine*, 116 (1992) 1009-16.

Dworkin S.F.: Behavioral and educational modalities: *Review. Oral Surgery, Oral Medicine, Oral Pathology, Oral Radiology, and Edodontics*, 83 (1997) 128-133.

Flor H. and Birbaumer N.: *Basic issues in the psychobiology of pain*. In: G.F. Gebhart, D.L.

Hammond and T.S. Jensen (Eds.). Progress in Pain Research and Management, 14, *Proc. VII World Congress on Pain*, IASP Press, Seattle, 1994, pp.113-125.

Fordyce W. E.: *An operant conditioning method for managing chronic pain*. Postgrad. Med., 53 (1973) 123-128.

Fordyce W. E.: Treating chronic pain by contingency management. *Adv. Neurol.*,(1974) 583-9

Fordyce W. E.: Behavioral *Methods for Chronic Pain and Illness*. Mosby, St. Louis, 1976.

Fordyce W. E.: Learning processes in pain. In: R.A. Sternbach (Ed.). *The Psychology of Pain*, Raven Press, New York, 1978, pp. 49-72.

Fordyce W. E., Fowler, R.S. and DeLateur, B.J.: An application of behavior modification technique to a problem of chronic pain. *Behav. Res. Therapy*, 6 (1968) 105-107.

Fordyce W.E., Fowler R., Lehmann J. and DeLateur, B.: Some implications of learning in problems of chronic pain. *J. Chron. Disability*, 21 (1968) 179-190.

Fordyce W.E., Fowler R., Lehmann J., DeLateur B., Sand P. and Treischmann, R.: Operant conditioning in the treatment of chronic pain. *Arch. Phys. Med. Rehab*, 54 (1973) 399-408.

Fries J.F.: The assessment of disability: from first to future principles. Br. *J. Rheumatol.*, 22.Suppl., (1983) 48-58.

Fries J.F.: The hierarchy of quality-of-life assessment, the Health Assessment Questionnaire (HAQ), and issues mandating development of a toxicity index. *Controlled Clinical Trials*, 12 (1991) 106S-117S.

Fries J.F., Singh G., Morfeld D., Hubert H.B., Lane N.E. and Brown B. W., Jr.: Running and the development of disability with age. *Annals of Internal Med*, 121 (1994) 502-509.

Gilson B.S., Gilson J.S. and Bergner M.: The sickness impact profile. Development of an outcome measure of health care. *Am. J. Publ. Hlth.*, 65 (1985) 1304-1310.

Grzesiak R.C.: Cognitive and behavioral approaches to management of chronic pain. *N.Y. State J. of Med.*, 82 (1982) 30-38.

Grzesiak R.C. and Ciccone D.S.: Relaxation, biofeedback and hypnosis in the management of pain. In: N. T. Lynch and S.V. Vasudevan (Eds.). *Persistent Pain: Psychosocial Assessment and Intervention*, Kluwer Academic Publishers, Boston, 1988, pp. 163-188.

Hahn M.B., Jones M.M., and Carron H.: Idiopathic pelvic pain: the relationship to depression. Postgrad. Med.: *Chron. Pain*, 85 (1989) 263-270.

Hansotia P.: Evaluation and treatment of headache: practical approach to a common symptom. Postgrad. Med.: *Headache*, 79 (1986) 75-84.

Hubert H.B. and Fries J.F.: Predictors of physical disability after age 50. Six-year longitudinal study in a runners club and a university population. *Annals of Epidemiology*, 4 (1994) 285-294.

Hupli M. Hurri H. Luoto S. Sainio P. and Alaranta H.: Isokinetic performance capacity of trunk muscles. Part I: The effect of repetition on measurement of isokinetic performance capacity of trunk muscles among healthy controls and two different groups of low-back pain patients. *Scandinavian J. of Rehab. Med.*, 28 (1996) 201-206.

Hurri H., Slatis P., Soini J., Tallroth K., Alaranta H., Laine T. and Heliovaara M.: Lumbar spinal stenosis: assessment of long-term outcome 12 years after operative and conservative treatment. *J of Spinal Disorders*, 11 (1998) 110-115.

Kalsher M.J., Cataldo M.F., Dear R.M., Traughber B. and Jankel W. R.: Behavioral covariation in the treatment of chronic pain. *J of Behavior Therapy and Experimental Psychiatry*, 16 (1985) 331-339.

Kames L.D., Nalihoff B.D., Heinrich, R.L. and Schag, C.C.: The chronic illness problem inventory: problem-oriented psychological assessment of patients with chronic illness. *Int. J. Psychiat. Med.*, 14 (1984) 65-75.

Kankaanpaa M., Taimela S., Laaksonen D., Hannienen O. and Airaksinen O.: Back and hip extensor fatigability in chronic low back pain patients and controls. *Archives of Phys Med and Rehab*, 79 (1998) 412-417.

Keefe F.J. and Crisson J.E.: Assessment of behaviors. In N.T. Lynch and S.V. Vasudevan (Eds.). *Persistent Pain: Psychosocial Assessment and Intervention*, Kluwer Academic Publishers, Boston, 1988, pp. 61-73.

Keefe F.J. and Hill R.W.: An objective approach to quantifying pain behavior and gait patterns in low back pain patients. *Pain*, 21 (1985) 153-161.

Kientz J.E., Fitzsimmons D.S. and Schneider, P.J.: Reducing medication use in a chronic pain management program. *Amer. J. of Hosp. Phar.*, 40 (1983) 2156-2158.

King J.C., Kelleher W.J., Stedwill J.E. and Talcott G.: Physical limitations are not required for chronic pain rehabilitation success. *Am. J. Phys. Med. Rehabil.*, 73 (1994) 331-337.

Klein M.J., Kewman D.G. and Sayama M.: Behavior modification of abnormal gait and chronic pain secondary to somatization disorder. *Arch. Phys. Med. Rehabil.*, 66 (1985) 119-122.

Leigh J.P. and Fries J.F.: Education, gender and the compression of morbidity. *International J. of aging and Human Dev*, 39 (1994) 233-246.

Linton S.J. and Gotestam K.G.: A controlled study of the effects of applied relaxation and applied relaxation plus operant procedures in the regulation of chronic pain. *British J. of Clinical Psychology*, 23 (1984) 291-299.

Linton S.J. and Gotestam K.G.: Controlling pain reports through operant conditioning: a laboratory demonstration. *Perpetual and Motor Skills*, 60 (1985) 427-437.

Linton S.J., Melin L. and Gotestam K.G.: Behavioral analysis of chronic pain and its management. In: M. Hersen, A. Bellack and H. Eisler (Eds.). *Progress in Behavior Modification*, Vol. 18, Academic Press, New York, 1984, pp. 1-42.

Little D.G. and MacDonald D.: The use of the percentage change in Oswestry Disability Index score as an outcome measure in lumbar spinal surgery. *Spine*, 19 (1994) 2139-2143.

Livengood J.M.: Biofeedback hypnosis in chronic pain management. In: P. Raj, D. Niv, S. Erdine, S. Raja (Eds.). *Management of Pain: A World Perspective*, Monduzzi Editore, Bologna, Italy, 1995, pp.577-582.

Livengood J.M.: Efficacy of psychological techniques used in pain management. In: P. Raj, D. Niv, S. Erdine, S. Raja (Eds.). *Management of Pain: A World Perspective*, Monduzzi Editore, Bologna, Italy, 1995, pp.563-568.

Livengood J.M.: Use of biofeedback with chronic pain patients: are there ever contraindications? *Pain Digest*, 5 (1995) 90-92.

Livengood J.M.: Psychological Intervention in Cancer Pain Management. In: W.C.V. Parris (Ed.). *Cancer Pain Management: Principles and Practice*, Butterworth-Heinemann, Boston, 1997, pp.245-252.

Livengood J.M.: Psychological techniques for chronic pain management: review. *Pain Digest*, 6 (1996) 77-82.

Muse M.: Stress-related, posttraumatic chronic pain syndrome: behavioral treatment approach. *Pain*, 25 (1986) 389-394.

National Institute of Health Report: NIH technology assessment panel on integration of behavioral and relaxation approaches into the treatment of chronic pain and insomnia. *JAMA*, 276 (1996) 313-318.

Osterbauer P.J., DeBoer K. F., Widmaier R., Petermann E. and Fuhr A.W.: Treatment and biomechanical assessment of patients with chronic sacroiliac joint syndrome. *J of Manipulative and Phys Therapeutics*, 16 (1993) 82-90.

Rainville J., Sobel J., Hartigan C., Monlux G. and Bean J.: Decreasing disability in chronic back pain through aggressive spine rehabilitation. J. Rehab Research and Development, 34 (1997) 383-393.amey D.R., Raynauld J.P. and Fries J.F.: The health assessment questionnaire 1992: status and review. *Arthritis Care and Research*, 5 (1992) 119-129.

Roberts A.H. and Reinhardt L.: The behavioral management of chronic pain: long-term follow-up with comparison groups. *Pain*, 8 (1980) 151-162.

Roberts A.H., Sternbach R.A. and Polich J.: Behavioral management of chronic pain and excess disability: long-term follow-up of an outpatient program. *Clinical J. of Pain*, 9 (1993) 41-48.

Silver A.I. and Greco T.S.: A comparison of the effects of vicariously instigated classical conditioning and direct classical conditioning procedures. *Pavlovian J. of Biological Science*, 10 (1975) 216-225.

Smith R.C.: A clinical approach to the somatisizing patient. *J. of Fam. Pract.*, 21 (1985) 294-301.

Soini J., Laine T., Pohjolainen T., Hurri H. and Alaranta H.: Spondylodesis augmented by transpedicular fixation in the treatment of olisthetic and degenerative conditions of the lumbar spine. *Clinical Orthopedics and Related Research*, 297 (1993) 111-116.

Sternbach R.A.: Psychological aspects of chronic pain. *Clin. Ortho. and Rel. Res.*, 129 (1977) 150-155.

Swanson D.W., Maruta T. and Swenson W.M.: Results of behavior modification in the treatment of chronic pain. *Psychosomatic Med.*, 41 (1979) 55-61.

Swanson D.W., Swenson W.M., Maruta, T. and McPhee M.C.: Program for managing chronic pain. I. Program description and characteristics of patients. *Mayo Clinic Proceedings*, 51 (1976) 401-408.

Tiusanen H., Hurri H., Seitsalo S., Osterman K. and Harju R.: Functional and clinical results after anterior interbody lumbar fusion. *European Spine Journal*, 5 (1996) 288-292.

Tiusanen H., Seitsalo S., Osterman K. and Soini J.: Anterior interbody lumbar fusion in severe low back pain. *Clinical Orthopedics and Related Research*, 324 (1996) 153-163.

Turk D.C.: Psychosocial and behavioral assessment of patients with temporomandibular disorders: diagnostic and treatment implications: review. *Oral Surgery, Oral Medicine, Oral Pathology, Oral Radiology, and Edodontics*. 83 (1997) 65-71.

Turner J.A. and Chapman C.R.: Psychological interventions for chronic pain: a critical review: operant conditioning, hypnosis, and cognitive-behavioral therapy. *Pain*, 12 (1982) 23-46.

Vlaeyen J.W., Groenman N.H., Thomassen J., Schuerman J. A., VanEek H., Snijders A.M. and van Houtem J.: A behavioral treatment for sitting and standing intolerance in a patient with chronic low back pain. *Clinical J. of Pain*, 5 (1989) 233-237.

Waschulewski-Floruss H, Miltner W., Brody S. and Braun C.: classical conditioning of pain responses. *International Journal of Neuroscience*, 78 (1994) 21-22.

White B. and Sanders S.H.: The influence on patients' pain intensity ratings of antecedent reinforcement of pain talk or well talk. *J of Behavior Therapy and Experimental Psychiatry*, 17 (1986) 155-159.

Williams R.C.: Review article: toward a set of reliable and valid measures for chronic pain assessment and outcome research. *Pain*, 35 (1988) 239-251.

In: The Handbook of Chronic Pain
Editors: S. Kreitler, D. Beltrutti, et al., pp. 335-357

ISBN 978-1-60021-044-0
© 2007 Nova Science Publishers, Inc.

Chapter 19

Hypnosis in the Management of Chronic Pain Conditions, and the Acute Pain Accompanying their Treatment

John F. Chaves

The effective management of chronic pain continues to present a serious challenge to the health professions. Even though we now have a wide array of medical therapies that are relatively safe and largely effective in managing many forms of chronic and acute pain, these therapies have significant limitations, especially in the management of chronic pain. The pain relief achieved with traditional biomedical and surgical therapies is often incomplete and sometimes ineffective (Stevens, Dalla Pozza, Cavalletto, Cooper, and Kilham, 1994). Moreover, relief too often comes at a high cost in terms of the patient's quality of life (Douglas, 1999). Adding to these considerations has been our growing awareness of the limitations of a narrow biomedical perspective on health and well-being and a recognition of the need to embrace a broader biopsychosocial perspective that encourages our examination of alternative approaches to pain management (Engel, 1977; 1987; 1997).

This chapter describes and evaluates the ways in which one such alternative, clinical hypnosis, has been used in the management of chronic pain, including the management of acute pain associated with the treatment of underlying medical conditions producing chronic pain. It describes the nature of hypnotic interventions and the manner in which they have been used in chronic pain management. It also considers the spectrum of application of hypnosis in chronic pain management and reviews systematically collected data as well as case studies pertaining to several chronic pain problems. The emphasis is placed on finding reported since recent critical reviews by Spanos (1989; Spanos, Carmanico, and Ellis, 1994) and Chaves (1989; 1993; 1994). My goal is to provide a framework for clinicians who may be unfamiliar with this modality to understand better the nature of hypnotic treatment, help them appreciate the empirical evidence supporting its use, and introduce some of the practical issues involved in its effective use in chronic pain management.

To put this topic in context, it is important to note that contemporary approaches to chronic pain management have increasingly coming to reflect an awareness of the significant contribution of psychosocial factors in the etiology, diagnosis, and treatment of many painful medical conditions. That fact is due, in part, to the reconceptualization of pain perception provided by the gate control theory of pain (Melzack and Wall, 1965) that offered new ways of understanding the neurophysiological mechanisms by which psychosocial factors could amplify or attenuate the pain experience. Although the basic observation that pain could be profoundly modulated by various psychological interventions was already well known, the articulation of a formal theory that provided explicit mechanisms by which this modulation of pain could be produced had an enormous impact on research and clinical practice and helped to encourage the development of multidisciplinary approaches to pain management (Kotarba, 1983). Soon, systematic efforts were underway to refine older therapeutic strategies and to develop new strategies for exploiting psychological resources that were already available to patients as well as assisting them in developing new skills that could be beneficially applied to reducing their symptoms (Fordyce, 1976; Turk, Meichenbaum, and Genest, 1983).

Although substantial gains in the clinical practice of pain management have been made since the Gate Control Theory was promulgated, the biomedical perspective has continued to dominate contemporary medical practice, even as more sophisticated psychological interventions for pain management were developed (Turk et al., 1983). In recent years, however, there has been substantial growth in the amount of research, including randomized clinical trials, being conducted on psychological interventions for chronic pain management. Favorable results have contributed to a growing acceptance of the notion that interventions like hypnosis, that can augment more traditional medical or pharmacological approaches, or reduce reliance on them, have the potential to play an important role in contemporary pain management (Chaves and Dworkin, 1997; Holroyd, 1996; National Institutes of Health, 1995).

A Brief Historical Overview of Clinical Hypnosis

Hypnosis is arguably one of the oldest forms of psychological therapy (Crabtree, 1993; Ellenberger, 1970). Although hypnotic-like phenomena have been observed throughout recorded history (Edmonston, 1986; Hilgard and Hilgard, 1983), the topic came to the serious attention of the health professions in the late 1700's and early 1800's. It was then that anecdotal reports began to appear in the medical literature suggesting that hypnosis, or Mesmerism, as it was then called, could be used to control the pain associated with various medical procedures. These reports described limb amputations, mastectomies, and dental extractions apparently completed with substantially less than the expected levels of pain (Deane, 1844; Delatour, 1826; Ward and Topham, 1842; West, 1836). By the time inhalation anesthetics had been discovered in the middle of the 19th Century, hypnosis had already attracted a substantial following in the medical community, led by John Elliotson, a well-known physician at the University of London (Chaves and Dworkin, 1997). Of course, these accounts predate the discovery of inhalation anesthetics, so it is not surprising that evidence that surgical pain could be controlled received considerable attention. It is also noteworthy that the initial clinical reports focused almost entirely on the mitigation of pain associated with medical and dental procedures, rather than with chronic pain.

Although we now accept the mitigation of chronic and acute pain as important and legitimate therapeutic goals, this was not always the case. For a variety of reasons, the health professions have, at times, expressed deep ambivalence about pain and its mitigation. During the Middle Ages, pain was seen both as a means of punishment and a means of redemption (Caton, 1985). Later, during the 17th and 18th Centuries, pain was thought to play an important facilitative role in the healing process (Rey, 1993). Some saw the induction of an unconscious state, by any means, as creating an ethical dilemma, because the unconscious patient would be unable to assess the speed, talent, and skill of the surgeon (Rey, 1993)! Even in colonial America, physicians, who were often members of the clergy, displayed complex attitudes toward pain that were influenced by both the Augustinian tradition that interpreted pain as the just punishment of the wicked, and the redemptive view that pain was a means of moral growth and salvation (Rey, 1993). Accordingly attitudes towards pain and its relief by techniques like hypnosis, and later by inhalation anesthesia, must be understood within the cultural context of the era (Caton, 1985).

That context probably served initially as a barrier to the adoption of inhalation anesthetics as well as the adoption of hypnosis (Chaves and Dworkin, 1997). Interestingly, as is probably true even today, the barriers to adopting new measures for pain relief seemed greater for professionals than for laymen. Indeed, Winter (1991; 1998) has provided us with a fascinating analysis of the brief but intense struggle between professionals who advocated the use of inhalation anesthetics and those who advocated the use of hypnosis in managing surgical pain. The superiority of inhalation anesthetics was not obvious at first, especially since its use was initially associated with high mortality rates. However, within a few years, inhalation anesthesia became a part of medical orthodoxy, while hypnosis was initially relegated to the margins of medical practice (Parssinen, 1979; Quen, 1973). Interest in hypnosis waxed and waned over the next several decades. Periods of heightened interest were most commonly associated with the appearance of clinical reports describing the successful use of hypnosis to control pain, such as that associated with battlefield injuries incurred during WW I and WW II, when pharmacological agents were unavailable, or in limited supply. Occasionally, other reports of the successful use of hypnosis in alleviating surgical pain appeared describing the fragile medical condition of patients that placed them at significant risk if pharmacological agents were employed (Chaves, 1989; Chaves and Barber, 1976).

In the 1950s and 60s interest in hypnosis grew rapidly and important research programs developed that investigated, among other topics, the use of hypnosis to control pain (Barber, 1959; Barber, 1963; Hilgard, 1969; Hilgard and Hilgard, 1975; Hilgard, 1967; Weitzenhoffer and Hilgard, 1962). By bringing this phenomenon into the laboratory, it was hoped that a better understand might be achieved concerning which aspects of the hypnotic intervention were effective in reducing pain, and to better understand how hypnotic interventions might be devised that optimized the clinical application of these techniques. That line of research has continued to the present and in recent years has been augmented by psychophysiological and electrophysiological studies intended to assess the physiological dimensions of the response to hypnotic procedure. The development of newer neuroimaging strategies have also added tools that have been applied in an effort to understand how hypnotic interventions reduce clinical and experimental pain (Chen, 2001; Crawford, Gur, Skolnick, Gur, and Benson, 1993; Hofbauer, Rainville, Duncan, and Bushnell, 2001; Rainville, Carrier, Hofbauer, Bushnell, and Duncan, 1999; Rainville et al., 1999). Before considering some of the chronic pain syndromes to which clinical hypnosis has been applied, it may be helpful to look at how hypnotic interventions are designed and implemented, with emphasis on some of the special issues that arise in its application in pain management.

THE CLINICAL APPLICATION OF HYPNOSIS IN PAIN MANAGEMENT

The typical treatment protocol for chronic pain management with hypnosis can be divided into six phases, each with its own specific issues: (a) Patient Selection and Preparation, (b) Induction, (c) Deepening, (d) Therapeutic Suggestions, (e) Post-hypnotic suggestion and (f) Termination. All patients come to hypnosis with expectations about the nature of hypnosis (Chaves, 1993; Johnson and Hauck, 1999; Kirsch, 1999). Sometimes these include elaborate notions about who can or cannot be hypnotized and how the process of becoming hypnotized occurs. Some of these beliefs can facilitate responding (e.g. the belief that good hypnotic subjects are intelligent and imaginative individuals) (Cronin, Spanos, and Barber, 1971). Other beliefs and expectations can inhibit responding (e.g. good hypnotic subjects are gullible, easily led individuals who lose control during the process (Barber and de Moor, 1972).

Special ethical and psychological complexities arise when hypnosis is employed for patients with cancer and patients or their family members express the belief that the disease might be cured by the use of hypnotic suggestion (Syrjala and Roth-Roemer, 1996). Under these conditions it is important to be clear about the lack of evidence that hypnosis can directly alter the course of the disease and, at the same time, encourage positive expectations about its impact on patient comfort and motivation. Although three randomized prospective studies have shown a survival differences favoring cancer patients who have been exposed to psychosocial interventions, two others have not (Spiegel, Sephton, Terr, and Stites, 1998). Although the possible influence of such psychosocial interventions on neuroimmune pathways is under active investigation, the present state of the evidence makes it inappropriate to offer hope of cure or even hope of prolonged survival to patients at this time. On the other hand, the case for success in enhanced comfort, decreased reliance on pharmacological agents, and improved quality of life is much more compelling, as we shall see.

The hallmark of the hypnotic intervention is often thought to be the induction process, although evidence indicates that suggestion, per se, can exert powerful effects in a wide variety of contexts (Spanos and Chaves, 1989). Although the nature, duration, and character of hypnotic inductions is highly variable, they typically include instructions to focus attention, suggestions for relaxation, and for entering a hypnotic state. They may also involve suggestions for overt responses that are often described by good hypnotic subjects as occurring effortlessly (e.g. automatic eye-closure in response to suggested drowsiness or movement of the arms in response to suggestions of lightness or heaviness). Such suggestions serve both as observable markers of the patient's subjective response to the procedure for the therapist, and to illustrate the involuntary character of hypnotic responding for the patient. Deepening suggestions follow the induction and are intended to help the patient have a more profound experience through various images, suggested alteration of breathing patterns, suggestions of bodily heaviness, and so forth (Chaves, 1979).

Eventually a point is reached where therapeutically relevant suggestions are administered. The nature of these suggestions is highly variable, even for chronic pain patients. Some of the considerations involved in developing these suggestions are discussed below. With chronic pain patients, post-hypnotic suggestions are generally administered to facilitate the continuation of treatment gains outside of the hypnotic context. This strategy is often augmented with further training in the use of self-hypnosis or by audiotaping the hypnotic intervention and asking the patient to listen to the tape on a regular basis at home. In working with chronic pain patients, significant issues arise with respect to the preparation, therapeutic suggestion, and post-hypnotic suggestion phases. Let is briefly consider some of these issues

SPECIAL ISSUES IN USING HYPNOSIS IN CHRONIC PAIN MANAGEMENT

One of the most important challenges clinicians face in using hypnosis in chronic pain management concerns the management of patient's expectations. Patients sometimes approach hypnosis with almost magical expectations regarding its efficacy. The dilemma facing the clinician is the decision about the extent to which to capitalize on initially positive expectations that may be unrealistic. While we often strive to assist patients in developing positive expectations about treatment outcomes, the failure to achieve unrealistically high initial expectations can make it difficult to pursue more modest, but attainable treatment goals. Patient expectations are known to play an important role in shaping treatment outcomes (e.g. Kirsch, 1999; Shutty, DeGood, and Tuttle, 1990; Shutty and DeGood, 1990). Indeed, neurophysiological evidence suggests that expectation of pain activates sites within the medial frontal lobes, insular cortex and cerebellum distinct from but close to sites activated during the pain experience (Ploghaus et al., 1999). In addition, evidence suggests that expectations can play an important role in shaping the hypnotic experience itself (Kirsch, 1990; 1999; Council, Kirsch, and Hafner, 1986).

The process of engaging a chronic pain patient in treatment typically entails a complex and often difficult negotiation in which the patient comes to relinquish the goal of seeking a "cure" and accept the legitimacy of the of the goal of pain management. This is particularly true for patients with chronic benign pain syndromes, or disorders whose pathophysiological basis has not been clearly established. Accordingly, such treatment sub-goals as increased up-time, decreased reliance on medication, and increased participation in family activities become legitimate treatment objectives. Indeed, the gains achieved with respect to these specific, measurable outcomes can serve as important markers of patient progress and help document success for these patients. As Dworkin and I have noted (Chaves and Dworkin,

1997), this "rehabilitation model" is not consonant with the way hypnosis has traditionally been used. This application requires an approach that encourages positive expectations, while minimizing magical expectations of immediate cure.

A second barrier encountered in preparing patient for the use of hypnosis for chronic pain, especially the chronic benign pain syndromes, is that these patients have often been told, "the pain is in your head." This diagnosis is frequently offered in a context in which psychological causes for pain are implied if not explicitly stated (Chaves, 1993). Although often offered to assuage patient concerns about more serious medical conditions, these statements have the unintended consequence of creating ambivalence, if not aversion, to psychological interventions like hypnosis. The obvious dilemma for the patient is that successful treatment will confirm the dismissive diagnosis that the pain only existed "in their head."

The successful use of hypnosis in chronic pain management requires that both of these issues be successfully managed before beginning treatment. That requires that patient attitudes and expectations regarding treatment be carefully elicited prior to treatment. Patients' views regarding the etiology and pathophysiology of their conditions, as well as their understanding of the views of the clinicians who have previously treated them, can be very helpful in developing a "heuristic model" for the patient that can help them understand the complex interplay between their cognitive and emotional life and their experience of pain. In turn, this model can provide a rationale for the hypnotic interventions to follow. This approach can be particularly important when patients are experiencing such subjectively puzzling phenomena as phantom limb pain, complex regional pain syndromes (e.g. reflex sympathetic dystrophies, causalgia, trigeminal neuralgia) or peripheral manifestations of central pain syndromes related to stroke or space-occupying lesions in the central nervous system).

The period of patient preparation for hypnosis also provides an important opportunity to explore the patient's phenomenology of the pain experience. This exploration provides a rich resource for the development of personally-relevant suggestions that may be therapeutically useful. My own clinical experiences, described elsewhere (e.g. Brown and Chaves, 1980; Chaves, 1981; 1985a; 1985b; 1989; 1993; 1996; 1997; 1999), indicate the importance of rejecting generic pain-relieving suggestions in favor of those that are shaped by the patient's own phenomenology of the pain experience. The careful and empathic listening that is required to elicit this information also helps establish rapport and confers an important therapeutic benefit for those patients who too often are surrounded by those who have become tired of listening.

Of course, commonly used suggestions for hypnotic analgesia, including suggestions that a painful part of the body is numb and insensitive, or that it is disconnected from the rest of the body, may be therapeutically valuable in chronic pain management. But their use can be enhanced when integrated with suggestive elements derived specifically from the patient's own experience of pain. For example, a patient of mine with phantom-limb pain was asked to describe her experience of pain. She said that when she thought of her pain, two images came to mind. One included little red ants that were nibbling at her stump. The other involved rubber bands that she could imagine being tied tightly around the end of her stump. An added feature of this patient's discomfort involved the vivid visual images she reported of her phantom limb when her pain was intense. The therapeutic suggestions derived to assist this patient included spraying her phantom limb with a powerful ant killer, cutting the rubber bands, and visualize her phantom being immersed in a dense fog that prevented her from seeing it, no matter how hard she tried. These brief examples illustrate how the clinician can assist the patient in developing cognitive strategies that may be idiosyncratically beneficial in reducing pain. Certainly, there is substantial evidence from the experimental pain literature supporting the value of this kind of approach (Chaves and Brown, 1987; Chaves and Barber, 1974; Spanos, Horton, and Chaves, 1975)

Patients do not readily admit us to their phenomenal world. Indeed, at times, they may have difficulty grasping what you are driving at when you ask about their pain phenomenology. Nevertheless, these explorations can be quite fruitful and, in my experience, can greatly enhance the efficacy of interventions for pain management. Preexisting cognitive coping strategies and metaphors that have guided efforts at pain-self management pain can also be very helpful. By the same token, knowledge of the patient's catastrophizing ideation, or other aspects of their phenomenology that limits their ability to cope can also be very helpful (Chaves, 2000). I view this phase of the hypnotic intervention as the most important in devising effective interventions. Properly conducted, it sets the stage for all other aspects of the hypnotic intervention and can play a vital role in its ultimate success.

THE SPECTRUM OF CLINICAL APPLICATION

Hypnotic techniques have been applied to a wide variety of medical conditions. Here I review some of the more important areas of application that have been explored. The intent is not to provide a comprehensive critical review of that literature. Instead, the goal is to provide some samples of the ways in which hypnotic interventions for chronic pain are being implemented and evaluated. Although the focus is on the use of hypnosis in chronic pain management, many chronic pain conditions are accompanied by significant acute pain associated with medical treatments. Where relevant, I have included a description of ways in which hypnosis has been used in reducing pain associated with these treatments.

CANCER

Cancer is often accompanied by pain associated with disease progression as well as with the implementation of uncomfortable diagnostic and treatment protocols. Hypnosis has been used in a multifaceted fashion for patients suffering from cancer. It has used as a tool for chronic pain management as well as to reduce the pain, discomfort, and anxiety associated with many aspects of cancer treatment (Chaves, 2000). Stam (1989) has provided a detailed critical review of much of the early literature. In recent years, other descriptive reviews have appeared (Genuis, 1995; Liossi and Mystakidou, 1996; Lynch, 1999). Steggles and his colleagues have provided useful annotated bibliographies of the relatively recent literature on the use of hypnosis in cancer in adults and in children and adolescents (Spanos, Steggles, Radtke-Bodorik, and Rivers, 1979; Steggles, Damore-Petingola, Maxwell, and Lightfoot,

1997; Steggles, Fehr, and Aucoin, 1986; Steggles, Maxwell, Lightfoot, Damore-Petingola, and Mayer, 1997; Steggles, Stam, Fehr, and Aucoin, 1987).

A number of early reports described the application of hypnosis with cancer pain (Cangello, 1961; 1962; Lea, Ware, and Monroe, 1960). Methodological limitations, poorly specified treatment interventions and outcome measures limit the usefulness of these early reports, although their positive findings were encouraging. In addition they seemed to indicate that the benefits of hypnotic intervention could be seen across the entire spectrum of hypnotizability, indicating that its use need not be restricted to very good hypnotic subjects. In more recent years, more detailed and complete reports have become available describing the use of hypnosis with cancer pain and the pain associated with medical procedures frequently used with children suffering from cancer, including lumbar punctures and bone marrow aspiration (LP/BMA) (Katz, Kellerman, and Ellenberg, 1987; Kuttner, Bowman, and Teasdale, 1988; Zeltzer and LaBaron, 1982; Wall and Womack, 1989), and hyperthermia (Reeves and Shapiro, 1983).

Zeltzer and LaBaron (1982) compared a hypnotic treatment that entailed therapist-assisted deep breathing and pleasant imagery with alternative behavioral intervention, including deep breathing exercises and non-imaginal distractions (e.g. counting, talking). Although both procedures were effective in reducing the pain of BMA and anxiety associated with LP, the hypnotic procedure was more effective in reducing pain and anxiety. The hypnotic technique employed in this study might be more accurately described as a guided imagery intervention, since the procedure was not defined as a hypnotic intervention to either the patients or their families.

Wall and Womack (1989) compared a hypnotic intervention to a distraction procedure in reducing pain associated with BMA and LP for children and adolescents. Both procedures were found to be effective in reducing pain, but not anxiety. Kuttner at al. (1988) randomized two groups of children receiving BMA, ages 3-6 and 7-10, to three treatment groups: hypnotic "imaginative involvement," distraction, and standard medical practice. Two intervention sessions were investigated. During the first session distress was reduced for the younger group using the hypnotic treatment, while both treatments reduced distress for the older patients. During the second intervention, all groups showed reduced distress. The authors concluded that hypnosis had an "all-or-none effect" while the response to distraction only developed with experience.

Katz et al. (1987) studied 12 female and 24 males aged 6-11 years with acute lymphoblastic leukemia who were undergoing repeated BMA. The patients were randomized to either a hypnosis or an unstructured play comparison group. The hypnotic intervention included eye fixation, relaxation, imagery, and coping suggestions. Both groups showed reduced self-reported fear and pain. Girls showed more distress than boys on 3 of 4 measures, and there was some suggestion of an interaction between gender and treatment.

Hilgard and LeBaron (1982) examined the role of hypnotizability and relief of BMA pain in children. They found that children identified as highly hypnotizable showed greater reductions in self-reported and observer-rated pain than low hypnotizables. This finding has not been confirmed in other studies by Wall and Womack (1989) and Katz et al (1987), although rapport seemed to predict pain reduction in the Katz et al study.

The use of hypnosis for pain management usually involves the administration of suggestions for relaxation as well as suggestions that are specifically intended to attenuate pain and discomfort. However, Spiegel and his colleagues have explored the benefits of a complex psychosocial intervention for patients with metastatic breast cancer that includes teaching them to use self-hypnosis. The intent of the intervention was to encourage patients to express and deal with strong emotions and also focuses on clarifying doctor-patient communication. Spiegel and his associates (Classen et al., 2001) studied the impact of this intervention on sixty four-women were randomized to the intervention group, while another 61 were assigned to a control condition. The intervention included weekly group therapy and educational materials in addition to a self-hypnosis exercise. Participants were assessed at baseline and every four months during a 12-month period. Results showed that the intervention reduced traumatic stress symptoms and mood disturbance. Spiegel and Moore (Spiegel and Moore, 1997) reported a 10-year follow-up of a randomized trial involving 86 women with cancer showing that this kind of intervention also conferred a survival benefit, significantly increasing survival duration and time from recurrence to death.

Syrjala and associates (Syrjala, Cummings, Donaldson, and Chapman, 1987) reported that hypnotherapy reduced oral pain secondary to chemotherapy and radiation treatment for cancer (caused by oral mucositis). In a later study (Syrjala, Cummings, and Donaldson, 1992) they compared the benefits of hypnosis, cognitive behavioral coping skills training, therapist contact, and usual treatment in 67 patients with hematological malignancies who were undergoing BMT. Hypnosis was effective in reducing treatment-related oral pain for these patients. The treatment groups did not differ with respect to nausea, emesis and opioid use. Interestingly, the cognitive-behavioral intervention was not effective in reducing symptoms in this study.

In related study (Syrjala, Donaldson, Davis, Kippes, and Carr, 1995) oral mucositis pain levels were compared in 94 patients receiving BMT. A cognitive-behavioral skills training and a hypnotic-like relaxation-imagery intervention were equally effective in reducing pain. However, adding behavioral skills training did not improve pain levels beyond the level achieved with the relaxation-imagery intervention alone.

HEADACHE

Hypnosis has often been applied to the management of headache. Complete or moderate success has been reported in relieving pain associated with migraine headache. Some reports used hypnotic imagery techniques (Davidson, 1987; Friedman and Taub, 1984; Harding, 1967; Milne, 1983); others used rational stage-directed hypnotherapy (Howard, Reardon, and Tosi, 1982) and still others employed suggested hand warming (Ansel, 1977; Graham, 1975; Milne, 1983).

Comparative studies of hypnotic and non-hypnotic treatment of migraine, tension or mixed migraine/tension headaches have appeared (Andreychuk and Skriver, 1975; Friedman and Taub, 1985; Friedman and Taub, 1984; Olness, MacDonald, and Uden, 1987; Schlutter, Golden, and Blume, 1980; Spinhoven, Van Dyck, Zitman, and Linssen, 1985; Mellis, Rooimans, Spierings, and Hoogdiun, 1991; Nolan, et. al., 1994 Spanos et al., 1993;

Spinhoven, 1988; Zitman, Van-Dyck, Spinhoven, and Linssen, 1992). Taken together, these studies suggest that hypnotic interventions seem to be consistently effective in treating these headaches, although they do not consistently demonstrate a superiority of hypnotic interventions over other cognitive-behavioral interventions.

Holden, Deichmann, and Levy (1999) reviewed 31 investigations of recurrent pediatric headache that have appeared since 1981 using predetermined criteria to evaluate the adequacy of research methodology. They concluded that sufficient evidence exists to support the conclusion that hypnosis/self-hypnosis is a well-established and efficacious treatment for recurrent headache.

Gysin (1999) compared the efficacy of five weekly hypnosis/self-hypnosis sessions with behavior therapy and physician counseling for children and adolescents suffering from chronic episodic headaches. Although both treatment interventions reduced headache frequency and intensity, hypnosis was thought to enhance patient control of headaches.

Spinhoven and ter Kuile (2000) explored the role of hypnotizability in the treatment of patients with chronic tension-type headaches. They allocated 169 patients to either a self-hypnosis or an autogenic training treatment. Pain reduction immediately following treatment and at later follow-up was significantly associated with hypnotizability. Moreover, early treatment responders had higher hypnotic susceptibility scores than non-responders. These findings confirmed those of an earlier study that also found a correlation between hypnotizability and response to hypnotic treatment or to autogenic training for recurrent headache (ter Kuile et al., 1994).

Although hypnotizability appears to predict treatment response for headache pain, many other personal and demographic variables do not seem to predict treatment outcomes. ter Kuile, Spinhoven and Linssen (1995) employed cognitive self-hypnosis training or autogenic training for 156 patients with chronic recurrent headache. At 6 month follow-up, 43 were classified as responders (greater than 50% pain reduction) while 113 were classified as non-responders. Although patients who expected more pain reduction at pretreatment achieved greater pain reduction, none of the other pretreatment differences predicted either immediate or long term pain reduction. This included demographic and medical status variables, measures of psychological distress, personality, coping strategy use and pain appraisals.

NEUROPATHIC PAIN

A variety of neurological conditions are associated with chronic pain. These include post herpetic neuralgia, diabetic neuropathy, complex regional pain syndrome, spinal cord injury, post amputation and AIDS-related neuropathy (Haythornthwaite and Benrud-Larson, 2001). While clinical reports of the use of hypnosis to manage the pain associated with these conditions have appeared, no clinical trials have been reported. Nevertheless, a few examples suggest some of the ways that hypnosis has been employed in these conditions.

Gainer (1993) employed hypnosis and self-hypnosis to treat a patient with reflex sympathetic dystrophy (RSD). Over a two year period, the patient reportedly achieved complete relief from her RSD symptoms. In this case, hypnosis was combined with other psychotherapeutic interventions.

Phantom limb pain is a common sequelae of surgical or traumatic amputation and is frequently unresponsive to conventional medical/surgical interventions (Chaves 1985b). A number of case reports describe the use of hypnosis with phantom limb pain. Muraoka and associates (Muraoka, Komiyama, Hosoi, Mine, and Kubo, 1996) describe the use of hypnosis in the treatment of severe lower limb phantom limb pain and an associated post-traumatic stress disorder. In this case, hypnosis was employed as one part of a more complex intervention that included antidepressants.

Rosen and colleagues (Rosen, Willoch, Bartenstein, Berner, and Rosjo, 2001) used hypnosis to modify the experience of phantom limb pain in two patients. Positron emission tomography (PET) was employed to study the central pathways by which the phantom limb was experienced and hypnotically modified in these patients. The authors concluded that hypnosis can be incorporated into treatment protocols for phantom limb pain. This finding was subsequently extended in a study with 8 patients where hypnosis was used to alternate between sensations of pain and movement (Willoch et al., 2000). They found that phantom limb pain sensations were associated with activation of the anterior and posterior cingulate cortex.

Chaves (1985b; 1993) described the hypnotic treatment of phantom limb pain in two different cases using a combination of suggestions designed to reduce pain sensations, reduce awareness of the phantom, and alleviate depressive symptoms. In both cases, deriving therapeutically relevant pain-relieving suggestions from the patient's pain phenomenology seemed important to achieving a successful outcome. Another important element was the use of audiotapes of clinical sessions to reinforce daily practice with the hypnotic intervention. One patient was successfully treated in three sessions (Chaves, 1985b), while for the other, hypnosis was only one part of a more complex intervention.

BURN PAIN

Patients who suffer burns experience pain associated with their injury as well as procedural pain associated with surgery and wound debridement. Patterson and his colleagues have made important contributions to this literature (e.g. Everett, Patterson, Burns, Montgomery, and Heimbach, 1993; Martin-Herz, Thurber, and Patterson, 2000; Patterson, 1992; Patterson, 1995; Patterson, Everett, Burns, and Marvin, 1992; Patterson, Goldberg, and Ehde, 1996; Patterson and Ptacek, 1997; Patterson, Questad, and Boltwood, 1987; Patterson, 1989; Patterson, Adcock, and Bombardier, 1997). The use of hypnosis in the management of burn pain is supported by numerous clinical reports as well as by controlled studies, although admittedly the former seem stronger than the latter (Patterson et al., 1997). Indeed, in one case, hypnosis proved effective in managing the pain of a 55-year old man with an extensive burn who had experienced significant respiratory depression due to low dosage of opiods that had been administered during wound care (Ohrbach, Patterson, Carrougher, and Gibran, 1998). An excellent outcome was achieved with little or no opioids, no anxiolytic medication and a shortened length of wound care.

Wright and Drummond (2000) asked 30 hospitalized burn patients to rate their levels of pain and relaxation for four burn care sessions. Hypnosis was employed twice on 15 patients while the remaining 15 patients served as controls. Self-reported ratings of the sensory and affective dimensions of pain decreased significantly during and after hypnosis. In addition, anticipatory anxiety prior to subsequent dressing changes decreased in the hypnosis group.

IRRITABLE BOWEL SYNDROME

Irritable bowel syndrome (IBS) is not always responsive to conventional medical therapies. A number of studies, mostly conducted in the UK, have suggested that hypnosis can be an effective intervention for patients who are unresponsive to conventional medical treatments for this condition, which generally includes dietary and pharmacological interventions (Camilleri, 1999; Wald, 1999). The evaluation of these findings is somewhat complicated by the fact that a comorbid psychiatric diagnosis is common in IBS. Moreover, many symptomatic individuals never seek treatment (Goldberg and Davidson, 1997). Nevertheless, it is instructive to review how hypnosis has been employed with this population.

Forbes et al. (Forbes, MacAuley, and Chiotakakou-Faliakou, 2000) compared gut-directed hypnotherapy with a specially-devised non-hypnotic audiotape in a randomized controlled trial involving 52 patients with established IBS who had not responded to dietary and pharmacological therapy. The patient-selection criteria included abdominal pain or discomfort. Their hypnosis treatment protocol followed that advocated by Whorwell in several important earlier investigations (Whorwell, 1990; Whorwell, Prior, and Colgan, 1987; Whorwell, Prior, and Faragher, 1984). Hypnotic induction employed eye-fixation with suggestions for closure. When patients displayed eye-closure and altered breathing pattern, additional deepening suggestions were administered, including suggestions for progressive muscle relaxation and hand levitation. Therapeutic suggestions were then administered that focused on the predominant IBS symptoms. Post-hypnotic suggestions form only a "modest" part of the therapy and regressive strategies (e.g. to uncover psychodynamic factors) were not used.

The non-hypnotic tape lasted approximately 30 minutes and consisted of background information about IBS, stress management strategies, and structured relaxation. Patients were encouraged to use the tape on a daily basis. Those assigned to hypnotherapy received 6 treatment sessions scheduled at two-week intervals. Sessions lasted about 30 minutes, with the hypnotic intervention consuming only about 15 minutes of that period. An audiotape was made of one of the sessions, generally the third, and this was provided to the patient for practice at home.

For the 45 patients who provided complete data, more than half of the patients in each group clinically improved, but those in the hypnotherapy group showed significantly greater symptom reduction. The authors concluded that, for economic reasons, the tape might be recommended as a second line of intervention for patients who had not responded to traditional IBS treatment, saving the more effective, but more expensive intervention with hypnosis for treatment failures.

Galovski and Blanchard (1998) confirmed the findings reported in the UK studies in a study with 6 pairs of matched IBS patients assigned to either a gut-directed hypnotherapy group or to a symptom-monitoring wait list control. Subjects in the control condition were later crossed into the treatment condition. On a composite measure of IBS symptoms, hypnotherapy was significantly better than the control condition. Treated patients also showed reduced state and trait anxiety scores. Interestingly, there was no correlation between hypnotic susceptibility and treatment gain.

The clinical gains achieved in using hypnosis with IBS patients do not seem restricted to disease-specific symptoms (e.g. abdominal pain, bloating, bowel habits, flatulence, backache, dyspareunia). Houghton, Heyman, and Whorwell (1996) found that IBS patients treated with hypnotherapy also demonstrated improvements on a number of measures of quality of life and had reduced absenteeism from work as compared to control patients with disease of comparable severity. They concluded that hypnotherapy was a good long-term investment, in spite of its higher initial cost. It is difficulty to say at this point whether it will be possible to achieve significant economies of scale in using hypnotherapy in treating IBS. Some of those who have reported successful use of the procedure are convinced that an individually-tailored approach is necessary to achieve the best treatment outcomes (Vidakovic-Vukic, 1999).

APPLICATION OF HYPNOSIS WITH OTHER PAINFUL SYNDROMES

Hypnosis has occasionally been applied with a variety of other painful disorders including arthritis (Nolan, 1983, Domangue, Margolis, Lieberman, and Kaji, 1985), recurrent aphthous stomatitis (Andrews and Hall, 1990), head, facial, and back pain, (Toomey and Sanders, 1983), sickle cell disease (Thomas, Koshy, Patterson, Dorn, and Thomas, 1984; Dinges et al., 1997), multiple sclerosis ((Dane, 1996), (Sutcher, 1997); temporomandibular disorder (Stam, McGrath, and Brooke, 1984); Oakley et al., 1994; Simon and Lewis, 2000); repetitive strain injuries (Moore and Wiesner, 1996; Karjalainen et al., 2000); ischemic pain associated with Burger's disease (Klapow, Patterson, and Edwards, 1996) and interstitial cystitis (Webster and Brennan, 1995). Support for these applications is generally based on case reports or small clinical studies. There is a need for more systematic data to be collected with respect to all of these applications to document more fully the efficacy of hypnotic interventions and specify the indications and contraindications for its use.

CONCLUSIONS

Those working with more conventional biomedical therapies for chronic pain need to be aware of the potential contribution of hypnotic interventions. Hopefully this may not only permit hypnosis to be considered when conventional interventions have failed, but also enable more prospective exploration of where hypnosis might be introduced earlier in the pain-management process to maximize its benefits. We also need additional information about how hypnotic interventions might be beneficially added to the array of service offered to patients during end-of-life care (Pan, Morrison, Ness, Fugh-Berman, and Leipzig, 2000).

In spite of the methodological limitations that apply to many of the studies cited here, taken together, they point strongly to the potential value of hypnosis as an effective intervention for the relief of clinical pain that is not or cannot be managed effectively with conventional medical therapies. This conclusion is supported not only by clinical case studies, but also meta-analyses of systematic studies that have evaluated the use of hypnosis for both clinical and experimental pain (Montgomery, DuHamel, and Redd, 2000).

Of course, a number of important questions remain. How can we select patients most likely to benefit from hypnosis as an intervention? What is the role of hypnotizability in determining treatment outcome? How can we best prepare patients for clinical hypnosis? What are the best treatment protocols for using hypnosis in pain management? What is the role of practice and training in optimizing clinical outcomes? What comorbid conditions are indications or contraindications for hypnotic intervention?

At present, the answers to these questions remain incomplete and ultimately will require more systematic data. In the meantime, however, hypnosis has demonstrated substantial promise and is sufficiently benign in the hands of properly trained professional health care providers, that it probably should be considered in any case where pain control is incomplete or unsatisfactory with conventional therapies. Evidence seems to suggest that the relationship between hypnotizability and clinical outcome is complex, and probably influenced by a complex array of factors. Accordingly, hypnosis should not be ruled out on the basis of apparent low hypnotizability alone. The presence of chronic pain or a life-threatening condition can change patient motivation, and make acceptable interventions that might not have been welcomed under other circumstance. For most clinical purposes, the assessment of hypnotizability is not necessary before conducting a clinical trial with hypnosis. Another advantage of the use of hypnosis is that its flexibility permits the simultaneous pursuit of a wide range of therapeutic targets. This makes it possible to address concurrent anxiety and depressive symptoms as well as other disease-related symptoms beside pain. Indeed, it is sometimes the improvements achieved in mitigating non-pain related symptoms that convinces patients that hypnosis can make it possible to reduce pain (Chaves, 1993).

REFERENCES

Andrews, V. H., and Hall, H. R. (1990). The effects of relaxation/imagery training on recurrent aphthous stomatitis: A preliminary study. *Psychosomatic Medicine, 52*(5), 526-535.

Andreychuk, T., and Skriver, C. (1975). Hypnosis and biofeedback in the treatment of migraine headache. *International Journal of Clinical and Experimental Hypnosis, 23*(3), 172-183.

Ansel, E. L. (1977). A simple exercise to enhance response to hypnotherapy for migraine headache. *International Journal of Clinical and Experimental Hypnosis, 25*, 68-71.

Barber, T. X. (1959). Toward a theory of pain relief: Relief of chronic pain by prefrontal leucotomy, opiates, placebos, and hypnosis. *Psychological Bulletin, 56*, 430-460.

Barber, T. X. (1963). The effects of "hypnosis" on pain: a critical review of experimental and clinical findings. *Psychosomatic Medicine, 25*, 303-333.

Barber, T. X., and de Moor, W. (1972). A theory of hypnotic induction procedures. *American Journal of Clinical Hypnosis, 15*(2), 112-135.

Brown, J. M., and Chaves, J. F. (1980). Hypnosis in the treatment of sexual dysfunction. *Journal of Sex and Marital Therapy, 6*(1), 63-74.

Camilleri, M. (1999). Review article: clinical evidence to support current therapies of irritable bowel syndrome. *Alimentary Pharmacology and Therapeutics, 2 Suppl.*, 48-53.

Cangello, V. W. (1961). The use of hypnotic suggestion for pain relief in malignant disease. *International Journal of Clinical and Experimental Hypnosis, 9*, 17-22.

Cangello, V. W. (1962). Hypnosis for the patient with cancer. *American Journal of Clinical Hypnosis, 4*, 215-226.

Caton, D. (1985). The secularization of pain. *Anesthesiology, 62*, 493-501.

Chaves, J. F. (1981). Tactics and strategies in clinical hypnosis. Audiotape series (6 cassettes). San Francisco, CA: Proseminar.

Chaves, J. F. (1985a). Hypnosis in the management of behavioral components of Prader-Willi Syndrome. E. T. Dowd, and J. M. Healy (pp. 301-310). NY: Guilford.

Chaves, J. F. (1985b). Hypnosis in the management of phantom limb pain. E. T. Dowd, and J. M. Healy (pp. 198-209). New York: Guilford.

Chaves, J. F. (1989). Hypnotic control of clinical pain (pp. 242-272). N. P. Spanos, J. F. Chaves, (eds.) Hypnosis-The cognitive behavioral perspective. Buffalo, NY, USA: Prometheus Books.

Chaves, J. F. (1992). Hypnotic analgesia: The social-psychological perspective. W. Bongartz (ed.) Hypnosis: 175 years after Mesmer-Recent developments in theory and application. Konstanz: Universitätsverlag Konstanz, Germany.

Chaves, J. F. (1993). Hypnosis in pain management (pp. 511-532). J. W. Rhue, S. J. Lynn, and I. Kirsch, (eds). Handbook of clinical hypnosis. Washington, D.C.: American Psychological Association.

Chaves, J. F. (1994). Recent advances in the application of hypnosis to pain management. *American Journal of Clinical Hypnosis, 37*(2), 117-129.

Chaves, J. F. (1996). Hypnotic strategies for somatoform disorders (pp. 131-151). S. J. Lynn, and I. Kirsch (eds) Casebook of clinical hypnosis. Washington, DC: American Psychological Association.

Chaves, J. F. (1997). Hypnosis in dentistry: Historical overview and current appraisal. *Hypnosis International Monographs, 3*, 5-23.

Chaves, J. F. (1999). Hypnosis in chronic pain management: Some pragmatic considerations in patient preparation. *Psychological Hypnosis, 8(2)*, 1, 4-5.

Chaves, J. F. (2000). Hypnosis in the management of anxiety associated with medical conditions and their treatment (pp. 119-142). D. I. Mostofsky, and D. H. Barlow (eds). The management of stress and anxiety in medical disorders. Boston: Allyn and Bacon.

Chaves, J. F., and Brown, J. M. (1987). Spontaneous cognitive strategies for the control of clinical pain and stress. *Journal of Behavioral Medicine, 10*(3), 263-276.

Chaves, J. F., and Barber, T. X. (1974). Cognitive strategies, experimenter modeling, and expectation in the attenuation of pain. *Journal of Abnormal Psychology, 83*(4), 356-363.

Chaves, J. F., and Barber, T. X. (1976). Hypnotic procedures and surgery: A critical analysis with applications to "acupuncture analgesia." *American Journal of Clinical Hypnosis, 18*(4), 217-236.

Chaves, J. F., and Dworkin, S. F. (1997). Hypnotic control of pain: Historical perspectives and future prospects. *International Journal of Clinical and Experimental Hypnosis, 45*(4), 356-376.

Chen, A. C. (2001). New perspectives in EEG/MEG brain mapping and PET/fMRI neuroimaging of human pain. *International Journal of Psychophysiology 42*(2), 53-65.

Classen, C., Butler, L. D., Koopman, C., Miller, E., DiMiceli, S., Giese-Davis, J., Fobair, P., Carlson, R. W., Kraemer, H. C., and Spiegel, D. (2001). Supportive-expressive group therapy and distress in patients with metastatic breast cancer: a randomized clinical intervention trial. *Archives of General Psychiatry, 58*(5), 494-501.

Council, J. R., Kirsch, I., and Hafner, L. P. (1986). Expectancy versus absorption in the prediction of hypnotic responding. *Journal of Personality and Social Psychology, 50*(1), 182-189.

Crabtree, A. (1993). *From Mesmer to Freud: Magnetic sleep and the roots of psychological healing.* New Haven: Yale University Press.

Crawford, H. J., Gur, R. C., Skolnick, B., Gur, R. E., and Benson, D. M. (1993). Effects of hypnosis on regional cerebral blood flow during ischemic pain with and without suggested hypnotic analgesia. *International Journal of Psychophysiology, 15*(3), 181-195.

Cronin, D. M., Spanos, N. P., and Barber, T. X. (1971). Augmenting hypnotic suggestibility by providing favorable information about hypnosis. *American Journal Clinical Hypnosis., 13*(4), 259-264.

Dane, J. R. (1996). Hypnosis for pain and neuromuscular rehabilitation with multiple sclerosis: case summary, literature review, and analysis of outcomes. *International Journal of Clinical and Experimental Hypnosis, 44*(3), 208-231.

Davidson, P. (1987). Hypnosis and migraine headache: Reporting a clinical series. *Australian Journal of Clinical and Experimental Hypnosis, 15*(2), 111-118.

Deane, J. (1844). Amputation of the leg in the mesmeric state. *Boston Medical and Surgical Journal, 32,* 194-197.

Delatour, M. (1826). untitled report. *L'Hermes, 25,* 144-146.

Dinges, D. F., Whitehouse, W. G., Orne, E. C., Bloom, P. B., Carlin, M. M., Bauer, N. K., Gillen, K. A., Shapiro, B. S., Ohene-Frempong, K., Dampier, C., and Orne, M. T. (1997). Self-hypnosis training as an adjunctive treatment in the management of pain associated with sickle cell disease. *International Journal of Clinical and Experimental Hypnosis, 45*(4),

Domangue, B. B., Margolis, C. G., Lieberman, D., and Kaji, H. (1985). Biochemical correlates of hypnoanalgesia in arthritic pain patients. *Journal of Clinical Psychiatry, 46* (6), 235-8.

Douglas, D. B. (1999). Hypnosis: useful, neglected, available. *American Journal of Hospital Palliative Care, 16(*5), 665-70.

Edmonston, E. E. Jr. (1986). *The Induction of Hypnosis.* New York: Wiley.

Ellenberger, H. F. (1970). *The Discovery of the Unconscious: The History and Evolution of Dynamic Psychiatry*. New York: Basic Books.

Engel, G. E. (1987). Physician-scientists and scientific-physicians. Resolving the humanism-science dichotomy. *American Journal of Medicine, 82,* 107-111.

Engel, G. L. (1977). The need for a new medical model. *Science, 196,* 129-136.

Engel, G. L. (1997). From biomedical to biopsychosocial. Being scientific in the human domain. *Psychosomatics, 38*(6), 521-528.

Everett, J. J., Patterson, D. R., Burns, G. L., Montgomery, B., and Heimbach, D. (1993). Adjunctive interventions for burn pain control: comparison of hypnosis and ativan: the 1993 Clinical Research Award. *Journal of Burn Care and Rehabilitation, 14*(6), 676-683.

Forbes, A., MacAuley, S., and Chiotakakou-Faliakou, E. (2000). Hypnotherapy and therapeutic audiotape: effective in previously unsuccessfully treated irritable bowel syndrome? *International Journal of Colorectal Disorders, 15*(5-6), 328-34.

Fordyce, W. (1976). *Behavioral methods for chronic pain and illness*. St. Louis: Mosby.

Friedman, H., and Taub, H. (1985). Extended follow-up study of the effects of brief psychological procedures in migraine therapy. *American Journal of Clinical Hypnosis, 28,* 27-33.

Friedman, H., and Taub, H. A. (1984). Brief psychological training procedures in migraine treatment. *American Journal of Clinical Hypnosis, 26,* 187-200.

Gainer, M. J. (1993). Somatization of dissociated traumatic memories in a case of reflex sympathetic dystrophy. *American Journal of Clinical Hypnosis, 36*(2), 124-131.

Galovski, T. E., and Blanchard, E. B. (1998). The treatment of irritable bowel syndrome with hypnotherapy. *Applied Psychophysiology and Biofeedback, 23*(4), 219-32.

Genuis, M. L. (1995). The use of hypnosis in helping cancer patients control anxiety, pain, and emesis: A review of recent empirical studies. *American Journal of Clinical Hypnosis, 37*(4), 316-325.

Goldberg, J., and Davidson, P. (1997). A biopsychosocial understanding of the irritable bowel syndrome: a review. *Canadian Journal of Psychiatry, 42*(8), 835-40.

Graham, G. W. (1975). Hypnotic treatment for migraine headaches. *International Journal of Clinical and Experimental Hypnosis, 23*(3), 165-171.

Gysin, T. (1999). [Clinical hypnotherapy/self-hypnosis for unspecified, chronic and episodic headache without migraine and other defined headaches in children and adolescents]. *Forschende Komplementarmedizin, 6 Suppl 1,* 44-6.

Harding, C. H. (1967). Hypnosis in the treatment of migraine. J. Lassner, (ed.) *Hypnosis and psychosomatic medicine* . New York: Springer-Verlag.

Haythornthwaite, J. A., and Benrud-Larson, L. M. (2001). Psychological assessment and treatment of patients with neuropathic pain. *Current Pain and Headache Report, 5*(2), 124-9.

Hilgard, E. R. (1969). Pain as a puzzle for psychology and psychophysiology. *American Psychologist, 24,* 103-113.

Hilgard, E. R., and Hilgard, J. R. (1975). Hypnosis in the relief of pain. Los Altos, CA: William Kaufmann.

Hilgard, E. R., and Hilgard, J. R. (1983). *Hypnosis in the Relief of Pain. 2nd Edition.* Los Altos, CA: William Kaufmann.

Hilgard, E. R., Cooper, L. M., Lenox, J., Morgan, A. H., and Voevodsky, J., (1967). The use of pain-state reports in the study of hypnotic analgesia to the pain of ice water. *Journal of Nervous and Mental Disease, 144*(6), 506-513.

Hilgard, J. R., and LeBaron, S. (1982). Relief of anxiety and pain in children and adolescents with cancer: Quantitative measures and clinical observations. *International Journal of Clinical and Experimental Hypnosis, 30*(4), 417-442.

Hofbauer, R. K., Rainville, P., Duncan, G. H., and Bushnell, M. C. (2001). Cortical representation of the sensory dimension of pain. *Journal of Neurophysiology, 86*(1), 402-11.

Holden, E. W., Deichmann, M. M., and Levy, J. D. (1999). Empirically supported treatments in pediatric psychology: recurrent pediatric headache. *Journal of Pediatric Psychology, 24*(2), 91-109.

Holroyd, J. (1996). Hypnosis treatment of clinical pain: understanding why hypnosis is useful. *International Journal of Clinical and Experimental Hypnosis, 44*(1), 33-51.

Houghton, L. A., Heyman, D. J., and Whorwell, P. J. (1996). Symptomatology, quality of life and economic features of irritable bowel syndrome--the effect of hypnotherapy. *Alimentary Pharmacology andTherapeutics, 10*(1), 91-5.

Howard, L., Reardon, J. P., and Tosi, D. (1982). Modifying migraine headache through rational stage directed hypnotherapy: a cognitive-experiential perspective. *International Journal of Clinical and Experimental Hypnosis, 30*(3), 257-69.

Johnson, M. E., and Hauck, C. (1999). Beliefs and opinions about hypnosis held by the general public: a systematic evaluation. *American Journal of Clinical Hypnosis, 42*(1), 10-20.

Karjalainen, K., Malmivaara, A., van Tulder, M., Roine, R., Jauhiainen, M., Hurri, H., and Koes, B. (2000). Biopsychosocial rehabilitation for upper limb repetitive strain injuries in working age adults. *Cochrane Database Syst Rev, (3)*, CD002269.

Katz, E. R., Kellerman, J., and Ellenberg, L. (1987). Hypnosis in the reduction of acute pain and distress in children with cancer. *Journal of Pediatric Psychology, 12*(3), 379-394.

Kirsch, I. (1990). *Changing expectations: A key to effective psychotherapy.* Pacific Grove, CA: Brooks/Cole.

Kirsch, I. (1999). *How expectancies shape experience.* Washington, DC: American Psychological Association.

Klapow, J. C., Patterson, D. R., and Edwards, W. T. (1996). Hypnosis as an adjunct to medical care in the management of Burger's Disease: A case report. *American Journal of Clinical Hypnosis, 38*(4), 271-276.

Kotarba, J. A. (1983). *Chronic Pain: Its Social Dimension.* Beverley Hills: Sage.

Kuttner, L., Bowman, M., and Teasdale, M. (1988). Psychological treatment of distress, pain, and anxiety for young children with cancer. *Developmental and Behavioral Pediatrics, 9*(6), 374-381.

Lea, P. A., Ware, P. D., and Monroe, R. R. (1960). The hypnotic control of intractable pain. *American Journal of Clinical Hypnosis, 3*(3-8).

Liossi, C., and Mystakidou, K. (1996). Clinical hypnosis in palliative care. *European Journal of Palliative Care, 3(2)*, 56-58.

Lynch, D. F. Jr. (1999). Empowering the patient: hypnosis in the management of cancer, surgical disease and chronic pain. *American Journal of Clinical Hypnosis., 42*(2), 122-130.

Martin-Herz, S. P., Thurber, C. A., and Patterson, D. R. (2000). Psychological principles of burn wound pain in children. II: Treatment applications. *Journal of Burn Care Rehabilitation, 21*(5), 458-72.

Mellis, P. M., Rooimans, W., Spierings, E. L., and Hoogdiun, C. A. (1991). Treatment of chronic tension-type headache with hypnotherapy: A single-blind control study. *Headache, 31*, 686-689.

Melzack, R., and Wall, P. (1965). Pain mechanisms: A new theory. *Science, 150*, 971-979.

Milne, G. (1983). Hypnotherapy with migraine. *Australian Journal of Clinical and Experimental Hypnosis, 11*(1), 23-32.

Montgomery, G. H., DuHamel, K. N., and Redd, W. H. (2000). A meta-analysis of hypnotically induced analgesia: How effective is hypnosis? *International Journal of Clinical and Experimental Hypnosis, 48*(2), 138-153.

Moore, L. E., and Wiesner, S. L. (1996). Hypnotically-induced vasodilation in the treatment of repetitive strain injuries. *American Journal of Clinical Hypnosis, 39*(2), 97-104.

Muraoka, M., Komiyama, H., Hosoi, M., Mine, K., and Kubo, C. (1996). Psychosomatic treatment of phantom limb pain with post-traumatic stress disorder: a case report. Pain, 66(2-3), 385-8.

National Institutes of Health (1995). Integration of behavioral and relaxation approaches into the treatment of chronic pain and insomnia. NIH Technology Assessment Statement, October-16-18, 1-34.

Nolan, M. (1983). A combination of hypnotherapy, megavitamins and "folk" medicine in the treatment of arthritis. *Australian Journal of Clinical Hypnotherapy and Hypnosis, 4*(1), 21-25.

Nolan, R. P., Spanos, N. P., Hayward, A. A., and Scott, H. A. (1994). The efficacy of hypnotic and nonhypnotic response-based imagery for self-managing recurrent headache. *Imagination, Cognition and Personality, 14*(3), 183-201.

Oakley, M. E., McCreary, C. P., Clark, G. T., Holston, S., Glover, D., and Kashima, K. (1994). A cognitive-behavioral approach to temporomandibular dysfunction treatment failures: a controlled comparison. *Journal of Orofacial Pain, 8*(4), 397-401.

Ohrbach, R., Patterson, D. R., Carrougher, G., and Gibran, N. (1998). Hypnosis after an adverse response to opioids in an ICU burn patient. *Clinical Journal of Pain, 14*(2), 167-175.

Olness, K., MacDonald, J. T., and Uden, D. L. (1987). Comparison of self-hypnosis and propranolol in the treatment of juvenile classic migraine. *Pediatrics, 79*(4), 593-597.

Pan, C. X., Morrison, R. S., Ness, J., Fugh-Berman, A., and Leipzig, R. M. (2000). Complementary and alternative medicine in the management of pain, dyspnea, and nausea and vomiting near the end of life. A systematic review. *Journal of Pain Symptom Management, 20*(5), 374-87.

Parssinen, T. M. (1979). Professional deviants and the history of medicine: Medical Mesmerists in Victorian Britain (pp. 103-120). In R. Wallis (ed.). On the margins of science:The social construction of rejected knowledge. Keele: University of Keele.

Patterson, D. R. (1992). Practical applications of psychological techniques in controlling burn pain. *Journal of Burn Care and Rehabilitation, 13*(1), 13-8.

Patterson, D. R. (1995). Non-opioid-based approaches to burn pain. [Review]. *Journal of Burn Care and Rehabilitation, 16.*

Patterson, D. R., Everett, J. J., Burns, G. L., and Marvin, J. A. (1992). Hypnosis for the treatment of burn pain. *Journal of Consulting and Clinical Psychology, 60*(5), 713-7.

Patterson, D. R., Goldberg, M. L., and Ehde, D. M. (1996). Hypnosis in the treatment of patients with severe burns. *American Journal of Clinical Hypnosis, 38(*3), 200-212.

Patterson, D. R., and Ptacek, J. T. (1997). Baseline pain as a moderator of hypnotic analgesia for burn injury treatment. *Journal of Consulting and Clinical Psychology, 65*(1), 60-7.

Patterson, D. R., Questad, K. A., and Boltwood, M. D. (1987). Hypnotherapy as a treatment for pain in patients with burns: research and clinical considerations. *Journal of Burn Care and Rehabilitation, 8*(4), 263-8.

Patterson, D. R. (1989). Hypnotherapy as an adjunct to narcotic analgesia for the treatment of pain for burn debridement. *American Journal of Clinical Hypnosis, 31*(3), 156-163.

Patterson, D. R., Adcock, R. J., and Bombardier, C. H. (1997). Factors predicting hypnotic analgesia in clinical burn pain. *International Journal of Clinical and Experimental Hypnosis, 45* (4), 377-395.

Ploghaus, A., Tracey, I., Gati, J. S., Clare, S., Menon, R. S., Matthews, P. M., Nicholas, J., and Rawlins, P. (1999). Dissociating pain from its anticipation in the human brain. *Science, 284,* 1979-1981.

Quen, J. (1973). Case studies in nineteenth century scientific rejection: Mesmerism, perkinism, and acupuncture. Presented at the Fifth Annual Meeting of Cheiron-The IInternational Society for the History of the Behavioral and Social Sciences, at Plattsburgh, N. Y., June 10, 1973.

Rainville, P., Carrier, B., Hofbauer, R. K., Bushnell, M. C., and Duncan, G. H. (1999). Dissociation of sensory and affective dimensions of pain using hypnotic modulation. *Pain, 82*(2), 159-71.

Rainville, P., Hofbauer, R. K., Paus, T., Duncan, G. H., Bushnell, M. C., and Price, D. D. (1999). Cerebral mechanisms of hypnotic induction and suggestion. *Journal of. Cognitive Neuroscience, 11*(1), 110-125.

Reeves, J. L. 2nd, and Shapiro, D. (1983). Heart-rate reactivity to cold pressor stress following biofeedback training. *Biofeedback and Self Regulation, 8*(1), 87-99.

Rey, T. (1993). *The history of pain.* Cambridge, MA: Harvard University Press.

Rosen, G., Willoch, F., Bartenstein, P., Berner, N., and Rosjo, S. (2001). Neurophysiological processes underlying the phantom limb pain experience and the use of hypnosis in its clinical management: an intensive examination of two patients. *International Journal of Clinical and Experimental Hypnosis, 49*(1), 38-55.

Schlutter, L. C., Golden, C. J., and Blume, H. G. (1980). A comparison of treatments for prefrontal muscle contraction headache. *British Journal of Medical Psychology, 53*(1), 47-52.

Shutty, M. S. Jr., DeGood, D. E., and Tuttle, D. H. (1990). Chronic pain patients' beliefs about their pain and treatment outcomes. *Archives of Physical Medicine and Rehabilitation, 71*(2), 128-132.

Shutty, M. S., and DeGood, D. E. (1990). Patient knowledge and beliefs about pain and its treatment. *Rehabilitation Psychology, 35*(1), 43-54.

Simon, E. P., and Lewis, D. M. (2000). Medical hypnosis for temporomandibular disorders: treatment efficacy and medical utilization outcome. Oral surgery, oral medicine, oral pathology, oral radiology, and endodontics, *90*(1), 54-63.

Spanos, N. P. (1989). Experimental research on hypnotic analgesia. In N. P. Spanos, and J. F. Chaves (eds). Hypnosis: The Cognitive-Behavioral Perspective (pp. 206-240). Buffalo, NY: Prometheus.

Spanos, N. P., Carmanico, S. J., and Ellis, J. (1994). Hypnotic analgesia. P. D. Wall, and R. Melzack (3rd ed., pp. 1349-1366). Edinburgh: Churchill Livingstone.

Spanos, N. P., Horton, C., and Chaves, J. F. (1975). The effects of two cognitive strategies on pain threshold. *Journal of Abnormal Psychology, 84*, 677-681.

Spanos, N. P., Steggles, S., Radtke-Bodorik, H. L., and Rivers, S. M. (1979). Nonanalytic attending, hypnotic susceptibility, and psychological well-being in trained meditators and nonmeditators. *Journal of Abnormal Psychology., 88*(1), 85-87.

Spanos, N. P., and Chaves, J. F. (1989). *Hypnosis: The cognitive-behavioral perspective* (Psychology series) . Buffalo, NY, USA: Prometheus Books.

Spanos, N. P., Liddy, S. J., Scott, H., Garrard, C., Sine, J., Tirabasso, A., and Hayward, A. (1993). Hypnotic suggestion and placebo for the treatment of chronic headache in a university volunteer sample. *Cognitive Therapy and Research, 17*(2), 191-205.

Spiegel, D., and Moore, R. (1997). Imagery and hypnosis in the treatment of cancer patients. *Oncology, 11*(8), 1179-1189.

Spiegel, D., Sephton, S. E., Terr, A. I., and Stites, D. P. (1998). Effects of Psychosocial Treatment in Prolonging Cancer Survival May Be Mediated by Neuroimmune Pathways. *Annals of the New York Academy of Sciences, 840*, 674-683.

Spinhoven, P., and ter Kuile, M. M. (2000). Treatment outcome expectancies and hypnotic susceptibility as moderators of pain reduction in patients with chronic tension-type headache. *International Journal of Clinical and Experimental Hypnosis, 48*(3), 290-305.

Spinhoven, P., Van Dyck, R., Zitman, F. G., and Linssen, A. C. G. Treating tension headache: Autogenic training and hypnosis imagery. *10th International Congress of Hypnosis and Psychosomatic medicine* .

Spinhoven, P. (1988). Similarities and dissimilarities in hypnotic and nonhypnotic procedures for headache control: A review. *American Journal of Clinical Hypnosis, 30*(3), 183-194.

Stam, H. J., McGrath, P. A., and Brooke, R. I. (1984). The treatment of temporomandibular joint syndrome through control of anxiety. *Journal of Behavior Therapy and Experimental Psychiatry, 15*(1), 41-45.

Stamm, H. J. (1989). From symptom relief to cure: Hypnotic interventions in cancer (pp. 313-339). In N. P. Spanos, and J. F. Chaves (eds) Hypnosis: The cognitive-behavioral perspective. Buffalo, NY: Prometheus Books.

Steggles, S., Damore-Petingola, S., Maxwell, J., and Lightfoot, N. (1997). Hypnosis for children and adolescents with cancer: an annotated bibliography, 1985-1995. *Journal of Pediatric Oncology Nursing, 14*(1), 27-32.

Steggles, S., Fehr, R., and Aucoin, P. (1986). Hypnosis for children and adolescents with cancer: an annotated bibliography 1960-1985. *Journal of the Association of Pediatric Oncology Nurses, 3*(1), 23-5.

Steggles, S., Maxwell, J., Lightfoot, N. E., Damore-Petingola, S., and Mayer, C. (1997). Hypnosis and cancer: an annotated bibliography 1985-1995. *American Journal of Clinical Hypnosis, 39*(3), 187-200.

Steggles, S., Stam, H. J., Fehr, R., and Aucoin, P. (1987). Hypnosis and cancer: an annotated bibliography 1960-1985. *American Journal of Clinical Hypnosis, 29*(4), 281-90.

Stevens, M. M., Dalla Pozza, L., Cavalletto, B., Cooper, M. G., and Kilham, H. A. (1994). Pain and symptom control in paediatric palliative care. *Cancer Surveys, 21,* 221-231.

Sutcher, H. (1997). Hypnosis as adjunctive therapy for multiple sclerosis: a progress report. *American Journal of Clinical Hypnosis, Apr;39(4),* 283-290.

Syrjala, K. L., Cummings, C., Donaldson, G., and Chapman, C. R. (1987). Hypnosis for oral pain following chemotherapy and radiation. *Pain, Supplement 4,* S171.

Syrjala, K. L., Cummings, C., and Donaldson, G. W. (1992). Hypnosis or cognitive behavioral training for the reduction of pain and nausea during cancer treatment: a controlled clinical trial. *Pain, 48(*2), 137-46.

Syrjala, K. L., Donaldson, G. W., Davis, M. W., Kippes, M. E., and Carr, J. E. (1995). Relaxation and imagery and cognitive-behavioral training reduce pain during cancer treatment: a controlled clinical trial. *Pain, 63*(2), 189-198.

Syrjala, K. L., and Roth-Roemer, S. (1996). Cancer pain (pp. 121-157). J. Barber (ed) Hypnosis and suggestion in the treatment of pain. New York: W. W. Norton.

ter Kuile, M. M., Spinhoven, P., and Linssen, A. C. (1995). Responders and nonresponders to autogenic training and cognitive self- hypnosis: prediction of short- and long-term success in tension-type headache patients. *Headache, 35*(10), 630-6.

ter Kuile, M. M., Spinhoven, P., Linssen, A. C., Zitman, F. G., Van Dyck, R., and Rooijmans, H. G. (1994). Autogenic training and cognitive self-hypnosis for the treatment of recurrent headaches in three different subject groups. *Pain, 58*(3), 331-340.

Thomas, J. E., Koshy, M., Patterson, L., Dorn, L., and Thomas, K. (1984). Management of pain in sickle cell disease using biofeedback therapy: a preliminary study. *Biofeedback and Self Regulation, 9*(4), 413-20.

Toomey, T. C., and Sanders, S. (1983). Group hypnotherapy as an active control strategy in chronic pain. *American Journal of Clinical Hypnosis, 26*(1), 20-25.

Turk, D., Meichenbaum, D. H., and Genest, M. (1983*). Pain and Behavioral Medicine.* New York: Guilford.

Vidakovic-Vukic, M. (1999). Hypnotherapy in the treatment of irritable bowel syndrome: methods and results in Amsterdam. *Scandanavia Journal of Gastroenterology: Suppl, 230,* 49-51.

Wald, A. (1999). Irritable Bowel Syndrome. *Current Treatment Options in Gastroenterology, 2*(1), 13-19.

Wall, V. J., and Womack, W. (1989). Hypnotic versus active cognitive strategies for alleviation of procedural distress in pediatric oncology patients. *American Journal of Clinical Hypnosis, 31*(3), 181-191.

Ward, W., and Topham, W. (1842). *Account of a case of successful amputation of the thigh during the mesmeric state, without knowledge of the patient.* London: H. Bailliere.

Webster, D. C., and Brennan, T. (1995). Self-care strategies used for acute attack of interstitial cystitis. *Urologic Nursing, 15*(3), 86-93.

Weitzenhoffer, A., and Hilgard, E. R. (1962). *Stanford Hypnotic Susceptibility Scale* (Form C ed.). Palo Alto, CA: Consulting Psychologists Press.

West, B. H. (1836). Experiments in animal magnitism. *Boston Medical and Surgical Journal, 14*, 349-351.

Whorwell, P. J. (1990). Hypnotherapy for selected gastrointestinal disorders. *Digestive Diseases and Sciences, 8(4)*, 223-225.

Whorwell, P. J., Prior, A., and Colgan, S. M. (1987). Controlled trial of hypnotherapy in the treatment of refractory irritable bowel syndrome. *Gut, 28*, 423-425.

Whorwell, P. J., Prior, A., and Faragher, E. B. (1984). Controlled trial of hypnotherapy in the treatment of severe refractory irritable-bowel syndrome. *Lancet, 2*(8414), 1232-1234.

Willoch, F., Rosen, G., Tolle, T. R., Oye, I., Wester, H. J., Berner, N., Schwaiger, M., and Bartenstein, P. (2000). Phantom limb pain in the human brain: unraveling neural circuitries of phantom limb sensations using positron emission tomography. *Annals of Neurology, 48*(6), 842-9.

Winter, A. (1991). Ethereal epidemic: Mesmerism and the introduction of inhalation anesthesia to early Victorian London. *Social History of Medicine, 4*, 1-27.

Winter, A. (1998). *Mesmerized: Powers of mind in Victorian Britain.* Chicago: University of Chicago Press.

Wright, B. R., and Drummond, P. D. (2000). Rapid induction analgesia for the alleviation of procedural pain during burn care. *Burns., 26*(3), 275-282.

Zeltzer, L., and LaBaron, S. (1982). Hypnotic and nonhypnotic techniques for reduction of pain and anxiety during painful procedures in children and adolescents with cancer. *Journal of Pediatrics, 101,* 1032-1035.

Zitman, F. G., Van-Dyck, R., Spinhoven, P., and Linssen, A. C. (1992). Hypnosis and autogenic training in the treatment of tension headaches: A two-phase constructive design study with follow-up. *Journal of Psychosomatic Research, 36*(3), 219-228.

Part VI:
Nursing and Palliative Approaches

In: The Handbook of Chronic Pain
Editors: S. Kreitler, D. Beltrutti, et al., pp. 361-377

ISBN 978-1-60021-044-0
© 2007 Nova Science Publishers, Inc.

Chapter 20

Chronic Pain: A Nursing Perspective

Wendy Lewandowski and Marion Good

This chapter discusses chronic pain from a nursing perspective. Nurses focus on acknowledging, valuing, and understanding the personal experiences of the chronic pain sufferer. Multidimensional models of the chronic pain experience are proposed and used by nurses, as well as innovative ways to conceptualize the pain experience within the context of health and well-being.

NURSING SCIENCE PERSPECTIVES OF PAIN

The Experience of Living with Pain

Pain is manifested in many ways, yet it has been likened to an "invisible ravager" that often leads to an isolating journey for the sufferer (Carson and Mitchell, 1998). Over thirty years ago, a visionary nurse defined pain in a way that highlights its private, subjective nature: "Pain is whatever the experiencing person says it is, existing whenever the experiencing person says it does" (McCaffery, 1968, p. 95). Nurses, as well as other clinicians, have typically tried to understand and manage pain from their own perspectives instead of realizing that the pain sufferer is the best authority on his/her own pain experience. Because providing skillful care to persons experiencing chronic pain starts with an appreciation of what it is like to live with it, nursing science has focused on acknowledging, valuing, and understanding the personal experiences of the chronic pain sufferer (Watson, 1985). According to Price (1996), "The provision of skillful care to patients suffering from chronic illness starts with an appreciation of what it is like to live with a chronic condition . . .Getting inside the experience of such illness may be key to understanding patient motivation, noncompliance with therapy, and altered patterns of social engagement" (p. 275).

Several nurse researchers (Bowman, 1991; Brown and Williams, 1995; Carson and Mitchell, 1998; Seers and Friedli, 1996; Thomas, 2000) used qualitative designs to study and understand the experience of living with chronic, nonmalignant pain. They identified and clustered global themes from patients' descriptions, and produced a thematic structure of this phenomenon. Themes related to loss of the physical and psychological self were evident in all studies. Persons with chronic pain revealed that they experienced a continuous awareness of their bodies, in contrast to the relative lack of consciousness of the physical self that is found in healthy individuals. Their bodies became the primary focus of their existence (Thomas, 2000). Pain often overtook the mind, blocking all other sensation or thought, and sufferers believed that their personalities were greatly influenced by the pain. Pain sufferers described pain as tiring, relentless, depressing, restrictive, and coloring most of their existence. Some participants expressed losing sight of what it was like to feel normal (Bowman, 1991; Seers and Friedli, 1996). The unit of time most important was the "moment," a concept that defined pain, not only in the present time, but also as a stopping of time. It was as if the moment and the pain would never end, raising the dispiriting possibility of endless suffering. Several pain sufferers spoke of extreme desperation and thoughts of suicide. Persons with chronic pain viewed the body as an obstacle rather than an enabler to action, and they expressed sadness about the loss of physical abilities and power. Several participants stated pain made them more aware of their aging (Thomas, 2000).

The experience of chronic pain was also associated with patterns of disengagement and isolation (Carson and Mitchell, 1998; Seers and Friedli, 1996; Thomas, 2000). Participants in these studies viewed pain as a physical problem that was invisible to people around them, and believed it isolated them both physically and emotionally. They often hid their condition to avoid adverse reactions from other people. Many perceived others to hold pejorative views of the pain, and expected skepticism and disinterest rather than support. Few participants mentioned a support person with whom they could freely talk about their pain. Pain closed up communication with family members, and pain sufferers were often very concerned over the effects it had on the family system. When pain sufferers tried to engage others, this occurred most often in the context of appointments with physicians, whom they approached with both hope and mistrust.

The experience of seeking help and of communicating with health professionals about pain were themes identified in several studies (Brown and Williams, 1995; Seers and Friedli, 1996). Overall, there was disparity between the expectations and perspectives of study participants and those of health professionals. It was common for participants to perceive that their pain was not believed. Being believed and having pain acknowledged as real, especially by the physician, was very important to participants. Some participants communicated insight that their pain was being treated within a model of acute care. When procedures or medications failed to relieve their pain, they perceived that blame was directed toward them; at times, participants indicated they too began to believe that the persistent pain may be of their own doing.

Chronic pain imposed diverse restrictions on daily living and role performance (Bowman, 1991; Brown and Williams, 1995). It affected sleep, mobility, work, finances, travel, recreation, and simple activities like cooking and cleaning. Participants searched for the cause and meaning of their pain; in fact, they were emphatic that the pain must be due to something. Not knowing the cause of their pain left them feeling helpless; many described how the pain controlled their lives. They indicated they were prepared to try anything that might help with pain relief. In this respect, participants spent a lot of time and money on alternative treatments. Most, however, did not give up hope for comfort and relief of their pain (Brown and Williams, 1995; Carson and Mitchell, 1998; Seers and Friedli, 1996).

Multidimensional Models of Pain

Through a concept analysis, guided by the research tradition of phenomenology, a model of pain was proposed by Mahon (1994). This method involved studying pain in a variety of literary forms; the purpose was to reveal the nature of pain as it is humanly experienced. Mahon delineated four defining attributes associated with the experience of pain. First, pain is a personal experience. If a person says that pain is present, it exists, and only the person experiencing pain is capable of describing it. Another attribute is that pain is an unpleasant experience. Third, pain is a domineering force; it rules over and controls a person's consciousness. Finally, pain has the attribute of being endless in nature. Persons experiencing pain are unable to imagine that the pain will ever end.

A stimulus and damage precede the experience of pain in Mahon's (1994) model. These two antecedents can be physical and/or psychological in nature. Three consequences were reported to arise from the experience of pain. Pain is ceaseless, unending, and tiring. It interferes with relationships with self and others. And, it gives meaning to life, either in a negative or positive way. The model depicts pain within a circle representing the unending qualities of pain. The pain encircles the person, indicating the dominating and separating nature of pain and how it impacts on interpersonal relationships.

Within the framework of stress and coping, pain is a stressor. Pain elicits attempts by the sufferer to reduce its effects through the use of cognitive and/or behavioral mechanisms. Coping with chronic pain is defined as the thoughts and actions that pain sufferers engage in to manage pain on a daily basis (Richardson and Poole, 2001). Researchers across disciplines have tried different ways to capture the process of coping with chronic pain (Brown and Nicassio, 1987; Carver, Schier, and Weintraub, 1989; Fernandez, 1986; Jensen, Turner, Romano, and Karoly, 1991). Difficulties abound in this area of research. First, it is difficult to isolate what a chronic pain sufferer does to cope with the pain as distinct from their coping with problems associated with the pain, i.e. financial difficulties or marital problems. Second, to be useful in pain management, knowledge of the coping mechanisms that each person perceives to be helpful is critical information that can lead to interventions to support and enhance their coping abilities. Third, nurses see an urgent need to develop a definition of coping with chronic pain that has usefulness and meaning for the individuals being served, rather than as a mechanism to classify adaptive and non-adaptive copers (Richardson and Poole, 2001).

To address these difficulties, Richardson and Poole (2001) propose that nurses assess coping using an activity-of-living model, such as the one set forth by Roper, Logan, and Tierney (RLT) (1996). This particular model identifies twelve activities of living, such as sleep, sexuality, safety, mobility, spirituality and communication. Each activity of living is assessed along five dimensions: biological, psychological, sociocultural, environmental, and politicoeconomic. Using the RLT model places the assessment of coping with the chronic pain experience back in the domain of the everyday practitioner and in terms that are familiar and understood by the pain sufferer. It is proposed that the use of such a model promotes earlier intervention, more efficient use of resources, and more effective service provision to persons experiencing chronic pain.

Health Within Illness

Living with chronic pain challenges health, or the person's "ability to realize aspirations, satisfy needs, and respond positively to the challenges of the environment" (World Health Organization, 1986, p. 73). Promoting health for the chronic pain sufferer is complex and multifaceted. Throughout the past several decades, linear models have been used to study chronic pain. These models were advanced through a reductionistic scientific approach evolving from a traditional worldview that perceives pain as negative and focuses research on causation and adaptation. Because of these influences, both health care professionals and the pain sufferers they treat have directed attention primarily on the pain and on preventing or minimizing associated limitations; the underlying assumption was that health would improve. Despite over 30 years of research, many questions about the genesis and course of chronic pain are unanswered, and linear models failed to capture the essence of this multifaceted phenomenon.

Although health and illness are inextricably part of the human experience, it is oftentimes viewed as a dichotomy. Within nursing science, health is a resource for everyday living, implying that health promotion for chronic pain sufferers must focus simultaneously on health and on illness (McWilliam, Stewart, Brown, Desai, and Coderre, 1996). Furthermore, many of the resources and strategies for addressing health and illness are the same. For instance, Miller (1992) identifies knowledge, coping, problem-solving, personal mastery, and motivation as factors that influence adaptation to chronic illness. Nursing strategies detailed in the chapters of her book are directed toward helping people overcome powerlessness, facilitating behavior change, enhancing self-esteem, and inspiring hope. If nurses are to promote the health of those living with chronic pain, then their efforts must be directed toward the person's larger life context, personal goals, aspirations, and patterns, rather than solely toward the person living with the limitations resulting from pain. Creating health within the chronic pain experience demands a different focus than does the idea of simply living with or adapting to chronic pain. Nurses who aim to promote the health of those experiencing chronic pain focus on the person's life and health, of which the chronic pain experience is merely one component.

Pain as a Manifestation of Human-Environmental Patterning

Nursing is concerned with the human being as a whole, the patterns of the human life process that relate to health, and identification of nursing actions and environmental conditions which best facilitate healing and health. The conceptual frameworks of Rogers (1970, 1986, 1989, 1990a, 1990b, 1992), Parse (1981), Fitzpatrick (1989), and Newman (1994) specify human energy field pattern as the primary unit of observation for nursing science. Each framework supports a worldview acknowledging a universe of open systems and an evolutionary view of human beings. Open systems, both human beings and their respective environments, are perceived to be in a process of negentropic unfolding in which traditional emphasis on adaptation, homeostasis, and equilibrium is rejected; instead, importance is placed on mutual process and unitary unfolding. Traditional views of causation are also discarded and replaced with the notion of non-causality, suggesting that change is continuously innovative and diverse. (Rogers, 1992; Sarter, 1988).

Wholeness implies that human behavior cannot be described or predicted by generalizing about or adding together particular characteristics in a linear fashion. Nor can a whole be understood when it is reduced to its particulars; rather, a whole is more than and different than the sum of the parts. Rogers' Science of Unitary Human Beings proposes that a human being and his/her respective environment are irreducible wholes. A human being is a dynamic energy field coexisting with an environmental energy field. Both human and environmental fields exist in a universe of open systems and are in a non-causal, continual, and simultaneous interaction with each other. Unitary human beings and their environments are continuously in a process of change into "increasing heterogeneity, differentiation, diversity, and complexity of pattern" (Sarter, 1988, p. 61). This conceptual system is supported by work in contemporary sciences (Bohm, 1980; Cushing and McMullin, 1989; May, 1989; Prigogine, 1980), and has been used extensively in nursing research.

Conceptualization of pain within the framework of Martha Rogers' Science of Unitary Human Beings offers a new perspective from which to study a complex, multidimensional phenomenon. In acknowledging the puzzling and complex nature of pain, the phenomenon lends itself to the study of the whole, and to the study of persons in process with their environments. Instead of adapting to the pain, Rogers' framework offers a vision of the pain sufferer evolving with the pain experience. Manifest health, encompassing illness and wellness, is viewed as an explication of the underlying pattern of person and environment; this infers that health is ultimately defined by human beings for themselves (Barrett, 1990). In this perspective, knowledge about the particulars of human structure and function, such as physiological factors underlying basic nociception, is not overlooked or devalued; however, from a unitary nursing perspective, "man is visible only as his particulars disappear from view. The characteristics of man are those that identify his wholeness, his unity" (Rogers, 1970, p. 47). The recognition of people as distinct from their parts and as irreducible wholes has characterized nursing since the time of Florence Nightingale.

Within a unitary context, pain and disease are information, or the way a person gets in touch with his/her pattern. Pain can also be an indicator of pattern change (Cowling, 1990). Chronic pain may represent an inability for the human energy field to evolve to increasing differentiation, diversity, and complexity of pattern. Prigogine's theory of dissipative structures makes clearer the process by which pattern evolves, and supports Rogers' assumption of increased complexity of pattern (Newman, 1994). Essentially, the human energy field operates in a rhythmic, predictable fashion until some critical event brings about a giant fluctuation that propels it into disorganized, unpredictable fluctuations in pattern.

Eventually, the human energy field emerges at a higher level of organization, and field patterning resumes at this higher level. During periods of disorganization of pattern, knowing participation in change, or choosing and executing behaviors that lead to maximum fulfillment of one's potential, promotes evolution to more diverse patterning. Chronic pain may manifest the period of chaos and fluctuation in the dissipative structure of the human energy field. Persons with chronic pain may get "stuck in" the chaotic fluctuations in pattern which precede evolution to higher levels (Matas, 1997).

Chronic pain often evolves into a lifestyle. It is characterized as having a progressive, changing nature marked by unpredictability in symptom development and prognosis. With chronic pain, there is a sense of failure to cure, and the pain sufferer is frequently confronted with limitations and reduction of choices. Literature describing the nature of chronic pain is replete with portrayals of chronic pain sufferers experiencing less power (Affleck, Tennen, Pfeiffer, and Fifield, 1987; Buckelew, Shutty, Hewett, Landon, Morrow, and Frank, 1990; Crisson and Keefe, 1988; Jensen and Karoly, 1991; Laborde and Powers, 1985; Wells, 1994). Within Rogers' conceptual framework, the phenomenon of chronic pain may indicate an inability of the human energy field to evolve to increased differentiation, complexity, and diversity of pattern which manifests in a greater sense of individual well- being. Chronic pain sufferers may not have the power or the capacity to participate in bringing about specific changes that will make a difference in their lives.

In the Science of Unitary Human Beings, the most important conceptual feature for nursing practice is the capacity of a person to participate knowingly in the process of change (Cowling, 1990). As described by Rogers (1990a), humans are continuously engaged with the environment in the mutual process of change, actualizing some of an infinite number of potentials in the process of becoming. Rogers makes the assumption that human beings are able to actively participate in the process of change by choosing which potentials to actualize. Continuous change is inevitable. Chronic pain is not an isolated event. It is a manifestation of the whole. Getting well entails resolving the issues that are present in all aspects of one's life. Nurses assist pain sufferers when old patterns of living no longer work and new ways are sought. The disequilibrium inherent in the mutual person-environment process is fundamental to increasing diversity of the human being. Out of the disequilibrium and disorder emerge new patterns. Such new patterns enable people to rise above perceived limitations of their bodies or environment and to actualize unique potentials for increased well-being. This is especially compelling given current chronic pain treatment approaches that emphasize self-management. With self-management, the pain sufferer is responsible for assessing and selecting management directions, including interpreting and reporting symptoms accurately, coping with emotional, social, and economic consequences, and/or changing behaviors to improve symptoms. Stated another way, "Health is the product of health care and the patient as principal caregiver is the producer of health" (Holman & Lorig, 2004, p. 242). This perspective shifts the focus of care from treatment of symptoms to cultivation of personal strategies to manage and live with pain. The pain sufferer's success in meeting these responsibilities has reverberating effects, and shapes his/her pain experience over a period usually gauged in years.

THE NURSE'S ROLE IN CARING FOR THE PERSON EXPERIENCING CHRONIC PAIN

Pain Assessment

Failure by clinicians to ask questions about a person's pain, to accept the person's report of pain as real, and to then act on these reports contribute significantly to inadequate pain management (McCaffery and Pasero, 1999). Overall, research in this area shows lack of adequate pain assessment across disciplines, and/or differences between the clinician's pain assessment and pain reported by the pain sufferer. For instance, findings in one study of 34 surgical oncology patients (Paice, Mahon, Faut-Callahan, 1991) revealed that only 28% of the sample indicated the nurse had asked questions about their pain during their hospitalization. In the same study, patients, nurses, and physicians were asked rate patients' pain. There were no significant correlations between nurse-patient, physician-patient, or nurse-physician pain ratings indicating inadequate pain assessment. Studies also show that nurses tend to underestimate severe pain (Bergh and Sjostrom, 1999; Zalon, 1993), and most physicians fail to appreciate the severity of a person's reported pain (Grossman, Sheidler, and Sweeden, 1991).

One of the most challenging aspects of caring for the person in pain is to accept that the experience of pain is completely subjective, and to let the pain sufferer be the authority of his/her private pain experience. When clinicians believe that patients exaggerate their pain, pain is inaccurately assessed, resulting in pain management strategies designed on the basis of the clinician's beliefs rather than what patients report. This is a major factor in patients' continued reports of unsatisfactory pain relief. Moreover, clinicians hold an array of misconceptions about pain that further impedes assessment and treatment (McCaffery and Pasero, 1999). McCaffery (1979) asserts that these misconceptions, or myths and prejudices, developed and proliferated over time because clinicians struggled with understanding the complexity of pain. Examples of common misperceptions involve beliefs that nurses and physicians are the best judges of a person's pain and about the truthfulness of the person's pain status, the need for objective evidence and validation of pain by physical causes, and fears of being duped by persons pretending to have pain (McCaffery, 1979; McCaffery and Pasero, 1999). Although these misperceptions have greatly influenced practice, they have undermined the goal of effective pain treatment, and contributed to mismanagement of pain sufferers.

Another issue in pain assessment is the tendency for clinicians to rely on an acute pain model to guide pain assessment. Lack of pain expression does not necessarily mean lack of pain. Clinicians tend to believe that chronic pain has characteristics of the acute pain model, i.e. physiological symptoms such as perspiration, elevated heart rate and blood pressure, and behavioral symptoms such as moaning, grimacing, and/or crying. There is a need to validate persons' reports of pain with another sign or symptom, and clinicians frequently validate reports of persistent pain using indicators of acute pain (McCaffery and Pasero, 1999). According to McCaffery and Pasero (1999), the acute pain model is of limited value in assessing chronic pain. Physiologic and behavioral indicators, if present, are so for short periods of time; then, pain sufferers adapt both physiologically and behaviorally. The essence of pain assessment is the person's self-report. Physiologic measures and behavioral observations misrepresent the pain experience and are not considered sensitive or specific indicators of pain (Acute Pain Management Guideline Panel, 1992; American Pain Society, 1992).

Assessing and managing pain has long been a core nursing responsibility. Now the Joint Commission on Accreditation of Healthcare Organizations (JCAHO) is requiring accredited facilities to develop policies and procedures that formalize this responsibility. Some key concepts underlying the new JCAHO standards are: (a) Patients have the right to appropriate assessment, (b) Patients will be treated for pain or referred for treatment, (c) Pain is to be assessed and regularly reassessed, (c) Patients will be taught the importance of effective pain management, (d) Patients will be involved in making decisions about their care, (e) Routine and p.r.n. analgesics are to be administered as needed, and (f) Discharge planning and teaching will include continuing care based on the patients needs at the time of discharge, including the need for pain management (Joint Commission on Accreditation of Healthcare Organizations, 1999).

A comprehensive, initial assessment of pain identifies new or ongoing pain problems. Components of an initial nursing pain assessment include: (a) location of the pain, (b) pain intensity, (c) pain quality, (d) onset, duration, variations, rhythms, (e) manner of expressing pain, (f) current pain relief strategies and their effectiveness, (g) activities that exacerbate pain, (h) effects of pain on activities of daily living, mood, and relationships with others, and (i) miscellaneous information. Pain rating scales, such as the Visual Analogue Scale (VAS), dual VAS (sensory and affective pain), Graphic Rating Scale (GRS), Simple Descriptor Scale (SDS), and Numerical Rating Scale (NRS), are also used by nurses to initially assess the intensity of pain, to reassess pain at regular intervals, and to assess the effectiveness of specific pain management strategies (Acello, 2000; Good, Stiller, Anderson, Stanton-Hicks, and Grass, 2002; Macklin, 1999; McCaffery and Pasero, 1999).

Implementing Pharmacological Pain Management

Persons experiencing pain are under medicated (Copp, 1993; Greipp, 1992; McCaffery and Pasero, 1999; Hazard Vallerand, 1991). Morgan (1985) coined the expression "American opiophobia," or the underutilization of opioid analgesics, and claims that physicians under treat severe pain to a significant degree based on an irrational and undocumented fear that the use of opioids will lead to addiction. Research findings also show that perhaps the most common reason why nurses do not accept and act on patients' reports of pain is the belief that the patient is or will become addicted to an opioid (McCaffery and Pasero, 1999). The fear of addiction is pervasive, not only affecting clinicians, but the pain sufferer and his/her family as well. Understanding the origins of this fear and educating health care professionals, patients, and families about pharmacological management of pain and addiction can help. Application of ethical models have also been proposed to assist nurses with decision-making related to pain management and with understanding issues related to under medication of pain (Copp, 1993; Greipp, 1992).

The most common method of pain relief is through the use of analgesic medication. Although pain medication has been used for hundreds of years, the perfect analgesic has yet to be discovered, and virtually all have undesirable side effects. Nurses are in the position to determine whether or not an analgesic is administered to patients, and if so, when it is given, to choose the appropriate analgesic when more than one is prescribed, to evaluate its effectiveness, to be alert for the possibility of side effects, to report to the physician the need for change in the analgesic, and to teach patients about the use of their pain medications (McCaffery, 1979). McCaffery and Pasero (1999) emphasize that effective pharmacologic management of pain requires application of two principles: individualizing the regimen and optimizing administration. Frequently, when analgesics are used to relieve pain, patients receive inadequate doses at intervals that allow the pain to return or persist.

Within an interdisciplinary context, individualizing the analgesic regimen involves initially choosing the pain medication most likely to meet the goal of immediate pain relief, and then to consider the long-range goals of pain management. The dose of the analgesic(s) is titrated to effect, that is, to optimize the balance between analgesia and side effects. The nurse's role in dosing is to accurately assess ongoing pain, pain relief and side effects, and to communicate this information back to the team. Optimizing administration of analgesic medication means staying on top of the pain. It is recommended that nurses give analgesics before pain occurs or increases, i.e. prior to a painful procedure and at regularly scheduled doses if pain continues (McCaffery and Pasero, 1999).

Analgesic regimens for chronic pain often include a number and variety of different medications. Teaching the patient and family about the analgesic regimen is crucial to its success and ensures adherence to the treatment plan. It is important that nurses discuss the harmful effects of unrelieved pain with patients and families. Written instructions listing all analgesics by name, dosage, and dose times are crucial. Patients and families need to know that different analgesics are used for different types of pain, and reassurance must be given that use of more than one analgesic is not dangerous. It is very important that patients learn and accept the importance of maintaining control of their pain through the use of regularly scheduled doses of analgesic medication (McCaffery and Pasero, 1999).

Complementary Therapies

Complementary therapies are non-pharmacologic ways of managing pain, and are designed to complement traditional medical approaches to pain management. Findings from a national survey on the use of complementary pain management therapies in the United States revealed an estimated 60 million Americans used these therapies in 1990 at an estimated cost of $13.7 billion (Eisenberg, Kessler, Foster, Norlock, Calkins, and Delbanco, 1993). Pain is best treated with an integrated approach, one that combines the optimal use of analgesics with a non-drug therapy, and is individualized for the pain sufferer. It is important that this integrative approach be used right from the start, especially for persons with chronic pain. Waiting years before offering a complementary therapy is often misinterpreted by patients, who assume clinicians are "giving up on them" or relegating them to "it's all in your head" status.

Relaxation. The experience of pain is often perceived as stressful. Chronic pain, by its very nature, is associated with day-to-day stress. A psychophysiologic model explains the cyclical nature of interactive events that occur with the chronic pain experience and lead to chronic stress. Relaxation provides a method to interrupt this cycle of events (Owens and Ehrenreich, 1991). When relaxation techniques are used for pain sufferers, anxiety is often reduced and sometimes, but not always, pain is lessened. In addition to reduced anxiety and possible pain reduction, potential benefits of relaxation may include promotion of sleep, improved ability to problem solve, reduced skeletal muscle tension, decreased fatigue, and increased confidence in the ability to handle pain. For patients who report severe, breakthrough pain, a brief and simple technique, such as centering on slow, deep breathing, is most appropriate. For chronic pain, a more involved technique, such as progressive muscle relaxation or combination of rhythmic breathing and peaceful imagery, may be indicated (McCaffery and Pasero, 1999). A large, randomized controlled trial showed that relaxation and soft music were effective for acute sensation and distress of pain at ambulation and rest following major abdominal surgery (Good, Stanton-Hicks, Grass, Anderson, Schoolmeesters, and Salman, 1999; Good, Stanton-Hicks, Grass et al., 2001). 2001). Reduction of acute pain lends support to findings that relaxation is also useful in managing chronic pain in a variety of conditions (Creamer, Singh, Hochberg et al., 2000; Graffam and Johnson, 1987; Pan, Morrison, Ness et al., 2000) (see chap. 19).

Guided imagery. An image is a mental picture, a representation of something that can be real or imaginary. An image can appear as a sight, a sound, a sense of movement, a smell, or a taste. Imagery is the purposeful development of an image or images through the use of one, several, or all of the five senses. When an image or images are suggested in part or whole to a person by a guide to achieve a specific, therapeutic goal, this is referred to as guided imagery. Guided imagery is an active process; the person is alert, concentrating intensely, and imagining sensory images (Dossey, 1988; McCafferty, 1979).

Conceptualizations of the usefulness of imagery in pain management center around four major schools of thought: Eastern philosophy, psychodynamic theory, cognitive-behavioral theory, and psychophysiologic theory (Nucho, 1995). The effectiveness of imagery in reducing pain has been studied widely. Most of this research is derived from pain induced in laboratory situations, and shows imagery to be effective in decreasing pain (Fernandez and Turk, 1989). The comparatively smaller number of studies using clinical pain reveals that guided imagery is effective in decreasing the intensity of reported pain (Baird & Sands, 2004; Fors, Sexton, & Gotestam, 2002; Lewandowski, 2004; Mannix et al., 1998; Moran, 1989; Raft, Smith, and Warren, 1986; Syrjala, Donaldson, Davis, Kippes, and Carr, 1995). In addition, Lewandowski, Good, & Draucker (2005) found that persons with chronic pain who used guided imagery described pain as changeable and less tormenting; descriptions of pain as never-ending also abated. The efficacy of imagery for pain management appears to be related to the person's motivation for using the technique, and the person's ability to create and become absorbed in the images (Kwekkeboom, Huseby-Moore, and Ward, 1998; Owens and Ehrenreich, 1991) (see chap.19).

Therapeutic touch. Therapeutic touch was originally developed by Kunz and Krieger as an energy field interaction between the nurse and patient (Krieger, 1975). Since the 1970's, further development and testing of this intervention occurred within Martha Rogers' Science of Unitary Human Beings. During the process of therapeutic touch, the nurse initially assumes a meditative state of awareness and a conscious intent to therapeutically assist the patient. Through movement of her hands over the patient, from head to toe, the nurse assesses the patient's energy field and facilitates balancing of the field. The nurse becomes attuned to the patient's condition by developing awareness of differences in sensory cues in her hands; then, she purposively patterns areas of accumulated tension through focused intent and movement of her hands (Meehan, 1993). Several studies explored the effectiveness of therapeutic touch in reducing anxiety (Heidt, 1981; Quinn, 1988; Randolph, 1984). Keller and Bzdek (1984) found a significant decrease in tension and headache pain in those individuals who received therapeutic touch. In another study with patients experiencing postoperative pain, Meehan (1993) found that therapeutic touch decreased patients' need for analgesic medication. Basic research designed to explicate and test the conceptual links between therapeutic touch and Roger's Science of Unitary Human Beings is needed, as well as the placebo effect of this intervention, and its' long term effectiveness as a adjuvant to traditional methods of pain management.

Music. Research indicates that music has an effect on all the major systems of the body, such as increased circulation to the brain, increased respiration, and increased muscle strength (Owens and Ehrenreich, 1991). McCaffery and Pasero (1999) state the value of music for pain sufferers is found in its relaxing and sleep promoting effects; music can also divert attention from pain. Schorr (1993) suggests that the use of music helps the pain sufferer move beyond his or her present shape, form, or way of being – such changes promote a shift consciousness and self-transcendence. A number of studies have shown music to be effective in reducing both acute and chronic pain (Good et al., 1999; Good et al., 2001; Locsin, 1981; Schorr, 1993; Siedlecki & Good, 2006; Zimmerman, Pozehl, Duncan, and Schmitz, 1989) (see chap. 19).

Massage. Massage can promote muscle relaxation, sleep promotion, and pain relief (Owens and Ehrenreich, 1991). McCaffery and Pasero (1999) suggest that massage can also be used to create an acceptable method of touch for certain patients and to communicate care and concern, especially if the patient is cognitively impaired. Several mechanisms are proposed to explain the effects of massage in modifying pain. It is postulated that massage may inhibit the transmission of noxious stimuli by stimulating large nerve fibers that have been shown to alter pain perception. The sensation of touch and the feelings related to a caring and empathetic touch may also affect the higher brain centers, further influencing the perception of pain (Melzack and Wall, 1988). Finally, based on the assumption that there is a relationship between anxiety and pain, massage promotes a relaxation response and reduction in anxiety, thereby facilitating pain relief (Ferrell-Torry and Glick, 1993). Research shows that brief massage is a safe and effective pain management strategy (Ferrell-Torry and Glick, 1993; Labyak and Metzger, 1997; Meek, 1993; Weinrich and Weinrich, 1990) (see chap. 24).

SUMMARY

In caring for the person with chronic pain, nurses are concerned with the person's unique experience and perspective of his/her pain, and its' meaning. Gaining an understanding of the effects of persistent pain on activities of daily living and role performance, as well as the ways the chronic pain sufferer copes with pain and loss, is crucial in helping the person live with and manage his/her pain. Along with developing pain management strategies, these insights also help nurses facilitate health with the goal of improving overall quality of life. Nurses have an important role in assessing pain, administering analgesic medication, advocating for the person in pain, and providing complementary therapies, helping to overcome patterns of powerlessness and inspiring hope.

From a unitary perspective, the essence and treatment of chronic pain lie in the concept of pattern. Chronic pain is viewed as a manifestation of the underlying patterning process of unitary human beings and their environments. Unitary human beings participate knowingly in the patterning process. Knowing participation means that people share in the creation of their human and environmental reality. Within Rogers' Science of Unitary Human Beings, knowing participation in change denotes power, and health is viewed as the process of actualizing potentials for well being by knowing participation in change. Nursing's aim is to assist people to achieve their own potentials and to help them participate knowingly in the process of change.

ACKNOWLEDGEMENTS

Support for this chapter was provided by an American Nurses Foundation grant #99-71 to Wendy Lewandowski, PhD RN CS (October1, 1999 to October 1, 2001).

REFERENCES

Acello, B., (2000). Meeting JCAHO standards for pain control. *Nursing 2000, 30*(3), 52- 55.

Acute Pain Management Guideline Panel. (1992). *Acute pain management in adults: Operative procedures. Quick reference guide for clinicians,* AHCPR Pub. No. 92-0019. Rockville, Maryland: Agency for Health Care Policy and Research, Public Health Service, U.S. Department of Health and Human Services.

Affleck, G., Tennen, H., Pfeiffer, C., and Fifield, J. (1987). Appraisals of control and predictability in adapting to chronic disease. *Journal of Personality and Social Psychology, 53,* 273-279.

American Pain Society. (1992*). Principles of analgesic use in the treatment of acute pain and cancer pain.* Skokie, IL: The Society.

Baird, C.L., & Sands, L. (2004). A pilot study of the effectiveness of guided imagery with progressive muscle relaxation to reduce chronic pain and mobiity difficulties of osteoarthritis. *Pain Management Nursing, 5,* 97-104.

Barrett, E.A.M. (1990). Rogers' science-based nursing practice. In E.A.M. Barrett (Ed.), *Visions of Rogers' science-based nursing* (pp. 31-45). New York: National League for Nursing.

Bergh, I., and Sjostrom, B. (1999). A comparative study of nurses' and elderly patients' ratings of pain and pain tolerance. *Journal of Gerontological Nursing, 25*(5), 30-36.

Bohm, D. (1980). *Wholeness and the implicate order.* Boston: Routledge and Kegan Paul.

Bowman, J.M. (1991). The meaning of chronic low back pain. *AAOHN Journal, 39,* 381-384.

Brown, G.K., and Nicassio, P.M. (1987). Development of a questionnaire for the assessment of active and passive coping strategies in chronic pain patients. *Pain, 31,* 53-64.

Brown, S., and Williams, S. (1995). Women's experiences of rheumatoid arthritis. *Journal of Advanced Nursing, 21,* 695-701.

Buckelew, S.P., Shutty, M.S., Hewett, J., Landon, T., Morrow, K., and Frank, R.G. (1990). Health locus of control, gender differences and adjustment to persistent pain. *Pain, 42,* 287-294.

Carson, M.G., and Mitchell, G.J. (1998). The experience of living with persistent pain. *Journal of Advanced Nursing, 28,* 1242-1248.

Carver, C.S., Schier, M.F., and Weintraub, J.K. (1989). Assessing coping strategies: A theoretically based approach. *Journal of Personality and Social Psychology, 56,* 267-283.

Copp, L.A. (1993). An ethical responsibility for pain management. *Journal of Advanced Nursing, 18,* 1-3.

Cowling, W.R. (1990). A template for unitary pattern-based nursing practice. In E.A.M. Barrett (Ed.), *Visions of Rogers' science-based nursing* (pp. 31-45). New York: National League for Nursing.

Creamer, P., Singh, B.B., Hochberg, M.C., and Berman, B.M. (2000). Sustained improvement produced by nonpharmacologic intervention in fibromyalgia: Results of a pilot study. *Arthritis Care and Research, 13,* 1198-204.

Crisson, J.E., and Keefe, F.J. (1988). The relationship of locus of control to pain coping strategies and psychological distress in chronic pain patients. *Pain, 35,* 147-154.

Cushing, J.T., and McMullin, E. (1989). *Philosophical consequences of quantum theory.* Notre Dame: University of Notre Dame.

Dossey, B.M. (1988). Imagery, awakening the inner healer. In B.M. Dossey, L. Keegan, C.E. Guzetta, and L.G. Kolkmeter (Eds.), *Holistic nursing* (pp. 223-261). Denver: Aspen Publishing.

Eisenberg, D.M., Kessler, R.C., Foster, C., Norlock, F.E., Calkins, D.R., and Delbanco, T.L. (1993). "Unconventional" medicine in the United States: Prevalence, cost, and patterns of use. *New England Journal of Medicine, 127,* 246-252.

Fernandez, E., and Turk, D.C. (1989). The utility of cognitive coping strategies for altering pain perception: A meta-analysis. *Pain, 38,* 123-135.

Ferrell-Torry, A.T., and Glick, O.J. (1993). The use of therapeutic massage as a nursing intervention to modify anxiety and the perception of cancer pain. *Cancer Nursing, 16,* 93-101.

Fernandez, E. (1986). A classification of cognitive behavioral coping strategies for pain. *Pain, 26,* 141-151.

Fitzpatrick, J.J. (1989). A life perspective rhythm model. In J.J. Fitzpatrick and A. Whall (Eds.), *Conceptual models of nursing Analysis and application* (2nd ed.) (pp. 401-408). Norwalk, CT: Appleton and Lange.

Fors, E.A., Sexton, H., & Gotestam, K.G. (2002). The effect of guided imagery and amitriptyline on daily fibromyalgia pain: A prospective, randomized, controlled study. *Journal of Psychiatric Research, 36,* 179-187.

Good, M., Stanton-Hicks, M., Grass, J.A., Anderson, G.C., Lai, H.L., Roykulcharoen, V., and Adler, P. (2001). Relaxation and music to reduce postsurgical pain. *Journal of Advanced Nursing, 33,* 208-215.

Good, M., Stanton-Hicks, M., Grass, J.M., Anderson, G.C., Choi, C.C., Schoolmeesters, L., and Salman, A. (1999). Relief of postoperative pain with jaw relaxation, music, and their combination. *Pain, 81,* 163-172.

Good, M., Stiller, C., Zauszniewski, J., Stanton-Hicks, M., Grass, J., and Anderson, G.C. (2002). Sensation and distress of pain scales: Reliability, validity, and sensitivity. *Journal of Nursing Measurement, 9*(3), 219-238.

Graffam, S., and Johnson, A. (1987). A comparison of two relaxation strategies for the relief of pain and its distress. *Journal of Pain and Symptom Management, 2,* 229-231.

Greipp, M.E. (1992). Undermedication for pain: An ethical model. *Advances in Nursing Science, 15,* 44-53.

Grossman, S.A., Sheidler, V.R., and Sweeden, K. (1991). Correlation of patient and caregiver ratings of cancer pain. *Journal of Pain and Symptom Management, 6,* 53-57.

Hazard Vallerand, A. (1991). The use of narcotic analgesics in chronic nonmalignant pain. *Holistic Nursing Practice, 6,* 17-23.

Heidt, P. (1981). Effect of therapeutic touch on anxiety level of hospitalized patients. *Nursing Research, 30,* 32-37.

Holman, H., & Lorig, K. (2004). Patient self-management: A key to effectiveness and efficiency in care of chronic disease. *Public Health Reports, 119,* 239-243.

Jensen, M.P., and Karoly, P. (1991). Control beliefs, coping efforts, and adjustment to chronic pain. *Journal of Consulting and Clinical Psychology, 59,* 431-438.

Jensen, M.P., Turner, J.A., Romano, J.M., and Karoly, P. (1991). Coping with chronic pain: A critical review of the literature. *Pain, 47,* 249-283.

Joint Commission on Accreditation of Healthcare Organizations. (1999). *Comprehensive accreditation manual for hospitals: The official handbook.* Oakbrook Terrace, Illinois: The Commission.

Keller, E., and Bzdek, V.M. (1984). Effects of therapeutic touch on tension headache pain. *Nursing Research, 33,*33-36.

Krieger, D. (1975). Therapeutic touch: The imprimatur of nursing. *American Journal of Nursing, 75,* 784-787.

Kwekkeboom, K., Huseby-Moore, K., and Ward, S. (1998). Imaging ability and effective use of guided imagery. *Research in Nursing and Health, 21,* 189-198.

Laborde, J.M., and Powers, M.J. (1985). Life satisfaction, health control orientation, and illness-related factors in persons with osteoarthritis. *Research in Nursing and Health, 8,* 183-190.

Labyak, S.E., and Metzger, E.L. (1997). The effects of effleurage backrub on physiological components of relaxation: A meta-analysis. *Nursing Research, 46,* 59-62.

Lewandowski, W.A. (2004). Patterning of pain and power with guided imagery. *Nursing Science Quarterly, 17,* 233-241.

Lewandowski, W. A., Good, M., & Draucker, C. (2005). Changes in the meaning of pain with guided imagery. *Journal of Pain Management Nursing, 6,* 58-67.

Locsin, R.G. (1981). The effect of music on the pain of selected postoperative patients. *Journal of Advanced Nursing, 1,* 19-25.

Macklin, E.A. (1999). Pain management – An overview. *Ohio Nurses Review 74,* 4-15, 12-16.

Mahon, S.M. (1994). Concept analysis of pain: Implications related to nursing diagnosis. *Nursing Diagnosis, 5,* 14-25.

Mannix, L.K., Chandurkar, R.S., Rybicki, L.A., Tusek, D.L., & Solomon, G.D. (1998). Effect of guided imagery on quality of life for paitents with chronic tension-type headache. *Headache, 39,* 326-334.

Matas, K.E. (1997). Human patterning and chronic pain.*Nursing Science Quarterly,10,* 88-96.

May, R. (1989). The chaotic rhythms of life. *New Scientist, 124,* 21-25.

McCaffery, M. (1968). *Nursing practice theories related to cognition, bodily pain, and man-environment interactions.* Los Angeles: UCLA Students' Store.

McCaffery, M. (1979). *Nursing management of the patient with pain.* Philadelphia: J.B. Lippincott Company.

McCaffery, M., and Pasero, C. (1999). *Pain clinical manual.* St. Louis: C.V. Mosby Company.

McWilliam, C.L., Stewart, M., Brown, J.B., Desai, K., and Coderre, P. (1996). Creating health with chronic illness. *Advances in Nursing Science, 18*(3), 1-15.

Meehan, T.C. (1993). Therapeutic touch and postoperative pain: A Rogerian research study. *Nursing Science Quarterly, 6*(2), 69-78.

Meek, S.S. (1993). Effects of slow stroke back massage on relaxation in hospice clients. *Image, 25,* 17-21.

Melzack, R, and Wall, P. (1988). *The puzzle of pain.* Middlesex, England: Penguin Books.

Miller, J.F. (1992). *Coping with chronic illness: Overcoming powerlessness.* Philadelphia: F.A. Davis.

Moran, K.J. (1989). The effects of self-guided imagery and other-guided imagery on chronic low back pain. In S.G. Funk, E.M. Tornquist, M.T. Champagne, L.A. Copp, and R.A. Wiese (Eds.), *Key aspects of comfort management of pain, fatigue, and nausea* (pp. 160-184). New York: Springer Publishing.

Morgan, J. (1985). Opiophobia: Customary underutilization of opioid analgesics. *Advances in Alcohol and Substance Abuse, 5,* 163-173.

Newman, M. (1994). *Health as expanding consciousness.* St. Louis: The C.V. Mosby Company.

Owens, M.K., and Ehrenreich, D. (1991). Literature review of nonpharmacologic methods for the treatment of chronic pain. *Holistic Nursing Practice, 6,* 24-31.

Pan, C.X., Morrison, R.S., Ness, J., Fergh-Berman, A., and Leipzig, R.M. (2000). Complementary and alternative medicine in the management of pain, dyspnea, and nausea and vomiting near the end of life: A systematic review. *Journal of Pain and Symptom Management, 20,* 374-387.

Parse, R.R. (1981). *Man-Living-Health: A theory of nursing.* New York: John Wiley and Sons.

Price, B. (1996). Illness careers: The chronic illness experience. *Journal of Advanced Nursing, 24,* 275-279.

Prigogine, I. (1980). *From being to becoming.* San Francisco: Freeman.

Quinn, J. (1988). Building a body of knowledge: Research on therapeutic touch. *Journal of Holistic Nursing, 6,* 37-45.

Raft, D., Smith, R.H., and Warren, N. (1986). Selection of imagery in the relief of chronic and acute clinical pain. *Journal of Psychosomatic Research, 30,* 481-488.

Randolph, G. (1984). Therapeutic and physical touch: Physiological response to stressful stimuli. *Nursing Research, 35,* 101-105.

Richardson, C., and Poole, H. (2001). Chronic pain and coping: A proposed role for nurses and nursing models. *Journal of Advanced Nursing, 34,* 659-667.

Rogers, M.E. (1970). *An introduction to the theoretical basis of nursing.* Philadelphia: F.A. Davis.

Rogers, M.E. (1986). Science of unitary human beings. In V.M. Malinski (Ed.), *Explorations on Martha Rogers' Science of Unitary Human Beings* (pp. 3-8). Norwalk, CT: Appleton-Century-Crofts.

Rogers, M.E. (1989). Nursing: A science of unitary human beings. In J.P. Riehl-Sisca (Ed.), *Conceptual models for nursing practice* (3rd ed., pp. 181-188). Norwalk CT: Appleton-Century-Crofts.

Rogers, M.E. (1990a). Nursing: Science of unitary, irreducible, human beings: Update 1990. In E.A.M. Barrett (Ed.), *Visions of Rogers' science-based nursing* (pp. 5-11). New York: National League for Nursing.

Rogers, M.E. (1990b). Space-age paradigm for new frontiers in nursing. In M.E. Parker (Ed.), *Nursing theories in practice* (pp. 105-113). New York: National League for Nursing.

Rogers, M.E. (1992). Nursing science and the space age. *Nursing Science Quarterly, 5,* 27-34.

Roper, N., Logan, W.W., and Tierney, A.J. (1996). *The elements of nursing. A model for nursing based on a model of living, 4th edition.* London, England: Churchill Livingstone.

Sarter, B.J. (1988). *The stream of becoming: A study of Martha Rogers' theory.* New York: National League of Nursing.

Schorr, J.A. (1993). Music and pattern change in chronic pain. *Advances in Nursing Science, 15*(4), 27-36.

Seers, K., and Friedli, K. (1996). The patients' experiences of their chronic non-malignant pain. *Journal of Advanced Nursing, 24,* 1160-1168.

Siedlecki, S., & Good, M. (2006). Effect of music on power, pain, depression and disability. *Journal of Advanced Nursing, 54*(5), 553-562.

Syrjala, K.L., Donaldson, G.W., Davis, M.W., Kippes, M.E., and Carr, J.E. (1995). Relaxation and imagery and cognitive-behavioral training reduce pain during cancer treatment: A controlled clinical trial. *Pain, 63,* 189-198.

Thomas, S.P. (2000). A phenomenologic study of chronic pain. *Western Journal of Nursing Research, 22,* 683-705.

Watson, J. (1985). *Nursing: Human science and human care: A theory of nursing.* Norwalk CT: Appleton-Century-Crofts.

Weinrich S.P., and Weinrich, M.C. (1990). The effect of massage on pain in cancer patients. *Applied Nursing Research, 3,* 140-145.

Wells, N. (1994). Perceived control over pain: Relation to distress and disability. *Research in Nursing and Health, 17,* 295-302.

World Health Organization. (1986). *Health promotion: Concepts and principles in action – A policy framework.* London, England: World Health Organization.

Zalon, M.L. (1993). Nurses' assessment of postoperative patients' pain. *Pain, 54,* 329-334.

Zimmerman, L., Pozehl, B., Duncan, K., and Schmitz, R. (1989). Effects of music in patients who had chronic cancer pain. *Western Journal of Nursing Research, 3,* 298-309.

In: The Handbook of Chronic Pain
Editors: S. Kreitler, D. Beltrutti, et al., pp. 379-398

ISBN 978-1-60021-044-0
© 2007 Nova Science Publishers, Inc.

Chapter 21

Palliative Care

*Diego Beltrutti, Aldo Lamberto, Mauro Nicosia
and Francesco Marino*

1. PALLIATION

1.1. A Working Definition of Palliative Medicine

Palliative care is a medical doctrine that reflects an underlying ideology and philosophy of life. It affirms that there is a time in the evolution of a chronic illness when expectations need to be focused less on curing and more on caring [1]. The purpose of palliative care is to improve the quality of the patient's remaining life by means of regular control of symptoms, such as pain, which is one of the most important of the symptoms requiring management.

Accordingly, the major components of palliative care are: affirming life and considering dying as a normal process, without hastening or postponing it; providing relief from pain and other distressing symptoms; integrating the physical, psychological and spiritual aspects of patient care; offering support to patients to live as well as possible until death; and help the family cope by providing information and support. In recent years palliative care has ceased to be limited to the terminal phases of disease and is increasingly considered as a system of symptom care supplementing any phase of medical practice, even in the early stage of disease [2].

1.2. Pain and Palliative Medicine

Palliative medicine focuses on the alleviating symptoms, rather than on curing. Palliation deals primarily with those symptoms that cause the patient the most distress and the greatest impairment in quality of life (see chapter 6, this book). Pain ranks highest among these.

Accordingly, pain relief plays a major role in the various palliative programs. So much so, that palliative care itself is sometimes defined primarily as specialized care designed to alleviate pain and suffering or alternately to improve the patient's quality and life by overcoming pain.

1.3. The Focal Characteristics of Palliation

Palliation is not a singular approach to therapy that merely provides basic care to terminally ill patients, but is a multifaceted technique that incorporates medical concepts in a humanistic way. This philosophy is evident in many ways that palliation may be considered.

(a) **Palliation is a way of overcoming the concept that there is nothing else that can be done.** The patient and the illness are two not equivalent aspects. Even though the illness may be incurable it is still possible to help the individual. Dying is in fact "the last stage of growth" [3].

(b) **Palliation is assistance**. Assistance is a personal commitment of the team to be present and provide the patient help by recognizing and meeting the patient's needs. For the patient it signifies the certainty of having somebody close by whatever happens and regardless of his/her physical or mental state. Palliative medicine is dynamic and flexible, being designed to be modified not according to the needs of the provider, but according to those of the patient In the palliative setting the patient is not only the object of care but continues to be the "subject-object" of the care.

(c) **Palliation is rehabilitation**. Palliation encourages the rehabilitation of those who are approaching death by restoring to them capabilities, that even if minimal, may be highly significant, such as sitting up for meals, visiting the toilet, or talking about one's condition. Thus, rehabilitation is not merely a matter of using an assisting device or of doing exercises, but is an emotional achievement. In this way it provides hope and faith at a time of great uncertainty. This palliation-rehabilitation concept does not decline with the physical deterioration of the patient, but provides new objectives to be assessed daily.

(d) **Palliation is diagnostic medicine**. There are various types of pain, in line with their sites or causes, e.g., compression of the roots of nerve endings, external pressure on hollow organs, bone erosion or joint capsule tension. The precise diagnosis of pain is important, because it will help in finding the right treatment. Only an efficient pain management program as well as comprehensive symptom management can help prevent a patient's request for euthanasia [4].

(e) **Palliation is communication**. During the advanced and terminal stages of an illness, the patient does not confide in everyone. Patients will open up and talk about their worries, fears, sadness for life coming to an end and their last wishes, to those whom they feel to be truly close to them. The messages are often unclear, cryptic and in need of decoding. This does not happen simply by a quick stop by the bed and a bland "How's it going? Everything all right?" which is typical of what occurs on ward rounds. Understanding these patients requires time and effort. The palliation team must be skilled in both verbal and nonverbal communication. Empathy, discretion, understanding, rising of the spirits and even silence are the non-pharmacological techniques with which palliative care providers need to be familiar.

(f) **Palliation is being present**. Palliation is a means of approaching the patient, a form of assistance, which precedes drug administration. More than a way of "doing things" or of symptom control, it is a means of approach in relation to the suffering patient, with bare hands without any needles or drugs. Palliation is a "form of being". It is a way of being present, without fear, prejudice or embarrassment in front of those, who may generate these feelings in the population at large.

(g) **Palliation is precision medicine**. Palliation is not approximate medicine that focuses on symptoms, but rigorous medicine that is patient-centered. The terminal disease stage is not the time for a "let's see if this works" approach. The patient's unfavorable prognosis should never prevent us from providing skilled, careful and precise assistance, using every means at our disposal to improve the patient's quality of life. Palliation cares more about "how" the process of death will come about rather than "when". Analgesic drugs should also be prescribed and administered in a precise manner: "as needed" administration is replaced by "around the clock" administration, since the pathogenic stimulus that causes the pain is also active around the clock.

(h) **Palliation is goal-oriented**. We do not expect the patient to scream out in pain. Rather we should regularly ask how he or she is feeling and observe his/her behavior. "Are you feeling any pain?" "Could you sleep last night?" "Are you feeling down today?" Our objectives are to determine the patient's comfort level, needs, and satisfaction in order to provide appropriate assistance. Pain relief, the control of insomnia and of depression are examples of realistic and attainable goals. Yet, pain control should be a primary goal for all palliative care patients.

It is crucial that the objectives not be over-ambitious. Also, they should be agreed upon with the patient, just as the proposed solutions. The objectives are targeted to meeting actual needs, so that when they are attained they provide satisfaction to the patient, the family and the care team.

The plan of action must be personalized and realistic, thereby avoiding the risk that failure to realize these objectives will lead to desperation and a sense of failure.

(i) **Palliation is continuous care**. The continuity of care until death is one of the primary characteristics of palliative medicine. A patient who enters a palliation program will not be discharged, and caring for that patient will last up to death. Palliative medicine does not consider excuses such as "We performed three surgeries already. Sorry, we can't do anything more, maybe you should see someone else".

The patients are followed-up by the team both in hospital and on their return home or their transfer to another health service facility. Family members are also fully integrated into the care program, and they will also be assisted later during the mourning and condolence stages.

(j) **Palliation is anti-dogmatic**. Palliative medicine does not provide a specific treatment but rather comprises a series of patient-specific and balanced interventions that take into account the clinical, mental and emotional states of the patients in relation to their cultural background and surroundings. Nothing needs to be imposed on the patient. For example, it is not necessary to establish a specific protocol for chemotherapy, rather, it may simply be used when and if required. Patients must be aware that they are an integral part of the decision making process and that it is they who select the main goals to be reached.

(k) **Palliation defines the roles, skills, and attitudes of the caregivers**. In palliative medicine there is awareness that there are many individuals with the capacity of helping the patient, including the family leader, doctors, psychologists, professional nurses, social workers, home care providers, voluntary workers, religious representatives, charity organizations, and friends. It is the responsibility of the palliative care team to designate a defined role to all individuals involved in the caring process according to their skills, attitudes, abilities, and desires. Yet, at all times, the role of the caregiver must be oriented both to the family structure and to the patient's needs and desires.

(l) **Palliation is analytic medicine**. To face a patient in the terminal disease phase may be discouraging because of the clinical complexity of the situation. Therefore it is crucial that each problem, regardless of how big it is, be broken down into its major elements, and then the most advantageous solution to each of these will be looked for. Finally, all the minor improvements can be summed to provide the global improvement in the quality of life that is being sought.

(m) **Palliation monitors results**. The life span of a patient in the terminal stage of a disease is unknown but is likely to be short. Therefore, results need to be obtained within an acceptable time limit. Hence, only objectives that can be attained with a minimum delay have to be selected.

(n) **Palliation is dynamic medicine**. In the terminal phase, the control of pain, like the treatment of any other symptom, requires regular and repeated reassessments. It is quite common that the treatment that produced good results a week before has to be modified in the present week because new clinical problems may have arisen. Palliative medicine attempts to use the least amount of analgesic drugs, while at the same time providing effective pain relief without negative effects on the quality of life. This difficult task can be realized only by constant monitoring of the various clinical parameters. The regular use of pain assessment scales is essential for accurate analgesic titration. Pain assessment, analgesic drug intake, side effects and quality of life are dynamic conditions that lead to dynamic clinical responses.

2. PALLIATIVE CARE SERVICES

A patient with chronic fatal disease progresses from a stage of relative well being to a stage of physical decline in the advanced and terminal stages. A patient's needs change rapidly during this progression. Therefore, the provided care should be flexible, anti-dogmatic, and attentive to the actual needs of the patient, who must be rapidly satisfied. Furthermore, focusing on satisfying the various needs of the palliative patients requires a multidisciplinary approach implemented by a team of physicians, nurses, psychologists, social workers, volunteers, and clergy, often reinforced by physical therapists, musical and art therapists, and dieticians.

It is evident that palliative care is difficult to provide in the hospital setting, which is standardized and based on rigid protocols. Therefore, different palliative services have been developed. The major ones are the following: (1) Palliative care units with beds: (a) a specialist unit (ward) that is part of a general hospital; (b) an autonomous department incorporated into a general hospital; and (c) a residence that is physically separated and at a distance from the hospital buildings, and is generally located in a peaceful setting; (2) Palliative care units without beds within a hospital, which can be autonomous or a branch of a larger department, and provide care to patients from other wards; (3) Home care service, providing assistance and consulting; (4) Rapid Response team, providing emergency interventions in crisis situations; (5) Respite Care team, providing care for the patient so that the family members get some free time; (6) Day Hospice, which take care of the patients during the day; (7) The out-patient consulting service.

3. The Continuing Role of "Cause Oriented" Therapies

3.1. Palliative Chemotherapy

It is well known that reduction or ablation of a tumoral mass can decrease pain and ameliorate collateral symptoms. It is not clear if such symptomatic relief can also occur in the absence of cancer regression. However, there are theoretical reasons why pain and other symptoms can be modified by chemotherapy apart from the cancer response.

The analgesic effects of chemotherapy can be related in part to the adjunctive use of steroids that have well-known co-analgesic potential. These drugs function by inhibiting or modifying the production of pro-inflammatory molecules, such as cytokines and eicosanoids that contribute to edema, inflammation, and nociception. For example, methotrexate has an inhibitory effect on interleukin-1 (IL-1) and prostaglandin biosynthesis [5]. These drugs can also reduce the production of cytokines as a result of their cytolytic effect on lymphoid cells: cytotoxic drugs have a strong effect on granulocytes, lymphocytes and monocytes that are associated with cancer and contribute to the tumor mass [6]. Cytotoxic chemotherapy has demonstrated efficacy and palliative benefit in patients with hormone-refractory prostate carcinoma. Its role in managing advanced prostate carcinoma patients is growing but remains an area of active investigation [7].

Cancer pain and other symptoms are not simply connected with the pressure of a tumor on an organ or surrounding tissues. Pro-nociceptive molecules can be released by cancer cells, especially during the vascularization process required to support the tumor. The presence of these algogenic molecules supports the concept that cancer pain is often out of proportion to the level of structural involvement. Some cytotoxic drugs alter the function of peripheral nerves and are able to cross the blood-brain-barrier, resulting in alteration of both central and peripheral neurotransmission.

3.2. Palliative Radiotherapy

In the context of palliative care, radiotherapy is used for controlling the local symptoms caused by the cancer at a specific site, particularly pain. Therapeutically, local irradiation of a tumor in a patient affected by metastatic progression will have an effect only on the site irradiated, and will not influence the pathology external to this area. Unlike radical radiotherapy treatment, the aim of palliative radiotherapy is to control local symptoms and minimize the acute reaction to the radiation [8]. The aims of radiotherapy (i.e. delay cancer growth, alleviate pain, and prevent hemorrhages), can usually be achieved with relatively low doses, given as a brief course treatment for one or two weeks. This approach both minimizes the collateral acute effects of the radiation, and controls the symptoms.

Collateral effects of radiotherapy include an acute toxicity that may be manifested by erythema, skin desquamation, mucositis, esophagitis, cystitis and gastrointestinal irritation [9].

Regeneration of the damaged epithelial surfaces can occur after the end of treatment, if stem cells have not been destroyed. Recovery usually occurs within a period of days to weeks. Only on rare occasions is the lesion persistent, particularly in vulnerable sites, such as the inferior part of the leg or the back or after and trauma. In these rare cases, radionecrosis can occur.

The long-term damage caused by radiation is potentially much more dangerous than the acute reaction. It can develop several months or years after treatment and is mainly caused by progressive vascular changes in small vessels (endoarteritis obliterans). Clinical signs include skin atrophy and telangiectasias at the site of irradiation, with more serious sequelae affecting the intestine and bladder (perforations and fistulae) and the central nervous system (necrosis).

Treating the symptoms helps to control the acute effects of radiotherapy and aids recovery of the affected area. The slight skin reactions don't require active treatment, and local irritation can be alleviated by the application of a 1% solution of hydrocortisone cream. Desquamation is generally treated by topical application of gentian violet, even though there is no evidence of its real value. Talcum powder and creams containing metal salts should be avoided since they can exacerbate the reaction to the radiation.

Nausea often occurs during irradiation of the abdomen and pelvis, but it usually responds to therapy with antiemetics such as metoclopramide. Prednisolone and/or ondansetron can prevent or alleviate more acute nausea. Diarrhea responds to codeine phosphate or loperamide. Radiation cystitis is more difficult to control. It is important to prevent concomitant infections and to induce diuresis.

Potassium citrate is sometimes prescribed but is generally useless. Parenteral analgesics are useful for pain relief. Relief from oropharyngeal mucositis can be obtained with aspirin or benzydamine, which can be dissolved in mouthwash. Maintain a high level of oral hygiene can be done by the regular use of a mouthwash containing chlorhexidine. Candidiasis can be treated with either a suspension of nystatin or clotrimazole gel.

Pneumonia may be suspected if there is a dry cough and dispend, and diagnosis is classically by thoracic radiogram. Treatment generally includes steroids as well as antibiotics.

It is important to inform the patients and their family in advance about the possibility of acute collateral effects of radiation, to explain their causes and provide reassurance about prompt resolution at the end of radiotherapy.

3.3. Palliative Surgery

Palliative surgery is used for alleviating serious pain and distress even under conditions that do not promote recovery and survival. There are several applications of palliative surgery: (a) "Cleaning" operations, such as the amputation of a limb or a breast, due to an ulcerated or bleeding tumor, or presence of metastasis; (b) Intestinal resections, such as in the case of hepatic symptomatic metastasis; (c) Atypical ablation of relapsing tumors in the presence of oral cavity radionecrosis; (d) Total laryngectomy instead of simple tracheotomy for stenosing tumors with concomitant lung metastasis; and (e) Removal of adenopathic masses causing ulceration or nerve root compression. In many situations, ethical considerations, have resulted in renouncing some useful operations whose benefits are considered to be too short lasting or too risky [10].

4. THE MANAGEMENT OF PAIN

The control of pain experience is crucial in any palliative care program [11, 12]. Although palliative care programs provide assistance to patients with all kinds of diseases, the majority of terminally ill patients in these programs are cancer patients. A level of pain requiring prompt and lasting treatment is experienced in as many as 45% of patients in the earlier phases of cancer and 75% of patients in the advanced phases. Factors that determine the prevalence of pain in cancer patients include the type of cancer, presence of metastases, the involvement of neural structures, bones, vessels, and hollow organs, as well as the production of pro-nociceptive substances by the tumor, the use of invasive diagnostic and therapeutic procedures, secondary effects of radiotherapy, toxic effects of chemotherapy, comorbidity and age.

Misconceptions on the part of health professionals and patients contribute to ineffective management of cancer pain. Yet, interventional pain techniques have proven to be useful in alleviating pain to some extent in as many as 90% of the patients (see Chap. 30, this book).

5. SYMPTOM MANAGEMENT

Symptom control and management, especially in those with disabling features, is a key goal of palliative medicine. Patients in the advanced and terminal phases of a disease may present with one or more of a variety of symptoms or problems affecting different organs or organ systems that may result in pain or be accompanied by pain.

5.1. Gastrointestinal Symptoms

(1) Nausea and vomiting. Emesis is a complex syndrome consisting of nausea, retching and vomiting, and is associated with anorexia. It is a frequent complication in terminal cancer patients or in those undergoing chemotherapy or radiotherapy (60-70%) [13]. Patients

consider emesis to be a disgusting and humiliating symptom. Excessive and repetitive vomiting may lead to electrolyte depletion, risk of dehydration and a hypothermic reaction.

The clinical approach to the care of patients suffering from emesis must consider the position of the patient as a determining factor in order to avoid gastric inhalation, especially in patients whose reflexes are depressed. Determining the stimulus that causes vomiting can provide a targeted approach for pharmacological therapy. A stimulus originating from the myenteric plexus responds better to anticholinergic drugs and antidopaminergic drugs with anticholinergic effects (e.g. cyclizine). A central stimulus originating from a trigger zone responds better to antidopaminergic agents, although domperidone and metoclopramide may also be effective [14].

Assessment through a visual analogue scale and recording in a diary may be necessary for controlling the symptom [15].

(2) Dysphagia and dyspepsia. The general incidence of dysphagia in terminal cancer patients ranges from 10% to 23 % [16]. In patients with head and neck tumors, the percentage rises to 40% at onset and to 80% in the terminal phase [17]. Dysphagia in terminal cancer patients is mainly the result of the presence of primitive head and neck, esophageal or stomach tumors.

Swallowing is a complex process involving the medulla oblongata, several of the cranial nerves, and 25 skeletal muscles including facial, pharyngeal and esophageal muscles.

While *dysphagia* refers to difficulty in swallowing and is not always accompanied by pain, *odynophagia* refers to painful swallowing. It occurs in patients with primitive neck tumors, and is also a common manifestation of infectious or non-infectious inflammatory syndromes (reflux esophagitis, radiation and chemotherapy-associated mucositis).

Problems in swallowing first develop with solid food and only later progress to problems with liquids. Liquid or saliva accumulating in the piriform fossa causes a physical obstruction often associated with a reduction of the nerve function that controls peristalsis. Prophylactic treatment is effective in about 60% of patients [18].

Dysphagia can cause a high level of anxiety not only to the patient, but also to the relatives. Consequently, accurate information needs to be provided to allow patients and their relatives to understand the situation. The act of eating is not identical with maintaining the nutritional state. For many patients the ability to eat is a factor contributing to quality of life. Management strategies and advice about enhancing the swallowing process are important. If progressive esophageal stenosis occurs, it is important to maintain a patent lumen, either with a week of treatment with dexamethasone to reduce the compression, or in refractory cases, surgery, palliative radiation, or insertion of an intraesophageal tube may be effective [19].

Dyspepsia refers to a complex of gastrointestinal symptoms that include retrosternal or epigastric pain, abdominal discomfort, nausea and vomiting [20]. Dyspepsia can be identified as organic when a specific cause can be recognized (gastroesophageal reflux, peptic ulcer, gastric carcinoma or cholelithiasis), or functional, when an organic cause cannot be defined (motility disorders, aerophagia, idiopathic dyspepsia).

During the course of a neoplastic disease, dyspepsia can result from the presence of gastric carcinoma, autonomic dysfunction, gastric paresis, post-surgical syndromes (small stomach syndrome, gastroesophageal reflux), radiation of the lumbar spine or epigastrium.

Dyspepsia may also be caused by the use of drugs (such as iron, NSAIDs, steroids, opioids, metronizadole, tranexamic acid, anticholinergic drugs, or cisplatinum).

Up to 50% of non-ulcer dyspepsia is associated with antrum hypomotility. Dyspepsia combined with persistent nausea and anorexia is present in patients affected by autonomic dysfunction and gastric over-inflation due to gastric paresis. Gastric over-inflation is present in 15% of patients who undergo total laryngectomy [21]. Instrumental diagnosis is rarely needed since an accurate case history can help to establish the different types of pathology.

Polypharmacy is common among patients in palliative care: they often combine drugs that delay gastric emptying, stimulate gastric secretion, and irritate the gastric wall. Dyspepsia associated with morphine use can be alleviated by prokinetic drugs. With NSAID-associated dyspepsia, an alternative drug with similar effects but improved tolerability should be used.

The use of antacids (dimethicone) is often not enough to control gastroesophageal reflux and acid-related disorders. In these cases, an inhibitor of gastric acid secretion (H_2-receptor blockers or proton pump inhibitors) or a cytoprotectant (sucralfate, misoprostol) may be recommended.

Ranitidine is the most widely use of the H_2-receptor blockers because of its greater efficacy and greater tolerability. A prokinetic drug to accelerate gastric emptying may also be used concomitantly with a gastroprotective agent [22, 23].

Omeprazole should be used in palliative care only if other agents have not been successful. In palliative medicine, pharmacological interventions targeted to symptoms are generally preferred. Yet, for patients with esophageal reflux of bile, surgery is the treatment of choice.

(3) Constipation and diarrhea. *Constipation* refers to the infrequent and difficult elimination of hard feces. It occurs in about 50% of terminal patients [24]. There are multiple causes. Apart from a direct pathogenic cause, poor nutrition, reduced mobility, and the use of opioid analgesics are contributory factors. An accurate case history that documents the beginning and duration of constipation can contribute to making an accurate diagnosis. The nature of the feces, the presence of abdominal pains, nausea and vomiting are the clearest signs of constipation or an obstruction. In doubtful cases, a radiologic exam can be helpful.

Prophylactic measures can help reduce the incidence of constipation. The aim of prophylactic therapy is to achieve comfortable regular elimination. Controlling symptoms, encouraging activity, adequate liquid consumption, a diet high in fiber, and use of laxative drugs as adjuncts to analgesic therapy are all effective prophylactic therapies. However, the choice of the laxative drug must be in agreement with patient's wishes with dosing based on the therapeutic response.

In contrast to constipation, *diarrhea* is the frequent passing of unformed feces and is generally defined as the passing of more than three unformed feces in a day. It is a less frequent problem than constipation, occurring in 7% to 10% of patients admitted to a hospice and in 6% of hospitalized patients [25].

Diarrhea is generally an acute event, lasting several days and often resulting from an intestinal infection, such as Salmonella, E. coli, Shigella, or Candida. In palliative care patients it may also result from viral infections, such as rotavirus or Norwalk-type virus. If diarrhea persists for more than three weeks it is considered chronic and implies the presence of a serious pathology.

The most frequent cause of diarrhea in palliative care patients is an imbalance in laxative therapy [17]. Consequently, a 24 – 48 hour interruption in administering laxatives followed by a decrease in dose can often resolve the problem. However, diarrhea may have other causes such as the use of certain drugs, radiation, obstructions, malabsorption, intercurrent diseases and diet. An accurate patient history can indicate the nature of the problem, which will determine the best approach to diagnosis and treatment.

Palpation or a rectal examination can help in determining the presence of abdominal masses, fecal impaction, or intestinal obstructions. Radiological techniques may assist in cases of uncertainty. In palliative care, diarrhea is rarely so acute and prolonged as to cause dehydration.

(4) Jaundice, ascites, hepatic encephalopathy, liver failure. In a terminal patient, *jaundice* represents a sign of progressive decay and imminent death. However, the causal mechanism should be investigated. In some cases, for example when it is associated with pruritus, symptomatic treatment may be adequate. In other cases, a more aggressive treatment, such as the positioning of a biliary stent, may be required. The appearance of jaundice is an event that patients and their family consider to be very serious, and its treatment and resolution can make them feel relieved and hopeful of recovery [26].

Three types of jaundice can be distinguished: (a) *Pre-hepatic jaundice:* this is a condition in which there is an imbalance in the liver's capacity to process hemolyzed red blood cells resulting in the excretion of excess unconjugated bilirubin into the plasma and tissues; (b) *Hepatic jaundice*: any condition interfering with or preventing the liver from releasing bilirubin into the general circulation. It is secondary to hepatocellular necrosis or a functional incapacity of biliary excretion (cholestasis); and (c) *Post-hepatic jaundice:* this is also known as obstructive jaundice and results from the significant obstruction of the bile duct outside the liver. It can be caused by a pancreatic tumor, carcinoma of the ampulla, or swelling of the portal lymph nodes.

Patient history and an objective exam are important for the differential diagnosis. Clinical jaundice is easily recognized, but in the patient already worn-out by disease, the state of latent jaundice, often accompanied by lymphoadenopathy and edema, must be accurately investigated.

Reducing serious *anemia* by means of blood transfusions improves cenesthesis, and the subsequent amelioration of the general condition can provide significant relief.

Confirming the presence of *pruritus* is an important step. Its exacerbation can be prevented by maintaining a low temperature, which has the added benefit of reducing perspiration and increasing patient comfort. Topical cortisone, other emollients, as well as systemic administration of antihistamines may also be advantageous.

The appearance of *ascites* in patients suffering from an advanced-phase tumor is considered a negative event both because it reduces the patient's comfort and because it limits therapeutic treatment options, which are associated with risks of both morbidity and mortality. Ascites is more frequent in some types of tumors than in others. In ovarian tumors, 30% of patients develop early ascites, and at the time of death it is present in more than 60%. It is also present in tumors of the large intestine, breast, stomach and pancreas [27].

For diagnostic and therapeutic purposes ascites can be divided into four subgroups: (a) *Central ascites* is present in about 15% of cases and results from the spread of the tumor throughout the hepatic parenchyma (causing compression of the portal vein) and lymphatic system; (b) *Peripheral ascites* is present in 50% of cases and is due to the presence of neoplastic metastasis in the visceral and parietal peritoneum [28]; (c) *Mixed ascites* results from a combination of the above two types and is present in about 15% of cases; and (d) *Chylous ascites* occurs when the retroperitoneal infiltration of the tumor produces a compression of the lymphatic nodes and pancreas consequently blocking the lymphatic flow.

Not all of the ascites in cancer patients are of neoplastic origin. Some pre-existing conditions like hepatosis, portal hypertension, portal vein thrombosis, congestive heart failure, nephrotic syndrome, pancreatitis, and intestinal perforations may be the primary cause of ascites. In the presence of excessive effusion, abdominal and inguinal hernias, scrotal edema and abdominal venous engorgement can occur [29].

Opacity on an abdominal radiogram is indicative of ascites. CT scans and echography can also help to establish the nature and source of the ascites [30]. Diagnostic paracentesis and removal of 15-100 ml of the ascites fluid for analysis can provide further information. The appearance of the liquid, the concentration of albumin, the types and numbers of cells present, and Gram staining and culture are generally used for characterizing the ascites [31].

Treatment of ascites is palliative in nearly all cases. However, notable exceptions include ovarian tumor, where surgery and adjuvant treatments can result in a longer expectancy of life, and lymphomas responding to chemotherapy and radiotherapy.

Medical treatment consists of rest, water restriction and diuretics [32]. Massive paracentesis seems to reduce the hospital stay significantly without increasing the complications, morbidity or mortality associated with treatment. However total paracentesis must be supplemented by infusions of albumin and dextrose [33]. Peritoneal venous shunting has also been demonstrated to be effective and to improve the patient's quality of life [34].

Hepatic encephalopathy, similar to ascites, is considered to be a terminal event in neoplastic disease. Its appearance corresponds to a period of anxiety and bed confinement. Choice of therapy is critical in this phase, and should be based on the considerations of prolonging survival and reducing the patient's suffering.

The most common signs of hepatic encephalopathy include continuous somnolence, inversion of the sleep-wake cycle, difficulty in concentration, and in the most advanced phases, confusion [35]. Other signs likely to be observed are fetor epaticus, tendon hyperactivity, and decerebrate posture. Patients with hepatic encephalopathy have problems speaking, resulting in a slow, monotonous and indistinct tone. Asterixis or "flapping wing fremitus" (defined as an arrhythmic and asymmetrical hyperextensions of the head and trunk extremities) develops in the phase preceding coma. The specific treatment is targeted to the removal or restriction of the causative factors such as reducing the levels of ammonia and toxic metabolites in the blood and limiting the absorption of proteins and nitrogenous compounds in the intestine [36].

(5) Intestinal obstruction. Intestinal obstruction is caused by occlusion of the intestinal lumen or by reduced motility of the smooth muscles. It is usually accompanied by pain. It can appear as one of the early symptoms in the onset of cancer or develop during the course of the disease [37]. Surgery is generally indicated, but there are advanced phase patients who are too weak to undergo a surgical operation. In these patients, alternative medical treatment is required. Obstruction can be characterized by the following pathologies:

(a) *Intraluminal obstruction:* may occur as the result of several different processes. The presence of polyps in the right colon can produce invaginations of the intestine resulting in occlusion. Heteroplastic localization may result in ring-shaped obstructions and lumenal restriction. Occasionally, metastatic formations protrude into the lumen, causing blockage;

(b) *Intramural obstruction:* the intestine may appear hard and contracted as a result of *linitis plastica* with involvement of the *tunica muscularis* of the ileum; diagnosis often requires histological evaluation;

(c) *Extramural obstruction:* the presence of an omental and/or mesenteric mass associated with abdominal and pelvic adhesions creates extrinsic compression and occlusion that can generally be diagnosed by a radiologic exam;

(d) *Intestinal motility disorder:* reduced or absent intestinal motility (pseudo-obstruction) may simulate a physical obstruction but without actual occlusion of the lumen. Pseudo-obstruction may also be present as a paraneoplastic syndrome of lung cancer;

(e) *Multiple sites:* obstruction of both the large and small intestine is mainly observed in the presence of ovarian tumors.

(f) *Other factors:* inflammatory edema, fealties, fibrosis, inelasticity and muscular stress, and a change in the intestinal flora can also contribute to intestinal obstruction

A differential diagnosis between constipation and obstruction is necessary. Yet, in advanced-phase patients, diagnostic examination of the intestinal obstruction should be performed only in cases where the evolution of the tumor may be affected.

The major alternatives for the treatment of intestinal obstruction are surgery, insertion of a gastrointestinal tube, gastrostomy, and symptomatic treatment.

The possibility of surgical treatment must always be considered in patients with intestinal obstruction, but the final decision is based on specific indications [38]. The most common surgery types are resection and anastomosis, decompression, colostomy, and enterostomy.

Aspiration to remove swallowed air reduces the potential for vomiting fluids from the stomach. The use of a nasogastric tube alleviates gastrointestinal compression in patients with a physical or functional obstruction. However, only 14% of the patients obtain some improvement with a nasogastric tube, and its use in the treatment of obstruction is controversial since it prolongs hospitalization, immobilization, and patient discomfort. Furthermore, it limits the patient's relationship with his or her family at a time when mutual support is needed [39].

Gastrostomy or jeujunostomy is a technique used to alleviate the symptoms of nausea and vomiting in patients affected by inoperable obstruction since it is better tolerated than a nasogastric tube [40]. In most patients nausea and vomiting are likely to decrease because of the reduction of intestinal obstruction.

5.2. Depression

Although depression can be a pre-existing condition in palliative care patients, it is generally correlated with poor pain control and a general physical deterioration that characterize advanced or terminal disease phases. In these patients, the incidence of depression varies from 20 to 25% while the prevalence varies from 23% to 58% [41]. Depression may be masked by the concurrent presence of symptoms, such as anorexia, weight loss, and fatigue.

The palliative care physician needs to inquire about feelings of hopelessness, helplessness, and mood modifications that can help in diagnosing depression. Pharmacological antidepressant therapy is the most widely used approach to treatment, although psychotherapy, relaxation techniques and cognitive behavioral therapy can also be extremely useful [42].

The older tricyclic antidepressants at low dosages are generally used as first-line treatment. Since the onset of action of these drugs often takes several weeks, it is not recommended that they be initiated as treatment in the last month of life. The serotonin-specific reuptake inhibitors (SSRIs) are used as second-line agents when there are secondary effects with the tricyclics. However, use of SSRIs can reduce appetite. When anxiety or panic attacks are present, psychotropic drugs such as benzodiazepines may be used.

5.3. Urinary Retention and Incontinence

There are no available data on the incidence and prevalence of urinary incontinence in terminal patients, although total, paradoxical, urge and stress incontinence can be identified. In the advanced disease stage, urinary incontinence is treated according to clinical practice guidelines. In the very late phase an indwelling urinary catheter can provide increased comfort and facilitate proper patient care [43]. In some cases an external urinary catheter (condom) may be preferred by the patient. Contractions of the bladder (detrusor muscle) should be treated with relaxants, such as oxybutynin (2.5 mg 3-4 times a day), or propantelin (15 mg 2-3 times a day).

5.4. Dyspnea, Cough, Hiccup, Hemoptysis and other Respiratory Symptoms

Respiratory symptoms represent a small part of palliative medicine, but in the terminal phase of the neoplastic disease they may become an increasing problem for patients and their families. The presence of moderate respiratory symptoms is present in up to 70% of advanced or terminal cases. Acute and severe dyspnea are evident in 10 – 63% of terminal cases, with frequency and severity increasing right before death [44].

Dyspnea is considered prognostic of short survival and may be associated with a variety of factors including the tumor itself, therapy, and concomitant diseases (chronic obstructive pulmonary disease, congestive heart disease, pleural effusion, bronchial pneumonia).

From the pathophysiologic and pathogenetic point of view, the following conditions occur: (a) An increase in the respiratory effort to overcome the mechanical burden (obstructive or restrictive pulmonary disease, pleural effusion); (b) An increase in the proportion of respiratory muscles required to maintain a normal respiratory burden in the presence of neuromuscular weakness, malnutrition, asthenia, or cachexia; (c) an increase in the respiratory frequency to compensate for hypoxemia, hypercapnia, metabolic acidosis, or anemia.

Pharmacologic and nonpharmacologic approaches are used for the therapeutic and symptomatic treatment of dyspnea. These approaches include:

- *General support and counseling* (supportive care): these can be effective relaxing techniques mainly if there is a component of anxiety in the genesis of dyspnea;
- *O₂ therapy:* oxygen therapy can alleviate symptoms in some patients, although its role is controversial and dyspnea may not necessarily be correlated with hypoxia. A general consensus has not been reached about the use or value of this treatment especially in non-hypoxic patients. When used, for a high flow rate for a brief period is recommended;
- *Blood transfusion:* the subjective improvement in well-being (which is not linked to the severity of dyspnea or exertion) resulting from transfusion has been reported in more than 50% of terminal cancer patients. Although there may not be a clear correlation with the pre-transfusion hemoglobin levels, its efficacy is doubtful in patients with hemoglobin levels >8 g/dl. In patients who respond, efficacy is observed one or two days after treatment and may be maintained for two weeks. Yet, the data are still poor and contradictory;
- *Erythropoietin:* recombinant human erythropoietin (r-HuEPO) is an effective treatment, mainly in patients undergoing chemotherapy with platinum-containing agents. However, its effectiveness in terminal patients is limited by the high treatment cost and by the long period before a significant improvement is observed (4 or 6 weeks);
- *Systemic opioids:* systemic opioids have a respiratory depressant effect and hence their use should be discontinued in the presence of respiratory problems. Yet clinical experience shows that often they cannot be substituted or interrupted due to the presence of persistent pain. When terminal dyspnea occurs in a conscious patient who experiences a feeling of suffocation and imminent death, terminal sedation may be appropriate. In this case sedation is obtained with continuous intravenous infusion of benzodiazepines (midazolam).

When terminal rales and tachypnea occur concomitantly with dyspnea, the anticholinergic drugs hyoscine methylbromide or hyoscine hydrobromide are recommended via continuous intravenous or subcutaneous administration.

Hiccups are a respiratory reflex caused by the spasmodic contraction of one or both hemidiaphragms, and resulting in a quick inhalation in the presence of closed vocal chords. Accessory respiratory muscles are sometimes involved [45]. The most frequent cause is gastric over-inflation. After excluding "squashed stomach syndrome", diaphragmatic or phrenic irritation resulting from a tumor should be considered [46]. Its incidence is not known, but in palliative medicine a small number of people seem to require symptomatic treatment. Occasionally it accompanies brain and esophageal tumors. Hiccups are considered a pathologic symptom since its functionality is not recognized. Its temporal association with eating suggests that its purpose may be to enhance esophageal motility. It is more frequent in adults than in children. The reflex arc that results in hiccups includes: (a) *Afferent nerves*: the phrenic nerve, vagal nerve, and/or thoracic sympathetic fibres; (b) *Central connectors:* although a specific center has not been identified, there appears to be an interconnection at the brainstem level which includes the respiratory centers and phrenic nerve nuclei, and the reticular substance and thalamic nuclei; and (c) *Efferent nerves*: the phrenic nerve seems to predominate.

Stimulation of the nasal part of the pharynx can produce symptom regression. It is most often done by inserting a nasogastric tube, but the same result can be obtained by stimulating the anterior part of the palate at the midline with a cotton wool for a minute. Chlorpromazine is also often used and acts as a depressor of the reticular brainstem without peripheral action on gastric distension [47].

5.5. Skin Problems

Ulcerations and decubitus represent the principal skin problems in cancer patients. These problems are usually associated with extension of the primitive tumor to the skin, side effects of surgery, radiotherapy and chemotherapy, long duration of bed confinement, and the presence of stomas.

Pressure ulcers are common in terminal cancer patients [48] and are caused by a combination of moisture, pressure, friction and shear. Further risk factors are fecal and urinary incontinence, bed confinement, and hypoalbuminemia. Adequate management consists in reduction of pressure on the affected area, debridement of necrotic tissue, regular wound cleaning and changing of dressing, and treatment of underlying factors if possible. In the late phase, applying a hydrocolloid dressing (e.g., Duoderm) can help prevent spreading and promote healing. If the wound is infected and life expectancy is short, basic maintenance with saline-soaked gauze applied loosely in the wound and changed three times daily is recommended.

The development and nature of both early and delayed cutaneous and subcutaneous lesions following radiotherapy depend on several factors concerning the characteristics of the treatment (i.e., absorbed dose, number of treatments, total duration, radiation quality, and field amplitude) and on the patient (i.e., anatomic site and individual sensitivity).

Concerning usual treatments, skin alterations are more frequent after X-ray therapy or techniques using quick electron beams, while they are rare after techniques involving high-energy photon radiation (telecobalt radiotherapy, linear accelerator).

There are two major types of reactions following radiotherapy:

a) *Precocious reactions* that include erythema, desquamation or dry epidermolysis, residual pigmentation, and temporary loss of hair. Although these are common phenomena, they are not clinically important since they are almost always reversible. In contrast, exudative epidermolysis (destruction of basal epithelium with exposure of the dermis) is of great clinical importance since restitution of the dermal layers takes several weeks during which the risk of infective complications is high. If such complications do occur, it requires additional treatment, prolongs the period required for restitution, and may result in dystrophic and retracting scars. Only with high doses of therapy do the irreversible alterations of the dermal adnexa arise: definitive depilation and destruction of sebaceous glands with subsequent dryness of the skin.

   b) *Delayed reactions* that include dyschromias, skin and adnexa atrophy, teleangiectasiae, edema, and subcutaneous fibrosis. Usually, these reactions represent manifestations that are not of clinical significance, but they can become important from the esthetic point of view.

Necrosis can develop after high doses of therapy, and may occur precociously or after some delay. Its presence is consistent with formation of easily removable eschars and with difficult and often incomplete dermal restitution. These reactions, however, are infrequent, but when they do occur they are extremely painful, tend to worsen, are prone to infection and relapse, and present a risk for secondary tumor development.

Reactions of hypersensitivity and release of intermediary inflammatory substances from narcotic cells can occur after chemotherapy or as a result of toxic drugs acting directly on the skin, and may cause alopecia, extravasation necrosis, ungual dystrophy, and folliculitis.

5.6. Bone Metastasis and Vertebral Fractures

Theoretically every malignant tumor can produce bone metastasis and consequently, according to the circumstances, can provoke pathologic fractures. The tumors that most often have these effects are breast cancer, multiple myeloma, lung cancer, prostate cancer, and kidney cancer. The bones most often affected are the femur, vertebral column (85% of spinal involvement is due to extradural spinal compression resulting from vertebral body metastasis), cranial theca, and the thoracic cage. Regardless of the radiologic characteristics of the lesion (lithic, thickening, or mixed), there is a weakening of the bone structure. Life expectancy after a bone fractures is associated with the type of tumor: bronchial cancer, 0 % to 6 months; prostate cancer, >50% survival at 24 months; breast cancer, as long as 3-5 years; cancer of any origin with spinal compression, 30-60 days.

There are three therapeutic approaches: (1) Orthopedic treatment – it is designed to prevent imminent fractures and control pain when a fracture does occur. It may include plaster casts, collars, corsets, prosthetic devices, and stabilization with endomedullary nailing, laminectomy, and corporectomy, depending on the site and type of lesion; (2) Localized radiotherapy – it consists of a brief cycle of low-dose radiotherapy and it is designed to obtain greater pain control, especially in cases of combined bone metastasis and bone pain [49]; (3) Pharmacologic therapy - is based on administring bisphosphonates (clodronate, pamidronate), which were shown to reduce and delay non-vertebral skeletal complications of bone metastasis caused by breast cancer and multiple myeloma. They also seem to have an analgesic effect and their use is associated with a reduction in the plasma calcium levels.

5.7. Care of the Oral Cavity

The risk, intensity and complications of stomatitis depend on poor oral hygiene, poor nutrition, previous radiotherapy especially in the cervico-facial region, chronic oral infections, smoking and excessive use of alcohol. Attention to symptoms reported by the patient can help to recognize the presence of oral problems. If odynophagy is reported at the pharyngeal-esophageal level, mucositis should also be considered. Any accurate objective exam of the oral cavity should refer to the state of the tissues and the level of oral hygiene and is to be done in the absence of prostheses. All patients must be informed about appropriate oral hygiene (toothbrush, dental floss, mouthwashes, care of prosthesis) in order to avoid mucositis.

The treatment of mucositis depends on its severity. In mild cases (erythema, irritation, burning sensation, dryness of oral cavity and increase in acid sensitivity), the usual oral hygiene regimen suffices and should be performed at least every 2-4 hours. In moderate or serious cases (ulcerations, pain, diffused mucosal phlogosis and decrease in salivation), it is essential to avoid infections, alleviate the patient's suffering and enable eating [50] by performing oral hygiene every two hours with a soft bristle toothbrush for as long as it is tolerated.

The choice of mouthwash depends on the state of the oral cavity tissues and on tolerability to the oral hygiene tools. A mouthwash composed of hydrogen peroxide dissolved 1:4 in water or normal saline, followed by a single mouthwash with only water or sodium bicarbonate is effective. Adding a teaspoon of sodium bicarbonate to 250-500 ml of normal saline or water produces a mouthwash that is particularly effective against mucus, scabs or other debris.

Washing with a jet of water or a sterile syringe is effective in patients who are unable to perform mouthwashes or gargling themselves. Other types of mouthwash currently used are solutions with lidocaine and nystatin; bicarbonate 5% (250 ml) plus nystatin (100 ml) plus nonalcoholic chlorhexidine 0.12% (100 ml); lidocaine 2% plus magnesium hydroxide plus difenidrina in equal parts. The lips should be kept moist and clean. If there are scabs on the lips, cleaning with small gauze tampons soaked in a solution of sodium bicarbonate or hydrogen peroxide is recommended. Gelatin, artificial saliva or vaseline can be used to keep lips moist.

Patience, precise information and active support are required to ensure compliance regarding oral care. A compromised nutritional state, poor oral hygiene, steroid therapy and neutropenia represent well-known factors that increase the incidence and severity of oral infections.

6. CONCLUSION

Palliative care is a developing discipline that while tagetting the patient as a whole deals with an ever-increasing set of problems and medical domains. Yet, pain alleviation remains at the core of its concerns from a medical and psychological points of view in their broadest sense.

7. REFERENCES

[1]   George RJ, Jennings AL. Palliative medicine. *Postgrad Med J* 1993;69:429-49.

[2]   Johnston G, Abraham C. The WHO objectives for palliative care: to what extent are we achieving them? *Palliat Med* 1995;9:123-37.

[3]   Kubler-Ross E. *Death – The final stage of growth.* Prentice Hall, inc. Englewood Cliffs, New Jersey, 1975.

[4]   Beltrutti D. A "pitiful death": is it the response to a "painful life"? *Panminerva Med* 1994;36:97-100.

[5]   Johnson WJ, DiMartino MJ, Meunier PC, et al. Methotrexate inhibits macrophage activation as well as vascular and cellular inflammatory events in rat adjuvant induced arthritis. *J Rheumatol* 1988;15:745-9.

[6]   Rosenberg SA, Packard BS, Aebersold PM, et al. Use of tumor-infiltrating lymphocytes and interleukin-2 in the immunotherapy of patients with metastatic melanoma. A preliminary report. *N Engl J Med* 1988;319:1676-80.

[7]   Oh WK. Chemotherapy for patients with advanced prostate carcinoma: a new option for therapy. *Cancer* 2000;88(12 Suppl):3015-21.

[8]   Konski A, Feigenberg S, Chow E. Palliative radiation therapy. *Semin Oncol* 2005;32(2):156-64.

[9]   Hoskin PJ. Radiotherapy in symptom management. In: Doyle D, Hanks GWC, MacDonald N (Eds.) *Oxford Textbook of Palliative Medicine*, 2nd ed. Oxford University Press, Oxford, 1999.

[10]   Baum M et al. Surgical palliation. In: Doyle D, Hanks GWC, MacDonald N. (Eds.) *Oxford Textbook of Palliative Medicine*, 2nd ed. Oxford University Press, Oxford, 1999.

[11]   Levin ML, Berry JI, Leiter J. Management of pain in terminally ill patients: physician reports of knowledge, attitudes, and behavior. *J Pain Symptom Manage* 1998;15:27-40.

[12]   Simon KM, Miller SA; Cancer Centers of Florida. Pain management at the end of life. *J Am Osteopath Assoc* 2001;101(10):599-608.

[13]   Von Roenn JH, Cleeland CS, Gonin R, et al. Physician attitudes and practice in cancer pain management. A survey from the Eastern Cooperative Oncology Group. *Ann Intern Med* 1993;119:121-6.

[14]   Ross DD, Alexander CS. Management of common symptoms in terminally ill patients: Part I. Fatigue, anorexia, cachexia, nausea and vomiting. *Am Fam Physician* 2001;64(5):807-14.

[15]   Willems JL, LeFebvre RA. Peripheral nervous pathways in nausea and vomiting. In: Davis CJ, Lake-Bakaar GV, Grahame-Smith DG (Eds.) *Nausea and Vomiting: Mechanisms and Treatment.* Berlin, Springer-Verlag, 1986:56-64.

[16]   Milne RJ and Heel RC. Ondansetron. Therapeutic use as an antiemetic. *Drugs* 1991;41:574-95.

[17]   Twycross RG, Lack SA. *Control of Alimentary Symptoms in Far Advanced Cancer* Edinburgh, Churchill Livingstone, 1986.

[18]   Aird DW, Bihari J, Smith C. Clinical problems in the continuing care of head and neck cancer patients. *Ear Nose Throat J* 1983;62(5):230-43.

[19] Logeman J. *Evaluation and treatment of swallowing disorders* San Diego, College-Hill Press, 1983.

[20] Barbara L, Camilleri M, Corinaldesi R, et al. Definition and investigation of dyspepsia. Consensus of an international ad hoc working party. *Dig Dis Sci* 1989;34: 272-6.

[21] Levitt MD. Gastrointestinal gas and abdominal symptoms. *Pract Gastroenterol* 1983;7:6-12.

[22] Mitchard M, Harris A, Mullinger BM. Ranitidine drug interactions-a literature review. *Pharmacol Ther* 1987;32:293-325.

[23] Somogyi A, Gugler R. Drug interactions with cimetidine. *Clin Pharmacokinet* 1982;7:23-41.

[24] Cartwright A, Hockey L, Anderson JL. *Life before death*. London, Routledge & Kegan Paul, 1973.

[25] Roston, KV, Rodriguez, S., Hernandez, M., Bodey, GP. Diarrhea in patients infected with the human immunodeficiency virus. *Am J Med* 1989;86:137-8.

[26] Cotton PB. Nonsurgical palliation of jaundice in pancreatic cancer. *Surg Clin North Am* 1989;69:613-27.

[27] Runyon BA, Hoefs JC, Morgan TR. Ascitic fluid analysis in malignancy-related ascites. *Hepatology* 1988;8:1104-9.

[28] Deraco M, Santoro N, Carraro O, et al. Peritoneal carcinomatosis: feature of dissemination. A review. *Tumori* 1999;85:1-5.

[29] Tabbarah IIJ, Casciato DA. Malignant effusions. In: Haskell CM (Ed.) *Cancer Treatment* Philadelphia, W.B. Saunders, 1990:815-25.

[30] Callen PW, Marks WM, Filly RA. Computed tomography and ultrasonography in the evaluation of the retroperitoneum in patients with malignant ascites. *Journal of Computer Assisted Tomography* 1979;3:581-4.

[31] Covey AM. Management of malignant pleural effusions and ascites. *J Support Oncol* 2005;3(2):169-73.

[32] Gines P, Arroyo V, Rodes J. Treatment of ascites and renal failure in cirrhosis. *Baillieres Clin Gastroenterol* 1989;3:165-86.

[33] Pinto PC, Amerian J, Reynolds TB. Large-volume paracentesis in nonedematous patients with tense ascites: its effect on intravascular volume. *Hepatology* 1988;8:207-10.

[34] Becker G, Galandi D, Blum H. Malignant ascites: systematic review and guideline for treatment. *Eur J Cancer* 2006;42(5):589-97.

[35] Jones EA, Skolnick P. Benzodiazepine receptor ligands and the syndrome of hepatic encephalopathy. In: Popper H, Schaffner F (Eds.) *Progress in Liver Diseases*, Vol.9. Philadelphia: W.B. Saunders, 1990:345-70.

[36] Albrecht J, Jones EA. Hepatic encephalopathy: molecular mechanisms underlying the clinical syndrome. *J Neurol Sci* 1999;170:138-46.

[37] Adler DG, Baron TH. Endoscopic palliation of colorectal cancer. *Hematol Oncol Clin North Am* 2002;16(4):1015-29.

[38] Walsh HP, Schofield PF. Is laparotomy for small bowel obstruction justified in patients with previously treated malignancy? *Br J Surg* 1984;71:933-5.

[39] Lau PW, Lorentz TG. Results of surgery for malignant bowel obstruction in advanced, unresectable, recurrent colorectal cancer. *Dis Colon Rectum* 1993;36:61-4.

[40] Cozzi G, Gavazzi C, Civelli E, et al. Percutaneous gastrostomy in oncologic patients: analysis of results and expansion of the indications. *Abdom Imaging* 2000;25:239-42.

[41] Breitbart W. Psycho-oncology: depression, anxiety, delirium. *Semin Oncol* 1994;21:754-69.

[42] Van Loon RA. Desire to die in terminally ill people: a framework for assessment and intervention. *Health Soc Work* 1999;24:260-8.

[43] Fainsinger RL, MacEachern T, Hanson J, Bruera E. The use of urinary catheters in terminally ill cancer patients. *J Pain Symptom Manage* 1992;7:333-8.

[44] Fainsinger RL, Miller MJ, Bruera E, et al. Symptom control during the last week of life on a palliative acre unit. *J Palliat Care* 1991;7:5-11.

[45] Friedman NL. Hiccups: a treatment review. *Pharmacotherapy* 1996;16(6):986-95.

[46] Ripamonti C, Fusco F. Respiratory problems in advanced cancer. *Support Care Cancer* 2002;10:204-216.

[47] Smiths HS, Busracamwongs A. Management of hiccups in the palliative care population. *Am J Hosp Palliat Care* 2003;20(2):149-54.

[48] Eisenberger A, Zeleznik J. Care planning for pressure ulcers in hospice: the team effect. *Palliat Support Care* 2004;2(3):283-9.

[49] Falkmer U, Jarhult J, Wersall P, Cavallin-Stahl E A systematic overview of radiation therapy effects in skeletal methastases. *Acta Oncol* 2003;42:620-33.

[50] Aldred MJ, Addy M, Bagg J, Finlay I. Oral health in the terminally ill: a cross-sectional pilot survey. *Spec Care Dentist* 1991;11:59-62.

Part VII: Physical and Complementary Approaches

In: The Handbook of Chronic Pain   ISBN 978-1-60021-044-0
Editors: S. Kreitler, D. Beltrutti, et al., pp. 401-421   © 2007 Nova Science Publishers, Inc.

Chapter 22

Use of Electricity and Other Physical Agents For Chronic Pain Relief[1,2,3]

Michaela Bercovitch and Abraham Adunsky

INTRODUCTION

Pain is one of the most widespread symptoms. It is estimated that one of every four people is affected by pain each year. When the pain state outlasts the initial trauma subsequent recovery period, the multidimensional aspects of the pain experience become evident. Pain as a chronic sign has both physical psychological manifestations, affects not only the individual but also his or her entire family close friends (Newton, 1987).

In 1979 the subcommittee on taxonomy of the International Association for the Study of Pain (IASP), defined pain as "a sensory emotional experience associated with actual or potential tissue damage or described in terms of such damage." (Merskey and Bogduk, 1994).

While acute pain is like a protective mechanism of some physical damage caused by a traumatic or presently occurring stimulus, chronic pain is a continuous feeling of an unpleasant sensation, even if the pathological cause has healed. The patients suffering from chronic pain are dominated by their pain. They are ready to use any medication or technical strategies to overcome their suffering. Chronic pain is the most difficult symptom to control not only because of the presence of physical damage but also because of its psychological implications.

---

[1] Michaela Berkovitch, MD. is senior physician and Information and Research Coordinator at the Hospice, Sheeba Hospital, Tel-Hashomer, Israel. Tel. +972-3-5341134 (office), +972-3-9772826 (home), +972-53-414494 (mobile).

[2] Abraham Adunsky, MD, is Director of Geriatric Institute, Sheeba Hospital, Tel-Hashomer, Israel; Tel. +972-3-5303411 (office), +972-3-5409224 (home), +972-58-546540 (mobile)

[3] The section on *Special Physiotherapy Methods* was written by Shulamith Kreitler, Department of Psychology, Tel-Aviv University, Tel-Aviv 69978, Israel; Tel. +972-3-6973874 (office), +972-3-5227185 (home), +972-544-526434 (mobile)

Even if drugs remain the first line in the treatment of chronic pain, the use of other pain relieving strategies is also essential, especially within the framework of a more comprehensive program of rehabilitation. As pain has always been a part of the human experience, trying to alleviate pain is part of being human (Meryl, 1992). This chapter is designed to present an overview of possible techniques and major physical interventions for the relief of chronic pain and for the patient's rehabilitation.

TRANSCUTANEOUS ELECTRICAL NERVE STIMULATION (TENS)

One of the earliest "recorded" methods for treating pain by electricity comes from Ancient Egypt. Drawings from the time of the Fifth Dynasty (2500 BC) depict the use of Malapterurus Electricus, a fish with electrical properties, for treating pain. The first written record of the use of electricity for pain treatment was attributed to Scribonius Largus (46 AD) (Schonoch, 1912-1913). In 1759 John Wesely described the use of electrotherapy for the pain of sciatica, headache, gout and kidney stones (Wesely, 1760). Two centuries later, Sarlandière applied the electrical stimulus to acupuncture points for treating rheumatic pain, pain of gout, neuralgia and migraine headaches (Sarlandière, 1825). Galvanic currents were used during the 18th and 19th centuries, but in the 20th century the electroanalgesic became very popular and was applied successfully in highly diverse situations, ranging from dental extractions to labor pain and even in amputations (Burton, 1975).

According to the prevalent view based on Descartes' approach, the body was considered as a machine that could be studied by Gallilean methods, the psychological aspects of pain were ignored and the brain was attributed only a "passive role" as a simple "receptor". This view was replaced by Melzack and Wall's (1965) new Gate Control theory, which considered the brain and the psychological factors acting as one unit and as dynamic and integral parts of the whole pain process. In line with this theory it was postulated that by a low electrical stimulus, the larger A delta fibers would be preferentially activated and because of their relatively low electrical threshold, would subsequently activate the small interneurons of the substantia gelatinosa Rolando. In this way the nociceptive input of the small fibers would be reduced (Shealy et al., 1967).

According to the conception of the "central control trigger" introduced by Melzack and Cassey (1968), dorsal column stimulation and spinothalamic stimulation may activate the descending inhibitory pathways from the reticular limbic system, and this may modify the sensory input at the level of dorsal horn.

The explanation provided for the action of transcutaneous electrical nerve stimulation (TENS) is the following: By stimulation of large afferent fibers of the "central control trigger" TENS may modulate the input through the descending pathways. The descending mechanisms can in turn modify the sensory input at the levels of dorsal horn. Basbaum and Fields (1978) described the opioid-mediated inhibitory pathways from the nucleus reticularis gigantocellularis through the periappeductal gray nuclei at the dorsal horn. The afferent input from small fibers is transmitted through ascending pathways to the thalamus and the nucleus reticularis gigantocellularis. By stimulating of the periapeductal gray it is possible to generate analgesia. Basbaum and Fields (1978) hypothesized that TENS may act by excitation of the brain stem nuclei.

Based on the Gate Control theory, Shealy tried in 1967 to control intractable back pain by stimulating the dorsal column in cats and in the same year successfully implanted the first cord stimulator in a patient's dorsal column (Shealy et al, 1967). This was the first time that a prototype of TENS was used for the treatment of pain. From this time began the worldwide development of TENS machines, operated by small batteries.

TENS Units

The simple TENS machine consists of a hand held battery-operated unit with an electrical pulse stimulator and electrodes. The commercial apparatus has three different pulse patterns: continuous, burst (pulsed) and modulated (ramped). Using these patterns can produce a cyclic variation of pulse, duration, frequency or amplitude. Nowadays there are many different models of TENS, some using single channel devices, some using multi-channels ones. The latter model requires an electrical outlet connection. TENS for pain treatment may use low frequency (LF) – 1-4 Hz or high frequency (HF) – 120-150 Hz.

The recommended TENS for a mobile patient is a small single or dual–channel unit (~5.5cm, weight ~60gr) equipped with clips that permit attachment of the apparatus to clothing. These types are less powerful and are recommended for chronic pain.

The area for the placement of electrodes is usually decided by the nature, location and structural source of the pain. There are charts indicating the dermatomal trigger points and acupuncture points.

Indications for Using TENS

Even though there are still not enough evidence-based indications regarding TENS efficacy, there are a lot of chronic pain conditions that TENS may alleviate (see Table 1). In some of these conditions TENS was used as a single agent or as complementary therapy.

Dysmenorrhea. Pain during menstruation is believed to be caused by the presence of prostaglandines in the menstrual fluid. That may cause hyperexcitability of the myometrium which in turn causes uterine ischemia. The recommended treatment may be the use of prostaglandines synthetic inhibitors. TENS may be considered a non-pharmacological alternative at least for those women who cannot use these drugs.

Manheimer and Wallen (1985) compared a group receiving conventional TENS with another group receiving placebo. The placement of the electrodes was at the level of the umbilicum and superior anterior spine. The used setup was an intensity of 125 Hz at a frequency of 30 microseconds. A significant and longer pain relief was observed in the group receiving TENS.

Kaplan et al. (1994) used conventional TENS by placing the electrodes in a triangle position T2 dermatome and T10 – T11 dermatome. They reported in 59% moderate pain relief, in 31.2% total pain relief and in only 10% of patients no response. Comparing the efficacy of TENS with that of Naproxen showed a significant pain relief for both (Milson et al., 1994).

Table 1. Chronic Pain Conditions

AFTER INJURIES
Whiplash injury
Extension flexion injury
Arthritis of cervical spine
Cervical root syndrome
Cord tumors
Joint pain of haemophilia

DEAFFERENTIATION PAIN
Phantom limb pain
Trigeminal neuralgia
Postherpetic neuralgia

CENTRAL PAIN
Injuries
Tumors of spinal cord, brainstem, thalamus

VASCULAR PAIN
Arterial insufficiency
Raynaud's syndrome
Thrombophlebitic pain
Headaches (from vascular origin - Migraine)

CANCER PAIN
Metastatic bone pain
Neuropathic pain
Visceral pain

BLADDER PAIN

PANCREATIC PAIN

PSYCHOGENIC PAIN

OTHER PAIN CONDITIONS
Contractures
Wounds
Fractures
Venous stases – treatment
Venous stases – prevention
Pruritus
Lymphoedema

Low back pain. This is one of the most common medical conditions that affects modern society because in addition to pain it involves disability, loss of working days and financial cost. In their study about the application of TENS for treating low back pain Deyo et al. (1990) used three randomized groups: one got TENS alone, another got TENS in association with exercise, and the third got sham TENS. The findings showed that true TENS and sham TENS did not differ significantly in their effects, and that exercise was a better treatment for reducing low back pain than TENS alone.

In another pseudo-randomized control trial, 42 patients with chronic low back pain were divided into three groups: one got TENS, another got placebo and a third group served as control. Pain severity was assessed by means of the VAS, 3 days after initializing the treatment. The electrodes were posed in a dermatomal position and the TENS was performed for 30 minutes, twice a week for ten weeks. The findings showed that in the TENS group reduction of pain and unpleasantness was significantly greater than in the other groups (March et al., 1993).

Diabetic neuropathic pain. Somers and Somers (1999) published a case report about a 73-years old woman with neuropathic pain in her left lower extremity. By placing electrodes of TENS in her lumbar area, pain reduction of 38% was obtained in the first day and pain reduction of 100% after 17 days of 20 minutes daily treatment.

A positive palliative effect of TENS was demonstrated in a study with 31 patients diagnosed with painful neuropathy of both lower extremities secondary to type 2 diabetes (Kumar and Marshal, 1997). The patients were randomly assigned to one of two treatments: true TENS and sham TENS. In the true TENS group all analgesic therapy was discontinued when using TENS. TENS treatment continued for 30 minutes daily for each leg during one month. There was a significant reduction in pain scores in the group that got true TENS. The differences between the groups of true TENS and sham TENS were strengthened by the findings that when sham TENS patients who had experienced no pain relief were switched to true TENS, they reported reduction in pain. However, upon discontinuation of true TENS in either group, pain increased again. The investigators concluded that because the disease process is ongoing TENS is merely a palliative method of treatment.

Myofacial pain syndrome. One study showed that applying four different forms of TENS to trigger points of patients with myofacial pain led to pain reduction after 10 minutes of treatment in all groups. The group whose response to treatment was largest was the one whose level of pain had been highest prior to treatment (Graft-Radford et al., 1998). In another study TENS and conservative therapy (i.e., ibufen, bite plate, self physiotherapy) were used as single blind trial with 10 patients suffering from myofacial pain. True TENS and sham TENS were compared during 14 weeks. Pain was assessed on the VAS before and after the TENS applications. The findings showed that TENS did not increase the syndrome release (Kruger et al., 1998).

Phantom limb pain. Katz and Melzack (1991) compared auricular low frequency and high intensity TENS with placebo in a controlled crossover study with three types of patients: patients with phantom limb pain, patients with phantom limb but no phantom pain, and patients with no phantom limb at all. In the group with a painful phantom limb the reduction in pain intensity following TENS was significantly higher than following placebo.

Orofacial pain. Metha et al. (1994) used TENS in stimulation of the Gasserian ganglion and tried to treat pain from central origin (stroke), trigeminal pain and post herpetic pain. The therapy was successful in those patients with central damage post stroke (in 5 out from 7 patients there was pain reduction).

Cancer pain. Applying TENS with low frequency in 3 patients with severe cancer pain in the head and neck, led to excellent pain control (Bauer, 1983).

Other Types of TENS

Following the successful implantation of the spinal cord stimulation by Shealy, different patterns of electrical stimulation for pain relief were developed. Major among these are acupuncture-like TENS, percutaneous electrical stimulation and deep brain stimulation.

Acupuncture-like TENS (ALTENS). This treatment technique is based on administering a low frequency and high intensity stimulus at the classical Chinese acupoint (Wang, 1997) without using needles. The electrical stimulus produces paraesthesia and muscle contraction. The mechanism of action is thought to be via descending inhibitory pathways. The onset of analgesia is delayed and lasts longer than in the case of conventional simple TENS (Paul et al., 1999). Gadsby and Floverdew (1996) selected out of the Cohrane data base 28 studies using TENS and ALTENS versus placebo in patients with low back pain. A review of these studies showed that the use of ALTENS for chronic back pain is seven times more effective than placebo in reducing pain.

Percutaneous electrical stimulation (PENS). PENS employs another technique of using electricity for pain treatment. By electrical stimulation of the spinal cord using percutaneously inserted electrodes in the epidural space (TOUHY NEEDLE) good control of intractable chronic low back pain and cancer pain was obtained (North et al., 1997). More recently, this technique consisted of inserting 32 gauge acupuncture needles into the soft tissues and muscles, and stimulating electrically the peripheral nerve fibers in the area of the sclerotomes, myotomes, or dermatomes corresponding to the patients' pain (Ahmed et al., 2000; Ghoname et al., 1999a; Ghoname et al., 1999b; Hamza et al., 2000).

The advantage of PENS seems to be the bypass of the skin resistance and transmission of the electrical stimulus to the immediate peripheral nerve endings located in the soft tissues, muscle and periosteum.

The pain generated by bony metastases may be an indication for the use of PENS in cancer patients (Ahmed, 1998). A good response to TENS treatment is affected by the location (White et al., 2000), frequency (Ghoname et al., 1999b) and duration of electrical stimulus application (Hamza et al., 1999). In conclusion, these studies demonstrate that the best combination for pain relief is a mixed frequency of 15 Hz with 30 Hz during 30–40 minutes.

Spinal cord stimulation. After 30 years of clinical use, even though still controversial, spinal cord stimulation may be considered as one of the most important techniques for alleviating a variety of intractable pain syndromes, such as pain in peripheral vascular disease (Kumar et al., 1998), peripheral neuropathy (Lang, 1997), intractable angina pectoris (Fanciuno et al., 1999), chronic pain caused by mesenteric ischemia (Ceballos et al., 2000), chronic regional pain syndrome (Lang, 1997), as well as pain after unsuccessful lumbar or cervical surgery (Kumar et al., 1998).

The proposed mechanism for electrical spinal cord stimulation is based on the gate control theory (Melzack and Wall, 1965). By closing the gate at the level of the dorsal column of the spinal cord no more impulses are transmitted via "C" fibers, so that "the pain transmission is blocked". Further mechanisms that were proposed more recently include, for example, inhibition of sympathetic afferents, or activation of the descending pain modulation pathways (Pomeranz, 1981).

The technique of spinal cord stimulation for the treatment of chronic pain consists of two stages (White et al., 2001): (a) Trial placement of electrodes and testing by use of an external stimulator; and (b) Permanent implantation of the electrical device.

Even though the technique is simple, some complications can occur, such as infections, bleeding, fibrosis and some technically related failures as electrode dislocation, breaking of leads, or battery failure. In addition, the possibility of tolerance development was described in the literaure (Kumar and Pineda, 1999).

However, a search of the literature shows that spinal cord stimulation may be a good alternative for patients with intractable chronic pain syndromes. Yet, one must remember that it is an analgesic procedure with potentially serious side effects. Hence, it should be reserved only for the most serious cases of severe pain.

Magneto Therapy

Magnetic stimulation could be considered as one of the methods of electrical stimulation for pain relief. Even if the pain inhibiting mechanism is not well known, it is thought that application of transcranial magnetic stimulation acts by inhibiting the cerebral blood flow in the ipsilateral thalamus, orbito frontal and cyngulate gyri and the upper brain stem (Peyron et al., 1995). In addition, Garcea et al. (1999) support the idea that by thalamic activation, a synaptic cascade is produced in pain related parts of the brain by receiving afferents. Moreover, by activation under magnetic effects of cyngulate and orbito frontal structures, descending inhibition is produced. In another study the effects of transcranial magnetic stimulation of the motor cortex at high frequencies (more than 1Hz) were compared with the effects of sham treatment. The participants were 12 patients with intractable chronic pain and controls. Magnetic stimulation produced pain relief, but the results were not statistically significant (Rolnic et al., 1999). Further studies are needed in order to demonstrate the therapeutic non-invasive action of the magnetic stimulation.

Concluding Remarks About Electrical Stimulation

In conclusion, after this short review of the use of electricity for treatment of chronic pain syndromes,we can affirm that even though the literature is not so rich is sometimes even contradictory, these techniques may be considered as valuable complementary options to drug therapy. There is a compelling need for future research to elucidate the mechanisms responsible for electroanalgesia as well as of well controlled methodological studies to prove the benefit of these methods and the best way of their application.

Thermal Therapy

Thermal therapy consists in the use of thermal agents for pain relief. Even though these agents are used in rehabilitation and for chronic pain treatment, the underlying mechanisms accounting for their effects are unknown. However, several techniques using high or low temperatures for treating chronic pain are known.

Heat Therapy

For centuries applying heat has been a modality for treating pain caused by trauma and muscle spasm. It is well known that warmth is associated with relaxation. Beyond that, heat entails physiological effects, such as increasing blood flow, altering metabolic activity, increasing neural response, improving skeletal muscle activity and acting on the physical properties of collagen-tissues (Abramson et al., 1961a).

Increasing the tissue temperature produces vasodilatation, thus raising the blood flow in one specific area. But there are different possibilities of accounting for the manner in which this change may have an effect at the level of skin or skeletal muscles. Since skin is the most important preserver of constant body temperature, it is known that it has a unique "architecture" of vessels and arterio-venous anastomoses. A reflex activation of temperature receptors may activate a circulation of warmed blood through vasodilated vessels to the preoptic region of the hypothalamus. Therefore, warmth may be a relieving possibility for pain in the areas of hands, feet, and face (Berne and Levy, 1981).

On the other hand,, changes of blood flow of the skin, by stimulation of thermoreceptors may conduct to a vassoactive relieving mediator (i.e., prostaglandines or histamine) and/or kallicreine from the sweat glands. Kallicreine may act on production of bradikinine. In this way it may produce an increased permeability of capillaries of smooth muscles, increasing the interstitial fluid and causing a mild local edema (Milnar, 1974). The vasodilating effect of the temperature may evoke a spinal cord reflex which causes a decrease of sympathetic nerve activity in the smooth muscles of the blood vessels. In this way the response is not only limited to the application area but may produce a response in other areas too. Thus, for example, in peripheral vascular disease, application of warmth in the area of the low back may have a positive effect on the feet (Abramson et al., 1961b)

The effect of heat on raising the pain threshold was first described by Lenman et al. (1958). In this way pain may be reduced before exercises active or passive joint mobilization techniques. Chastain (1978) demonstrated that by using a deep heating agent isometric strength may be decreased.

The therapeutic action of heat applications depends on the intensity, duration the nature of the theramal medium used.

It is indicated to use thermal techniques in chronic pain after neurological trauma, joint pain or painful muscle spasms.

Heat Agents

Therapeutic hear agents differ in whether they act through deep heating or superficial warmth. Deep heating modalities increase temperature to depth of 3-5 cm and consist in converting another form of energy to heat, for example, electrical currents in shortwave diathermy, and coustic vibration in ultrasound heating. All these modalities require special equipment and trained professionals.

Superficial heating modalities increase temperature of tissues and produce the largest effect at 0.5 cm ior less from the skin's surface. The common means are hot pack, hot water bottle, moist compress, heating pads (electric, chemicals or gel pack), hydrotherapy (e.g. heated pool or whirlpool), infrared lamps (sunlamps), and paraffin wax. The superficial heating means are by far more common and can readily be used at home.

Paraffin. Paraffin is one of the most commonly used techniques for heat application. Paraffin is usually mixed with mineral oils that act to lower its melting point (54.5C). Paraffin treatment is used for application on the distal extremities. In such cases some indications are to be respected: (1) removing jewelry; (2) washing and drying the area; (3) spreading apart of the fingers; (4) dipping the hand or foot 8-10 times into the tank containing paraffin wax until they are covered by a solid paraffin glove; (5) wrapping the extremity in a plastic bag to prevent the heat from going out. If edema appears, it is recommended to elevate the extremity until the end of the treatment (6). Daily treatment for 3 weeks is recommended.

The hands or the feet are dipped into the liquid paraffin immediately removed to enable a cool of vax to form. Thus, 8-10 coats are created; then the hands or feet are wrapped first in a plastic bag, then in a blanket to contain the heat for about half an hour.

Paraffin wax heating is contraindicated in cases of wounds and infected skin.

Cold Therapy (or Cryotherapy)

Cold is another well-known agent for relieving pain not only in the acute phases of pain but also in chronic pain. Applying cold may be uncomfortable in the first few moments but soon leads to pain relief.

The most common indication for cryotherapy is musculo-skeletal pains following traumas. The first trial of treating pain with ice was done with patients who have undergone orthopedic procedures. Shaubel (1946) comared a group receiving ice packs over their soft caste for a 48 hour period with a group that had no ice packs. The findings showed a reduction in pain and also in analgesic intake following cold.

The underlying mechanism of cold therapy is not fully understood. It is assumed that localized disturbances in the blood flow lead to hypoxia and thus to accumulation of toxic metabolites. Lund et al. (1986) demonstrated a decrease in oxygen partial pressure in trapezius and brachioradialis muscles in those patients suffering from chronic muscle pain. All three proposed mechanisms are thought to be under sympathetic control (Bengtson and Bengtson, 1988).

Use of a cold pressor is a well recognized method of activating the sympathetic system (Maekawa et al., 1998; Shobel et al. 1995; Victor et al., 1987). Ice massage having as cold pressor a vapocoolant spray with fluori-methane was tried for alleviating pain in trigger point, myofacial and other different muscle pains.

Although it is a well-known utilized method in all pain centers, in recent years there has been little research of cold as a pain therapeutic modality.

Laser Therapy

Another accepted adjunct treatment in chronic pain is laser therapy. This method appears to be effective in treating myofacial pain, post traumatic joint pain, chronic low back pain, rheumatoid arthritis, etc. (Walker et al., 1987). Despite the worldwide use of low level laser therapy as a rehabilitation method and for the treatment for pain, the real mechanism of action remains unknown. Its beneficial action may be attributed to a photochemical effect that produces a biostimulatory action rather than to a temperature action on the treated tissues (Backsford, 1986). In vitro, Herbert et al. (1989) demonstrated that the use of a laser light at 820 nm may increase ATP levels, this action may be the trigger of re-energization of the cells. They pointed out that the ischemia of swollen points is caused by a decrease of adenosin triphosphate in the tissues which in turn may reduce capacity for biosynthesis.

There are some techniques known as lower gallium-aluminium-arsenide laser biotherapy 3 (Omega Universal Technologies), Q-switch neodymium laser, infrared laser, and He-Ne laser, which differ in parameters of wave lengths, energy density and time of exposition, but until today it is not clear which one is best.

To date there are only few studies of laser therapy. One study reported that a low energy laser therapy applied in the low back region may be effective for pain relief (Klein and Eek, 1990). But due to the limited number of participants the results are inconclusive.

So far the results of using different types of Laser with different doses and for very different pathologies have not been conclusive and the beneficial effect of this kind of therapy is still to be demonstrated by clinical research.

Hydrotherapy, Balneotherapy and SPA Therapy

The use of water as a therapeutic agent has been known already in antiquity. During the Hypocratic era water was considered a therapeutic measure for most diseases (Jakson, 1990). The Romans recommended it as an efficient therapeutic treatment for various orthopedic illnesses. Since the beginning of the 20th century the term hydrotherapy has become analogous with Bather therapy or spa therapy and comprises all the therapeutic measures using water.

The use of water as a therapeutic agent is based on principles similar to those underlying thermal therapy. Hydrotherapy differs from thermal therapy in that it covers a larger area of the body. Exposure of the whole body to water varying in temperatures has not only local effects but also systemic ones, for example, on the cardiovascular, renal and other systems.

The use of water as a therapeutic agent is based on the Archimedes principle of buoyancy: a body immersed in a liquid experiences an upward force equal to the weight of the displaced liquid (Nave and Nave, 1980) The hydrostatic force brings about relative pain relief by reducing loading and the water reduces the forces of gravity acting on painful and rheumatic joints (Simon Blotman, 1981).

The treatment is performed using whirlpool. All tanks require an ample supply of cold and hot water that may be mixed by a thermostatic control valve until the desired temperature is attained. The tanks may be of different sizes as a function of the treatment area – upper or lower extremities or full body immersion.

The main indications for hydrotherapy are in cases of arthritis, psoriatic rheumatoid arthritis, low back pain, and fibromyalgia.

Rheumatoid arthritis is one of the principal indications for full water therapy as complementary to pharmacological treatment because of its impact on the patients' quality of life. The pain is excruciating and disabling. Balneotherapy seems to be effective in significantly reducing their pain and enabling pain free movement (Elkayam et al., 1991; Sukenic et al., 1990, 1994).

Chronic low back pain remains a big yet unresolved medical and social problem Despite the development of pharmacological treatment, it seems to be inadequate in relieving the disabling pain improving the functional ability of these patients. A randomized controlled study of patients with low back pain found that spa therapy may reduce the pain and improve functional ability as well as the well being of the patients (Constant et al., 1998). Another study showed that these beneficial effects may last up to one year (Strauss-Blashe et al., 2000). However, a later conclusional work on effects of spa therapy on chronic pain concluded that the active therapies, such as exercise have a positive effect on pain and well-being but only for a short or medium term; the spa treatments, such as mud applications and massages have only short-term effects; only the spinal traction in thermal water appears to have a positive medium term effect in back pain (Strauss-Blashe et al., 2002).

Another indication for spa therapy may be ankylosing spondylitis. A randomized controlled trial in patients with ankylosing spondilitis showed that a three weeks' course of spa therapy combined with standard drug therapy and weekly group physical therapy has significant long term benefits as compared with standard treatment with drugs and weekly group physical therapy alone (Van Tubergen et al., 2001).

In conclusion, hydrotherapy and/or spa therapy remain controversial in the literature. More research is needed to understand the principal factors that bring about pain relief.

Physical Therapy and Rehabilitation

Chronic pain is considered nowadays as an illness because in addition to the physical injury it involves further factors, such as avoidance of activity, loss of self esteem, depression and fears of re-injury (Hazard, 1997). In addition to drug treatment for pain relief, it is thought today that one of the greatest challenges in treating chronic pain patients is returning them to normal activity (Deyo, 1998). If in previous years extended bed rest was the first therapeutic indication in pain management, today it is thought that a well-coordinated series of exercises and functional restoration programs will be the best addition to the drug therapy for returning the patient to his or her normal activity.

It is well-known that the positive influence of exercise activity on pain cannot be explained only through their physical effects. Physical activation of the patient brings about psychological benefits by way of improving transmission of noradrenaline, serotonin dopamine (Meeusen and De Meirleir, 1995) which are vital for control of mood. Gradually by improving the patient's sense of control and self-sufficiency, there is an increase in social reinforcement and diversion from pain anxiety, all of which benefit the patient's psychological status (Weyerer and Kupfer, 1994).

Koes et al. (1991) found that the majority of the studies reviewed (11 randomized controlled trials) used a combination of exercise and other therapies. Only two of these studies referred to exercise alone, as compared to placebo, and these studies concluded that single exercise therapy was not more efficacious than other conservative treatments but it was not shown to be ineffective (Manniche et al., 1988; Somers and Somers, 1999). In contrast, a review of 16 trials concluded that there is strong evidence that exercise is effective in the management of low back pain (Van Tulder, 1997). Comparing individual physiotherapy treatments and group exercises in patients with shoulder and neck pain showed that patients in both groups experienced improvement of symptoms, but preferred individual therapy (Wasseljen et al., 1995). Another review of studies showed no significant differences between groups receiving only exercise therapy in contrast with other forms of therapy (Aker et al, 1996).

Chronic shoulder pain may be another indication for exercise therapy. A search of the literature reveals controversial findings. A review of studies by Green et al. (1998) showed no difference between the use of active exercise alone other treatments in the management of adhesive capsulitis. By contrast, comparing a group with shoulder pain that got exercise as treatment with a non-treatment control group showed an improvement of pain in the treated group in contrast to deterioration in motion in the control group (Ginn et al., 1997).

Fibromyalgia is a syndrome defined by generalized pain accompanied by various symptoms in multiple body systems (Clauw, 1995). We found three studies that analyzed the role of exercise in the management of fibromyalgia. All studies showed positive effects in terms of pain assessment, functional status disability measures of the patients during the treatment period, but these achievements were not maintained over time (Burckhardt et al., 1994; McCain al., 1988; Wigers et al., 1996).

Massage

Massage is another therapeutic technique for pain management that has been known used in China Egypt for thousands of years (Ramsey, 1997). It is thought that massage provides a relaxation of muscles, increases endorphin release, enhances the blood flow to the affected area. Increasing blood flow in a painful area is assumed to decrease the concentration of pain mediators (Ernst and Fialka, 1994). Despite the common assumption of the beneficial results of massage, research support of these effects is scant. A systematic review of the literature on massage therapy for low back pain located four randomized clinical trials in which massage was used as a single therapy for low back pain (Ernst, 1999). According to one of these studies, massage was superior to no treatment; according to two of the studies, massage was equal to spinal manipulation and TENS; according to one study, massage was less effective than spinal manipulation. Further, an interesting demonstration project about massage in a geriatric population used a twice weekly touch massage for 12 weeks, assessing pain by the authors' own tools, on basis of weekly before and after massage. There was a slight decrease in pain scores of different etiologies as manifested in diminished requirements of analgesic drugs. Moreover, an analysis of the role of touching in reducing anxiety or agitation showed decrease of these symptoms but not for a long time period (Sansone and Schmitt, 2000)

Even though evidence based medicine is not sufficiently rich in data, it is generally thought that the effectiveness of massage therapy as a complementary method of treatment for pain control is unquestionable (Harris and Clauw, 2002). Yet, double blind randomized controlled studies are badly needed in this domain.

Special Physiotherapy Methods

In the framework of Western and Eastern cultures different specific methods have been developed and are currently applied for treating chronic pain. Some of the better known ones are the Feldenkrais method (Feldenkrais, 1977), chiropractice (Bergman and Peterson, 2002), the Alexander technique (Barlow, 1986), Pilates (Blount and McKenzie, 2003), Ring Muscles technique (Garbourg, 1994), osteopathy (Digiovanna and Dowling, 1997), reflexology (Kunz, 2003) and Shiatzu (Turk, 2001). Several principles are shared by these and similar techniques. First, they do not use drugs for treatment but only specific physical manipulations done by the individual passively or actively or actively-assisted, mostly without the application of mechanical devices. Secondly, the practitioners base themselves on a specific theory of the body, accounting for chronic pain by focusing on a specific location or organ of function in the body. Accordingly, therapy consists in correcting the specific malfunction. Thus, chiropractors focus on the spine, osteopaths on the joints, Pilates practioners on breathing and the torso musculature, reflexologists on the feet and hands, Shiatsu practitioners on blocked energy (Qi), and ring muscle therapists on the sphincter muscles all over the body. Thirdly, the specified malfunction is considered as the source not only of pain but also or mainly of many other ailments of body and soul. Thus, most of these techniques address a whole array of diverse disorders, some of which are not related to pain in any obvious way (e.g., eating disorders). Hence, correcting the malfunction is expected to bring about improvement in the individual's whole state and well-being. In this sense these approaches are holistic. Finally, a fourth characteristic shared by most of these techniques is that so far they are supported more by reputation and case reports than by studies that qualify as evidence. Three representative treatment methods will be described in some detail.

The Feldenkrais Method. Its major objective is to reduce pains originating in the skeletal muscles. It assumes that chronic pain is not a necessary evil but develops because of the loss of the innate capacity to move adequately, namely, in line with the requirements and structure of the body. Moving adequately entails considering (a) the dynamic relations between different parts of the body (mainly, pelvis vs. legs, pelvis vs. torso) and (b) the flow (mainly, moving in line with the natural path or trajectory vs. skipping phases straight to the goal).

There are several reasons why we have lost the capacity for proper movement:

1. Culture dictates specific forms of movement appropriate, for example, for particular age and gender groups while prohibiting others (e.g., moving the pelvis is considered indecent).
2. The structure of the environment imposes specific movements, for example, by means of furniture (e.g., sitting on chairs) and clothing.
3. Modeling and imitations of others.
4. The individuals' beliefs (e.g., minimizing movements because the body is inferior and deserves as little attention as possible) and emotions (e.g., constant fear causes contractions).
5. Problems and malfunctioning in any of the domains of life – social, behavioral, emotional or cognitive – which affect the functioning of the organism, viewed as a total bio-psycho-motional whole.

Improper movement requires more effort and leads to increase of tension first in the proximal muscles and later in the distal ones. The result is distorted effortful motion and constricted movement repertory that persevere and generate constant pain. Reinstating proper movement cannot occur by conscious decision but only through directed learning which will help to establish a simple and efficient organization of the body. It is useless to focus on the aching spot without attending to the underlying faulty organization. Recovery entails, for example, learning to distribute weight properly, attending not only to the aching body part but also to all body parts down to the tongue and the eyelids, considering the total organization, and exploring ways of moving easily, freely, and comfortably.

Healing and getting rid of pain are regarded as the result of learning and not of treatment. Learning is targeted toward enabling the construction of a new "correct" dynamic organization of the body. The learning-healing process starts with overcoming the bad movement habits (by relaxation and breathing exercises) and by minimizing gravity (i.e. lying on the floor which reduces greatly proprioceptive stimulation). The major part of the process consists in learning to move properly. The key terms are attaining "functional integration", using "awareness through movement" and pursuing exploratory variations constrained and facilitated by functional demands of the body and the environment.

Some of the principles of learning are demonstrating to the body the right movement by passive movement or by handling the other non-aching part of the body; letting the aching organ explore by trial and error the right way by initial tiny steps, in a context detached of any goal attainment; concentrating full awareness on the movement and analyzing it to uncover its components, which are then trained separately under different variations of contexts, sequences and spatial orientations; exploring the whole range of potentialities of an aching organ, when it moves alone but in unusual ways or in combination with other organs.

There are many studies, mostly descriptive of the method and its effects in specific cases (e.g., Jackson-Wyatt, 1992; Ruth et al., 1992).

The Alexander technique. Chronic pain is considered as the direct result of habitual muscular tension, caused by improper movements. Maintaining unnecessary muscular tension causes unbalance, distortion, compression and fatigue of the body. Healing consists in re-education designed not to learn new ways of movement but merely to unlearn the improper ways of moving. The basic principle is subtracting previously assumed required effort from movements one does in any context. The major tool of the learning is feeling oneself and one's body, while considering oneself as a total co-coordinated whole. The major emphasis is on unlearning the wrong habit, mainly by stopping to think and sense before responding by habitual movements to common stimuli. Habitual reactions are overcome by techniques, such as sidestepping, stalling, fatiguing the old reaction or otherwise tricking it. The key terms are "sensory adaptation" through habits, "inhibition" of habits, attention to "direction" as revelatory of physical functionality and performing with ease (or "do-lessness"). The result is regaining the natural ease, balance, support and motional freedom that children have.

Chiropractic treatments. Pain is assumed to be the result of biomechanical and structural derangements of the spine that affect the nervous system. When an injury, such as a fall or over-exertion occur, the inability of the spine to compensate may bring about a minor displacement or derangement of one or more vertebrae, which would cause irritation to spinal nerve roots through pressure or indirectly through reflexes. Hence, the goal of the treatment is to re-instate normal spinal mobility, which in turn reduces the irritation to the spinal nerve and/or re-establishes reflexes that may have undergone change.

"Subluxation" is the term used to denote the partial abnormal separation of the articular surface of the joint, which involves an alteration of the physiological and mechanical dynamics of contiguous structures, such as hyperemia, minute hemorrhages, atrophy, local ischemia, congestion, edema, and eventually rigidity and adhesions in the joint capsules themselves and also in ligaments, tendons and muscles. These changes can cause neural disturbances. Chiropractics identifies several types of subluxation, for example, static intersegmental subluxation (e.g., flexion or extension malposition) and kinetic intersegmental subluxation (e.g., hypomobility or aberrant motion). Since subluxation is a dynamic developing process, pains should be treated as early as possible after their occurrence.

Treatment consists in first identifying by palpation and other methods (e.g., X-rays) spinal segments that are hypomobile or fixated or otherwise function abnormally, and then applying "adjustment" designed to reduce subluxation. Adjustment consists of a high velocity, short lever arm thrust applied to a vertebra, often accompanied by an audible release of gas which reduces joint pressure (joint cavitation). The immediate response is often relief, but discomfort may also occur. Three types of treatment effects have been reported: (a) Sensory and motor effects (e.g., reduction of pain, reduced muscle spasm); (b) Sympathetic nervous system effects (e.g., increased blood flow, reduced blood pressure); and (c) Blood chemistry changes (e.g., increased secretion of melatonin and of plasma beta endorphines).

There are many studies, mostly descriptive of the method and its effects in specific cases (Hoffman et al., 1995) or assessing the benefits of chiropractics in conjunction with other treatments. Thus, a recent pilot study of 28 patients with neck pain showed that chiropractic spine manipulation together with prescription medications and self-care education led to over 75% improvement by self-report in 61% of the participants (Evans et al., 2003).

SOME CONCLUSIONS

The various reviewed methods share several characteristics. They have have been used for centuries and are still popular in different countries. This is all the more surprising because they do not adhere to the criteria of evidence-based medicine. There are many anecdotal and other reports of their beneficial effects, but little if any controlled studies supporting them. The effects seem often to be short-term, which may account for the continued application of the methods. They are non-invasive and mostly do not seem to be injurious or harmful. Moreover, in many cases it is possible to relate the methods to known or assumed physiological and medical effects, studied in other contexts. An important characteristic is that some of the methods and others at least in some form may be applied at home by the patients themselves. This turns them into a kind of self-help therapies that get easily assimilated into the recent cultural trends of patient empowerment, mobilization of so-called natural healing processes and cultivating "bodily intelligence". Needless to mention, serious controlled trials of these methods are badly in need.

REFERENCES

Abramson DI et al. (1961). Changes in blood flow – Oxygen uptake and tissue temperatures produced by the topical application on wheat heat. *Arch of Physical Medical Rehabilitation.* 42, 305.

Abramson DI, et al. (1961b).changes in blood flow, O2 uptake and tissue temperatures produced by therapeutical physical agents. Effect of indirect or reflex vasodilatation. *American Journal of Physical Medicine.* 404-405.

Ahmed HE, White PF, Craig WF et al. (2000). Use of percutaneous electrical nerve stimulation (PENS) in the short term management of headaches. *Headache. 40.* 311-315.

Ahmed HE, Craig WF, White PF, Hubert P.(1998) percutaneous electrical nerve stimulation (pens): a complimentary therapy for the management of pain secondary to bony metastasis. *Clinical Journal of Pain. 14,* 320-323.

Aker PD, Gross AR, Goldshmidt CH et al. (1996) Conservative management of mechanical neck pain : systematic overview and metaanalysis . *BMJ. 313,* 1291-1296.

Baksford JR. (1986). Low energy lasser-therapy treatment of pain and wounds : hype, hope or hokum. *Mayo Clin Proc.* 61, 671-675.

Basbaum AI, Fields HL (1978). Endogenous pain control mechanisms: review and hypothesis. *Annual Journal of Neurology.* 4.451.

Bauer W (1983) Electrical treatment of severe head and neck cancer pain. *Archives of Otolaryngology.109,* 382-383.

Bengtsson A, Bengtsson M (1988) Regional sympathetic blockade in primary fibromyalgia. *Pain. 33,* 161-167.

Berne R, Levy MN. (1981). Cardiovascular physiology. Ed 4. *Mosby CV, St Louis.*

Burckhardt CS, Mannercorpl K, Hedenbert L et al. (1994) A randomized, controlled clinical trial of education and physical training for women with fibromyalgia . *Journal of Rheumatology* . *21*,714-720.

Burton C (1975). Dorsal column stimulation: optimization of application. *Surgical Neurology. 4*, 169-177.

Ceballos A, Cabezudo L, Bovaira M et al. (2000). Spinal cord stimulation: a possible therapeutic alternative for chronic mesenteric ischemia. *Pain.87*, 99-101.

Chastain PB.(1978).The effect of deep heat on isometric strengh. *Physical Therapy*. 58-43.

Constant F, Gillemin F, Collin JF, et al . (1998). Use of spa therapy to improve the quality of life of chronic low back pain patients. *Medical Care. 36*, 1309-1314.

Clauw DJ. (1995). Fibromyalgia more than just a musculoskeletal disease. *American Family Physicians. 52*(3),843-851.

Deyo RA, Walsh NE, Martin DC, Schoenfield LS, Ramamurthy S. (1990). A controlled trial of transcutaneous electrical nerve stimulation (TENS) and exercise for chronic low back pain. N*ew England Journal of Medicine. 322*(23),1627-1634.

Deyo RA. (1998). Low back pain. *Sci Am. 279.* 48-53.

Digiovanna E, Dowling DD (1997)An ostheopathic approach to diagnosis and treatmant (2nd ed). Philadelphia, PA: Lippincott Williams and Wilkins.

Elkayam O, Wigler I, Tishler M et al. (1991). Effect of spa therapy in Tiberias in patients with rheumatoid arthritis and osteoarthritis. *Journal of Rheumatology. 18.* 1779-1803.

Ernst E, Fialka V. (1994). The clinical effectiveness of massage therapy – A critical review. *Forshe Komple Mentarmedicine. 1*, 226-232.

Ernst E. Massage therapy for low back pain: A systematic review. (1999). *Journal of Pain and Symptom Management. 17*(1), 65-69.

Fanciullo GJ, Robb JF, Rose RJ, Sanders JM Jr. (1999). Spinal cord stimulation for intractable angina pectoris. *Anesth Analg. 89,* 305-306.

Feldenkrais M (1977). The case of Nora: Body awareness as healing therapy. New York: Harper and Row.

Gadsby JG, Flowerdew MW. (1996). The effectiveness of Transcutaneous electrical nerve stimulation (TENS) and acupuncture like TENS (ALTENS) in the treatment of patients with low back pain. In Bombardier C, Nachemson A, Deyo Et Al, Eds GMSG *Book Module Of The Cohrane Data Base Of Systematic Review: Oxford : The Cohrane* .

Garbourg P (1994). Self healing "The secret of the ring muscles"(2nd ed). Fort Lauderdale, FL:Peleg Publishers.

Garcea L, Peyron L, Mertens P, Gregoire MC, Lavenne F, Laurent B. (1999). Electrical stimulation of the motor cortex for pain control: a combined PET scanand electrophysiological study. *Pain. 83,* 259-273.

Gemigniani G. (1991) Chronic low back pain in patients with ankylosing spondylitis a double blind study. *Arthritis Rheumatology 34,.* 788-789.

Ghoname EA, White PF, Ahmed HE, et al. (1999a).Percutaneous electrical nerve stimulation: An alternative to TENS in the management of sciatica. *Pain. 83.(2),* 193-199.

Ghoname EA, Craig WF, White PF et al. (1999b). The effect of stimulus frequency in the analgesic response to percutaneous electrical nerve stimulation in patients with chronic low back pain. *Anesth Analg. 88,* 841-846.

Ginn KA, Herbert RD, Knouw W et al. (1997). A randomized, controlled clinical trial of treatment for shoulder pain. *Physical Therapy.77*.802-a.

Graft-Radford SB, Reevers JL, Baker RL,Chiu D. (1989). Effects of transcutaneous electrical nerve stimulation on myofacial pain and trigger point sensitivity. *Pain . 37,* 1-5.

Green S, Buchbinder R, Glazzier R,et al. (1998). Systematic review of randomized controlled trials of interventions for painful shoulder: selection criteria, outcome assessment and efficacy. *British Medical Journal. 316,* 354-360.

Hamza MA, White PF, Craig WF et al.(2000).Percutaneous Electrical Nerve Stimulation (PENS): A novel analgesic therapy for diabetic neuropathic pain. *Diabetes Care. 23,* 365-376.

Hamza MA, Ghoname EA, White PF et al. (1999) Effect of the duration of electrical stimulation on the analgesic response in patients with chronic low back pain. *Anestiology*; *91.* 1622-1627.

Harris RE, Clauw D.(2002) The use of complimentary medical therapies in the management of myofacial pain disorders. In *Current Pain and Headache Reports, 6.* 370-374.

Herbert KE, Bhusate LL, Scott DL Diamantopoulos C. Perrt D. (1989). Effect of lasser light at 820nm on adenosine nucleotide levels in human lymphocytes. *Lasser Life science 3.* 37-45.

Hoffman, LE, Taylor JA, Price D, Gertz G. (1995). Diffuse idiopathic skeletal hyperostosis: a review of radiographic features and report of four cases. *Manipulative Physiology, 18,* (8), 547-553

Jakson R. Waters and spas in the classical world. (1990) *Medical History.(suppl) 10.* 1-13.

Kaplan B, Peled Y, Pardo J, et al . .(1994)Transcutaneous electrical nerve stimulation (TENS) as a relief for dysmenorrhea. *Clinical and Experimental Obstretics and Gynaecology. 21,* 87-90.

Katz J, Melzack R.(1991). Auricular transcutaneous electrical nerve stimulation (TENS) reduces phantom limb pain. *Journal of Pain and Symptom Management. 6, 20,* 73-83

Klein RG, Eek BC. (1990). Low energy lasser therapy exercise for chronic low back pain: Double –Blinded controlled trial. *Arch of Physical and Medical Rehabilitation .71,* 34-37.

Koes BW, Buter LM, BekermanH et al. (1991). Physiotherapy exercises and back pain: A blinded review. *British Medical Journal. 302,* 1572-1576.

Kruger LR, Van der LidenWJ, Cleaton-Jones PE. (1998). Treatment of myofacial pain dysfunction. *South African Jounal of Surgery. 36,* 35-38.

Kumar K, Toth C, Nath RK, Laing P. (1998). Epidural spinal cord stimulation for treatment of chronic pain: some predictors of success – A 15 years experience. *Surg Neurol 50,* 110-120.

Kumar K, Pineda A. (1999).Complications of dorsal column stimulation. *Journal of Neurosurgery Sciences, 43,* 285-293.

Kumar K, Marshall H. (1997) Diabetic peripheral neuropathy:amelioration of pain with Transcutaneous elecrostimulation. *Diabetes Care, 20,* 1702-1705

Lang P. (1997). The treatment of chronic pain by epidural spinal cord stimulation: A 15 years follow up-present status. *Axone, 18,* 71-73.

Lehman JA, Brunner JD, Stow RW. (1958). Pain threshold measurement after therapeutic application of ultrasound, microvawes infrared. *Arch Physical Medicine and Rehabil.* 39,560.

Lund N, Bengtsson A, Thobotg P. (1986) Muscle tissue oxygen pressure in primary fibromyalgia. *Scandinavian Journal of Rheumatology. 15.* 165-173.

Maekawa K, Kuboki T, Clark GT, Shinoda M, Yamashita A. (1998). Cold pressor stimulus temperature and resting masseter muscle haemodynamics in normal human subjects. *Archoral Biology.*43. 849-859.

Manheimer JS, Wallen EC. (1985).The eficacy of transcutaneous electrical nerve stimulation in dysmenorheea. *Clinical Journal of Pain .1,:*75-83.

Manniche, Hesselsoe G, Bentzen L, Christenzen I, Lundberg E.(1988). Clinical trial of intensive muscle training for chronic low back pain. Lancet. 2(8626-8627):1473-1476.

Marchand S, Charest J, Li J, Chenard RG, Lavignolle B, Laurencelle L (1993). Is TENS purely a placebo effect? A controlled study on chronic low back pain. *Pain 54*:99-106

Mc Cain GA, Bell DA, Mai KM ,Halliday PD (1988). A controlled study of the effects of a supervised cardiovascular fitness training program on the manifestation of primary fibromyalgia. *Arthritis and Rheumatism 31.(9),* 1135-1141.

Meeusen R.,,De Meirleir K (1995). Exercise and brain transmission. *Sports Medicine*, 20, 160-188.

Melzack R, Casey KL (1968). Sensory motivational and central control determinants of pain. In: Kenshalo DR, ed. *The skin senses.* Charles C Thomas, Springfield, Ill.

Melzack R, Vetere P, Finch L , (1983) . Transcutaneous electrical nerve stimulation for low back pain. *Physical Therapy. 63*(4):489-93

Melzack, R., Wall, P. D. (1965). Pain mechanisms: a new theory. *Science*, 150, 971-979.

Merskey, H., Bogduk, N. (Eds.) (1994). *Classification of chronic pain (2nd ed., pp. 209-214).* IASP Task Force on Taxonomy, Seattle, USA: IASP Press.
Meryl RG. (1992). Transcutaneous electrical nerve stimulation for management of pain sensory pathology. In: *Electrotherapy in rehabilitation* (pp. 149-196). Philadelphia, PA: Davis Co.

Metha N, Kugel G, Al Shuria A, Ss M, Forgione A.(1994). Effect of electronic anesthesia TENS on TMJ orofaringeal pain. *Journal of Dental Rresearch 73.* 358

Milnor WR. (1974). Autonomic and peripheral control mechanisms. In Mountcastle VB (ed): *Medical Physiology*, 2,ed 13.Mosby CV, St. Louis.

Milson I, Hedner N, Mannheimer C. (1994). A comparative study of the effect of high intensity transcutaneous electrical nerve stimulation and oral naproxen on intrauterine pressure and menstrual pain in patients with dysmenorrhea. *American Journal of Obstretics and Gynecology 170.*(1),123-29.

Nave CR, Nave BC. (1980). *Physics For The Health Sciences, ed 2* WB Saunders, Philadelphia.

Newton RA. (1987) *Thermal agents in rehabilitation.* Eds: Michlovitz FA Davis Company, Philadelphia.(pp.18-42).

North RB, Fishell TA, Long DM. (1977) Chronic stimulation via percutaneousely inserted epidural electrodes. *Neurosurgery 1,*215-8

Paul FW, Philips J, Thimoty BS, Proctor J,Wiliams BA, and Craig F. (1999) *Bulletin of the American Pain Society.*

Peyron R, Garcia-Larrea L, Deiber MP, Cinotti L, Convers P Sindou M, Mauguiere F, Laurent B. (1995). Electrical stimulation of parenteral cortical area in the treatment of central pain. Electrophysiological and PET study. *Pain* 62,275

Pomeranz BA. (1981) Natural mechanisms of acupuncture analgesia. In: Lipton S Ed. *Persistent Pain.* New York: Academic Press 271-5.

Ramsey SM. (1997) *Holistic Manual Therapy Techniques.. Primary Care* 24(4).759-786.

Rolnic JD, Wustefeld S, Dauper J. Karst M, Fink M, Kossev A, Dengler R. (2002) Repetitive transcranial magnetic stimulation for the treatment of chronic pain. A pilot study. *European Neurology. 48*,6-10.

Ruth S, Kegerreis S (1992). Fcilitating cervical flexion using a Feldenkrais method: Awareness through movement. *Journal of Sports and Physical Therapy, 16*, 25-29.

Sansone P, Schmitt L. (2000) Providing tender touch massage to elderly nursing home residents- A Demonstration Project *Geriatric Nursing 21*(6),303-308.

Sarlandiere JB (1825). *Memoires sur l'electro-puncture.* Delaumay, Paris.

Schonoch W (1912-19130: Die Rezept Sammlung des Scribonius. Jena: Baken Museum of Electricity in Life. Minneapolis MN.

Shaubel HH. (1946). Local use of ice after orthopedic procedures. *American Journal of Surgery 72*,711.

Shealy CN, Mortimer JT, Reswich JB (1967). Electrical inhibition of pain by stimulation of the dorsal column: preliminary clinical reports. *Anesthesia and Analgesia*, 46:489-491.

Shobel HP, Schmieder RE, Hartmann S, Schachinder H, Luft FC. (1995). Effects of Bromcriptine on cardiovascular regulation in healthy humans. *Hypertension 25,1075-1082*

Simon L, Blotman F. (1981) Exercise therapy and hydrotherapy in the treatment of rheumatic diseases. *Clinical Rheumatology Disease 17*:.337-347.

Somers DL, Somers MF. (1999)Treatment of neuropathic pain In a patient with diabetic neuropathy using transcutaneous

Electrical nerve stimulation applied to the skin of the lumbar region. *Physical Therapy 79*(8).767-775.

Strauss-Blashe G, Ekmekcioglu C, Klammer N et al. (2000) The change of well being associated with spa therapy. *Forh Komplementarmed Klass Naturheilkd 7*. 269-274.

Strauss-Blashe G, Ekmekcioglu C, Vacariu G, Melchart H, Fialca-Moser V, Marktl W. (2002) Contribution of individual spa therapies in the treatment of chronic pain. *Clinical Journal of Pain 18*(5).302-309.

Sukenic S. Neuman NL, Buskila D, Kleiner-Baumgarten A, Zimlichman S, HorovitzJ,(1990) Dead Sea salt bath for the treatment of rheumatoid arthritis. *Clinical Experimental Rheumatology* 8. 353-357.

Sukenic S, Gires H, Halevy S, Neumann L, Fluser D, Buskila D. (1994) Treatment of psoriatic arthritis at the Dead Sea. *Journal of Rheumatology 21*. 1305-309.

Turk, M. (2001). Pain's healing secret. Chico, CA: *Acu Press*

Victor RG, Wayne N, Leimbach J, Seals DR, Wallin BG, Mark AL. (1987) Effect of the cold pressor test on muscle sympathetic nerve activity in humans. *Hypertension 9*. 429-436.

Van Tubergen A, Landewe R, Van Der Heijde D, Hidding A, Wolter N, Assher M,Falkenbach A, Genth E, Goeithe H, Van Der Linden S. (2001) Combined Spa exercise therapy in patients with ankylosing spondylitis – A randomized controlled trial. *Arthritis-Rheumatology 45*(5).430-438.

Van Tulder MW, Koes BW, Bouter LM. (1997) Conservative treatment of acute and chronic non specific low back pain. *Spine 22*,2128-2156.

Walker J, Akhanjee L, Cooney M, Goldstain J, Tamayoshi S, Sgal-Gidan F. (1987). Laser therapy for pain of rheumatoid arthritis *Clinical Journal of pain 3*. 54-59.

Wang BG, Tang J, White PF et al. (1997). Effect of the intensity of transcutaneous acupoint electrical stimulation on the postoperative analgesic requirements. *Anesth.analg 85*. 406-413.

Wasseljen O Johansen BM, Westgaard RN,(1995) The effect of pain reduction on perceived tension and EMG – recorded trapezius muscle activity in workers with shoulder neck pain. *Scandinavian Journal of Rehabilitation Medicine 27*. 243-252.

Wesley J (1760). The desideratum: or electricity made plain and useful. W Flexney, London

Weyerer S, Kupfer B. (1994) Physical exercise and psychological health. *Sparta Medicine 17*,108-116.

White PF, Craig WF, Wacharia AS et al. (2000) Percutaneous Neuromodulatory Therapy: does the location of electrical stimulation affect the acute analgesic response? *Anesthesia Analgesia 91*. 949-954.

White PS, Fanzca, Shitong Li, Jen W Chiu. (2001) Electroanalgesia: its role in acute and chronic pain management. *Anesthesia Analgesia 92*. 505-513.

Wigers So, Stiles TC, Vogel PA. (1996) Effects of aerobic exercise versus stress management treat study. *Scandinavian Journal of Rheumatology 25*. 77-86.

In: The Handbook of Chronic Pain
Editors: S. Kreitler, D. Beltrutti, et al., pp. 423-430

ISBN 978-1-60021-044-0
© 2007 Nova Science Publishers, Inc.

Chapter 23

Herbal Therapy for Pain Control

F. Barak, L. Ostrowsky and S. Scharf

INTRODUCTION

Evidence about the therapeutic use of herbs has come down to us from ancient Egypt, China, India, Arab countries, Greece, Rome, Northern Europe, Africa, Native American Indians and the Maya. A number of famous historical books describing herbal medicines were written by ancient physicians, such as Chen-Nong from China; Ibn Cenna, from Asia; Diascorides (100 BC) and Hippocrates (370 – 460 BC) from Greece; Paracelsius and Galen from Europe etc. They described some 300-400 medicinal herbs, some of which are still in use in various forms. Famous Jewish physicians have made great contributions to this store of knowledge. Assaf Harofeh (1135 – 1204 AD), who compiled "The Book of Medicines", used a variety of medical herbs in the 12th century. The mediaeval Jewish doctor Maimonides described not only the curative effects of medical herbs but also their toxic characteristics, including opioides and poisons. This knowledge has been gathered from experience and observation throughout the centuries. Concerning herbal medicine it is apt to quote Sir William Oster's famous saying: "The philosophies of one age become the absurdities of the next, and the foolishness of yesterday becomes the wisdom of tomorrow".

Current information about herbs is based not only on past experience but also on chemical analytic tests and experiments carried out by professionals, pharmacists and doctors.

Many modern medicines have been developed on the basis of herbal studies. Initially the herbs themselves were used as medicines, but later some were replaced by medicines that had been chemically synthesized in laboratories. In fact, the synthesized medicines are more efficacious and less toxic than the original herbal remedies, since the synthetic drugs mostly contain only the required active components without the unnecessary toxic ones.

In using natural herbs and herbal remedies we must keep in mind that herbs are indeed medicines. This implies that like any other medicine, apart from the effective beneficial drug components that they contain, in a natural unprocessed or pure processed form, they also have other properties, which may cause negative side effects.

For the purpose of this chapter, a number of popular books recommended to the general public on the use of herbs were reviewed. Surprisingly, it was found that few of the popular books published the necessary precautions that need to be observed prior to using herbal treatments. Some books did not mention any precautions at all, and the overall impression given was that any usage in any form and in any amount was beneficial. It seems as if herbs, being a part of nature, enjoy the aura of health, virtue and goodness that attach to so-called natural things in the collective cultural mythology.

However, this approach corresponds neither to the fact that some highly potent poisons are perfectly "natural" (viz. arsenic) nor to the observation that all drugs are benefcial only when used in the proper amount and form. Furthermore, this chapter must not be regarded as a recommendation for the use of herbal medicines, gained from the authors' personal experience, but only as a professional statement on the medical therapeutic components of the plant's materials and composition. The presentation of each drug or plant is accompanied by a presentation of the contra-indications for the general use of the herbs, extracted from a number of recognized and approved medical books and internet sites.

PLANTS AND DRUGS

This section presents the major herbs used for pain relief and about which there exists reliable information concerning usage and restrictions on usage (e.g., contra-indications, drug interactions).

Name: Aloe, Aloevera

Pharmacology

Active ingredient: mucilage, resin, anthraquinones, glycosides (aloin), aloe-emolin; aloin A and B; aloinside; sterols; saponins and vitamins,

Usage: External-the gel: antiseptic, antifungal, burn and wound treatment.

Internal - Anticonstipational, and against asthenia.

Useful section: Leaves.

Comments:

Contra indications: Internal Usage: during menstruation (possible stimulation of endometrial activity), abdominal pain (of unknown cause); Crohn's disease, ulcerative colitis; appendicitis, or any other Inflamed Intestinal disease; for patients taking medication containing cardiac glycosides or anti arrhythmic (a possible side effect is potassium loss which can affect the action of cardiac drugs), thiazide diuretics, licorice or corticosteroids (potassium loss may be aggravated by these drugs), pregnant women, or those trying to get pregnant; breast-feeding and administration to a child.

Do not use for longer than 8 to 10 days or more than the prescribed dose.

Side effects: (relatively rare)

Overdose and long term enteral usage- loss of electrolytes (potassium, albuminuria and hematuria) and fluid imbalance; hyperaldosteronism; inhibition of intestinal motility and enhancement of cardioactive steroid. Potassium deficiency can lead to muscular weakness, (especially with concurrent use of cardiac glycosides, diuretics, and corticosteroids), heart arrhythmias, nephropathies, edemas, accelerated bone deterioration, albuminuria and hematuria.

Side effects that usually do not require medical attention: red coloring of urine and intestinal cramps (harmless and usually vanish when usage is discontinued).

Name: Salix Alba (Willow; White Willow)

Pharmacology

Active ingredient: salycin, tannins, flavonoids, phenolic glycosides; picein, triadrin with ethers of salicylic acids and coumarins.

Usage: anti – inflammatory, antipiretic, perspiration enhancement, analgesic, anti-rheumatic and antiseptic.

Useful section: In modern times, the cork of the tree has been found to be more useful but sometimes the fresh leaves are used for making an infusion (tea) to be taken after meals.

Comments:

Contra indications: gastro - duodenal ulcers.

Side effects: causes allergies, anaphylaxis, erosion of teeth and abdominal pains.

Name: Peppers (Including Capsicum Annuum L., Black Pepper, Arabidopsis Thaliana and Cayenne Pepper - Capsicum Frutescens (Solanaeae), Capsicum Minimum; Chili; African Chili.

Pharmacology

Active ingredients: Flavonoids, alkaloids, fatty acids, Vit. B_1, Vit. C (ascorbic acid), tocopherols (Vit. E), Vit. A, beta – carotene, sugars, etheric and phenolic acids; saponins (capsaicinoids), volatile oil.

Usage: External: skin ointment, improves blood circulation; massage and bath oil- for local analgesia, in small amounts as a gargle; anti-rheumatic, lower back pain and antiseptic,.

Internal: enhances perspiration, improve digestion, prevents flatulence and has anti-oxidant activity.

Useful section: The entire fruit.

Comments:

Contraindications: skin ulcers, ulcerative and inflammatory gastro intestinal diseases, hypothermia, high blood pressure and pregnancy.

Avoid: Eye and mucous membrane contact, and the use of capsicum seeds, due to their toxicity.

Exact dosage of fruit is essential, oral overdose may cause gastric and hepatic toxicity and over long skin contact may cause serious skin irritation.

Side effects: intensification of pain, irritation of mucous membrane and skin, irritation of the nervous system and local hyperthermia.

Name: Harpagophytum Procumbemce. (Pedaliaceae) Devil's Claw

Pharmacology

Active ingredient: Iridoid glycosides, harpogoside, harpogide, and procumbide; flavonoids, especially kaemferol and luteolin glycosides; phenolic acids

Usage: anti-inflammatory, anti-rheumatoid, analgesic and sedative.

Useful section: bulbs only.

Side effects: not known.

Comments:

Avoid in pregnancy

Name: Hypericum Perforatum – St John's Wort. (Hyperforen, Hyperaceae)

Pharmacology

Active ingredient: Essential oil containing cariophyllene, pinene, limonene and myrcene; hypericins flavonoids resin.

Usage: Internal: Anti depressant (light, moderate); chronic pain and anxiety relief; anti - inflammatory; antiseptic. External: wounds, burns and infections.

Useful section: Dried tops, including flowers.

Comments:

Side effects: Photosensitivity or photoallergy; acute neuropathy; dizziness, gastrointestinal irritation, nausea, tiredness, restlessness, headaches.

Drug interaction: with anti-depressants , narcotics, chemotherapy (irrinotecan) and cyclosporine.

Avoid : Alcohol consumption. It has been suggested that foods or substances that contain tyramine (present in some foods s.c. as wine, yogurt, cheese, ripe bananas, yeast, meat extracts, smoked or pickled meats) should be avoided. Should not be used for children under the age of 2 years old as there is no clinical data available. Solutions of St. John's Wort may stain clothing and skin.

Name: Kava , Kava, Cava Root (Piper Methysticum Rhizoma)

Pharmacology

Active ingredient: Kava pyrones

Usage: For treatment of pain; for relief of nervous anxiety, stress, restlessness, and insomnia; asthma; as sedative, anti-convulsive, antispasmodic, and central muscular relaxant; anti-septic; stimulant, tonic, diuretic, diaphoretic, and aphrodisiac.

Useful section: Root.

Comments:

Side effects: Scaly yellowing of the skin, nails and hair (suggestive of ichthyosis and brought on by excessive or extended continuous use .This condition is reversible if usage is discontinued); eye irritation, tiredness and a tendency to sleep, impairment of motor reflexes, equilibrium, and judgment; rash; gastrointestinal problems; pupil dilation and tiredness in the morning; liver damage; dizziness; stupor.

Drug interaction: alprazolam or other bensodiazepine drugs; barbiturates, psychopharmacological medicines CNS depressants (may enhance effects); substances that act on the nervous system (may potentiate effectiveness)

Contraindications: Endogenous depression(may increase the risk of suicide), interacts with barbiturates and psychopharmacological substances; drinking alcohol; nor to take this herb for longer than three months; pregnancy (may cause loss of uterine tone); breast-feeding; administration to a child.

Notes: Should not be taken for longer than three months without consulting your health care physician. Do not overdose with this herb! If you miss a dose, take it as soon as you can. If it is almost time for your next dose, take only that dose. Do not take double or extra doses.

Caution: As Kava usage may impair motor reflexes and judgment.- Do not operate heavy machinery or drive.

On February 22, 1998, the FDA announced that it had identified 16 dietary supplements as risky; Kava was listed with a warning that it "can potentiate the effects of alcohol and certain psychological drugs."

Name: Canabis Sativa (Cannabaceae) CANNABIS, GAJA, HEMP, HASHISH

Pharmacology

Active ingredient: Canabioids (60 kinds); volatile oil; flavonoids.

Usage: Moderate to severe analgesic, muscle relaxation; anti spasmatic; central sedative; neuralgia; inhibits spasmodic coughing and migraine; chemotherapy induced nausea and vomiting.

Useful section: Leaf, resin, seeds.

Comments:

Side effects: Constipation, nausea and vomiting; psychological addiction; impairment of motor reflexes, equilibrium, and judgment; rash; gastrointestinal problems; pupil dilation and somnolence.

Drug interaction: Opioids, psychopharmacological medicines CNS tranquilizers (may enhance effects); substances that act on the nervous system (may potentiate effectiveness)
Contraindications: Drinking alcohol; pregnancy; breast-feeding; administration to a child.

Caution: Possession of cannabis is illegal in most countries.

Name: Papaver Somniforum (Papaveraceae) OPIUM POPPY, WHITE
POPPY, MAWSEED

Pharmacology

Active ingredient: Alkaloids, especially morphine, codeine, papaverine, opioides.

Usage: Pain relief; muscle relaxation; anti spasmatic; central sedative; neuralgia; inhibits coughing; antidiarrhoeal.

Useful section: Latex and leaves.

Comments:

Side effects: Constipation, nausea and vomiting; psychological addiction; impairment of motor reflexes, equilibrium, and judgment; rash; gastrointestinal problems; pupil dilation and somnolence.

Drug interaction: Opioids, psychopharmacological medicines CNS tranquilizers (may enhance effects); substances that act on the nervous system (may potentiate effectiveness)

Contraindications: Drinking alcohol; pregnancy; breast-feeding; administration to a child.

Notes: Use only under guidance of a qualified physician. (De Smet, 2002; Ernst and Chrubasik, 2000)

CONCLUSIONS

Because herbs, like conventional medicines, contain powerful chemical substances they are effective in treating medical conditions or affecting favorably medically-relevant states like pain. Treatment with herbs is efficacious due to the powerful chemical substances they contain which are similar to those used in conventional medicine. For example, the analgesic effect of Salix alba is due to its salicylic acid content, which is a well-known modern medicament (aspirin), largely used for pain control and anti coagulation treatment. In fact, many of our modern medicines have been originally extracted from plants, but only the active ingredient is extracted or synthesized. However, some important facts must be kept in mind.

Home-prepared infusions, extractions and other preparations from medical herbs may also contain or be often polluted by dangerous bye-products, which may cause reactions, such as severe allergies, liver toxicity, or renal toxicity. When the herb medications are professionally produced, the exact quantity of the active ingredient can be controlled and a safe dose recommended for treatment. This kind of accuracy cannot be assured under non-professional conditions.

Belladonna, for instance, is a plant containing atropine in differing amounts per plant. Levels of atropine are affected by seasons and the time of year and even the time of day the plant is harvested. When processed or synthesized under controlled conditions, an exact dose is prepared, something which is impossible to achieve under amateur non-professional conditions. Atropine, when given in the correct dose, is a very efficacious drug, but can prove fatal when the dose is increased even by milligrams. Thus, "natural" is not synonymous with "safe". Many allergic reactions are caused by our daily contact with flowers, fruits, trees, etc.

However, in our contact with the patient we must be careful to maintan a logical and understanding approach when we do not approve of or do not recommend herbal medicine in place of conventional drugs. In each instance, the points for and against the use of the herbal medicine should be explained in detail. The patient should be aware of the precise active ingredients in herbal medicines, their frequent side effects and possible interactions between herbal medicines, conventional medications, and even food intake.

For example, St. John's Wort contains anti-depressant substances from the group of anti mono-aminooxidase. This group of anti-depressants is no longer in use in psychiatric practice due to its many side effects and its known interaction with tyrramin, which is found in such simple foodstuffs as, chocolate, yellows cheese, wine, and bananas.

The indications for natural medications are often over- simplified and do not take into account a precise diagnosis or other medicines taken. Moreover, the prepared herb is often lacking a precise listing of contents and an annotation (often giving the impression that the preparation is innocuous), in comparison to conventional medicines where a detailed annotation is always supplied. It is the physician's task to make the patients aware of the problems attending the use of the herbal medicine, and to alert them to the precautions that need to be taken so as not to expose themselves to any damage, that may accompany the possible benefits accruing from the use of the herb.

REFERENCES

[1]   Massey. P. B., Dietary supplements. In, *Medical Clinics of North America* 2002; 86: 1. W.B. Saunders.

[2]   Cohen M. R., Herbal and complementary and alternative medicine therapies for liver disease. A focus on Chinese Traditional Medicine in Hepatitis C Virus .In, *Clinics in liver disease* 2001; 5: 2. W.B. Saunders Company.

[3]   Marcia L. B., Robert S. M., Talking with families about herbal therapies, grand rounds. *Journal of pediatrics* 2000; 136: 5. Mosby , Inc

[4]   Kramer N. Complementary and alternative therapies for Rheumatic diseases 1.Why I not recommend complementary or alternative therapies: A. Physician's perspective. In: *Rheumatic Diseases Clinics of North America.* 1999; 25:4

[5]   Ernst E., Chrubasik S. Phyto-Anti-Inflammatory. A Systematic Review of Randomized, Placebo - Controlled, Double - Blind Trials. *Rheumatic Disease Clinics of North America.* 2000; 26 (1), 13-27.

[6]   Foster D.F., Phillips R.S.,. Hamel M.B.,. Eisenberg D.M. Clinical Investigation. Alternative Medicine Use in Older Americans. *Journal of the American Geriatrics Society.* 2000; 48 (12)

[7]   Steyer T.E. Complementary and Alternative Medicine. A Primer.You may be surprised by the number of your patients using CAM therapy. This primer provides the background and tips you'll need to have a productive conversation about it .*Family practice management* , 2001; 8 (3)

[8]   Gallagher R.M. 1999. Treatment Planning in Pain Medicine. Integrating Medical, Physical, and Behavioral Therapies. *Medical Clinics of North America,* 83(3)

[9]   Ziment I, Tashkin D.P. Current reviews of allergy and clinical immunology. In: Alternative medicine for allergy and asthma. *Journal of allergy and clinical immunology*, 2000; 106(4)

[10]   Chivato T., Juan F., Montoro A., Laguna R. Anaphylaxis induced by ingestion of a pollen compound. *J Investig Allergol Clin Immunol*. 1996; 6 (3): 208 - 9.

[11]   Dubois P., Pereira da Silva L. Towards a vaccine against asexual blood stage infection by Plasmodium falciparum .*Res. Immunol*. 1995; 146 (4-5): 263 - 75.

[12]   Soulimani R., Younos C., Jarmouni - Idrissi S., Bousta D., Khalouki F., Laila A. Behavioral and pharmaco - toxicological study of Papaver rhoeas L. in mice . *J Ethnopharmacol*. 2001; 3:74 (3): 265 - 74.

[13]   Fleming L.W. A medical bouquet. Poppies, cinchona and willow.*Scott med J*. 1999; 44 (6): 176 – 9.

[14]   Chen Y.F., Tsai H.Y., Wu T.SAnti - inflammatory and analgesic activities from roots of Angelica pubescens. *Planta Med*, 1995; 61 (1): 2- 8

[15]   Chrubasik S., Thanner J., Kunzel O., Conradt C., Black A., Pollak S. Comparison of outcome measures during treatment with the proprietary Harpagophytum extract doloteffin in patients with pain in the lower back , knee or hip. *Phytomedicine* 2002; 9 (3): 181 – 94.

[16]   Chrubasik S., Junck H., Breitschwerdt H., Conradt C., Zappe H. Effectiveness of Harpagophytum extract WS 1531 in the treatment of exacerbation of low back pain a randomized, placebo - controlled, double - blind study. *Eur J Anaesthesiol*. 1999; 16 (2) : 118 - 29 .

[17]   Polunin M., Robins C., *The natural pharmacy. An encyclopedic illustrated guide to medicines from nature*. Dorling Kindersley Ltd, London. 1994

[18]   P. A.G.M. De Smet , Herbal Remedies, *N Eng J Med 2002*; 347 , 25 : 2046 - 2056

Part VIII:
Particular Pain Syndromes:
Medical and Psychological Aspects

In: The Handbook of Chronic Pain
Editors: S. Kreitler, D. Beltrutti, et al., pp. 433-464

ISBN 978-1-60021-044-0
© 2007 Nova Science Publishers, Inc.

Chapter 24

Headache

Aldo Lamberto, Alfredo Fogliardi, Mauro Nicoscia,
Francesco Marino and Diego Beltrutti

1. BACKGROUND

Headache is one of the most common pains. It occurs in all cultures and in people of all ages, and can present either as a unique manifestation or as a symptom of an underlying pathology. Variability in pain intensity results not only in different levels of disability, but also in the approaches used for treatment. In many cases, a few minutes of rest or sleep may suffice for alleviating the pain, and preventive measures, such as use of sunglasses or keeping the head covered, may successfully prevent the onset of headache. However, for many people, especially those in whom headache is a chronic problem, stronger measures are needed, such as pharmacological interventions or a combination of therapeutic treatments.

Along with several of the gastrointestinal pathologies (e.g. ulcers, irritable bowel syndrome, etc.), headache is a syndrome that has been demonstrated to be highly correlated with psychological states. The causes of headache can often be associated with psychological components, such as stress, anxiety and emotions. The identification of these components as causal mechanisms provided one of the first collaborations between physicians and psychologists. The presence of the psychological factors results in a complex physiological reaction culminating in the painful response. This physiologic response, and the ability to correlate the onset of headache with the stresses of everyday life, suggests the continued importance of cooperation between medicine and psychology in the diagnosis and treatment of headaches.

2. PSYCHOLOGICAL FACTORS IN HEADACHE

Two approaches have been used for corroborating the empirical correlation between psychological factors and the onset and persistence of headache. The first relies on evaluations using the Diagnostic and Statistical Manual of Mental Disorders, currently in the fourth edition (DSM-IV)[1]. The second and more commonly used approach uses the Minnesota Multiphasic Personality Inventory (MMPI) to identify and evaluate psychopathologic problems which may be present in patients with headache.

Using the MMPI, Kudrow et al. [2] determined three profiles among patients with headache. The first profile is not associated with significant changes in MMPI and is characteristic of patients with migraine or cluster headache. The second profile is characterized by moderate somatization and some signs of depression, and is found among patients with tension or mixed headache. Patients with posttraumatic headache or transformed migraine have increased evidence of depression and somatization, and are included in the third profile. In correlating the profiles with the neurotic subscales for hypochondria, depression and hysteria, it has been shown that the first group differs from the other two groups in having a lower elevation of these scales.

Sternbach et al. [3] used the MMPI to evaluate three groups of patients, those with vascular, mixed, and tension type headache. The results were comparable to those of Kudrow in that they confirmed that patients with vascular headache have only minor elevations of the neurotic scales compared to the other two groups.

It can be hypothesized that these observed differences are a consequence of headache chronicity. In headaches of vascular origin, unlike the other two forms, there are many periods of pain remission. Consequently there is only minor psychological involvement compared to the more chronic pain and disability caused by persistent headaches. Andrasik et al. [4], using the MMPI, compared psychological involvement of patients with headache to controls without headache. While there were significant differences between the two groups, the levels of depression, anxiety, and somatization in patients with headache were moderate, without the characteristics of a psychopathologic state.

Psychological involvement was found to be a major component of headache in a study by Pradelier et al. [5] In 294 patients suffering from headache, stress was present in 68% of the cases, anxiety in 43%, worry in 32%, emotional factors in 18%, and depression in 18%. A subsequent study of 217 patients suffering from muscular tension headache determined that 42% of the patients had a combination of psychological factors, while the incidence of individual psychological factors such as anxiety, depression, and stress was 19%, 10%, and 7%, respectively [6]. This study also compared tension headaches with and without muscular contraction in order to determine psychological involvement in the two headache forms. In 20% of the patients with muscular contraction it was not possible to demonstrate the presence of psychological factors. In contrast, only 9% of the patients without contraction appeared to be without psychological factors. From these studies, it is evident that one of the major challenges in diagnosis and therapy of headache is to distinguish between patients with and without psychological problems. However, it should also be considered that in many patients, the problems of stress, anxiety, and depression do not reach psychopathologic levels.

2.1. Anxiety and Headache

The survival function of the anxiety response is to allow us to evaluate the difficulty inherent in a situation or behavior. In this way behavioral countermeasures can be activated that will allow us to face or avoid the problem. If the difficulties appear to be overwhelming, the anxiety response becomes exaggerated, resulting in additional psychological and physiologic responses that may be detrimental to a person's physical and mental health. One of these psychophysiological responses is muscular tension that may cause the frequent headaches that are reported in patients predisposed to anxiety. However, there are currently no data that demonstrate a clear correlation between anxiety levels measured by psychological tests and contraction of the pericranial muscle, suggesting that a more complex cause/effect mechanism exists. Additionally, while anxiety is often a causal mechanism of headache, the converse is also possible. Headache can cause anticipation anxiety, especially in the more acute and painful conditions such as cluster headache or certain migraines. In these cases, the patient feels the warning symptoms of the crisis and starts to worry and get anxious about not being able to resist or alleviate the headache.

2.2. Depression and Headache

It is almost unavoidable that a patient's psychological state will be affected by persistent chronic headache. Depression is one of the most frequent manifestations that accompany headache. However, it should be recognized that there are different levels of depression, ranging from minor depression that does not reach psychopathological levels, to that recognized as severe clinical depression. When a patient who has been suffering headaches for many years has not been able to find a remedy that meets their expectations, it is almost unavoidable that the sense of inadequacy and futility will negatively affect their mood. In this case, depression is a consequence of the headache and of the feeling of helplessness. Interpersonal relationships may be significantly affected by the presence or expectation of the crisis, since the patient often withdraws into an inner world of pain, anxiety, and depression. The understanding of the role of depression in headache is further complicated by the fact that different manifestations of depression (anorexia, sleep disorders, lack of energy, etc.) can be attributed to headache. Therefore, when evaluating patients with comorbid headache and depression, it is important to establish which is the cause and which is the effect [7]. Several psychological tests are available that can be used to determine if depression precedes headache or vice versa. In addition to the MMPI, other assessment tools that have been developed include the Beck Depression Inventory [8] and the Zung Self-Rating Depression Scale [9].

From a therapeutic viewpoint, it is important to be cautious in determining the appropriate treatment of headache in depressed patients. Symptomatic treatment is often inefficient because the headache may represent somatization of anxiety or depression. Therefore, it is necessary to balance the therapy so that the underlying causes of the problems are addressed. In those cases where migraine is comorbid with depression, daily pharmacological treatment with antidepressants is recommended. Although the tricyclic antidepressants (TCAs) have been a standard treatment because of their established efficacy in patients having both depression and migraine, their use is often limited by safety and tolerability issues. The new selective serotonin reuptake inhibitors (SSRIs) are as effective for depression as the TCAs and have fewer side effects [10]. Some of these agents, such as sertraline, have also demonstrated efficacy for the treatment of anxiety disorders [11].

2.3. Stress and Headache

The correlation between stress and headache is generally established by the patients themselves, often during the initial medical consultation when it is confirmed that the headache is a consequence of a stressful period. The definition of tension headache implies that the pain is caused by specific muscular involvement during tension. This muscular tension may be an early sign of daily stress. For vascular headaches, the cause/effect relationship is less clear than in muscular tension headaches, although daily stress can be a frequent cause of this headache type. Nevertheless, it can be hypothesized that people with a biologic predisposition to vascular or tension headaches are particularly sensitive to stress as an initiator of these conditions.

In addition to initiating a headache, stress can potentiate or intensify a pre-existing headache. The migraine caused by stress usually does not peak concomitantly with the peak of the stress, but rather during subsequent alleviation of the stress. It has therefore been suggested that stress is only one of the multifactorial components that affect the headache, and that it acts by increasing the vulnerability of the subject.

Another consideration in the relationship between stress and headache relates to how the prolonged presence of a headache provokes a vicious cycle of pain. The presence of a continuous or intermittent pain, and the expectation of a crisis, are both situations that increase the stress that becomes the starting point for the headache, which in its turn primes the cycle of stress and pain. Psychophysiological studies using biofeedback (BFB) show the difficulty in evaluating stress tolerance in patients with headache. Analysis of such studies demonstrates the importance of evaluating each of three fundamental phases: 1) first relaxation phase, 2) stress generated by mathematic or linguistic exercises resulting in annoying noises in the case of mistakes, 3) second relaxation phase. During these phases, different parameters are measured including heart rate, muscular tension (frontal, brachial, and nuchal), the amplitude of the cephalic pulse, and the intensity of the headache. Significant changes have been observed in the different parameters, but the magnitude of these changes relates to the type of experimentally induced stress.

These observations are important from both a diagnostic and therapeutic point of view. They suggest that it is not the stress characteristics that determine a specified reaction for each individual. Rather, what is fundamental are the individual's perception of the stress and its subsequent elaboration. External factors are psychologically filtered by each individual in order to determine the importance of the factor and the capacity of the individual to manage the stress. If the filter has a mesh that is too large, so that the stressful factors are too many, and/or the individual's capacity for handling it is perceived as limited, the physiologic reaction is of alarm, with all the correlated psycho physiological consequences.

The correlation between stress and headache has been presented by Bischoff and True by a model very similar to the diathesis-stress model proposed for lumbar problems of muscular origin [13, 14]. The model of Bischoff and True is composed of three separate elements that are strongly correlated:

- increase in muscular tension
- physiologic relationship between muscular tension and pain
- conditioning of the dysfunctional muscular activity

During the initiation and maintenance of tension-type headaches, there is a circular relationship among tension, biochemical processes, and pain.

Behavior therapy, in which learning occurs through the mechanism of classic operant conditioning, provides the theoretical basis for this model.

2.4. Headache and Emotions

The relationship between headache and emotions has benefited by a wide variety of studies that sought to confirm the common experience in which a headache attack immediately follows a deep emotional experience. Support for this was also suggested by experiences in which emotional factors cause an increase in intensity in a pre-existing headache. However, this empiric relationship cannot be established by anecdotal observations, and additionally, there are many cases in which the headache attack starts at the point when the emotional factors stop. This is typical of the weekend headache, characteristic of people who are deeply involved in their work and have headache attacks only during the weekend. Other experiences further show that, following an intense emotion, a headache pain may stop completely. In this regard perception of pain is often reduced or absent during a sports activity or in a war, where the subject does not feel the pain until after the event when attention is paid to the injury. In the specific context of the headache, it has been hypothesized that intense and repetitive emotional stimulation could reduce the antinociceptive response, with resultant hyperalgesia and pain [15].

Generally the antinociceptive system is stimulated by emotions that potentiate it. In patients with headache, this antinociceptive system is not properly activated and the decreased pain level would facilitate the causal mechanism through which the emotions could cause the headache.

3. Evaluation of the Headache

Diagnosis and evaluation of headache should consider the complexity of the cephalalgia as well as the interaction between psychological and physical factors. To facilitate these objectives, the International Headache Society (IHS) has established a set of criteria that have helped standardize the definition, diagnosis, and evaluation of headache [16].

These diagnostic criteria are especially useful for the specialist who studies and treats headache and whose purpose is twofold: 1) to provide an accurate diagnosis that takes both the physical and psychological factors into account, and 2) to formulate therapeutic strategies and provide an appropriate evaluation of therapeutic efficacy. Toward these objectives, a diagnostic paradigm has been developed that contains 5 fundamental elements: patient interview, medical evaluation, psychological evaluation, headache diary, and psychophysiological profile.

3.1. Patient Interview

The patient interview should incorporate discussion of critical areas such as the history and chronicity of the headache, previous lab exams and specialist visits, prior therapies and their efficacy or outcome, psychosocial profile, and reasons for further investigation and/or therapy.

The psychosocial profile includes information of the patient's job, quality of life, family, sexuality, leisure activities, self-sufficiency in the tasks of daily living with and without the presence of headache, the social consequences of the headache, the expectations of therapy, and the availability and utilization of pharmacological and no pharmacological therapy.

In some cases relatives of the patient may also be interviewed. This can provide further information on perception of pain, disability, and causal mechanisms/emotional reactions that provoke and/or accompany the headache. It may also be useful to request the cooperation of relatives in the various phases of therapy.

A standardized semi structured interview is generally used to obtain all relevant information. However, even the best standardized instrument cannot substitute for the sensitivity of the interviewing doctor and/or psychologist in catching important details that may be necessary for appropriate diagnosis and treatment.

3.2. Medical Evaluation

Although a general clinical exam is part of the overall medical evaluation, the primary objective of this evaluation is to provide a neurological assessment of the patient. Other specialists such as dentists, ophthalmologists, gynecologists, or internists should be consulted only if further investigations are indicated.

The case history, general clinical exam, and neurological exam are the basic evaluations that are subsequently used to determine if further medical assessments or tests are needed. Often, it is the patients themselves who request additional but useless procedures in an attempt to establish an organic basis for the headache.

A medical evaluation will usually include one or more of the following tests:

- Electroencephalogram (EEG)—used to study the loss of consciousness that occurs in some patients with migraine. It is only moderately useful since changes in EEG patterns are not specific and may be reversible.

- Evoked visual potentials—results in characteristic tracings during the time between attacks.

- Computed tomography (CT) scan of the head—generally reserved for patients who are suspected of having an underlying organic lesion.

- Nuclear magnetic resonance (NMR) imaging—it has been observed that patients with headache have larger hyperintense lesions compared to controls without headache.

- Cerebral angiography—since cerebral aneurysms almost never cause migraine-type headaches, this test is not generally recommended as first line, however, it is useful if the clinical exam shows cranial contusions or if a CT scan suggests cerebrovascular abnormalities.

- Positron-emission tomography (PET)—this procedure uses short half-life radioisotopes to follow metabolic pathways and can provide important information on the localized cerebral physiology, metabolism, and blood flow. Knowledge of blood flow patterns is especially useful since it has been noted that in migraine with aura, a wavelike reduction of the blood flow spreads ahead of the occipital pole. In contrast, migraine without aura is not associated with measurable modifications of the cerebral blood flow.

3.3. Psychological Evaluation

The objective of the psychological evaluation of a patient with headache is to determine the personal factors that result in the induction and persistence of the condition and influence perception of pain. Patients with headache are generally willing to undergo diagnostic psychological testing because they feel that their behaviors, beliefs, and cognitive functions play an essential role in the pathophysiology of their condition. While the psychological evaluation does not challenge the supposition that organic elements may be responsible for many types of headaches, it can provide additional information on the sources and chronicity of the pain states. In some cases, psychological factors can be the exclusive cause of headache, as in the somatization of anxiety. However, in many cases psychological and biological factors interact in initiating, maintaining, and/or exacerbating the headache.

The psychological evaluation for headache is not substantially different from that for benign chronic pain. In both cases the same instruments are used to evaluate levels of anxiety, depression, and general personality. It is also important to evaluate the thoughts of the patient regarding the disease, the expectations of the therapy, and the role of social or environmental factors in initiating and maintaining the crisis. Pain is evaluated using several patient assessment tools including the McGill Pain Questionnaire (MPQ) and the visual analogue scale (VAS).

3.4. Headache Diary

The headache diary is a patient-maintained daily report that can provide information and insight to both the patient and the health care provider into the causes and outcomes of headaches and their treatment. The diary is generally a standardized form that must be filled in daily by the patient and includes the date and the starting time of the headache, its intensity, the grade or stage of induced disability, and the duration, kind and quantity of drugs taken. Depending on the objectives, other kinds of data may be requested, such as the situation that initiated the crisis, prodromal symptoms, accompanying symptoms, associated thoughts, and subsequent behavior. This diary can then be presented during a subsequent visit or exam, when it can be used for various assessments including pharmacological compliance and treatment efficacy. The diary can also form a basis for discussion of problems or concerns that the patient may have with the disorder or its treatment.

Many patients tend to take drugs in excess of their medical prescriptions in what is often a useless attempt to diminish or eliminate the crisis. Through the use of the diary it is also possible to determine the kinds and dosages of drugs that are used by the patient, whether prescribed or not.

3.5. Psychophysiological Profile

A psychophysiological profile is an important first step that should be performed prior to initiating therapy in patients with headache. The purpose is to obtain information on the physiologic background and responses of the patient to determine the most appropriate biofeedback training program, and the physiologic functions that need to be monitored. The psychophysiological profile consists in measuring a predetermined set of parameters that may include muscle activity using electromyography (EMG), and thermal and skin conductivity using the galvanic skin response (GSR).

Since stress is always accompanied by generalized activation of the autonomic nervous system, central nervous system, and neuromuscular system, these tests are used to define a "stress profile." Patients with anxiety or with psychosomatic problems have difficulty in recovering from stress; there is an increase in the time required to return to the psychophysiological level preceding the stress compared with patients not having these problems [17].

The heartbeat, arteriolar pressure, and muscular tension all increase during stress, and there is sweating of the palms. The muscular tension in particular has been thought to be one of the causes of tension-type headaches, especially when the muscular tension is protracted beyond the period of the presence of the stressful factor. Fuller [18] measured peripheral temperature, electrodermal response and muscular electropotential in patients with stress undergoing biofeedback training. Patients with headache had difficulty in returning to the values obtained during relaxation, suggesting that subsequent stress provokes a continuous state of tension in various muscles, particularly the frontal muscle.

Although there is some variation, a stress profile has been proposed that is composed of six sequential phases of recording muscular tension: baseline, non-specific stress, recovery phase, induction of a specific stress state, and a final recovery phase. In the two recovery phases it is important to measure the time required to return to the baseline recorded prior to the stress.

Beltrutti and Lamberto evaluated [19] the psychophysiological profile of 21 patients (16 females, 5 males) suffering from tension-type headaches for more than 1 year using EMG and thermal BFB. The approximate 3:1 ratio of female:male patients in this study was similar to what has generally been reported to be the gender prevalence of tension-type headaches. Those authors reported a progressive reduction in the average values of the EMG and thermal BFB during the first 10 minutes in the absence of any instructions, and a further reduction during the subsequent 5 minutes when the patient was told to relax. This stable profile was maintained until the application of the first stress, which resulted in a peak that dropped immediately after the end of the stress and the beginning of the first recovery phase. The second stress produced another peak that did not return to the relaxation value of obtained during minutes 11-15. Within this group of patients the greatest differences were found in the recovery phases after the stress, especially for EMG BFB compared with thermal BFB. In the thermal BFB, there was a remarkable ability to recover after the stress, with greater interpatient variability than intrapatient variability. In contrast, EMG BFB was shown to present specific characteristics of patients with tension-type headache, with high levels of both interpatient and intrapatient variability, suggesting that there is difficulty in recovery among several the patients. The authors concluded that it is not the absolute values of the measurements that are important, but the overall pattern of response is typical of tension-type headache.

The *a priori* establishment of certain values to define a particular pathology would result in the error of starting all patients on biofeedback who exceed the pre-established threshold. A better approach takes into consideration not only the actual values, but the overall pattern of the profile, evaluating the observed changes not only during the phase of stress but also during recovery.

4. NON-PHARMACOLOGICAL THERAPY OF HEADACHE

Two elements characterize the majority of patients who suffer of headache: 1) the presence of one or more psychological problems such as anxiety, stress or depression, and 2) the lack of a specific physiologic event that accounts for the onset of the crisis. Nonpharmacological therapy is a useful approach by itself or in combination with pharmacological therapy for both preventive and symptomatic treatment of these patients. Nonpharmacological therapy can include modalities such as relaxation training, biofeedback training, cognitive behavioral techniques, and hypnosis.

4.1. Biofeedback Training

The evidence that pain in tension-type headaches is provoked by the contraction of various muscles suggested specific therapy that would rapidly reduce the prolonged contractions. BFB, starting from its first application, had positive results especially with EMG biofeedback by recording the value of the tension of the frontal muscle and training the patient to reduce it. The theoretical principle that supports this approach is that tension-type pain is related to an increase in muscular tension, and therefore a reduction in EMG activity measured (in micro volts) results in decreased pain [20, 21]. This technique has been promising, especially in headaches that were called muscle tensive in the old classification [22] and which are now referred to as "headaches of the tension type." In those headaches characterized by bilateral effects, lack of prodromal symptoms, and extended chronicity, the reduction in the contraction of the frontal and pericranial muscle obtained through EMG BFB training coincides with reductions of the crisis and in the intensity of pain.

The other muscular zones that are hypothesized to be responsible for headaches of the tension type are the trapezius and neck muscles. Traue et al. [23] carried out a series of studies that confirmed the importance of the trapezius muscle especially in tension-type headaches. Further confirmation came Arena et al. [24] that demonstrated that applying electrodes to the trapezius muscles provides better results than application to the frontal muscles.

With respect to the neck muscles, both the posterior bilateral and the posterior frontalis are used [25]. However, in the absence of further evidence, the position of the electrode in the neck muscles is recommended only in those patients who show specific problems in the masseter muscle.

The use of BFB in migraines had a serendipitous beginning and emphasizes the role that chance plays in many scientific discoveries. A patient undergoing measurement of peripheral temperature in the Menninger clinic had a sudden migraine. However, the ability of the patient to increase the peripheral temperature had an almost immediate effect in the reduction of the crisis and of its intensity [26]. Starting from this initial observation, further studies confirmed that the vasoconstrictive component of the vasomotor reaction can be controlled through feedback [27].

Training in thermal BFB consists in progressive exercises designed to promote the ability for vasomotor control that can reduce and eliminate the migraine attack. These actions can be used prophylactically as well as for symptomatic relief.

The possibility of modifying the intensity of the blood flow through appropriate training has opened new therapeutic horizons for headaches of the vascular type. Unfortunately, the method is complex and the patient needs to be trained through a series of controlled attempts. The patient learns to control the intensity of the blood flow in the temporal artery, which provides a response similar to that obtained with the pharmacological use of ergotamine.

The mode of action of BFB has not been completely elucidated. However, this therapy has been shown to provide positive results and is indicated as the most efficient no pharmacological therapy, although there may be some overlap with relaxation techniques.

According to Andrasik [28] relaxation and biofeedback are two techniques that are not interchangeable but can offer different advantages for different groups of patients. McGrady et al. [29] compared two groups of patients with migraine diagnosis. The first group was trained using BFB, whereas the second group carried out relaxation by themselves without the assistance of an apparatus. The results demonstrated a significant difference in the reduction of pain and the consumption of drugs that favored BFB training.

There are three variables that tend to improve the efficacy of BFB. The first is related to the personality of the patient and in particular to the patient's sense of self-sufficiency and expectations of therapy. The second is more technical and relates to the importance of the continuity of daily practice of the techniques. Third, it is necessary to consider the role of the therapist, who can provide a positive influence by encouragement and reinforcing the firm belief that the patient can achieve resolution of the headache.

4.2. Relaxation Training

Similar to BFB, the purpose of relaxation training is to reduce muscular tension. This simple and natural method makes it readily accepted by patients.

The most frequently used methods are progressive relaxation according to the method first propounded by Jacobson in 1938 [30], and the autogenous training method by Schultze [31]. The meditative relaxation method by Benson [32] and the guided imagery method by Horan [33] are not used as frequently. This latter technique, compared with biofeedback and a combined technique of biofeedback and guided imagery, seems to provide a greater ability in countering the pain and a stronger sense of control during migraine attacks [34]. From the point of view of efficacy, relaxation training overlaps with biofeedback [35]. The advantage of this latter technique is the rapidity of learning and a reliance on an instrument that appears to the patient to offer scientific validity.

4.3. Cognitive Behavioral Techniques

Headache pain, like pain in general, is an alarm signal that often is perceived in the early phases before becoming fully developed with resulting disability. The purpose of cognitive behavioral techniques is to alleviate painful sensations before they become intense. The patient learns to recognize the initial symptoms that signal the onset of muscular tension and headache. Various techniques are used including stress inoculation [36], rational-emotive therapy (RET)[37], mixed techniques with EMG biofeedback [38], and mixed techniques using thermal biofeedback, relaxation techniques and cognitive strategies [39]. Often, it is useful to more broadly evaluate headache by placing it in the more general category of chronic pain. Thus, modifying the cognitive factors likely to be associated with pain may provide an effective approach to treatment [40].

4.4. Hypnosis

As with chronic pain, the use of hypnosis for the treatment of headache is sporadic and is rarely used systematically. Goals of an hypnotic session can be nonspecific (improving self-control, building self-confidence, reinforcing the possibility of symptomatic) or specific (responses to anxiety, muscle relaxation, hemodynamic equilibration, symptomatic pain relief) [41].

5. PHARMACOLOGICAL THERAPY OF HEADACHE

As is well known, many classes of drugs have been shown capable to guarantee pain relief in different types of headache, such as beta blockers, antidepressants, calcium channel blockers, antiserotoninergic drugs, NSAIDs, steroids, lithium carbonate, sumatriptans, and others. The diversity of the drugs is a clear indicator of the fact that we do not have yet "the drug".

Indeed, each class of drug, and each specific compound seem to be more useful in specific types of headache and in different situations, for example, in case of episodic treatment, in the prophylactic phase or in chronic administration. Nevertheless we have to consider the high risk of abuse and dependence typical of these clinical conditions. In many cases side effects and complications outweight the theoretical positive clinical effects of these drugs.

6. PHARMACOLOGICAL VERSUS NO PHARMACOLOGICAL TREATMENT: A USELESS CONTROVERSY

One of the most frequent errors that occurs in the treatment of headache is to search for a definitive therapy, whether it be pharmacological or no pharmacological. While clinical practice has shown that this approach may be valid for specific kinds of headache, e.g. cluster headache or headaches of low intensity and frequency, most headaches seen by specialists are complex and need to be evaluated and treated accordingly.

Maintaining the separation of the therapeutic domains of the psychologist and the physician is no longer realistic given the multidisciplinary approach to pain therapy. The patient with headache can benefit from psychological treatment even when using a pharmacological therapy. Single treatments by themselves, whether pharmacological or biofeedback, have similar efficacy [42] that can be enhanced in combination. According to a study by Mathew [43] biofeedback alone results in only a 35% improvement. In mixed headaches the best results (improvement of 76%) were obtained with a combination of biofeedback, propanolol, and amitriptyline. However, one caveat is that the combination used should be appropriate, since some combinations, such as BFB and propanolol, may attenuate the respons [44].

When headache is accompanied by problems of mood, a combination of cognitive behavioral therapy and pharmacological therapy may be indicated [45]. Synergy between psychological and pharmacological treatments may effectively reduce fear of the crisis [46].

7. MIGRAINE (IHS CLASSIFICATION 1)

The pathogenesis of migraine has yet to be determined, although two different theories have been proposed. The first, referred to as the dry theory, hypothesizes that the pain is a manifestation of altered vasoregulation of the external carotid artery, while the prodromal symptoms are attributed to a similar alteration of the internal carotid artery [47]. Consequently, the painful symptoms and the collateral neurologic phenomena result from a vasoregulatory dysfunction; vasoconstriction followed by vasodilatation.

The second hypothesis is referred to as the wet theory. It assumes that during vasoconstriction, ischemia causes structural alterations in the cellular membranes, rupturing the membranes and releasing lysosomal enzymes (i.e. proteases) which activate vasodilatory bradykinins [48]. Thus, the pain is provoked by a double action, the first is an interaction with the pain receptors, and the second is a massive vasodilatation and increase in vascular permeability.

Vasoregulation is the basis of both theories, and research has shown that in most patients, the same pathophysiological situations result in a migraine that initiates with a reduction of the cerebral arterial flow [49]. Furthermore, it has also been observed that some intracranial arteries, especially those in the dura mater, dilate and become inflamed during the headache [50].

It is also likely that additional regulatory factors, such as prostaglandins, estrogens, and central and peripheral neurotransmitters (serotonin, dopamine, and noradrenaline) are involved in the initiation of the headache.

There are two main forms of migraine, with aura and without aura, and there are also many minor forms. The difference between migraine with aura and migraine without aura has been explained from a pathogenetical point of view.

Through the analysis of cerebral arterial flow, it has been noted that during aura there is a reduction of the blood flow in some areas of the brain. It is still not clear, however, whether this reduction leads to local ischemia that might correspond to the start of the aura.

7.1. Clinical Characteristics of Migraine

The primary characteristic of a migraine is a pain that is localized on one side of the head. To this pain is added the perception of an intense pain of the temple, or of the eyeball. Often the painful phase is preceded by prodrome of variable duration lasting between 5 and 60 minutes. In migraine with aura, the prodromal phase can include a numbness or tingling in the skin, characteristic eye problems, and occasionally dysphasia. However, the main phenomena are nausea or photophobia.

The migraine attack can be divided into 4 phases:

1. *Prodrome*: Greater than 50% of patients with migraine report prodromal symptoms prior to an acute attack. The experience of previous attacks facilitates recognition of the prodrome which, even if weak, may precede the real crisis by 24 hours. The patient may experience mood alterations, irritability, a feeling of lightness and/or torpor or sluggishness, sensations of boredom and annoyance with associated yawning, and a difficulty speaking. Some cases show variation in the appetite with a desire for specific foods such as sweets, or an unusual thirst.

2. *Aura*: Manifestation of the aura is very acute with a strong feeling of stress. The sense of sight is particularly affected; the patient has the feeling of seeing lightning

and vision is confused. Teichopsia can occur, which appears as flashes around a blind spot. A sensation of "pins and needles" is common, with loss of tactile response and dysphasia. The duration of the aura varies from 5 to 60 minutes, and precedes the migraine by a maximum of 60 minutes.

3. *Headache*: The start of the headache is often gradual. The pain becomes pulsating or penetrating, is typically unilateral, and may be accompanied by nausea, vomiting, photophobia, and photophobia. In general the pain corresponds to a temporal region but often spreads to the orbital area or to other areas on the same side of the head. The migraine can extend to the face, toward the neck, or to the opposite side of the head. In order to limit the intensity of the pain many patients stay in bed in a room isolated from noise and light.

4. *Remission*: At the end of the crisis, many patients describe asthenia, mealier, a feeling of emptiness, and great mental and physical fatigue. In some patients, however, the disappearance of the headache is accompanied by a sense of euphoria.

7.2. Epidemiology of Migraine

Although epidemiological studies confirm that many people throughout the world suffer from migraine, results from these studies are not homogeneous. However, one characteristic that does appear to be consistent is a 2-3-fold greater prevalence of migraine among females compared with males. The reason for this difference has not yet been determined, but it has been proposed that genetic factors at least partially account for it. Migraine most often develops between the ages of 25-34, with less common development in pediatric patients and in those greater than 40 years of age.

8. MIGRAINE WITHOUT AURA (IHS CLASSIFICATION 1.1)

Eighty-five percent of the patients who suffer migraine do not have aura, and 60-70% of patients are undiagnosed. According to the diagnostic criteria of the IHS, a diagnosis of migraine without aura is considered when the patient has shown at least 5 attacks which satisfy the following criteria:

1) Headache attacks which if not treated or treated without success have a duration of 4-72 hours (2-44 hours in those younger than 15 years of age).
2) Headache with at least 2 of the following characteristics:

- monolateral localization
- pulsating pain
- medium or high intensity pain that limits or prevents activities of daily living
- worsening with routine physical activity

3) Presence of at least one of the following symptoms during headache:

- nausea and/or vomiting
- photophobia and/or phonophobia

While it is not always possible to determine the specific factor that initiates the headache, every attempt should be made to do so since it can provide important information regarding susceptibility and therapeutic approaches. The following should be considered as potential contributors:

- Physical factors: tiredness, work, sexual intercourse
- Psychological factors: stress, anxiety or depression during a period of stress or during the relaxation period that follows an exacting task, e.g. relaxation during nonworking days (what is often called "weekend migraine")
- Medical factors: hypertension, allergic rhinitis, paranasal sinus abnormalities or dysfunction, therapeutic modifications
- Hormonal factors: premenstrual phase (catamenial migraine), estro-progesterone usage, menopause
- Dietary factors: tyramine (found in certain cheeses), caffeine, red wine, coffee, chocolate, fasting
- Climatic factors: changes in temperature, intense sunlight, cold, wind
- Migraine is often accompanied by nausea and a general hypersensitivity affecting the senses of sight, hearing and olfaction. It should also be noted that migraine often disappears during the last two trimesters of pregnancy, further suggesting the importance of hormonal factors.

9. MIGRAINE WITH AURA (IHS CLASSIFICATION 1.2)

As previously mentioned, migraine with aura occurs in only small proportion of patients, generally older individuals although it can also start during pregnancy.

According to the diagnostic criteria of the IHS, a diagnosis of migraine with aura is considered when the patient has shown at least 5 attacks with at least 3 of the following characteristics:

1) One or more symptoms of the aura are completely reversible, indicating a dysfunction of the focal cortex and/or of the encephalic trunk
2) Gradual development of at least one symptoms during a 4 minute period or development of 2 or more successive symptoms
3) None of the symptoms of the aura lasts more than 60 minutes, with a tolerated duration of symptoms proportionally increased if multiple symptoms are present
4) The headache follows the aura after a symptom-free interval of less than 60 minutes, although the headache may also start before the aura.

9.1. Treatment of Migraine

A comprehensive program of treatment for migraine incorporates the following 4 elements [51]:

- Therapy of acute attacks with drugs such as dihydroergotamine (DHE), Isomeheptene mucate, oxygen, nerve bloks of the sphenopalatine ganglion or sumatriptan
- Prevention through avoiding factors that can initiate the headache
- Long-term prophylactic therapy with beta adrenergic blockers, antidepressants, calcium channel blockers, serotonin antagonists, anticonvulsants, and/or nonsteroidal anti-inflammatory drugs (NSAIDs)
- Nonpharmacological therapy

9.2. Pharmacological Treatment of the Acute Phase

Analgesics have been shown to be effective in the earliest phase of the attack. The most common drugs are simple analgesics (acetylsalicylic acid, paracetamol) which are usually sufficient to reduce or eliminate the pain in most patients. Nonsteroidal anti-inflammatory drugs (NSAIDs) such as ibuprofen and naproxen, are not often used in the acute phase.

Ergotamine tartrate is generally used when analgesics fail. The ergots produce a vasoconstriction of the extracranial vessels involved in the progression of the migraine attack. Ergotamine is generally associated to caffeine in different combinations. Some patients prefer the rectal or sublingual administration since nausea and vomiting generally limit the oral administration. However, due to interpatient variability in ergotamine bioavailability, it does not provide symptomatic relief in all patients.

Oxygen (5-10 L/min) can be inhaled with a mask. The home treatment may present some risks in patients used to smoke.

Isomeheptene mucate has stopped the migraine attack in some patiets and for this reason the drug has been included in the first line abortive therapy. Recently, sumatriptan, an analog of 5 hydroxytryptamine (5-HT; serotonin) has been introduced into widespread use as a first line drug for symptomatic therapy of migraine both with and without aura in patients who suffer moderate or serious crises. Sumatriptan selectively inhibits dilation of intracranial cerebral arteries. Using a dose of 6 mg 70% of patients experience a marked pain relief. Some potential serious side effects limit the use of the drug in patients with coronary arthery diseas and periphaeral vascular insufficiency .

Measurement of changes in patient quality of life can provide a good indication of drug efficacy [52], although a baseline measurement prior to starting therapy is generally required for a more valid evaluation of this outcome [53].

While headache therapy is often combined with anti-depressive therapy, caution should be exercised when using concomitant medications, since certain drug classes can result in undesirable interactions [54].

9.3. Prophylactic Pharmacological Treatment

Prophylaxis is indicated in those patients who suffer from at least 2 attacks a month and who are refractory to conventional therapy. In general, prophylaxis is carried out as necessary rather than continuously.

Prophylactic drugs reduce the frequency and/or the intensity of the crises in 60-80% of patients, and it is important that they be used during serious and frequent attacks (more than twice a month). Onset of action is usually 2-4 weeks, with a peak in efficacy after two months. Their use does not preclude the concomitant use of drugs for symptomatic treatment, which may be prescribed in limited doses. Prophylactic treatment should be continued for at least 3-4 months and then interrupted to verify the necessity of its continuation.

Beta blockers are viewed as first line therapy for migraine profilaxys since Rabkin accidentally discovered the efficacy of these drugs in a patient with cardiac disease who was suffering from migraine [55] These include the selective beta blockers (metapropolol, bispropolol), non selective beta blockers (timolol, propanolol), and the tricyclic antideperessant amitryptyline. Second line agents include the vasodilator flunarazine, serotonin inhibitors (ciproheptadine, pizotyline), dopamine agonists (lisuride), serotonin precursors (5-hydroxytryptophan) and clonidine, a sympatholytic alpha adrenergic agonist-antagonist. In some cases a calcium channel blocker could be tried. Varapamil (80 mg three times a day) is generally used even if sustained release formulations will probably reduce the side effects that are consistent with hypotention, flushing, and g.i. problems.

9.4. Nonpharmacological Treatment

Despite much research and the variety of available options, the ideal therapy for migraine still has not been determined [56].

Results from several sources including studies performed at some of the largest research centers for the study of headache suggest an important role for nonpharmacological modalities in the treatment of migraine.

The Canadian Headache Society recently published guidelines for the management of migraine [57] which recommend a wider application of nonpharmacological therapies. Nonpharmacological therapies are not only of benefit to patients, but also have economic advantages.

Patients often prefer to try a nonpharmacological therapy before resorting to drug administration, and will frequently try little tricks to limit the pain. These tricks can include application of cold bandages or pressure to the temporal artery, although the relief is limited only to the time of the action and does not provide long-term benefits. The patient can also avoid staying in places with high noise levels or strong lights. Knowing the factors that initiate the headache can significantly contribute to a nonpharmacological approach.

Diet too can influence the initiation and outcome of headache. It is advisable to limit caffeine, avoid alcohol (mainly red wine), aged cheeses, chocolate, nuts, monosodium glutamate, and food rich in nitrites. Meals should be eaten at regular intervals, and fasting should be avoided.

Additionally, a regular sleep schedule avoids the modification of sleep rhythms that can provoke migraine. Pharmacological agents that that affect hormones, such as oral contraceptives, should also be avoided. Those headaches caused by symptomatic drug abuse, especially related to ergotamine, should be identified and can be treated by behavior modification.

Biofeedback (BFB) is one of the best-known nonpharmacological therapies. It is particularly recommended for young patients, pregnant or breastfeeding women, and patients who prefer not to use drugs or do not tolerate them. Patients who suffer frequent and/or severe episodes of headache often ingest large quantities of caffeine-based drugs. When starting BFB therapy, it is not necessary to interrupt these drugs, but one can gradually eliminate them as the nonpharmacological therapy proceeds.

Thermal BFB is commonly used although the exact mechanisms for its action are not clear [58]. Combination therapies that include BFB are becoming increasingly important, especially use of relaxation techniques or physical therapy [59].

Cognitive behavioral therapy is a method that can be used to train the patient to identify the thoughts, sensations, and beliefs present at the start and during the migraine attack [60]. It can also be used adjunctively with pharmacological therapy to improve patient compliance, which can have a significant effect on treatment outcomes.

Patient compliance is often related to the prescribing pattern, as has been shown in a study by Mulleners et al. [61] who evaluated the effects of compliance in 38 patients taking prophylactic therapy for migraine. In their study, while pill counts suggested that the quantity of drug taken corresponded to what was prescribed, they determined that the average compliance rate was only 66%. Variables were identified that potentiated the risk of treatment failure. These variables included the times and rates of consumption. Importantly, they observed that compliance was significantly better when the drug was prescribed once a day rather than two or three times daily. These data suggest that a pill count is inadequate to evaluate patient compliance, and that consumption of drug occurs irregularly and may contribute to treatment failure.

10. TENSION-TYPE HEADACHE (IHS CLASSIFICATION 2)

Tension-type headaches are characterized by a dull constant pain localized in the occipital or posterior cervical regions, often extending to the frontal region. This pain develops frequently after mental or physical stress and its initiation can often be associated with a specific stressful factor. The headache can subsequently autonomize and become a daily companion that only remits during sleep. In recent years an attempt was made to establish if tension-type headaches and migraine are part of a continuum in which the migraine symptoms such as nausea and vomiting, initiates only upon an increase in intensity of the headache. However, in the absence of confirming evidence for this hypothesis, the predominant opinion is that there are two distinct pathologies, each with its own diagnostic criteria and therapeutic regimens.

On the pathogenetic level, there appear to be differences between the episodic and chronic forms. In the former case, evidence suggests that psychological problems activate a contraction of the skeletal muscles of the face, scalp, neck and shoulders. However, there is currently no satisfactory theory that explains the chronic form.

Among the pathogenetic factors that are considered important in initiating the crisis are mood, oromandibular dysfunction, secondary muscular stress, remaining in an awkward or abnormal position, lack of sleep, and the abuse of, or dependence on, analgesics or anxiolytics.

10.1. Clinical Characteristics

The pain has been described as a pressure, a heaviness of the head, a vise, a constriction, and a ring around the head. The pain is dull and constant although with there are variations in intensity during the day. This pain is often referred to as lateral localized pain, but sometimes it may be characterized by a band of pain extending bilaterally. It can be felt at the temples, in the back of the head and the neck, or a combination, with movement from one part of the head to another; it may also affect the whole head.

Onset of pain is classically gradual rather than sudden. In the chronic forms it develops during the day so that it is present upon waking and continues until evening with variations in intensity. It often worsens toward the end of the day, but at night the patient does not wake up with headache. Activities of daily life are not generally impeded, and do not decline with physical effort. Collateral symptoms are often absent, although nausea, phonophobia, and photophobia have been reported in some cases. These associated symptoms are less frequent than in migraine, and their presence in an episodic form occurs only in the most acute phases. The neurologic exam is completely normal.

Correlated psychological symptoms can be anxiety, difficulty in concentration, and depressed mood. Work and spare time are greatly affected. The duration of the headache can vary from 30 minutes to 7 days. However, tension-type headache can be a transitory event, or have a duration of weeks, months or years with varying intensity.

10.2. Epidemiology

It is estimated that 90% of headaches are of the tension-type. Onset is at an early age, within the first 10 years in about 15% of the patients, but almost always occurring by years of age. Chronicity develops very early, and the headaches are often refractory to the common therapies. The incidence is higher in females than in males (3:1 ratio), and is considered hereditary in about 40% of cases.

10.3. Forms

Tension-type headache is considered episodic if it occurs with a frequency less than 15 days/month. It the headache is present 15 or more days a month for a period of at least 6 months, it is considered to be the chronic form.

10.4. Masked Headache

The differential diagnosis of tension-type headache should include consideration of other specific problems which may mask it. Cervical arthrosis can provide one example of masking, especially in an older patient. From the fifth decade of life, about 50% of people have some type of degenerative spinal problem, and during the sixth decade, the percentage increases to 75% with subsequent increases in further years. X-rays show skeletal alterations in the region of pain. Consequently, a diagnosis of cervical arthrosis is often made since psychological evaluation is rarely performed and the patient is reluctant to talk about such problems if not properly questioned. In reality, stress and daily problems may be producing a persistent contraction of the muscles of the neck, shoulder, and head which results in the complaint of pain.

Another example of masking is posttraumatic headache. A person suffering a head injury may have a local pain or stiffness in the specific region for a duration of hours or days. If the pain continues for a significant time after the accident, explanations other than an organic basis for the pain should be considered, such as anxiety or personality structure, which can play a decisive role in the continuity of the problem. In this case, it would not be called a posttraumatic headache, but rather a tension-type headache, because the trauma would cause recurrence resulting from an a previous psychological problem such as anxiety or depression.

10.5. Pharmacological Treatment

The patient who requests a specialist for tension-type headache often has a long history of administration of analgesics, NSAIDs, and/or caffeine-based drugs. The tricyclic antidepressant amitryptaline has proven to be effective independently of the presence of depression, especially as preventive therapy in those patients called "big chronics" and in those over age 60. In view of the fact that they act on the underlying depression, and normalize sleep and mood, antidepressants can be considered the drugs of choice in the tension type headache. Antidepressants have also some side effects and patients have to be informed about the possibility of sedation, dry mouth, blurred vision, and urinary retention. Patients must be informed also about the delay of the positive effects that will start in two-three weeks. Amytriptiline could be administered initially at bedtime (25 mg) increasing to two pills after a week and according to side effects. Salicylates and/or NSAIDs in association with a muscle relaxant may be prescribed in the most acute phases. An alternative therapy is injection of local anesthetics and steroids into the areas known as trigger points for the headache. Cervical steroids and epidural blocks with local anesthetics have been shown to provide long term pain relief.

Drug abuse can be a frequent problem in headache sufferers that arises from their constant attempt, and inability, to interrupt the pain. The chronic use and abuse of ergotamine or analgesics can produce a worsening in the frequency of the headache, that can turn into a daily problem.

10.6. Nonpharmacological Treatment

The preferred nonpharmacological therapy is electromyographic BFB. This method is particularly useful when the components of muscular contraction that cause the pain are evident. When this technique is used, the electrode is often positioned on the frontal muscle even when the position on the trapezius would appear to be more convenient or advantageous [24].

A complete evaluation with confirmed diagnosis and explanation on the part of the physician can also be of considerable therapeutic benefit by alleviating the patient's fears that the headache might hide a more serious pathology such as a tumor [62].

In addition to treating the muscular pathogenesis (such as by electromyographyic BFB), a certain level of relief can be obtained by therapies based on relaxation techniques such as progressive relaxation [30], autogenic training[31], or transcendental meditation [63]. In selected cases, cognitive behavioral therapy alone or associated with hypnosis may be effective[64].

11. CLUSTER HEADACHE (IHS CLASSIFICATION 3.1)

Cluster headache is characterized by its intensity, which is higher than in other types of chronic headache. It is also known as paroxysmal night headache because those who suffer from it wake up 2-3 hours after falling asleep at night due to the intense pain caused by the crisis. Other names are Horton's syndrome, histamine headache, or migrainous neuralgia, but the popular term "suicide headache" better expresses the dimension of this pain.

The pain starts with periorbital localization, with a partial syndrome of Horner consisting of ptosis and myosis, and proceeds with expansion to the proximal intracranial region of the internal carotid artery. Pathogenesis involves various vascular structures and neurogenic mechanisms. The remarkable regularity with which the crises take place suggests a role for the hypothalamic structures that are connected to the regulation of the circadian cycle.

Epidemiologically, there is a clear prevalence in males with a further clinically relevant observation of low testosterone levels in patients presenting with this type of headache. This suggests that there may be hypothalamic involvement as a consequence of the changes in the biological cycle caused by the headache.

11.1. Clinical Characteristics

Cluster headache is characterized by paroxysmal attacks of sharp pain (the clear definition of paroxysmal night headache) of variable duration from 15-180 minutes.

Localization is usually in the retro- or para-orbital regions. The patient often feels as if the pain starts from the inside of the eye. Sometimes the eye is red, the pupil contracts (myosis), the eyelid droops (ptosis), and although there can be a monolateral feeling of a clogged nose with an increase in nasal secretions (rhinorrhea) and a monolateral feeling of clamminess in the skin, the effect may also be bilateral. The pain radiates toward the temple,

454 Aldo Lamberto, Alfredo Fogliardi, Mauro Nicoscia et al.

the forehead, the neck, the jaw, the dental arch, and the chin, and is accompanied by intense monolateral lacrimation, conjunctival irritation, and nasal congestion.

The pain is sharp, pressing, unbearable. It starts suddenly and reaches its peak in a few minutes.

The crisis has a duration of 15 minutes to half an hour, and often starts at fixed times that correspond to the meals (circadian rhythm at fixed hours). The crises can be daily, single or multiple, and cyclic throughout the year. The word cluster refers to the alternation of multiple crises in a period of time that can last from 3 to 16 weeks. These periods do not have fixed boundaries and show variability from 6 months to 5 years. However, there is frequently a regular recurrence of two epicrises during a period of 12 months that is strictly connected to the seasons of spring and autumn. During the epicrisis the attacks occur from one to 3 times within a 24 hour period, with a nocturnal prevalence 2-3 hours after falling asleep. There are no prodromic symptoms and neither nausea nor vomiting. Due to pain intensity the person who is suffering takes antalgic positions and it is not infrequent to see patients hitting their head with their arms, or against a wall. Other times there may be an incessant swinging or undulation of the head or an appearance of a continuous tremor. The movements can become violent during states of extreme agitation that may be reached by the patient. Among the initiating factors are stress, alcohol, histamine, glaring lights, exposure to temperature extremes, REM sleep, and vasodilatory substances, such as nitrates that may be an ingredient in certain foods.

11.2. Epidemiology

Although there are few epidemiologic studies, it appears that the incidence of this type of headache is rare, about 0.5% of the male population and less than 0.1% of the female population (a 5:1 male:female ratio). Onset usually occurs between 20 and 30 years of age, and heredity does not appear to play a significant role.

11.3. Forms

Episodic cluster headache is characterized in untreated patients by at least 2 periods of headache of variable duration from 7 to 365 days separated by remission phases lasting longer than 14 days. In the chronic form, the attacks occur for more than 365 days without remission or with remission of less than 14 days. This form is difficult to treat, especially when the attacks are frequent or when there are problems of pharmacological abuse and/or neurotic personality.

11.4. Diagnosis

According to the diagnostic criteria of the IHS, a diagnosis of cluster headache is made when at least 5 attacks occur with the following criteria:

1) Monolateral pain, of severe intensity, localized in the orbital region, supraorbital region, and/or temporal region, of 15-80 minutes duration when not treated.

2) The headache must be associated with at least one of the following symptoms on the same side as the pain: Conjunctival congestion, Lacrimation, Nasal congestion, Rhinorrhea Hyperhidrosis (excessive perspiration) on the forehead and face, Myosis, Eyelid ptosis, and Eyelid edema.

3) Frequency of attacks varies from 1 every other day to 8 per day.

11.5. Pharmacological Treatment

The characteristics of cluster headache suggest urgent treatment. The inhalation of oxygen is probably the safest and most effective mean s to stop the acute cluster headache. Patients must be adequately instructed about the risks of explosions of oxygen in the presence of flames (i.e., smoke). Ergotamine, either inhaled, rectally, or sublingually, is considered the first-line agent. In difficult cases oxygen inhalation may be required [65]. Steroids demonstrated prophylactic efficacy, and prednisone was shown to be the most effective drug for prophylactic therapy in both chronic and episodic forms [66, 67] Some success was also obtained with lithium, especially in the chronic form [68, 69]. Calcium antagonists [70, 71] and sodium valproate [72] have also been used, and the serotonin antagonist methysergide has demonstrated good therapeutic efficacy in episodic forms and in young patients [73]. Methysergide ia a antiserotoninergic compound that is considered a medication of choice for episodic cluster headache. The drugs has heavy side effects, such as retroperitoneal and cardiac fibrosis, and for this reason the treatment must be often discontinued, the dosage is low and the use cannot exceed 6 months a year.

A recent epidemiologic study showed that the most common interventions are oxygen inhalation and sumatriptan injection, with injection of dihyroergotamine used less frequently [74]. A new therapeutic approach has been proposed based on the similiarity between cluster headache and seasonal affective disorder [75]. In both cases there are changes in the mechanisms in secretion of melatonin. The normalization of the melatonin secretory cycle could open new avenues of treatment using both phototherapy and melatonin administration.

11.6. Nonpharmacological Treatment

Personality evaluation using the MMPI in patients with cluster headache does not generally show any significant changes. Occasionally there is an elevation of the Depression and Hysteria subscales, and this may justify the further use of psychological diagnostic methods. Cognitive behavioral treatment in these patients is primarily based on reassurance and prevention, since patients demonstrate anxiety and anguish during the cluster period. Educational programs are recommended to relieve the fear that the problem is of a malignant nature.

One third of the patients having a first attack are likely to have a future attack of moderate or intense severity. For the other two-thirds, one third will not have further attacks, and one third are likely to have attacks of minor intensity. About half of the patients with the chronic form have difficulty finding an effective therapy. Preventive therapy may reduce the intensity of the crises but will not eliminate them. The avoidance of certain foods (especially alcohol) as well as of other vasodilatory substances, such as certain medications, hydrocarbons, and solvents, can help prevent onset of a crisis. A regular daily schedule without a midafternoon nap can also help prevent headache onset.

12. HEADACHE DURING THE DEVELOPMENTAL YEARS

Headache is the most prevalent of the benign chronic pain syndromes that are associated with the years of development (i.e. prior to adulthood). This period of life is characterized by frequent somatic disturbances that may especially become evident when a child begins school. Children complain mainly about headaches, stomach cramps and, less often, skeletal muscle disturbances. The causes of these discomforts can generally be correlated with the emotional responses to the everyday problems characteristic of this stage of life, particularly school difficulties and problems in interpersonal relationships with adults, most often parents and teachers. The effects of what is known as "peer pressure" are also evident at this stage. Gender has been correlated with the types of symptoms and the types of affective or behavioral problems that may be present [76]. Stomach disturbances in boys have been associated with oppositional defiant disorder and with attention deficit hyperactivity disorder (ADHD). In girls, anxiety has been associated with the presence of either musculoskeletal problems alone, or stomach problems in the presence of headache.

The approach to therapy has focused on prophylactic and symptomatic treatment of the pathology itself. A primary goal has been to limit the progression of headache into adulthood, as often happens. In a study by Bille et al., 40% of the patients who had headache during the years of development went on to have problems with headaches as adults [77].

In addition to being a medical problem, headache can become a scholastic problem when it becomes apparent that headache is one of the main causes of absence or withdrawal from school [78]. In many young patients, headache is evident primarily during the school year, and it is not infrequent to find that some of these patients also have memory and attention deficits.

The focus should not be exclusively on the headache itself, since there appears to be a strong correlation between "pain" as a principal symptom and depression as consequence. This correlation suggests a greater likelihood for the development of depressive syndromes in adulthood in younger patients whose problems remain unresolved.

The early administration of drugs, however, could lead to a greater propensity for drug abuse with its unavoidable side effects as well as the possibility of developing rebound headaches.

12.1. Risk Factors

Among the identified risk factors for the development of headache during the early years are the family history, the presence of sleep disorders, and the presence of headache warning syndromes [79] .The latter may start as early as the first month of life and may be identified by the presence of specific symptoms such as hyperactivity, kinetosis, and recurrent abdominal pains.

Within the family history, learning has a very important role. Early conditioning may be initiated by the presence of a parent with a headache or who complains about other types of pain. The child receives this imprint and responds in a similar manner. A controlled study compared 96 children 6 years of age having migraine or tensive muscular headache with a control group without headache [80]. The children with headache were observed to have behavioral problems that were not present or were reduced in the controls. For example, during play, there was a greater tendency to express fear, as well as a higher incidence of injury in the group with headache compared with the control group.

Among children with headache, there is also a greater tendency to complain of abdominal pains and to cry during vaccinations or upon drawing blood. According to the parents, such children are more sensitive to pain. An evaluation of the family environment, and how the parents face pain, can provide insight into the conditioning behavior patterns. The fathers of children who suffer from headache seem more sensitive to pain, and the mothers have an even greater sensitivity. A stressful familial environment can also be a direct cause of headache.

12.2. Initiating Events

General stress and school stress are the two factors most closely related to onset of headache during the developmental years.

Moscato reported a 27% incidence of headache among 15,806 children 6-16 years of age [81]. Another study evaluated the effect of school stress on headache development by comparing the frequency of headache after the first 12 months of school (children between 6 and 7 years of age), with previous and subsequent time periods [82]. The frequency of headache increased in 20% of the children who had headache in the six months prior to the start of school. It can be suggested that the starting of the school stress may be one of the factors which subsequently influences the development of the headaches in adulthood.

Usually, episodic headaches tend to diminish during the second school year, but a percentage of children will still continue to have headaches, and the presence of unsatisfactory conditions at home can provide a concomitant cause of migraine in these children [83].

12.3. Accompanying Factors

Children who suffer headaches often present with other problems such as an increased prevalence of sleep disorders (insomnia and nocturnal awakening), parasomnias (somnambulism, somniloquy, enuresis), or nocturnal snoring.

12.4. Therapy

During this stage of development, if the headache reaches an intensity or frequency such that it requires intervention, it is generally preferable to choose a non-pharmacological therapy. This avoids potential abuse and rebound effects [84]. Sartory et al compared psychological and pharmacological therapy in 43 children between the ages of 8 and 16 (mean age 11.3 years) who suffered from migraine [85]. The 6-week program of nonpharmacological therapy consisted of stress management training combined with either progressive relaxation or cephalic vasomotor biofeedback. The 10-week pharmacological therapy consisted of metoprolol administration. The most effective therapy for reducing both headache frequency and intensity was the combination of relaxation and stress management training. Good efficacy was also obtained in the group receiving BFB, which also had a positive effect on mood.

Duckro [86] reviewed seven studies published between 1984 and 1988 that used relaxation with or without biofeedback for the treatment of headache in children and adolescents. The types of headache were different but the results were all in agreement in affirming the efficacy of biofeedback. Headache during the developmental years has a strong anxiety component that likely plays a determinant role in causing tension of the neck muscles in these patients [87]. Thus, the efficacy of biofeedback therapy results from training the patient to reduce the negative effects caused by the anxiety [88].

Several studies tried to determine which were the best nonpharmacological treatments. One study compared biofeedback training with autogenous training in patients 8-18 years of age [89]. The study also considered a control group of patients not undergoing training. The results were evaluated during 6 months of followup. The BFB group had the greatest efficacy as measured by percent of symptom-free patients (80%), with 50% efficacy obtained with autogenous training, and no symptom-free patients in the control group.

Because of the simplicity of the relaxation method, it has generally been considered an important method of treatment in children and young adults. School programs of relaxation training have been developed for helping children with anxiety problems and headaches. These programs use muscle relaxation techniques adapted from adult programs, but no encouraging results were found [90]. The clinical and educational significance of the program are uncertain. More specific individualized interventions may be indicated. Generalized relaxation cannot be considered as prophylaxis for anxiety and pediatric headache.

Other nonpharmacological therapeutic proposals have found behavioral assessment with subsequent behavioral therapy to be a useful approach to headache diagnosis and treatment during the years of development [91]. Less promising are group therapies for children between the ages of 7 and 12 years which use a combination of relaxation, distraction, visualization and acquisition of ability of stress management techniques [92]. Recently, a portable apparatus for thermal BFB has been developed which may make this technique more readily available for home use. Evaluation of BFB at home with the assistance of the parents [93] has shown that the parents not only encourage the use of BFB but can also directly influence behavioral by avoiding the reinforcement of negative behaviors. The advantage of BFB is that efficacy has been correlated with the frequency of the practice at home. It has also been noted that the home-based therapy has a similar efficacy as an intensive in-hospital program [94], with the advantage of being more cost-effective [95].

However, the level of home-based BFB therapy also depends on child-related variables, such as the level of psychosomatic problems, the tendency to externalize behavior, and the age. On the other hand, variables related to the family do not seem to influence home-based BFB therapy [96].

13. REFERENCES

[1] Association AP. *Diagnostic and statistical manual of mental disorders*. 4th ed. Washington, DC: American Psychiatric Press; 1994.

[2] Kudrow L, Sutkus BJ. MMPI pattern specificity in primary headache disorders. *Headache* 1979;19(1):18-24.

[3] Sternbach RA, Dalessio DJ, Kunzel M, Bowman GE. MMPI patterns in common headache disorders. *Headache* 1980;20(6):311-5.

[4] Andrasik F, Blanchard EB, Arena JG, et al. Psychological functioning in headache sufferers. *Psychosom Med* 1982;44(2):171-82.

[5] Pradalier A., Mavre D., Serviere R., et al. Le minagreux: recherche des charateristiques psychologiques. *Rev Med. Interne*. 11: 410-413, 1990.

[6] Puca FM, Prudenzano AMP. Stato dell'arte sulle cefalee tensive. Paper presented at: IV Congresso Nazionale SICD, 1994; Bressanone.

[7] Luborsky L, Docherty JP, Penick S. Onset conditions for psychosomatic symptoms: a comparative review of immediate observation with retrospective research. *Psychosom Med* 1973;35(3):187-204.

[8] Beck AT, Ward CH, Mendelson M, Mock J, Erbaugh J. An inventory for measuring depression. *Arch Gen Psychiatry* 1961;4:561-71.

[9] Zung WW, Richards CB, Short MJ. Self-rating depression scale in an outpatient clinic. Further validation of the SDS. *Arch Gen Psychiatry* 1965;13(6):508-15.

[10] Silberstein SD. Comprehensive management of headache and depression. *Cephalalgia* 1998;18 (Suppl 21):50-55.

[11] Hirschfield RMA. Sertraline in the treatment of anxiety disorders. *Depression Anxiety* 2000;11:139-57.

[12] Bischoff C. Traue H.C.: Myogenic Headache. In Holroyd K.A. Schlote B., Zenz H. (Eds.). *Perspectives in research on headache*. Hogrefe. Toronto, 1983.}

[13] Turk DC, Flor H. Etiological theories and treatments for chronic back pain. II. Psychological models and interventions. *Pain* 1984;19(3):209-33.

[14] Flor H, Turk DC, Birbaumer N. Assessment of stress-related psychophysiological reactions in chronic back pain patients. *J Consult Clin Psychol* 1985;53(3):354-64.

[15] Sicuteri F.: Headache: disruption of pain modulation. In : J.J. Bonica e D. Albe-Fessard (Ed.) *Advances in Pain Research and Therapy*. Vol.1 Raven Press, New York. 871-880,1970..

[16] Classification and diagnostic criteria for headache disorders, cranial neuralgias and facial pain. Headache Classification Committee of the International Headache Society. Cephalalgia 1988;8 (Suppl 7):1-96.

[17] Malmo RB. *On Emotions, Needs, and Our Archaic Brain*. New York: Holt Rinehart & Winston; 1975.

[18] Fuller GD. *Biofeedback: Methods and Procedures in Clinical Practice*. New York: BMA; 1977.

[19] Beltrutti, D., Lamberto, A: *Aspetti psicologici nel dolore cronico: dalla valutazione alla terapia*. Edizioni CELI, Faenza, 1997, 307-335.

[20] Cohen RA, Williamson DA, Monguillot JE, et al. Psychophysiological response patterns in vascular and muscle-contraction headaches. *J Behav Med* 1983;6(1):93-107.

[21] Prima A, Agnoli A, Tamburello A. A review of the applications of biofeedback to migraine and tension headaches. *Acta Neurol* (Napoli) 1979;1(6):510-21.

[22] Basmajian JV. *Biofeedback - Principles and practice for clinicians*. Baltimore: Williams and Wilkins; 1978.

[23] Traue HC Mahoney A.M. Bischoff C.: Toward a new understanding of tension headache. In D. Papakostopoulos, S. Butler, I. Martin (Eds.) *Clinical and experimental Neuropsychophysiology*. Croom Helm, London, 1985, 558-577.

[24] Arena JG, Bruno GM, Hannah SL, Meador KJ. A comparison of frontal electromyographic biofeedback training, trapezius electromyographic biofeedback training, and progressive muscle relaxation therapy in the treatment of tension headache. *Headache* 1995;35(7):411-19.

[25] Schwartz MS. Headache: Selected issues and considerations in Biofeedback Evaluations and Therapies. *Biofeedback*. New York: Guilford Press; 1987.

[26] Snyder C, Noble M. Operant conditioning of vasoconstriction. *J Exp Psychol* 1968;77(2):263-68.

[27] Green EE, Green AM. Biofeedback: rationale and applications. *Intern.Encyclopedia of Neurology, Psychiatry, Psychoanalysis and Psychology*. New York: Van Nostrand Reinhold; 1977.

[28] Andrasik F. Relaxation and biofeedback for chronic headaches. In: Holzman AD, Turk DC, editors. *Pain Management: A Handbook of Psychological Treatment Approaches*. New York: Pergamon Press; 1986.

[29] McGrady A, Wauquier A, McNeil A, Gerard G. Effect of biofeedback-assisted relaxation on migraine headache and changes in cerebral blood flow velocity in the middle cerebral artery. *Headache* 1994;34(7):424-8.

[30] Jacobson E. *Progressive Relaxation*. Chicago: University of Chicago Press; 1938.

[31] Schultz, J. H. *Das Autogene Training* G.T. Verlag , Stuttgart 1932.

[32] Benson H. Your innate asset for combating stress. *Harvard Business Review*. 1983;52:49-60.

[33] Horan JJ. "In vivo" emotive imagery: a technique for reducing childbirth anxiety and discomfort. *Psychol Rep* 1973;32(3):1328.

[34] Ilacqua GE. Migraine headaches: coping efficacy of guided imagery training. *Headache* 1994;34(2):99-102.

[35] Holroyd KA, Penzien DB. Client variables and the behavioral treatment of recurrent tension headache: a meta-analytic review. *J Behav Med* 1986;9(6):515-36.

[36] Meichenbaum DH, Genest MA. A cognitive-behavioral approach: an illustration in the group treatment of anxiety. In: Harris GG, editor. *The Group Treatment of Human Problems: A Social Learning Approach.* New York: Grune and Stratton; 1977.

[37] Ellis, A :The basic clinical Theory of Rational-Emotive Therapy" in: A. Ellis and R. Grieger (Eds.) *Handbook of Rational-Emotive Therapy*, New York Springer 1977.

[38] Bakal DA, Demjen S, Kaganov JA. Cognitive behavioral treatment of chronic headache. *Headache* 1981;21(3):81-86.

[39] Blanchard EB, Ahles TA. Biofeedback therapy. In: Bonica JJ, editor. *The Management of Pain.* Malvern: Lea and Febiger; 1990.

[40] Schwartz SM, Gramling SE. Cognitive factors associated with facial pain. *Cranio* 1997;15(3):261-66.

[41] Sargent JD, Green EE, Walters ED. Preliminary report on the use of autogenic feedback training in the treatment of migraine and tension headaches. *Psychosom Med* 1973;35(2):129-35.

[42] Holroyd KA, Penzien DB. Pharmacological versus non-pharmacological prophylaxis of recurrent migraine headache: a meta-analytic review of clinical trials. *Pain* 1990;42(1):1-13.

[43] Mathew NT. Prophylaxis of migraine and mixed headache. A randomized controlled study. *Headache* 1981;21(3):105-09.

[44] Jay GW, Renelli D, Mead T. The effects of propranolol and amitriptyline on vascular and EMG biofeedback training. *Headache* 1984;24(2):59-69.

[45] Van Hook E. Non-pharmacological treatment of headaches--why? *Clin Neurosci* 1998;5(1):43-49.

[46] Saadah HA. Headache fear. *J Okla State Med Assoc* 1997;90(5):179-84.

[47] Wolff HG. *Wolff's Headache and Other Head Pain.* New York: Oxford University Press; 1963.

[48] Sicuteri F. Headache: disruption of pain modulation. In: Bonica JJ, Albe-Fessard D, editors. *Advances in Pain Research and Therapy.* New York: Raven Press; 1970. p. 871-80.

[49] Friberg L, Olesen J, Lassen NA, Olsen TS, Karle A. Cerebral oxygen extraction, oxygen consumption, and regional cerebral blood flow during the aura phase of migraine. *Stroke* 1994 May;25(5):974-9

[50] Friberg L, Olesen J, Iversen HK, Sperling B. Migraine pain associated with middle cerebral artery dilatation: reversal by sumatriptan.. *Lancet* 1991 Jul 6;338(8758):13-7

[51] Young WB, Silberstein SD, Dayno JM. Migraine treatment. *Semin Neurol* 1997;17(4):325-33.

[52] Mannix LK, Solomon GD. Quality of life in migraine. *Clin Neurosci* 1998;5(1):38-42.

[53] Litaker DG, Solomon GD, Genzen JR. Using pretreatment quality of life perceptions to predict response to sumatriptan in migraineurs. *Headache* 1997;37(10):630-34.

[54] Joffe RT, Sokolov ST. Co-administration of fluoxetine and sumatriptan: the Canadian experience. *Acta Psychiatr Scand* 1997;95(6):551-52.

[55] Diamond S, Dalessio DJ. *The Practining Physician's Approach to Headache. 3rd Ed.* Baltimore, William and Wilkins, 1982..

[56] Bic Z, Blix GG, Hopp HP, Leslie FM. In search of the ideal treatment for migraine headache. *Med Hypotheses* 1998;50(1).

[57] Pryse-Phillips WE, Dodick DW, Edmeads JG, Gawel MJ, Nelson RF, Purdy RA, et al. Guidelines for the nonpharmacologic management of migraine in clinical practice. *Canadian Headache Society. CMAJ* 1998;159(1):47-54.

[58] Blanchard EB, Peters ML, Hermann C, Turner SM, Buckley TC, Barton K, et al. Direction of temperature control in the thermal biofeedback treatment of vascular headache. *Appl Psychophysiol Biofeedback* 1997;22(4):227-45.

[59] Marcus DA, Scharff L, Mercer S, Turk DC. Nonpharmacological treatment for migraine: incremental utility of physical therapy with relaxation and thermal biofeedback. *Cephalalgia* 1998;18(5):266-72.

[60] Passchier J, Mourik J, Brienen JA, Hunfeld JA. Cognitions, emotions, and behavior of patients with migraine when taking medication during an attack. *Headache* 1998;38(6):458-64.

[61] Mulleners WM, Whitmarsh TE, Steiner TJ. Noncompliance may render migraine prophylaxis useless, but once-daily regimens are better. *Cephalalgia* 1998;18(1):52-56.

[62] Smeets G, de Jong PJ, Mayer B. If you suffer from a headache, then you have a brain tumour: domain-specific reasoning 'bias' and hypochondriasis. *Behav Res Ther* 2000;38(8):763-76.

[63] Hassed, C. Meditation in general practice. *Aust Fam Physician* 1996, 25 (8): 1257-60.

[64] Reich BA : Non-invasive treatment of vascular and muscle contraction headache: a comparative longitudinal clinical study. *Headache* 1989;29(1):34-41.

[65] Kudrow L. *Cluster Headache: Mechanisms and Management.* New York: Oxford University Press; 1980.

[66] Kudrow L. Response of cluster headache attacks to oxygen inhalation. *Headache* 1981;21(1):1-4.

[67] Fogan L. Treatment of cluster headache. A double-blind comparison of oxygen v air inhalation. *Arch Neurol* 1985;42(4):362-63.

[68] Ekbom K. Lithium in the treatment of chronic cluster headache. (editorial). *Headache* 1977;17(1):39-40.

[69] Mathew NT. Clinical subtypes of cluster headache and response to lithium therapy. *Headache* 1978;18(1):27-29.

[70] Meyer JS, Hardenberg J. Clinical effectiveness of calcium entry blockers in prophylactic treatment of migraine and cluster headaches. *Headache* 1983;23(6):266-77.

[71] Meyer JS, Nance M, Walker M, et al. Migraine and cluster headache treatment with calcium antagonists supports a vascular pathogenesis. *Headache* 1985;25(7):358-67.

[72] Hering R, Kuritzky A. Sodium valproate in the treatment of cluster headache: an open clinical trial. *Cephalalgia* 1989 Sep;9(3):195-8

[73] Curran DA, Hinterberger H, Lance JW. Methysergide. *Res. Clin. Stud. Headache* 1967;1:74.

[74] Riess CM, Becker WJ, Robertson M. Episodic cluster headache in a community: clinical features and treatment. *Can J Neurol Sci* 1998;25(2):141-45.

[75] Costa A, Leston JA, Cavallini A, Nappi G. Cluster headache and periodic affective illness: common chronobiological features. *Funct Neurol* 1998;13(3):263-72.

[76] Egger HL, Costello EJ, Erkanli A, Angold A. Somatic complaints and psychopathology in children and adolescents: stomach aches, musculoskeletal pains, and headaches. *J Am Acad Child Adolesc Psychiatry* 1999;38(7):852-60.

[77] Bille B. Migraine in childhood: a 30 year follow-up. In: Lanzi G, Balottin U, Cernibori A (Eds.) *Headache in Children and Adolescents*: Proceedings of the First International Symposium on Headache in Children and Adolescents, Pavia, Italy, 19-20 May 1988.: Elsevier Science; 1989.

[78] Collin C., Hockaday J. M., Waters W E: Headache and school absence. *Arch Dis Child* 1985; 60 (3):245-7.

[79] Di Prospero S, Gallo M. La cefalea in età pediatrica: studio clinico-epidemiologico. Comunicazizone preliminare: il rischio di cefalea. *Minerva Med* 1987 ;78 (16):1251-4.

[80] Aromaa M, Sillanpaa M, Rautava P, Helenius H. Pain experience of children with headache and their families: A controlled study. *Pediatrics* 2000;106(2 Pt 1):270-75.

[81] Moscato D. Incidenza della cefalea essenziale nelle scuole della USL RM18. *Impegno Ospedaliero* 1987;2:101-107.

[82] Anttila P, Metsahonkala L, Sillanpaa M. School start and occurrence of headache. *Pediatrics* 1999;103(6):e80.

[83] Anttila P, Metsahonkala L, Helenius H, Sillanpaa M. Predisposing and provoking factors in childhood headache. *Headache* 2000;40(5):351-56.

[84] Jensen VK, Rothner AD. Chronic nonprogressive headaches in children and adolescents. *Semin Pediatr Neurol* 1995;2(2):151-58.

[85] Sartory G, Muller B, Metsch J, Pothmann R. A comparison of psychological and pharmacologica treatment of pediatric migraine. *Behav Res Ther* 1998;36(12):1155-70.

[86] Duckro PN, Cantwell-Simmons E. A review of studies evaluating biofeedback and relaxation training in the management of pediatric headache. *Headache* 1989;29(7):428-33.

[87] Pritchard D. EMG levels in children who suffer from severe headache. *Headache* 1995;35(9):554-56.

[88] Bussone G, Grazzi L, D'Amico D, Leone M, Andrasik F. Biofeedback-assisted relaxation training for young adolescents with tension-type headache: a controlled study. *Cephalalgia* 1998;18(7):463-67.

[89] Labbe EE. Treatment of childhood migraine with autogenic training and skin temperature biofeedback: a component analysis. *Headache* 1995;35(1):10-13.

[90] King NJ, Ollendick TH, Murphy GC, Molloy GN. Utility of relaxation training with children in school settings: a plea for realistic goal setting and evaluation. *Br J Educ Psychol* 1998;68 (Pt 1):53-66.

[91] King NJ, Tonge BJ. Behavioural assessment and treatment of chronic headaches in children. *J Paediatr Child Health* 1996;32(5):359-61.

[92] Barry J, von Baeyer CL. Brief cognitive-behavioral group treatment for children's headache. *Clin J Pain* 1997;13(3):215-20.

[93] Allen KD, McKeen LR. Home-based multicomponent treatment of pediatric migraine. *Headache* 1991;31(7):467-72.

[94] Guarnieri P, Blanchard EB. Evaluation of home-based thermal biofeedback treatment of pediatric migraine headache. *Biofeedback Self Regul* 1990;15(2):179-84.

[95] Burke EJ, Andrasik F. Home- vs. clinic-based biofeedback treatment for pediatric migraine: results of treatment through one-year follow-up. *Headache* 1989;29(7):434-40.

[96] Hermann C, Blanchard EB, Flor H. Biofeedback treatment for pediatric migraine: prediction of treatment outcome. *J Consult Clin Psychol* 1997;65(4):611-16.

In: The Handbook of Chronic Pain   ISBN 978-1-60021-044-0
Editors: S. Kreitler, D. Beltrutti, et al., pp. 465-488   © 2007 Nova Science Publishers, Inc.

Chapter 25

Low Back Pain

Diego Beltrutti, Aldo Lamberto, Mauro Nicoscia
and Francesco Marino

1. EPIDEMIOLOGY

Approximately 50% of the patients with benign chronic pain attending pain centers complain of pain in the lumbar region [1]. LBP is a problem that can affect people of all ages but is most common between the ages of 30 and 40 years. It is the primary cause of occupational disability among people younger than 45, and the third leading cause in those older than 45 years [2].

The reason for the age prevalence has not been identified. One hypothesis blames the sedentary life style, but the percentage of LBP patients in sedentary and active occupations is almost identical [3]. It has also been difficult to establish a consistent correlation between LBP and specific occupations [4] possibly due to the involvement of psychosocial risk factors that may correlate more with lifestyle than with an occupation [5].

2. PATHOGENESIS

Despite the well-established effects of LBP on functional ability, its origin and development are still not fully characterized. It has been estimated that in 80% of the cases the etiology results from postural problems and mechanical causes, with obesity, weakness and poor elasticity of specific muscles, as well as stress being further potential causal factors [6-7]. One of the most common causes of LBP is trauma, which refers not only to sudden events, but also to prolonged events, especially in regard to posture, body position, or a continuous occupational activity. Despite the hypothesized correlation between LBP and lifestyle, the role of single behaviors in the initiation, maintenance, or reinforcement of these pathologies has not been ascertained [8].

The presence of organic or traumatic factors is often insufficient to justify the persistence of pain that is transformed from acute to chronic. For this transformation to occur, additional elements related to the social and psychological characteristics of the patient need to be involved. The presence of these psychosocial factors requires the diagnostic and therapeutic intervention of psychologists and psychiatrists, in addition to the orthopedists, neurologists, neurosurgeons, and physical therapists who may be consulted for LBP.

2.1. The Significance of Waddell's Signs in LBP

The increase in studies on chronic pain and the importance ascribed to the psychological aspects of pain have resulted in more research designed to identify common elements shared by the physical and the psychological factors.

In accordance with investigations in regard to other diseases, it is important, especially in the diagnostic stage, to try to determine which physical symptoms hide psychological problems and, conversely, which psychological symptoms hide a physical pathology. For example, headache often expresses both the physical and psychological characteristics, whereby the latter may include stress or well-defined personality traits. In such cases the patients themselves are generally able to tell the physician about the psychological origins of their condition. In contrast, patients with LBP are less likely to be able to tell the physician about stress factors that are potentially responsible for the pain, and may even be less willing to accept psychological factors as a primary or secondary cause of the pain. As a result, also the physician faces a diagnostic dilemma because in addition to the presence of organic factors that justify diagnostic tests, there may be psychosocial factors that may exacerbate the problem or increase the risk of therapeutic failure. However, psychological tests should not be used instead of a search for an organic cause, but rather as a supplement to the physical findings, regardless of whether an organic basis for the diagnosis can be found.

The lack of specific instruments to evaluate the nonphysical component of LBP was a gap that has been filled by Waddel et al. [9] His initial study involved 350 patients with LBP who were selected on the basis of the presence of "*nonorganic physical signs*". These signs were evaluated with respect to psychological parameters and were found to be different from those of the clinical pathology, which are generally used as the basis for diagnosis of LBP. Based on this study, assessment instruments were developed to distinguish pathologies of exclusively physical origin from those that needed further psychological evaluation.

A subsequent study [10] that further evaluated "nonorganic physical signs" identified the following symptoms that are more closely associated with stress than with a physical pathology:

a) Pain that is described at the highest possible levels according to each evaluation scale proposed to the patient, without correlation with the effect on activity.
b) Pain that is described as being persistent for long periods, in some cases for years without any periods of remission.
c) A lack of response to previously tried interventions. In some cases the pain is described as being aggravated by therapy, which has to be suspended.

d) Excessive use of emergency services including emergency home visits, phone calls, and spontaneous visits to pain clinics for worsening condition of chronic pain.

e) History of drug abuse.

The following specific parameters have also been characterized as part of the overall pattern of "nonorganic physical signs":

1. Non-anatomic and superficial pain
2. Positive responses to simulation of a physical examination
3. Different responses when patient is distracted from the focus of the examination
4. Nonphysiologic local disturbances of sensation, distribution of pain or weakness.
5. Overreaction to examination or stimuli.

The statistical relationships among the elements of behavior and chronic LBP were calculated in order to determine the significance of the symptoms. The results show that the objective physical findings constitute only about 50% of the total disability, whereas the other 50% results from psychological factors, such as emotional stress, which can be measured with specific psychological instruments. Applying these assessment tools showed poor understanding of our own body and its response to depression.

It has also been observed that LBP patients, with symptomatology highly indicative of attribution to psychological factors, often supply an inaccurate description of the symptoms and tend to do so at the time of the physical exam. This suggests the need for a complex assessment of LBP resulting in a diagnosis that should not be based on a single reported symptom.

Waddell further demonstrated that stress and illness behavior, rather than the physical problem, influenced the amount of therapy patients were getting. Patients who were observed to have a high percentage of illness behaviors were getting more therapy than those with fewer signs of illness behavior [11].

In a study with Pilowsky, who developed the Illness Behavior Questionnaire (IBQ), Waddell and Bond showed that "abnormal illness behavior" results from symptoms that express psychological and behavioral modifications [12]. Further, behavioral signs and symptoms can be directly correlated with the physical severity of LBP, the patient's report of pain and disability, and the efficacy of surgical interventions. The IBQ scores provided a good indication of the extent of affective disturbances and psychological stress, with the scales 'illness belief' and 'general hypochondriasis' being indicators of behavioral signs and symptoms. "Abnormal illness behavior" is often characterized by personal beliefs about the illness and mistrust of physician reassurance. Hence, the authors concluded that these behaviors are not only an expression of physical discomfort but a behavioral mechanism used by some patients for coping with stress.

Recently, Main and Waddell [13] suggested the need to provide a more accurate perspective on the identification and use of the nonorganic signs since they have been inappropriately used clinically as well as in the medico-legal field. In their review, they point out that although behavioral responses can supply useful clinical information, they should not be over-interpreted on the basis of the presence of isolated signs, but rather should be considered as an indication of the presence of psychological and social components of a physical problem. It may thus be suggested that the presence of behavioral signs in patients with LBP signals the need for a multidisciplinary approach to therapy that would include the physical aspects as well as the social and psychological ones.

Moreover, the presence of nonorganic signs should not be used as a discriminatory test to determine the patient's sincerity of effect in the course of the clinical diagnosis. In this regard, Lechner et al. [14] reviewed studies and methods that have been used to evaluate the sincerity of patient response in the course of the clinical assessment. They specifically focused on the validity and reliability of Waddell's nonorganic signs, patient description of pain and symptoms, musculoskeletal evaluation and function, measurement of grip strength, and the relation between heart rate and pain intensity. They concluded that since none of these assessment methods has been adequately studied to validate its use as a measure of patient sincerity, clinicians might be misled by using a test for a purpose other than the one for which it has been originally intended.

Another misconception is that Waddell's signs constitute evidence of the presence of psychological problems. These nonorganic signs should be considered merely as indicators of the need for subsequent administration of psychological tests and do not in themselves represent a discriminatory event identifying patients attempting to gain secondary gains (i.e. disability) from the physical pathology [15].

Often nonorganic signs may be concomitant with organic symptoms without necessarily suggesting the presence of psychological factors. For those patients who demonstrate nonorganic signs, it is important to closely monitor the rehabilitation stage in order to eliminate or reduce any illness behavior that can play a role in the maintenance of the pathology [15].

Another aspect that should be considered is the correlation between Waddell's signs and psychological test results. The best known and most often used psychological test in the field of pain therapy is the Minnesota Multiphasic Personality Inventory (MMPI). Novy et al. [16] used the MMPI-2 validity scales to examine the correlation between Waddell's signs and physical pathology, limitations in performance, depression, and anxiety. In a study of 75 patients with chronic back pain, 64% of the patients did not have Waddell's signs. In the remaining 36%, the number of Waddell's signs was significantly correlated with depression, functional limitations, somatic problems, and subjective pain intensity. However, a statistically significant correlation with anxiety and the physical pathology could not be demonstrated. These data suggest that there are a variety of factors that may lead to a sub optimal treatment response.

Pain drawing is one example of an assessment method of pain that has been psychometrically validated and is often used in pain therapy. Its advantage resides in its simplicity: the patient is merely requested to point out on a stylized figure which part of the body hurts. In a study by Chan et al. [17], 651 patients with chronic LBP performed the pain drawing test. A significantly greater proportion of patients with high Waddell scores produced drawings with nonorganic pain than patients without Waddell's signs. No significant differences were observed based on gender or kind of health plan. Despite using evaluators with and without experience in this technique, there was a high inter-evaluator reliability of 73%-78% in the test results.

Another assessment method uses derivative scales such as the Waddell Equivalency Scale (WES) developed by Dirks et al. [18], based on the correlation between the Pain Presentation Inventory and the nonorganic signs described by Waddell. Their objective was to apply the results obtained in studies of Waddell's signs in LBP to the evaluation of nonphysiologic factors that contribute to pain in other pain pathologies. However, the predictive capacity of Waddell's signs has not been consistently demonstrated.

Bradish et al. [19] observed that nonorganic signs were not correlated with either return to activity or with symptom resolution in 120 patients with an initial episode of LBP. A similar lack of correlation was observed in a study by Polatin et al. [20] whose goal was to determine whether behavioral signs could be used for predicting therapeutic success in patients enrolled in a functional rehabilitation program. Despite previous reports of the prognostic potential of Waddell's signs in patients with LBP of recent origin, they found no correlation in patients with long-term LBP. They concluded that in patients with long-term LBP, the use of functional rehabilitation represents a multidisciplinary therapeutic approach that manages physical and psychosocial factors, thus lowering the barrier to recovery. An important corollary to this conclusion is that appropriate therapy is likely to result in treatment success, and that Waddell's signs may be indicative more of the type of therapy required (i.e. inclusive of psychosocial factors) than of the success of the therapy itself.

2.2. Occupational Factors

Patients with LBP of long duration have a high rate of occupational absenteeism, and often request to be moved to a less strenuous activity. This suggests the need for a more effective approach to the treatment of LBP. Although the physicians provide what they believe to be the best possible treatment, it may not be adequate or appropriate to enable the patients to return to work. It therefore becomes necessary in the diagnosis of LBP to recognize the signals that may predispose patients to continued absenteeism.

Van der Weide et al. [21] investigated the potential factors that may predict the transformation of acute LBP into chronic disability. Their study evaluated 120 workmen at an occupational health unit who were absent from work for at least 10 days. The factors most highly correlated with absenteeism were radiating pain, severe functional disability, interpersonal problems with colleagues, and a high rate and quantity of work. These data suggest that both physical and psychosocial components need to be targeted in management strategies of occupational LBP.

In this respect, it is important to re-evaluate Waddell's work regarding nonorganic signs in order to determine if these signs can predict continued absenteeism or a return to work. Such an understanding can then be used on a per case basis to decide on an adequate treatment program.

Werneke et al. [22] investigated the correlation between Waddell's scores and return to work in 183 LBP patients with an average duration of disability of 8.7 months. The study center used an approach exclusively targeted to physical rehabilitation without applying psychological or social programs. On completion of the program, Waddell's scores were significantly reduced in those patients who subsequently returned to work, whereas there were no significant changes in those with continued absenteeism. These data suggest that a reduction in behavioral signs may be prognostic of treatment success in a rehabilitation program targeted to physical therapy. However, the continued presence of behavioral signs is indicative of a need for a comprehensive approach to treatment that takes into account psychosocial factors too.

Studies by Kummel [23] and Karas [24] showed that the number of nonorganic signs was highly and significantly correlated with absenteeism, thus providing support for the prognostic value of nonorganic signs in predicting return to work. Similarly, a study of 55 patients with acute occupational LBP showed that 25.5% had one or more nonorganic signs at the first examination [25]. Although this may be considered atypical, since Waddell's signs are generally identified in patients with chronic pain, it is to be noted that in these patients return to work was delayed significantly longer than in 74.5% of the patients without Waddell's signs (median of 58.5 days versus 15.0 days, respectively). Further, the patients with nonorganic signs underwent more frequent physical therapy and diagnostic tests such as lumbar CAT scans than the rest of the study population.

The significance of Waddell's signs during the three progressive phases of LBP (sub acute, acute, and chronic pain) was studied by Vallfors [26]. His study population included 220 patients: 50 with sub acute pain; 50 with acute pain; 70 with chronic pain and an absence from work for at least 3 months; and a control group of 50 patients who had not been absent from work in the previous year. In 51% of the patients who had been absent from work, it was impossible to identify objective physical signs during physical examination. They had an increased frequency of Waddell's signs as compared with those patients who had objective signs. Importantly, the percentage of patients without physical signs increased with the increasing duration of absence from work; 34% of patients with sub acute pain, 40% of patients with acute pain, and 70% of patients with chronic pain. Further, in the groups with greater absenteeism and higher Waddell scores there was evidence for the involvement of more psychological factors, such as psychiatric disturbances, alcoholism, and anticipated retirement problems.

A comprehensive prospective study by Gallagher et al. [27] took into account the three components of LBP: physical, psychological and social. The study was performed in two groups: 87 patients receiving treatment at a specialized university medical center, and 63 patients waiting for social security compensation for LBP and who were not receiving treatment. The study consisted of an initial assessment including a medical history, physical examination, biomechanical testing, psychiatric interview, MMPI evaluation, and a follow-up at 6 months to verify return to work. Statistical analysis determined that the psychosocial variables were the most significant predictors of return to work, with the physical and biomechanical factors having poor predictive value. Hence, an exclusively physical diagnosis does not provide an adequate evaluation of disability, and as previously reviewed studies, suggest that the psychosocial aspects are crucial for the diagnosis and should be incorporated into subsequent therapy.

Another indicator of the social impact of LBP is represented by the activity changes that take place after therapy. Results of a study by Fishbain et al. [28] suggest that the annual percentage of changes in employment is higher in those patients who are treated for LBP than in the general population. Furthermore, the work status of these patients at 24 months after treatment was an accurate indicator of both final employment status and disability.

A person's occupation has also been hypothesized to influence LBP. Several studies examined the magnitude of the effect that type of work could have on the risk of LBP. Smedley et al. showed that nurses had a high prevalence of LBP, that was perhaps associated with their manual handling of patients [29]. Although no gender differences were found, there was a greater likelihood of LBP among those who often reported non-musculoskeletal symptoms. Two follow-up studies evaluated predictors and the course of LBP in nurses [30, 31]. In the first study, the strongest predictor of new LBP was a prior history of symptoms, with a particularly high risk if the previous pain lasted for over a month and had occurred within the 12 months prior to study entry [30]. The presence of a psychological component was suggested by the observation that frequent low mood at baseline was strongly associated with subsequent absence from work. The longitudinal study which examined the natural history of LBP in 1165 nurses showed that duration of LBP was a good predictor for further pain; the longer the pain was consistently reported, the more likely it would be present at the next follow-up examination [31]. Other predictors of future LBP were the presence of sciatica and disability reported at baseline.

Xu et al. [32] focused on associations between the prevalence of LBP and occupational activities, by interviewing a random sample of 5185 Danish employees 19 to 59 years of age. After adjusting for age, gender, education, and employment duration, the predominant occupational risk factors were vibrations affecting the whole body, physically demanding work, frequent twisting or bending, standing up, and intense concentration. Prevalence of LBP increased with increasing exposure time to these factors.

Airline ground staff were also found to be at high risk for LBP compared with the general occupational setting, although specific factors contributing to this increased risk were not identified [33].

In contrast, several studies have identified specific occupational risk factors. In order to determine the risk of first onset and subsequent course of LBP associated with occupational stressors, Burton et al. [34] studied two different police forces that differed only in one known physical stressor - wearing body armor weighing approximately 8.5 kg. The study showed that exposure to occupational physical stress was detrimental, and was associated with reduced survival time to first onset of LBP. Recurrence was associated with time since onset, but persisting pain was not. Sports participation was also a risk in those who had a higher occupational risk.

A Finnish study comparing the risk of blue-collar and white-collar occupations [35] found that LBP could be predicted by exposure to harmful biomechanical loads among both white- and blue-collar workers, stress among white-collar workers, and draft among blue-collar workers. In these patients, psychosocial factors were also found to contribute to absenteeism in the form of lack of recognition and respect toward workers who were reported to have LBP.

A Japanese study [36] determined the occupational risk of LBP among 3,042 workmen in the same factory but with different work activities. The prevalent risk factor found was the physical burden of the job. In particular, the risk of onset and maintenance of LBP increased from a moderate physical activity to a more intense activity. Furthermore, a family history of back pain was also identified as a risk factor, with a higher incidence of this pathology among workers with a family history of LBP as compared to those without such a history.

A British study [37] of 1412 people, 18-75 years of age, correlated physical occupational factors with the onset of LBP. Significant risk was observed for occupational activities involving the handling of weights of at least 25 pounds or those activities that included long duration of moving or standing. Although there was a higher risk in women than in men, no clear correlation was observed between duration of exposure and level of risk.

The above examples support the claim that occupational risk factors for LBP can be identified, and consequently, appropriate management can reduce these risks, in some cases by instituting ergonomic regulations as has been done in the United States by the Occupational Safety and Health Administration (OSHA).

The social and economic implications of LBP have been demonstrated also in studies on the contribution of this pathology to loss of productivity.

A Norwegian study on the incidence and duration of LBP in the general working population (with at least 2 weeks of compensated absence from work) sought to determine the duration of job absenteeism [38]. Almost 90,000 workers were identified with LBP, with a 1-year incidence that was higher in women (2.72%) than in men (1.91%). Among these workers it was observed that 35% were back to work after one month, 70% after 3 months, and 85% after 6 months. However, those with radiating pain had a longer median duration of absence from work as compared with those who did not have radiating pain (59 days versus 38 days; $P < 0.001$). Importantly, those who were not back to work after 6 months had a high probability of obtaining permanent disability status and receiving disability pension or other social assistance. This shows how the burden of disease is not only increased by loss of productivity due to absenteeism, but also how the costs to society are increased by the social welfare programs used to support these individuals.

3. TRANSITION FROM ACUTE TO CHRONIC PAIN

In some patients, acute LBP will often recur periodically and become chronic. In other patients, the first episode initiates a pain that persists with periods of major or minor intensity. The organic etiology often does not support the patient's report of the maintenance of the pain, and hence other factors should be investigated. Intensity of the initial pain was one of the first variables to be investigated for its potential contribution to development of chronicity. Data from a study by Epping-Jordan et al. [39] suggest that while pain intensity was not correlated with chronicity, functional disability may be a predominant factor in the transition from acute to chronic pain resulting in a "failure to adapt" on the part of the patient. Another recent study by Lampe et al. suggested that stressful life events can contribute to chronicity of LBP, especially in cases of uncertain etiology [40].

Occupational factors, as noted earlier, may also be associated with transitions from acute to chronic pain. These factors can include job satisfaction, which has been shown to be a risk factor for new episodes of back pain, high work load, and absenteeism due to LBP [41,42].

The identification and recognition by physicians of factors that may predispose the transition from acute to chronic pain can be an important diagnostic tool. If the problem persists after 4-5 weeks following the first episode of acute pain, the potential presence of psychosocial factors that could interfere with a return to work should be evaluated.

4. PSYCHOLOGICAL ASPECTS OF LBP

General practitioners as well as specialists frequently detect a correlation between the onset of an illness and significant psychological events. However, patients are often reluctant to discuss problems of a nonorganic nature and may consult many specialists of both traditional and alternative medicine to look for a cause that is rarely found. As in other illnesses, this problem occurs in LBP too. Often no correlation can be found between a patient's description of pain and the presence of degenerative and/or structural abnormalities of the dorsal spine. Consequently, abnormal anatomical or physiologic structures should not be considered as the only cause or maintenance of LBP despite the patient's reluctance to discuss psychosocial factors [43]. Several psychological factors and theories have been investigated to determine the role of a psychological component in the onset and maintenance of LBP.

4.1. The Role of Operant Conditioning

Operant conditioning is one of the best known concepts accounting for the interaction between objective physical (physician-diagnosed) and psychological (subjective-patient) components in chronic pain in general and back pain in particular. It was emphasized by Fordyce [44] and served as the basis for the establishment of many pain clinics.

As in the case of other pain pathologies, the social environment reinforces pain behavior in LBP. For example, when patients in pain get help from others so that they do not have to do something that may involve pain, the patients are actually reinforced in their attempts to avoid unpleasant or stressful situations. Caldwell and Chase [45] suggested that a tendency toward physical immobility and difficulty in starting a rehabilitation program are mainly due to a) primary reinforcement to remain immobile, thereby avoiding immediate pain and b) secondary reinforcement to avoid situations which could cause pain. Although this model can explain the role of operant conditioning in the maintenance of pain, it does not adequately explain the initiation of the phenomenon.

4.1.1 Biopsychosocial Factors (Diathesis-Stress Model)

In the late 1980's, an explicative model of LBP was developed that incorporated evidence of the presence of biological, psychological, and social factors. This model was first presented by Levi [46], who used it to explain the relationship between psychosocial stress and disease, and was further elaborated by Flor et al. [47], who developed a biopsychosocial model of chronic low back pain (CLBP). These authors applied to LBP the concept of diathesis-stress that had been used to characterize other disease states, especially those with psychological involvement. The fundamental assumption of this model is that CBLP results from an interaction between environmental events and an organic predisposition. The physiologic or psychological diathesis may vary from person to person and can include health status, physical constitution, and psychological profile. Specific physical or psychological events can trigger the predisposing factors, causing a hyper-activation of the muscles in the lumbar region and resulting in the sensation of pain. The inability to overcome this stress may cause a permanent activation of the muscles, and consequently ischemia and pain develop. Three conditions are necessary for hyper-activation of the lumbar muscles: (a) The existence of a general response in the lumbar region; (b) The existence of significant intermittent or continuous personal stress; (c) The inability of the individual to overcome the stress.

These physical and psychological stress factors can promote a vicious cycle that increases the muscle tension as a natural response to the stress. The increasing muscle tension closes the vicious cycle because the resulting ischemia promotes muscle spasms in the affected area. Another vicious cycle can occur when ischemia, caused by sympathetic activation, produces vasoconstriction which consequently causes muscle spasms. The model may be complicated when long-term ischemia results in a release of substances that promote pain, such as bradykinin and substance P. This pain constitutes a new stress that contributes to increasing tension and pain, especially if the individual cannot adequately cope with either the stress or the pain. Movement may aggravate the pain, and the person becomes afraid of the pain, tends to limit movement, and thereby develops a negative conditioning response. The patient believes that starting an activity could exacerbate the pain or result in further damage, especially if the problem originated from traumatic back injury. Other factors that may be important in the maintenance of the pain include reinforcement of inactivity by family members or by insurance problems.

Three other interactive processes should be considered. The first is related to chronic pain and to its influences on quality of life. Since movement and activity may provoke pain or increase it, the patient tends to avoid any situation, even if potentially pleasant, that could start the pain. Consequently, there is an overall decrease in quality of life. The second process is related to the state of immobility, which paradoxically, facilitates the possibility of muscle spasms that may further increase the pain. Third, protective muscle spasms in reaction to back injury sensitize the muscles to a hypertensive state that may be exacerbated by stress.

The above description demonstrates that psychological and sociocultural factors may contribute to the development or maintenance of LBP, even when a precise organic cause has been established.

This model demonstrates the complexity of LBP, and suggests that even if physiologic factors are the first to be evaluated, diagnosis of this chronic pain condition should include other aspects in the life of the patient, such as psychological, social, cultural, and occupational conditions.

4.2. Depression

It is known that chronic diseases in themselves do not have a strict correlation with depressive states. In contrast, chronic pain has clearly been associated with depression.

The suspicion that pain, in the absence of an organic cause, may be masking a depressive state has been noted [48], with a general prevalence that may be as high as 83% [49].

However, in patients with lumbar pathology, Sternbach et al. [50] reported a prevalence of depression that approaches 100% based on elevation of the Depression scale of the MMPI. Further support for the high prevalence of depression comes from Krishnan et al. [51] who reported that 68% of 50 consecutive patients admitted to their pain clinic presented characteristics classifiable as major depression, as indicated by the DSM-III. Lefebvre [52], using questionnaires without specific depression scales but which evaluated cognitive distortion in depressed and non-depressed patients with and without pain, determined that depression is not a corollary to pain, but rather an integral part of it.

The question of whether psychological disorders precede the onset of musculoskeletal pain and disability, or whether the pain and disability are antecedent to the psychological disturbances was recently addressed in a large study by Dersh et al. [2]. Using the DSM-IV, they determined that, although the overall prevalence of psychological disturbances was significantly higher in patients with musculoskeletal pain and disability as compared with the general population, the prevalence of these disorders was significantly higher than the lifetime prevalence in the general population only after onset of the musculoskeletal condition. However, it was also observed that prior to onset, a third of the patients could be diagnosed with a DSM-IV Axis I condition. Significantly, major depression was present in 48.5% of the patients after onset of musculoskeletal pain.

Magni [53] had previously suggested that the correlation of depression with chronic back pain is more frequent than with other types of chronic pain. Numerous studies have characterized pain-prone personalities (chapter 8, this book), which may be considered a variation of hidden depression. Patients with chronic lumbar pain could be described as belonging to this personality type [54].

These considerations are supported by the observation that depression and chronic pain, in particular lumbar pain, could have a common anatomical-functional basis.

Basbaum and Fields [55] described the existence of an inhibitory control of nociception at the level of the encephalic trunk. Further, the gate control theory [56] hypothesizes that in chronic pain the spinal gate remains open to nociceptive stimulation due to a functional deficit of central inhibitory control pathways. Such a deficit could be caused by an alteration in the regulation or levels of serotonin, noradrenalin, and enkepahalins. It is not surprising, and has long been known, that many states of depression are characterized by similar alterations of these neurochemicals [57].

On a cognitive level it is important to establish the role of depression in connection with three other factors: cognitive distortion, perceived interference with instrumental activities, and self-control. These elements often appear simultaneously and provide a complex model of depression and chronic pain [58].

4.3. Psychophysiologic Aspects

The hypothesis that onset of LBP is caused by factors associated with muscle tension has been explored in several studies.

In this context, "tension" refers to the presence of musculoskeletal contractions that could be a result of psychological stress.

In many people, the increase in muscle tension associated with psychological stress does not remain localized but spreads to different body areas. The whole body becomes progressively tense, and neural feedback helps maintain the vicious cycle of tension and pain.

People with anxiety or stress are generally characterized by increased muscle tension even when at rest. Although these people have the capability to relax the muscles, their general response is one of increasing musculoskeletal tension.

In order to characterize the role that musculoskeletal tension plays in LBP, many studies have made use of the technique of electromyographic (EMG) biofeedback using surface electrodes. Nouwen and Bush [59] reviewed the results of such studies and summarized them in the form of the following five characteristics: (a) The EMG activity of paravertebral muscles at rest in patients with LBP is higher than in controls without pain; (b) The EMG activity of paravertebral muscles in various positions and during movement is higher in patients with LBP than in controls without pain; (c) EMG activity of paravertebral muscles in LBP is more reactive to stress compared to controls without pain; (d) The reduction of EMG activity of paravertebral muscles is correlated with a reduction in pain; (e) The EMG of paravertebral muscles in LBP is higher than in other muscle groups. However, these results were not found to be consistent in all reviewed studies. Consequently, better studies are needed to determine the individual roles of the physiological and psychological components as well as their interaction. The use of EMG activity has not been fully validated. The reason is that according to some authors the reduced range of vertebral motility or the activation of regional muscles, that may provide antalgic activity, can interfere with the accuracy of the results [60].

5. TREATMENT

5.1. Psychological Therapy

According to Rowlingson et al. [61], the evaluation of lumbar pain should include both the physical qualities of the pain as well as its impact on lifestyle, work capacity, and social relations. Treatment is to be initiated only after proceeding with such an evaluation and determining the importance and contribution of the psychosocial factors to the condition [62].

One of the most common characteristics of CBLP is its resistance to somatic therapy [62, 63]. This resistance suggests the need for other therapeutic strategies including the use of psychological approaches based on behavioral and biopsychosocial models. These psychological interventions focus on the painful symptoms as well as on the cognitive and learning structures that maintain and reinforce the painful symptomatology. The goals of psychological intervention are to acquire a general control of pain, to learn specific relaxation techniques and to improve the quality of life of the patient despite residual pain [64]. The validity of psychological interventions is suggested by the presence of specific psychological problems, by difficulty in coping with chronic pain, and by the efficacy of the interventions in reducing these problems.

Turner [65] compared the efficacy of some common psychological therapies. One group of patients received cognitive-behavioral therapy to modify negative responses and to increase the capacity for the control of pain. A second group was trained in relaxation with Jacobson's technique, and a third served as controls and did not receive any specific therapy. The results confirmed the efficacy of psychological therapies not only in regard to cognitive and depressive components but also in reducing the pain. Notably, the cognitive-behavioral therapy was found to be the most efficacious, even at follow-up.

5.1.1. Group Therapy

Although rarely used in the context of pain, within pain management programs, group therapy has been demonstrated to be as effective as individual therapy [66]. When applied to LBP, it focuses mainly on the understanding of the etiology of the pain and on what the patient can do to confront the pain, prevent its onset and/or limit its maintenance.

5.1.2. Behavioral Cognitive Techniques

Studies showed that behavioral cognitive techniques improve the efficacy of traditional therapies [67]. Cognitive strategies are based on behavioral therapies, but in addition to emphasizing the behavioral component they focus also on the cognitive aspect that concerns understanding the pain and the possibility of adequately coping with it.

LBP is an irregular pain that may be uncontrollable. For the patient, it is incomprehensible that such a strong pain cannot be medically resolved. Hence, the pain becomes more mysterious than the therapies used to treat it, and the lack of a precise explanation by the physician increases the patient's stress and confusion that often turn into anxiety and depression. According to Turk and Rudy [68], the cognitive behavioral perspective assumes that behavior and emotions are affected by interpretations of events rather than only by the characteristics of the event itself. They argue that when pain is interpreted as indicating ongoing tissue damage or life-threatening illness, it is likely to produce more suffering and behavioral dysfunction than when it is presented as the result of a minor injury, even though no change has taken place in the nociceptive input itself.

The initial objective of the therapy is to promote the ability to cope with pain by encouraging activities compatible with the pathology. It is also necessary to eliminate or reduce the cognitive characteristics that promote lack of hope or a sense of helplessness in regard to LBP. During cognitive-behavioral therapy, it is necessary to identify and resolve several obstacles that may impede an adequate patient response. One obstacle is the patient's conviction of the physician's ability to diagnose and treat each kind of pain. However, if in the course of examination and treatment of LBP there are either no objective findings or no apparent alleviation of the pain, this contradicts the patient's expectations and becomes a barrier to the patient's understanding of the problem. Another obstacle is the conviction that the pain must be a direct result of an injury, lesion, or illness. Both conceptions result in passivity on the part of the patient because they attribute to the medical staff the therapeutic diagnosis and treatment, or its failure. A third related impediment is the conviction that the pain is an obvious sign of a serious disease or illness, and therefore it is necessary to identify the illness for otherwise the pain will continue.

These convictions are responsible not only for the patient's passivity but also for the patient's rejection of psychological intervention as unacceptable and refusal to cooperate in it.

In fact, the patient often interprets the mere suggestion of psychological intervention as a sign that the medical staff consider his or her pain as psychogenic.

A cognitive-behavioral program includes a series of steps that usually start by supplying adequate information on the nature of the pain. Subsequently, the cognitions of the patient should be evaluated to determine how they differentially affect pain. The patient should be made aware that the sensation of pain, passivity, and avoidance behaviors are also a result of the above convictions. Further explanations concerning the pain and correlated thoughts should be provided and incorporated into the patients' views. At this stage, the patient is expected to be better able to understand his or her own pain and to implement a new explicative model.

The patients themselves may have different cognitive views about the pain that support different styles. Crombez et al. [69] compared avoidance and confrontational styles. As may be expected in view of the relatedness of avoidance to passivity, those patients with LBP who manifested avoidance behavior had a greater frequency and duration of pain as well as greater disability compared with patients who confronted their pain.

Cognitive behavior therapy makes it possible to start appropriate behavioral exercises with the goal of re-initiating the patient's physical activity, while providing the necessary information that will make it easier for the patient to understand and accept the explanation for the origins of the pain. These programs are generally concluded with a discussion on the nature and implications of the new cognition.

5.1.3. Hypnosis

The technique of hypnosis was initially used for acute pain, but recent applications have included its therapeutic use for LBP with the purpose of diminishing the pain and improving general well-being and the quality of sleep [70].

A more complex approach is hypno-behavioral pain management psychotherapy, which has been defined as "the therapeutic utilization of trans-induction techniques, along with cognitive and behavioral strategies, for purposes of improving a patient's self-management of pain and coping," [71].

The goal of hypnotic techniques in general, and of hypno-behavioral pain management psychotherapy in particular, is to produce relaxation, distraction, alleviation of pain, modification of painful sensations, transformation of painful perceptions, and hypnoanalgesia. It can also be used for cognitive purposes, such as overcoming periods of depression and increasing motivation for continuing therapy and for resumption of daily activities.

Hypno-behavioral pain management psychotherapy is not indicated when the symptoms have not yet been treated, or when medical therapies may prove effective. Nor is its use suggested if the patient has a low hypnotizability level or presents with concomitant psychiatric problems. Pending legal or insurance controversies represent a further exclusion criterion.

5.1.4. Relaxation Training

In general, relaxation training is used in combination with other methods within a comprehensive program of pain management. The objective is to reduce the muscle tension that could be responsible for the pain. By improving the patients' active role it is also possible to improve their ability of coping with the pain.

5.1.5. Biofeedback

The basic use of biofeedback in the treatment of lumbar pain is to improve the patients' knowledge about their own body and its physiology. More specifically, there are three major goals of biofeedback therapy:

a) Enhancement of relaxation therapy by reducing autonomic arousal and anxiety levels. The patient learns specific techniques to relax in stressful situations as well as in a daily program designed to limit stress and anxiety.
b) Increasing awareness of specific peripheral factors associated with pain (e.g. paravertebral muscles). During treatment when relaxation is controlled, the patient is made aware of the change of muscle tension.
c) Facilitation of psychosomatic therapy to include the inseparable and interdependent psychosocial and biological factors. During this process, the patients learn to become more fully aware of the functioning of their body.

Biofeedback is used as part of a global approach to the treatment of LBP, integrated with other methods, rather than as a unique or specific method. Since it is not temporally restricted, it can be continued once or twice weekly after the patient's release. This enables carrying out follow-up evaluations that can reinforce specific behaviors and abilities and focus the patients' attention on the importance of their own role in the treatment and resolution of the problem.

Although there are no specific indications that make this method preferable to others, EMG-biofeedback can be useful when the diagnosis indicates the presence of muscle spasms. In this situation, biofeedback can be used to interrupt the vicious cycle of tension-pain-tension.

From a strictly technical point of view, the positioning of electrodes can be either directly on the paravertebral muscles or on other significant muscles such as the trapezius.

When electrode placement is not on the painful muscles, the objective is to take advantage of the capacity for generalizing the relaxation over a wide area. However, Johnson and Hockersmith [72] reported poor results when electrode placement was on the paravertebral and trapezius muscles. They preferred placement on the flexor muscle of the forearm in order to monitor tension of the entire upper body. Their rationale for placement was that the forearm and the hand are extensively represented in the motor cortex, and therefore a relaxation of these areas has a more generalized effect. Learning to relax the upper body produces also an effect on the non-diaphragmatic respiratory muscles that expands to the muscles connected to the lumbar pain.

Burns et al. [73] determined the validity of the assumption that symptom-specific reactivity to stress (i.e. lower paravertebral muscle reactivity) among CLBP patients may exacerbate chronic pain. They found that that there was a correlation between lower paravertebral muscle reactivity during stress and intensity of pain only in those patients who have high levels of depression.

5.2. Pain Management Programs

Pain management programs originated in the United States and were rapidly accepted in other industrialized countries. These programs can be applied to all types of pain but have proved to be especially effective in headache and lumbar pain [74]. The prevalence of pain in lumbar and neck muscles among patients enrolled in pain management programs is especially high, varying from 35% to almost 100%, depending on the clinic [75]. This high prevalence is due to the fact that these pathologies often demonstrate resistance to conservative management with traditional pharmacological or surgical interventions.

Patients undergo an intensive program during a 2-3 week period, according to the needs of the patient and the protocols of the pain center. Usually, after an initial phase of assessment, treatment is provided using a multi-disciplinary therapeutic approach that includes various specialists, such as pain clinicians, physical therapists, rehabilitation therapists, and psychologists. The psychological programs vary from biofeedback to various relaxation-training methods, and they usually include educational programs and family involvement.

These programs generally have a favorable cost-benefit relationship. In particular CLBP rehabilitation programs, that include cognitive-behavioral rehabilitation, have been shown to be efficacious in reducing psychological stress, providing cognitive modifications, and improving daily activities. The inclusion of a motivational program can increase overall compliance and provide significant efficacy in reducing pain and disability in the first year of follow-up [76].

5.3. Interventional Pain Therapy

Surgery can solve the problem in many cases. The first surgery helps in 80% of back pain. However there are risks, the procedure is invasive, patients have to interrupt their activities, a recovery period is necessary, and above all there is some possibility that the pain may get worse and that a second surgery might be needed. Nowadays surgery seems to be limited to those cases where there is a strong risk of neurological sequelae of the motor activities in the limbs after nerve root compression.

Recently new minimally invasive techniques, such as intra discal electro thermo coagulation anuloplasty (IDET), and nucleoplasty, appeared on the medical stage. According to Saal and Saal [77] an aggressive non operative approach leads to success in patients with herniated disk. The authors reported a 90% of pain control and that 92% of patients were able to return back to work.

On the other hand, according to Waddel, we have to consider that 97% of patients receiving compensation after laminectomy have a persistent pain condition. The impairment of function in this group of patients was as high as 72% [78]. It is to be considered that when the patient has experienced a pain condition for a long time, neuro plasticity phenomena can interfere heavily with surgery causing more pain at the time of tissue recovery processes.

Nerve blocks could be another option. They can be used for diagnostic or therapeutical reasons with good chances of positive results. Epidural steroids have been used for many decades in the management of LBP. On this topic there are only a few RCT but the fact that this procedure has been widely used and accepted by millions of patients is a good reason to consider it an effective procedure for CLBP.

For those patients with small (<6-mm) contained disc herniations, whose annular integrity is documented by computed tomography discography and corresponding radicular symptoms confirmed by either selective nerve root blocks or electromyography and nerve conduction studies, nucleoplasty might be an effective long-term treatment for lumbar radiculopathy, either alone or with inradiscal electro thermal anuloplasty (IDET) [79].

According to Karasek and Bogduk [80], in carefully selected cases anuloplasty (IDET) can eliminate or dramatically reduce the pain of internal disc disruption in a substantial proportion of patients and appears to be superior to conventional conservative care for internal disc disruption. In a long-term study the same authors confirm that results of IDET are stable and enduring. The outcome is not a total success, but 54% of patients can reduce their pain by half, and one in five patients can expect to achieve complete relief of their pain [81].

6. FAILED BACK PAIN

Failed back pain occurs in a group of patients with LBP who despite repeated conservative pharmacological and surgical interventions do not obtain pain relief. Although they do not represent a high percentage of the total population of patients with LBP, they constitute a significant presence in ambulatory pain clinics. Few clinical signs are present and organic as well as non-organic factors contribute to the etiology.

(a) Psychological factors: Studies with the MMPI (82, 83) found that patients with poor treatment response are characterized by elevation of the hysteria and hypochondria scales as compared with patients who benefit from therapy. Burton et al. [84] showed that the psychological status of the patients in the acute phase has a major influence on subsequent outcomes, and in particular, coping strategies seem to be important in the progression to chronic pain. Coste et al. [85] used the DSM-III to evaluate 330 ambulatory patients with nonspecific LBP. Of these patients, 41% presented with Axis I psychiatric disorders. More recently Dersh et al. [2] also found not only a high prevalence of Axis I disorders in patients with chronic work-related musculoskeletal pain disability, but also a high prevalence of Axis II disorders. Although in a third of the patients these disorders were present prior to the injury, the prevalence of these disorders increased following the injury [2]. Personality and pathology seem to interact in determining the impact of psychological stress on the pathology. Patients with high levels of pain and disability show major levels of psychological stress connected to the disease. During therapy, there is less association between neuroticism and psychological stress, whereas the intensity of pain and the disability continue to be strongly connected to the psychological stress, possibly due to the modification of cognitive processes during therapy [86].

Some studies found significantly more stressful events in LBP patients than in controls [87, 88]. Furthermore, a significantly higher proportion of patients with idiopathic CBLP had a stressful life event preceding their last reported episode of pain than patients having an organic cause of their pain [40].

(b) Self-reports: One of the basic features in the diagnosis and therapy of LBP is the patients' self-reports of their symptoms and pain. Although these reports provide the physician with an image of the pathology from the patients' perspective, this information is sometimes distorted in such a way that the diagnosis as well as the report of therapeutic outcomes are liable to be incorrect.

A comparison of LBP patients who provided inconsistent descriptions of their behavior and pain with those who provided consistent ones showed that the "inconsistent" group had more pending insurance problems, higher pain focalization, less compliance, less involvement in maintaining physical activities and poorer therapeutic outcomes [89].

(c) Cultural factors: A comparison of CLBP in six cultures (American, Japanese, Mexican, Colombian, Italian, and New Zealand) showed significant cross-cultural differences in the perceived levels of disability, with the American patients manifesting the greatest dysfunction [90]. Brena et al. [91] compared American and Japanese patients with LBP on the Sickness Impact Profile (SIP) and a Standardized Medical Examination Protocol for Pain. For each cultural population, a control group without LBP was also considered. Patients with LBP demonstrated significant differences compared to their respective controls with regard to objective findings regardless of the cultural setting. However, differences in disability and psychosocial factors were observed between the cultural populations; the Japanese had significantly less disability in psychosocial, occupational, and daily functions compared with the Americans. It seems that the traditional stoicism of the Japanese population and the limited psychosocial support in the American culture contribute to these cultural differences. Similar significant cultural differences were observed between American and New Zealander LBP patients, with the American patients reporting more disability and dependence on medical intervention [92, 93].

(d) Occupational factors: Unfavorable pre-injury job perceptions could contribute to lower motivation for rehabilitation [95]. Since the ability to resume work becomes increasingly difficult with time, the therapy of LBP should target acute pain in order to prevent chronicity, and should include an early return to full rather than restricted work [94].

(e) Litigation and compensation: LBP is the main source of litigation between patients and insurance or compensation agencies. Since it is often impossible during diagnosis to determine the presence of physical components justifying the pain or disability, it is difficult to verify the basis for the disability. Patients often feel penalized by the healthcare system that may fail to recognize their problem. The litigation process itself was shown to impact negatively quality of life outcomes even when function improved [96]. It has also been suggested that compensation issues may have a negative effect on self-reported pain, disability, and depression even after rehabilitation programs [97], possibly because patients may be attempting consciously or subconsciously to obtain greater benefits [98].

7. CONCLUSION

It is well known that in the majority of cases acute LBP resolves on its own in a few weeks. In this chapter we showed how in many cases of chronic LBP it is difficult to demonstrate a sure, unequivocal and precise cause of the patient's complaint. In general 6 weeks are considered as a limit for conservative approach. If pain persists longer, there is an indication for the patient to be evaluated in an interdisciplinary pain center. Chronic LBP is another example of the poor correlations that in many cases occur between a mild pathology and a high pain behavior.

8. REFERENCES

[1]   Katon W, Egan K, Miller D. Chronic pain: lifetime psychiatric diagnoses and family history. *Am J Psychiatry* 1985;142:1156-1160.

[2]   Dersh J, Gatchel RJ, Polatin P, Mayer T. Prevalence of psychiatric disorders in patients with chronic work-related musculoskeletal pain disability. *J Occup Environ Med* 2002; 44:459-468.

[3]   Garofalo JP, Polatin P. Low back pain: An epidemic in industrialized countries. In: RJ Gatchel and DC Turk (Eds.) *Pychosocial factors in pain: Critical perspectives.* New York, Guilford, 1999 (164-174).

[4]   Brulin C, Gerdle B, Granlund B, et al. Physical and psychosocial work-related risk factors associated with musculoskeletal symptoms among home care personnel. *Scand J Caring Sci* 1998;12:104-110.

[5]   Papageorgiou AC, Croft PR, Thomas E, et al. Psychosocial risks for low back pain: are these related to work? *Ann Rheum Dis* 1998;57:500-502.

[6]   Hollinghead WH. *Functional Anatomy of the Limbs and Back.* Philadelphia: W. B. Saunders; 1976.

[7]   Cailliet R. *The Low Back Pain Syndrome.* Philadelphia: Davis; 1979.

[8]   Leboeuf-Yde C, Kyvik KO, Bruun NH. Low back pain and lifestyle. Part I: Smoking. Information from a population-based sample of 29,424 twins. *Spine* 1998;23:2207-2213.

[9]   Waddell G, McCulloch JA, Kummel E, Venner RM. Nonorganic physical signs in low-back pain. *Spine* 1980; **5**: 117-125.

[10]   Waddell G, Main CJ, Morris EW, et al. Chronic low-back pain, psychologic distress, and illness behaviour. *Spine* 1984; **9**: 209-213.

[11]   Waddell G, Bircher M, Finlayson D, Main CJ. Symptoms and signs: physical disease or illness behaviour? *Br Med J (Clin Res Ed)* 1984; **289**: 739-741.

[12]   Waddell G, Pilowsky I, Bond MR. Clinical assessment and interpretation of abnormal illness behaviour in low back pain. *Pain* 1989; **39**: 41-53.

[13]   Main CJ, Waddell G. Behavioral responses to examination. A reappraisal of the interpretation of "nonorganic signs". *Spine* 1998; **23**: 2367-2371.

[14] Lechner DE, Bradbury SF, Bradley LA. Detecting sincerity of effort: a summary of methods and approaches. *Phys Ther* 1998; **78**: 867-888.

[15] Scalzitti DA. Screening for psychological factors in patients with low back problems: Waddell's nonorganic signs. *Phys Ther* 1997; **77**: 306-312.

[16] Novy DM, Collins HS, Nelson DV, et al. Waddell signs: distributional properties and correlates. *Arch Phys Med Rehabil* 1998; **79**: 820-822.

[17] Chan CW, Goldman S, Ilstrup DM, et al. The pain drawing and Waddell's nonorganic physical signs in chronic low-back pain. *Spine* 1993; **18**: 1717-1722.

[18] Dirks HF, Wunder J, Reynolds J, et al. A scale for predicting nonphysiological contributions to pain. *Psychother Psychosom* 1996; **65**: 153-157.

[19] Bradish CF, Lloyd GJ, Aldam CH, et al. Do nonorganic signs help to predict the return to activity of patients with low-back pain? *Spine* 1988; **13**: 557-560.

[20] Polatin PB, Cox B, Gatchel RJ, Mayer TG. A prospective study of Waddell signs in patients with chronic low back pain. When they may not be predictive. *Spine* 1997; **22**: 1618-1621.

[21] van der Weide WE, Verbeek JH, Salle HJ, van Dijk FJ. Prognostic factors for chronic disability from acute low-back pain in occupational health care. *Scand J Work Environ Health* 1999; **25**: 50-56.

[22] Werneke MW, Harris DE, Lichter RL. Clinical effectiveness of behavioral signs for screening chronic low-back pain patients in a work-oriented physical rehabilitation program. *Spine* 1993; **18**: 2412-2418.

[23] Kummel BM. Nonorganic signs of significance in low back pain. *Spine* 1996; **21**: 1077-1081.

[24] Karas R, McIntosh G, Hall H, et al. The relationship between nonorganic signs and centralization of symptoms in the prediction of return to work for patients with low back pain. *Phys Ther* 1997; **77**: 354-360.

[25] Gaines WGJ, Hegmann K. Effectiveness of Waddell's nonorganic signs in predicting a delayed return to regular work in patients experiencing acute occupational low back pain. *Spine* 1999; **24**: 396-400.

[26] Vallfors B. Acute, subacute and chronic low back pain: clinical symptoms, absenteeism and working environment. *Scand J Rehabil Med Suppl* 1985; **11**: 1-98.

[27] Gallagher RM, Rauh V, Haugh LD, et al. Determinants of return-to-work among low back pain patients. *Pain* 1989; **39**: 55-67.

[28] Fishbain DA, Cutler RB, Rosomoff H, et al. "Movement" in work status after pain facility treatment. *Spine* 1996; **21**: 2662-2669.

[29] Smedley J, Egger P, Cooper C, Coggon D. Manual handling activities and risk of low back pain in nurses. *Occup Environ Med* 1995; **52**: 160-163.

[30] Smedley J, Egger P, Cooper C, Coggon D. Prospective cohort study of predictors of incident low back pain in nurses. *BMJ* 1997; **314**: 1225-1228.

[31] Smedley J, Inskip H, Cooper C, Coggon D. Natural history of low back pain. A longitudinal study in nurses. *Spine* 1998; **23**: 2422-2426.

[32] Xu Y, Bach E, Orhede E. Work environment and low back pain: the influence of occupational activities. *Occup Environ Med* 1997; **54**: 741-745.

[33] Froom P, Cline B, Ribak J. Disease evaluated on return-to-work examinations: aviation ground personnel compared to other workers. *Aviat Space Environ Med* 1996; **67**: 361-363.

[34] Burton AK, Tillotson KM, Symonds TL, et al. Occupational risk factors for the first-onset and subsequent course of low back trouble. A study of serving police officers. *Spine* 1996; **21**: 2612-2620.

[35] Wickstrom GJ, Pentti J. Occupational factors affecting sick leave attributed to low-back pain. *Scand J Work Environ Health* 1998; **24**: 145-152.

[36] Matsui H, Maeda A, Tsuji H, Naruse Y. Risk indicators of low back pain among workers in Japan. Association of familial and physical factors with low back pain. *Spine* 1997; **22**: 1242-1247.

[37] Macfarlane GJ, Thomas E, Papageorgiou AC, et al. Employment and physical work activities as predictors of future low back pain. *Spine* 1997; **22**: 1143-1149.

[38] Hagen KB, Thune O. Work incapacity from low back pain in the general population. *Spine* 1998; **23**: 2091-2095.

[39] Epping-Jordan JE, Wahlgren DR, Williams RA, et al. Transition to chronic pain in men with low back pain: predictive relationships among pain intensity, disability, and depressive symptoms. *Health Psychol* 1998; **17**: 421-427.

[40] Lampe A, Sollner W, Krismer M, et al. The impact of stressful life events on exacerbation of chronic low-back pain. *J Psychosom Res* 1998; **44**: 555-563.

[41] Hoogendoorn WE, Bongers PM, de Vet HC, et al. High physical work load and low job satisfaction increase the risk of sickness absence due to low back pain: results of a prospective cohort study. *Occup Environ Med* 2002; **59**: 323-328.

[42] Williams RA, Pruitt SD, Doctor JN, et al. The contribution of job satisfaction to the transition from acute to chronic low back pain. *Arch Phys Med Rehabil* 1998; **79**: 366-374.

[43] Magora A, Schwartz A. Relation between the low back pain syndrome and x-ray findings. 3. Spina bifida occulta. *Scand J Rehabil Med* 1980; **12**: 9-15.

[44] Fordyce WE. *Behavioral methods for chronic pain and illness*. St. Louis, MO: C.V. Mosby; 1976.

[45] Caldwell AB, Chase C. Diagnosis and treatment of personality factors in chronic low back pain. *Clin Orthop* 1977; **129**: 141-149.

[46] Levi L. Psychosocial stress and disease: a conceptual model. In: Gunderson EKE, Rahe RH (Eds.) *Life Stress and Illness*. Springfield, IL: Charles C. Thomas Publishers; 1979.

[47] Flor H, Turk DC, Birbaumer N. Assessment of stress-related psychophysiological reactions in chronic back pain patients. *J Consult Clin Psychol* 1985; **53**: 354-364.

[48] Freedman DX, Smith RJ, Lehmann H, et al. Depression today, part one. Recognizing and diagnosing depression. In: 31st Winter Scientific Meeting of the American Medical Association; 1977 1978; New York: CME Communications, Inc.; 1977.

[49] Blumer D, Heilbronn M. The pain-prone disorder: a clinical and psychological profile. *Psychosomatics* 1981; **22**: 395-397, 401-402.

[50] Sternbach RA, Wolf SR, Murphy RW, Akeson WH. Traits of pain patients: the low-back "loser." *Psychosomatics* 1973; **14**: 226-229.

[51] Krishnan KR, France RD, Pelton S, et al. Chronic pain and depression. II. Symptoms of anxiety in chronic low back pain patients and their relationship to subtypes of depression. *Pain* 1985; **22**: 289-294.

[52] Lefebvre MF. Cognitive distortion and cognitive errors in depressed psychiatric and low back pain patients. *J Consult Clin Psychol* 1981; **49**: 517-525.

[53] Magni G. On the relationship between chronic pain and depression when there is no organic lesion. *Pain* 1987; **31**.

[54] Maruta T, Swanson DW, M SW. Pain as a psychiatric symptom: comparison between low back pain and depression. *Psychosomatics* 1976; **17**: 123-127.

[55] Basbaum AI, Fields HL. Endogenous pain control systems: brainstem spinal pathways and endorphin circuits. *Annu Rev Neurosci* 1978.; **7**: 309-338.

[56] Melzack R, Wall PD. Pain mechanisms: a new theory. *Science* 1965; **150**: 971-979.

[57] Riederer P, Birkmayer W. A new concept: brain area specific imbalance of neurotransmitters in depression syndromes. Human brain studies. In: Usdin E, Youdim MB, Sourkes TL (Eds.) *Enzymes and Neurotransmitters in Mental Disease.* Based on a Symposium Held at the Technion Faculty of Medicine, Haifa, Israel August 28-30 1979: John Wiley & Sons; 1980, 261-280.

[58] Maxwell TD, Gatchel RJ, Mayer TG. Cognitive predictors of depression in chronic low back pain: toward an inclusive model. *J Behav Med* 1998; **21**: 131-143.

[59] Nouwen A, Bush C. The relationship between paraspinal EMG and chronic low back pain. *Pain* 1984; **20**: 109-123.

[60] Ahern DK, Follick MJ, Council JR, et al. Comparison of lumbar paravertebral EMG patterns in chronic low back pain patients and non-patient controls. *Pain* 1988; **34**: 153-160.

[61] Rowlingson JC. Lombalgia. In: Warfield CA (ED.) *Trattamento del dolore. Teoria e pratica.* Milano: McGraw-Hill; 1994.

[62] Flor H, Turk DC. Etiological theories and treatments for chronic back pain. I. Somatic models and interventions. *Pain* 1984; **19**: 105-121.

[63] Nachemson A. A critical look at the treatment for low back pain. *Scand J Rehabil Med* 1979; **11**: 143-149.

[64] Hobbs WR, Yazel JJ. Psychological management. In: Carron H, McLaughlin RE (Eds.) *Management of Low Back Pain.* Littleton: John Wright-PSG Inc.; 1982, 181-187.

[65] Turner JA. Comparison of group progressive-relaxation training and cognitive-behavioral group therapy for chronic low back pain. *J Consult Clin Psychol* 1982; **50**: 757-765.

[66] Rose MJ, Reilly JP, Pennie B, et al. Chronic low back pain rehabilitation programs: a study of the optimum duration of treatment and a comparison of group and individual therapy. *Spine* 1997; **22**: 2246-2251.

[67] Laborde JM. Cognitive-behavioral techniques in the treatment of chronic low back pain: preliminary results. *J South Orthop Assoc* 1998; **7**: 81-85.

[68] Turk DC, Rudy TE. Cognitive factors and persistent pain: a glimpse into Pandora's box. *Cognitive Ther Res* 1992; **16**: 99-112.

[69] Crombez G, Vervaet L, Lysens R, et al. Avoidance and confrontation of painful, back-straining movements in chronic back pain patients. *Behav Modif* 1998; **22**: 62-77.

[70] Crawford HJ, Knebel T, Kaplan L, et al. Hypnotic analgesia: 1. Somatosensory event-related potential changes to noxious stimuli and 2. Transfer learning to reduce chronic low back pain. *Int J Clin Exp Hypn* 1998; **46**: 92-132.

[71] Eimer BN, Freeman A. *Pain Management Psychotherapy: A Practical Guide*. New York: John Wiley and Sons; 1998.

[72] Johnson HE, Hockersmith V. Therapeutic electromyography in chronic back pain. In: Basmajian JV (Ed.) *Biofeedback: Principles and Practice for Clinicians*. Baltimore: Williams & Wilkins; 1978.

[73] Burns JW, Wiegner S, Derleth M, et al. Linking symptom-specific physiological reactivity to pain severity in chronic low back pain patients: a test of mediation and moderation models. *Health Psychol* 1997; **16**: 319-326.

[74] Flor H, Fydrich T, Turk DC. Efficacy of multidisciplinary pain treatment centers: a meta-analytic review. *Pain* 1992; **49**: 221-230.

[75] Maruta T, Swanson DW, McHardy MJ. Three year follow-up of patients with chronic pain who were treated in a multidisciplinary pain management center. *Pain* 1990; **41**: 47-53.

[76] Friedrich M, Gittler G, Halberstadt Y, et al. Combined exercise and motivation program: effect on the compliance and level of disability of patients with chronic low back pain: a randomized controlled trial. *Arch Phys Med Rehabil* 1998; **79**: 475-487.

[77] Saal JA, Saal JS.: Nonoperative treatment of herniated lumbar intervertebral disk with radiculopaty : an outcome study. *Spine* 14: 431-437, 1989.

[78] Waddel G: failed lumbar disk surgery following indistrial injuries. *J Bone Joint Surgery* (Am.) 1979;61: 201-207.

[79] Cohen SP, Williams S, Kurihara C, et al. Nucleoplasty with or without Intradiscal Electrothermal Therapy (IDET) as a treatment for lumbar herniated disc. *J Spinal Disord Tech.* 2005 Feb;18:S119-S124

[80] Karasek M, Bogduk N. Twelve-month follow-up of a controlled trial of intradiscal thermal anuloplasty for back pain due to internal disc disruption. *Spine.* 2000 ;25(20):2601-7

[81] Bogduk N, Karasek M. Two-year follow-up of a controlled trial of intradiscal electrothermal anuloplasty for chronic low back pain resulting from internal disc disruption. *Spine J.* 2002 ;2(5):343-50.

[82] Pheasant HC, Gilbert D, Goldfarb J, Herron L. The MMPI as a predictor of outcome in low-back surgery. *Spine* 1979; **4**: 78-84.

[83] Dzioba RB, Doxey NC. A prospective investigation into the orthopaedic and psychologic predictors of outcome of first lumbar surgery following industrial injury. *Spine* 1984; **9**: 614-623.

[84] Burton AK, Tillotson KM, Main CJ, Hollis S. Psychosocial predictors of outcome in acute and subchronic low back trouble. *Spine* 1995; **20**: 722-728.

[85] Coste J, Paolaggi JB, Spira A. Classification of non specific low back pain. I. Psychological involvement in low back pain. A clinical, descriptive approach. *Spine* 1992; **17**: 1028-1037.

[86] BenDebba M, Torgerson WS, Long DM. Personality traits, pain duration and severity, functional impairment, and psychological distress in patients with persistent low back pain. *Pain* 1997; **72**: 115-125.

[87] Leavitt F, Garron DC. Psychological disturbance and pain report differences in both organic and non-organic low back pain patients. *Pain* 1979; **7**: 187-195.

[88] Feuerstein M, Sult S, Houle M. Environmental stressors and low back pain: life events, family and work environment. *Pain* 1985; **22**: 295-307.

[89] Chapman SL, Brena SF. Patterns of conscious failure to provide accurate self-report data in patients with low back pain. *Clin J Pain* 1990; **6**: 178-190.

[90] Sanders SH, Brena SF, Spier CJ, Beltrutti D, et al. Chronic low back pain patients around the world: cross-cultural similarities and differences. *clin J Pain* 1992; **8**: 317-323.

[91] Brena SF, Sanders SH, Motoyama H. American and Japanese chronic low back pain patients: cross-cultural similarities and differences. *Clin J Pain* 1990; **6**: 118-124.

[92] Tait R, DeGood D, Carron H. A comparison of health locus of control beliefs in low back patients from the U.S. and New Zealand. *Pain* 1982; **14**: 53-61.

[93] Carron H, DeGood D, Tait R. A comparison of low back pain patients in the United States and New Zealand: psychosocial and economic factors affecting severity of disability. *Pain* 1985; **21**: 77-89.

[94] Burton AK, Erg E. Back injury and work loss. Biomechanical and psychosocial influences. *Spine* 1997; **22**: 2575-2580.

[95] Fishbain DA, Cutler RB, Rosomoff H, Khalil T, Steele-Rosomoff R. Impact of chronic pain patients' job perception variables on actual return to work. *Clin J Pain* 1997; **13**: 197-206.

[96] Blake C, Garrett M. Impact of litigation on quality of life outcomes in patients with chronic low back pain. *Ir J Med Sci* 1997; **166**: 124-126.

[97] Rainville J, Sobel JB, Hartigan C, Wright A. The effect of compensation involvment on the reporting of pain and disability by patients referred for rehabilitation of chronic low back pain. *Spine* 1997; **22**: 2016-2024.

[98] Pearce JM. Aspects of the failed back syndrome: role of litigation. *Spinal Cord* 2000; **38**: 63-70.

In: The Handbook of Chronic Pain
Editors: S. Kreitler, D. Beltrutti, et al., pp. 489-499

ISBN 978-1-60021-044-0
© 2007 Nova Science Publishers, Inc.

Chapter 26

Perineal and Pelvic Pain

Diego Beltrutti, Aldo Lamberto, Mauro Nicoscia
and Salvatore Di Santo

Chronic pelvic and perineal pain is a frequent source of frustration to both physician and patient. Few specialists are aware of the complexity and multifaceted nature of these complaints or are able to offer relief to the patients suffering from them. For example, in men, the urogenital tract represents only one of the five major sources of pelvic/perineal pain, which may also arise from psychological, myofascial, musculoskeletal, and gastrointestinal causes. A comprehensive evaluation of each of these components through a careful history and physical examination is crucial for determining appropriate therapy.

Perineal pain may be caused by various pathologies originating in the anorectal and/or pelvic regions. In the anorectal region, pain may result from rectal rhagades, hemorrhoids, carcinoma, ulcers, anal abscesses and fistulas, or Crohn's disease. Perineal pain of pelvic origin may be due to proctalgia fugax or anorectal neuralgia. Further, non-anorectal factors such as coccygodynia, neurologic, gynecologic or urogenital problems may also cause or exacerbate perineal pain [1]

1. ESSENTIAL ANAL PAIN

Essential anal pain may arise from osteoarticular lesions as well as colic, urogenital or pelvic pathologies, and even neuropsychological causes. Essential anal pain is a common functional disorder causing anorectal and perineal pain. It is classified as coccygodynia, proctalgia fugax, or anorectal neuralgia [2].

1.1. Coccygodynia

Coccygodynia is more prevalent in women than in men and is characterized by coccygeal pain that radiates to the perineal or inferior sacral area. The most frequent cause of coccygodynia is trauma to the coccygeal or sacral area following a fall. Although an idiopathic form may arise without any obvious causal event, many of the idiopathic forms are actually a delayed consequence of repeated microtrauma resulting from extended sitting, long-term use of a bicycle seat or horse saddle, or protracted non-relaxation of the elevator muscles of the anus (levator ani). One of the most common causes of coccygodynia is a lesion of the sacrococcygeal ligament during a difficult childbirth [3]. The pain is localized to the coccyx and may be especially pronounced following external pressure on the coccyx or during rectal examination.

Spasms or high tension of the levator ani occurs in more than half of these patients. The pain increases during defecation and when sitting. Hence, these patients have problems sitting in armchairs and on regular seats. They generally eat standing up, are not able to drive, and often carry a special cushion with a hole in the middle for work and other situations that require sitting.

Non-invasive therapy such as local anesthesia, ultrasound, laser therapy, and local massage can be used to treat most cases of coccygodynia. Only about 1% of patients are referred for coccygectomy because of failure of non-invasive therapy. Appropriate determination of a candidate's suitability for the surgery and the expertise of the surgeon are key factors determining the success of this operation.

Psychotherapeutic intervention is often provided to limit the negative effects of anxiety and tension that characterize many of the patients with perineal pain.

1.2. Proctalgia Fugax (Anorectal Spasms)

Proctalgia fugax is more prevalent in young males, and is characterized by a very strong episodic pain that lasts from several seconds to 15-20 minutes. The pain results from muscle spasms in the anorectal region, most often involving the coccygeal and levator ani muscles. The underlying pathology effecting these spasms may include anorectal infections, fractures of the coccyx, chronic prostatitis, and ischemia at the level of the pelvic and rectal vessels.

Proctalgia fugax often occurs at night, especially toward the early morning hours. Its frequency is intermittent, and it may occur every 4-5 months. Although its origins are not clear, episodes tend to diminish with age.

Patient reassurance is an important component of treatment but pharmacological and behavioral/physical interventions may also be provided, even in cases of pain of short duration. The drugs most often used include nitroglycerin, papaverine, and beta-blockers. The pain can also be limited by antalgic positions that provide pressure to the perineal region, or by intra-anal massage.

1.3. Anorectal Neuralgia

Anorectal pain is generally classified as anorectal neuralgia if the diagnosis is not consistent with the above two categories. The pain is usually difficult to define, with subjective variation that may be related to the performance of activities of daily life. Onset generally occurs in the morning and increases in intensity during the day. In many cases the patient needs to go to bed to obtain relief. The origins of anorectal neuralgia are unclear. It is possibly for this reason that there is a more pronounced tendency to attribute this pain to a psychological origin as compared with the two previous manifestations pf essential anal pain [2]. From an epidemiologic point of view, pain consistent with this diagnosis is more commonly reported among women over 50 years of age, who have a history of pelvic surgery or interventions than among other patients.

Non-pharmacologic treatment, including physiotherapy and massage of the levator ani muscle may be used but often has poor results. Common analgesic drugs may be prescribed to help relieve pain, and antidepressants and anxiolytics may be used to provide overall relief of anxiety, tension, and depression.

1.4. Essential Orchiodynia (Orchialgia)

This pathology is not generally included among the essential anal pains but should be included in discussions of perineal pain because of its peculiar characteristics. Pain may be described in either or both testicles and clinical and instrumental examination may not find any pathology of organic origin, even when the patient reports presumed local trauma.

The presence of a severe persistent pain in the testicular area in the absence of inflammatory, vascular or heteroplastic pathology suggests that orchiodynia may have a strong psychological component.

Symptomatic treatment is not always effective. However, a psychological evaluation may provide the opportunity to understand the determining factors in the onset and maintenance of the pain and enable psychological therapy.

2. EVALUATION OF PERINEAL PAIN

Patient evaluation should include an accurate case history, rectal examination, and proctoscopy. These basic tests can be integrated with other examinations, such as endorectal echography, electromyography, and anorectal manometry. During the first examination it is very useful to use pain assessment instruments, such as the McGill Pain Questionnaire (MPQ) developed by Melzack [4]. This tool assesses the sensory, affective, and evaluative dimensions of pain.

When using the MPQ for evaluating perineal pain, it is important to consider the words that the patients use to express their pain, especially with the groups of words that refer to the sensory dimension. For example, the type of pain referred to by the groups of words having a thermal connotation may suggest an inflammatory process or ulcerative lesions. In contrast, use of words relating to a feeling of pressure may refer to abscess, edema or hematomas, while words suggesting pressure by constriction may indicate a lesion of the anal channel.

3. PSYCHOLOGICAL ASPECTS OF PERINEAL PAIN

The hypothesis that perineal pain, and coccygodynia in particular, may have a psychological origin is not recent [5]. A medical history of patients who do not have an organic pathology usually shows some characteristic psychological elements suggestive of depression or related symptomatologies.

Approximately 60% of depressed patients suffer from some form of pain, and it has been suggested that 80-90% of pain center patients are also depressed. It has been established that depression lowers the tolerance to pain, increases the need for analgesics, and contributes to what is known as the vicious cycle of chronic pain (chronic pain leading to depression which leads to more pain). The large number of patients attending ambulatory proctology clinics who also show depressive characteristics suggests the need for cooperation between proctologists and psychologist during diagnosis and treatment.

According to Lopez-Ibor [6], coccygodynia is very often depression-based and can be treated with an appropriate choice of antidepressants. Using the Minnesota Multiphasic Personality Inventory (MMPI), the observed profile of the patient with perineal pain without organic causes shows the greatest elevation in the depression scale (the D scale), indicating that these patients are seriously depressed and have a pessimistic outlook.

Patients with perineal pain can be divided into two groups. The first group includes those patients who have pain as the primary condition and secondarily manifest a depressive state as a consequence of their suffering. In the second group, the pain is a key aspect of a pre-existing psychological state or disease. In these cases, the perineal pain is probably the expression of an underlying depressive syndrome that may be hidden by the physical pain, and pain upon rectal digital examination (RDE) can be used as an objective sign of masked depression [7].

There are no systematic studies on depression in patients with anorectal pathologies. Only a few publications have dealt with coccygodynia-associated depression that was treated with anti-depressants [7, 8]. In patients with anorectal pain, the second most elevated scale on the MMPI is the social introversion scale (SI scale), indicating reduced social interest, few friendships and a refusal of interpersonal relationships. These patients often report childhood problems of parental separation or death or feelings of being unwanted or unloved. The current family may also be a cause of conflict or tension, and in some cases occupational difficulties or a lack of social capacity may exacerbate the problem.

The personality structure of patients having perineal pain without an organic basis is often characterized by elevation of the schizophrenia scale (SC scale) on the MMPI. These patients tend to fantasize rather than react, and the reduction in social interests, that was already noted by elevation of the SI scale, becomes accentuated focusing of the patients towards themselves and their problems.

In perineal pain the psychological component is much more salient than in other pain pathologies and its identification is much easier. The patient's history is often characterized by psychiatric consultations and systematic use of psychotropic agents. In such cases, pain may be considered a symptom necessary for maintaining an equilibrium in regard to distress. However, eliminating the symptom without appropriate patient management may break this equilibrium, with a consequently increased risk of developing psychopathological tendencies.

Anxiety diminishes the pain threshold and reduces pain tolerance. Externalization is increased and from a cognitive point of view it anticipates the response to pain.

The MMPI profile suggests that anxiety may result in a physical obsession, with the patient becoming excessively concerned about his or her health and frequently going for medical examinations with different specialists, none of whom can solve the patient's problems. This sets up a vicious cycle because pain causes anxiety and as a result anxiety increases pain.

3.1. Anorectal Pain of Psychiatric Origin

According to Merskey [9], 10% of psychiatric patients who suffer pain report that it occurs in the rectal and perineal region. In the majority of these patients, the pain is described as secondary, and in only a small proportion (2%) is it considered primary.

The schizophrenic patient may complain of hallucinatory pain confined to the perineal or genital area, or may refer to the presence of an object that initiates the pain. In hysterical syndromes, the pain is often reported to affect other parts of the body, lasting only during the waking hours and without causing awakening at night.

Very seldom is a detailed description provided of the pain, and it can be associated with neurological dysfunction such as numbness and paralysis without showing an organic cause. In some cases the painful syndrome may be correlated with an early history of sexual abuse, incest or physical abuse [10].

3.2. Psychological Consultation

Many studies on anorectal pain have demonstrated the importance of psychological factors in the genesis and maintenance of anorectal neuralgia. The physician and the psychologist should not be misled into continuing to try to determine an organic cause in the absence of documented clinical or instrumentally visible lesions. In the past, we have begun to consider a diagnosis with a psychosomatic or psychological basis only when we were sufficiently certain that the disease is not organic.

The patients who are sent to a psychologist for anorectal neuralgia are often difficult to evaluate. The fact that the referring physician did not establish the origin or cause of the pain may make the patients suspicious and think that they are not being believed when they mention their disease. During psychological consultation, the patients may avoid answering questions related to the symptomatology, since they believe that the psychological aspect is a consequence of the pain that they are suffering rather than the converse.

In contrast to other pathologies, such as headache, tachycardia, and colic that may be associated with psychosomatic problems, patients with anorectal neuralgia rarely admit the presence of psychological components. The family relatives of the patient also reinforce the search for an organic cause since they may also be reluctant to consider the possibility of psychological components. Although it is not possible to determine a specific psychological profile among the neurotic behaviors, one common characteristic is the fear of a tumor.

In general, obsessive patients are very precise in describing their pain and also in explaining everything in minute detail to try to obtain a diagnosis and therapy. These patients will often ask questions about the origin of their disease and about its future effects.

Patients with hysteria syndromes are not very clear in their descriptions and tend to use many superlatives in their descriptions. They often describe their problem as a terrible one that causes great insomnia.

It is also easy to interpret the problem from a psychodynamic point of view because of the proximity of the anal area to the genital organs and due to the fundamental role that anality plays in the evolution of the libido. Therefore, it is often accurate to assume the involvement of sexual problems in the symptom and in its antecedents.

3.3. Perineal Pain and Sexuality

Patients with chronic pain tend to demonstrate reduced sexual activity that is often attributed to the intake of drugs as well as to anxiety and depression. In the case of perineal pain, its anatomical location suggests a strong association with the sexual response.

According to the psychosomatic concept, pelvic or perineal pain is often part of hysterical conversion symptoms in women, and serves as a means of expressing their sexual discomfort and their desire to be cared for. This mechanism is reinforced by the traditional approach of physicians who are often more willing to treat the pain than problems of sexual dysfunction. Further, the perineal pain may sometimes be an expression of auto-aggression or guilt.

Many gynecologists have observed that these patients may confuse the anal, urethral, and genital areas due to their anatomical proximity. In some cases the sexual pathology is the tip of the psychosomatic iceberg that is actually a global problem of self.

However, the perineal pain can also have an organic basis, with the psychosexual reactions as secondary components. Regardless of the source of perineal pain, both physical and psychological components should be appropriately addressed in the course of the therapeutic process. . Health professionals should educate and prepare patients; be trained to identify problems; and be competent to deal with them openly and sympathetically [11]. It has been noted that pain causes a reduction in sexual intercourse, but normal sexual activity will restart when the pain disappears. In fact, the resumption of sexual activity can be considered as an indicator of the efficacy of antalgic (anti-pain) therapy.

4. PELVIC PAIN

In men, diseases in the pelvis and perineal region may not only cause pain but also disturbances and problems in erection, ejaculation and micturition. From the pathophysiologic point of view, pelvic and perineal pain in men is often correlated with the presence of urogenital disorders that may encompass the bladder, urethra, prostate, seminal vesicle, penis and scrotal sac.

Men often describe urogenital pain as a severe, burning sensation associated with urination which can occur at the beginning, at the end (persisting even after voiding), or throughout urination. About 75% of patients seeking treatment for urinary symptoms present with an infection, which in some cases may be sexually transmitted. Initial dysuria is frequently related to herpetic lesions or gonococcal infections in the urethra. When total dysuria is present, lesions of the bladder and urethra are generally responsible for the pain sensation. Sometimes the discomfort is only present at the end of micturition, in which case the lesion may involve the urethra, bladder or prostate. The presence of a severe inflammation is responsible for a persistent and excruciating pain, spasms of the urethra and bladder, strangury and sometimes tenesmus.

The bladder can be responsible for a burning sensation that may extend to the distal urethra and penis. Stressful conditions as well as infections, cardiac problems with nocturnal mobilization of fluids, inflammations and bladder obstruction may cause urinary frequency, during the day and/or at night. Differential diagnosis should be used to eliminate acute and chronic cystitis or cancer and its recurrence as possible etiologies, especially if there is weight loss or persistent bleeding that can result from renal adenocarcinoma, carcinoma of the bladder, carcinoma of the prostate or penile carcinoma. Other potential considerations in differential diagnosis should include post-radiation cystitis, post-radiation contracted bladder, specific cystitis, and parasitic infections.

Over-distention of the bladder produces a severe painful suprapubic sensation and an urgent need to void. This condition can occur in paraplegic patients. The presence of a bladder stone induces painful sensations that may vary according to the position and the activity of the patient.

Chemical irritants, foreign bodies and traumata (e.g., medical instruments, self-inflicted lesions) can initiate a painful sensation that is perceived in the perineum, distal urethra, and glans penis. The presence of discomfort, rectal fullness, tenesmus, perineal pain, difficulty in voiding, reduction in stream size, changes in frequency and retention of urine are generally correlated with inflammation of the prostate. Hemorrhoidectomy may precipitate a severe perineal discomfort and spasm of the levator or perineal floor muscles with urinary retention. When seminal vesicles are associated with prostate disease, the patient may develop groin pain, lower abdominal pain or pain in the perineum, testicles, and penis.

Infections of the epididymis may also result in a painful condition. In this case, the patient presents with extreme tenderness and pain in the testicles. However, pain in the epididymis is difficult to interpret because this pain can mimic renal colic resulting from a similar embryonic origin and nerve supply to that of the kidney and renal pelvis.

Retrograde urine flow in the ejaculatory ducts can cause a chemical inflammation. Pain originating in the testicles can be caused by an infection, usually of viral origin, or may be due to an extension of epididymal pain resulting from a sexually transmitted disease. Differential diagnosis should be used to eliminate the possibility of a hematoma, rupture of the testicle, or infarction from torsion. Prolonged sexual stimulation can also produce an acute and painful congestion of the testicles.

Pain in the penis is often associated with the presence of pathologies in the bladder (neck and trigone), urethra, prostate or seminal vesicles. Other painful conditions in the penis can be due to paraphimosis, priapism, Peyronie's disease and herpetic infection (herpes progenitalis). Last but not least, pelvic and perineal pain can result from the presence of emotional and sexual problems.

Among women, pelvic pain is one of the most frequently cited reasons for a gynecology visit and examination. If this pain is prolonged, it can develop into a chronic pelvic pain syndrome (CPPS) which often requires surgical intervention.

The clinical causes of pelvic pain may vary, but the psychological and social implications are of particular importance. As already mentioned for perineal pain, the sexual component plays a very important role especially since there are possible problems related to both procreation and physical desire. Consequently, pelvic pain may have a strong psychosomatic component as an alarm signal for reduced arousal of the patient's spouse or partner. Therefore, it may often be necessary to determine if there are emotional or sexual problems such as those related to separation or divorce. In some cases, pelvic pain in women may be an expression of their desire for maternity or of their inability to become pregnant.

Pelvic pain is also accompanied by anxiety and depression, which can be the expression of social or psychological problems. In the case of CPPS, a high incidence of sexual abuse has also been noted.

In addition to CPPS, chronic pain in the pelvic region may also be due to vulvodynia or chronic vulvar discomfort [12]. Vulvodynia, as a chronic pain, differs from acute vaginal pain in its resistance to therapy [13]. Although in the acute form there is generally a quick therapeutic response, vulvodynia is often resistant to therapy. Unfortunately, there are not yet any accurate studies on the psychosocial characteristics of this pathology, which, nevertheless, may be expected to resemble chronic pain in general. Therefore, a multidisciplinary approach is needed, that would take into account not only the possible underlying pathology but also aspects of female sexuality.

5. THERAPEUTIC APPROACHES

From the point of view of diagnosis and therapy, evaluation of the psychological aspects suggests that the treatment of pelvic-perineal pain should consider the person as a whole, encompassing both physical and psychological components [14]. With this goal in view, pharmacological therapy should include drugs targeted to reducing the pain as well as antidepressants and anxiolytics for controlling depression and anxiety.

It has often been claimed that the most important component of treatment is the physician himself or herself. It is not only the bottle of syrup or the box of pills that counts, but also the way in which the physician has proposed them to the patient. The approach and attitude of the physician toward the prescription and administration of the drugs are as important as that which is being prescribed. The behavior of patient may be out of proportion to the degree of objective pathology, and as usually happens in chronic pain, the pain and behavior may continue for a longer period even after the effects of a possible trauma have been are resolved. Consequently, the pain has the potential to become a real disease by itself, and the life of the patient begins to revolve around his or her suffering, affecting work and social life.

While explanation and reassurance provided by the physician are an integral part of therapy, they do not suffice by themselves for modifying the patient's pain-maintaining behavior. Therefore psychological therapy should be initiated and can play an important role in treatment and recovery. Yet, according to Morel-Maroger [15], even in the presence of known psychological problems, the treatment of anorectal pain should not be assigned solely to the psychiatrist or the psychologist. In most cases it is the proctologist who can appropriately intervene by considering also the psychological component and initiating cooperation with a mental health specialist.

The role of the psychologist is to intervene and modify or limit the anxiety and depressive factors. Classical medical and antalgic therapies should be supplemented by cognitive-behavioral therapies, especially when depressive factors are involved. Other therapeutic approaches include the use of classical relaxation training techniques (16, 17). The evident presence of muscle tension in specific areas makes these relaxation techniques particularly useful. The patient learns to relax the peripheral muscles with a consequent reduction in pain.

The more technological approach based on biofeedback may overlap with the two previous methods. Biofeedback has been used for pain caused by vulvodynia instead of or in addition to topical, systematic and surgical therapies. Presuming that muscular tension is the cause of the chronic pain of vulvodynia, electromyographic biofeedback therapy has been used to monitor appropriate exercises to reduce tension and pain in the pelvic floor musculature [18].

Furthermore, the sexual implications of vulvodynia can result in the development of anxiety and depression, for whose treatment the intervention of the psychologist or psychiatrist may be required. In contrast to women, male patients suffering from orchialgia less frequently report sexual problems. However, problems of depression are similar for both genders.

Neurolitic blockade can be performed to relieve a variety of painful pelvic conditions, mostly of non oncologic origin (presacral neurectomy or superior hypogastric plexus block) (19). Another treatment option is the Ganglion impar procedure with local anesthetic for diagnostic purposes or with phenol for therapeutic neurolitic procedure. Indications are perineal pain in patients with cancer of the cervix, colon bladder rectum and endometrium.

Neuroaxial blocks should be considered only in patients with pre existing colostomy and urinary diversion. In the past, in this group of patients subdural phenolic saddle blocks have been used in severe perineal pain, having in mind the risk of limb paresis.

In cases of severe perineal pain due to cancer, coccygodynia and sciatic pain a bilateral S4 block may be applied. Cryoneurolysis or neruroablative RF procedure can be used at this level to avoid bladder denervation. Treatment at S1 and S2 may be very helpful when pain is experienced also in the sciatic distribution. However, this procedure very often leads to a bladder dysfunction.

It should be kept in mind that diagnostic blocks with local anesthetics of the ilioinguinal and iliohypogastric nerves provide good results. This procedure can be used to predict the clinical effects of cryoneurolysis even in pregnant women. This simple procedure has been shown to be useful for avoiding exploratory laparatomies designed to rule out acute abdominal diseases (20) .

Continuous intrathecal opioid administration with or without local anesthetics and clonidine is an option for patients that are refractory to oral administration of conventional medications.

6. CONCLUSION

Further research, development and application of therapy to problems of pelvic-perineal pain are needed since patients suffering from these pains, both acute and chronic, do not receive adequate diagnosis and treatment. Efforts are required for both the specific pathophysiologic mechanisms of pain that contribute to these syndromes and diseases, and the appropriate approaches to treatment, including the use of multidisciplinary therapies. In this context, the psychological and educational support of the patient should be of primary concern, regardless of the origin of the pain, in order to avoid undertreatment or overtreatment. The interdisciplinary approach seems to offer better opportunities of treatment since conservative and more invasive treatments are integrated in specific pain algorithms that can be used even in more enigmatic pain syndromes.

7. REFERENCES

[1]   Mazza L, Formento E, Fonda G. Anorectal and perineal pain: new pathophysiological hypothesis. *Tech Coloproctol.* 2004;8(2):77-83.

[2]   Segre D, Balestrino E, Menardo V, Beltrutti D, Quaranta L. Idiopathic anorectalgias. In: Beltrutti D, Gestin Y (Eds.) *Clinical Issues on Chronic Pain Management.* Borgo San Dalmazzo: 1993.

[3]   Johnson JG. Gynecologic pain. In: Tollison CD, (ED.) *Handboook of chronic pain management.* Baltimore: Williams and Wilkins; 1989.

[4]   Melzack R. The McGill Pain Questionnaire: major properties and scoring methods. *Pain.* 1975;1(3):277-299.

[5]   Holmes TH. Back muscle spasm, professional cramp and backache. In: Cecil RL, Loeb RF (Eds.) *Textbook of Medicine.* Philadelphia: W. B. Saunders; 1951.

[6]   Lopez-Ibor JJ. Depressive equivalents. In: Kielholz P, ed. *Masked Depression.* Bern: Hans Huber; 1973:97-121.

[7]   Maroy B. Spontaneous and evoked coccygeal pain in depression. *Dis Colon Rectum.* 1988;31(3):210-215.

[8]   Schultze G. Steissebeinschmertz and larviete depression. *ZFA (Stuttgart).* 1983;59:998-2000.

[9] Merskey H. Classification of chronic pain: description of chronic pain syndromes and definition of pain terms. *Pain*. 1986(Suppl 3):45-46.

[10] Gross RJ, Doerr H, Caldirola D, Guzinski GM, Ripley HS. Borderline syndrome and incest in chronic pelvic pain patients. *Int J Psychiatry Med*. 1980-81;10(1):79-96.

[11] Glazener CM, Sexual function after childbirth: women's experiences, persistent morbidity and lack of professional recognition. *Br J Obstet Gynaecol*. 1997, 104(3): 330-5.

[12] Bodden-Heidrich R, Kuppers V, Beckmann MW, et Al. Psychosomatic aspects of vulvodynia. Comparison with the chronic pelvic pain syndrome. *J Reprod Med*. 1999; 44(5):411-416.

[13] Masheb RM, Nash JM, Brondolo E, Kerns RD. Vulvodynia: an introduction and critical review of a chronic pain condition. *Pain*. 2000;86(1-2):3-10.

[14] Lamberto A, Beltrutti D. Benign perineal pain: psychological aspects. In: Beltrutti D, Gestin Y (Eds.) *Clinical Issues on Chronic Pain Management*. Borgo San Dalmazzo: Martini; 1993.

[15] Morel-Maroger MA. Aspect psychologique des névralgies ano-rectales. *Arch Fr Maladies de l'Appareil Digestif*. 1966;55:43-46.

[16] Schultz JH, Luthe W. *Autogenic training*. New York: Grune and Stratton; 1969.

[17] Jacobson E. *Progressive Relaxation* Chicago: University of Chicago Press; 1938.

[18] McKay E, Kaufman RH, Doctor U, Berkova Z, Glazer H, Redko V. Treating vulvar vestibulitis with electromyographic biofeedback of pelvic floor musculature. *J Reprod Med*. 2001;46(4):337-342.

[19] Kent E, De Leon Cassasla OA, Lema M: Neurolytic superior hypogastric plexus block for cancer related pelvic pain. *Reg Anesth* 1992;17 (suppl)19.

[20] Racz G, Hagstrom D: Iliohypogastric and ilioinguinal nerve entrapment: diagnosis and treatment. *Pain Digest* 1992;2:43-48.

In: The Handbook of Chronic Pain
Editors: S. Kreitler, D. Beltrutti, et al., pp. 501-531

ISBN 978-1-60021-044-0
© 2007 Nova Science Publishers, Inc.

Chapter 27

Rheumatic Pain

M. Zoppi and E. Beneforti

JOINT PAIN

The term "arthritis" is not specific enough to be considered as a diagnosis. Many patients believe that any joint pain is due to arthritis, but understanding of the term can be vague because local and systemic factors may induce pain in one or more joints. It is impossible to review the enormous amount of diseases in which joint pain is a symptom or the main symptom. The cause of joint pain is unknown in many ailments, such as rheumatoid arthritis, but in most of these diseases its early pathophysiologic mechanisms are known [1].

OVERLOAD ARTHRITIDES

Repeated microtraumas in the workplace or those observed in sport medicine may induce pathologic changes in joints, bones and supporting structures. This pain may become chronic and worsen if proper therapeutic measures are not applied early. Worsening of pain may develop even if the joint is rested, because of a series of vicious cycles starting from the joint.

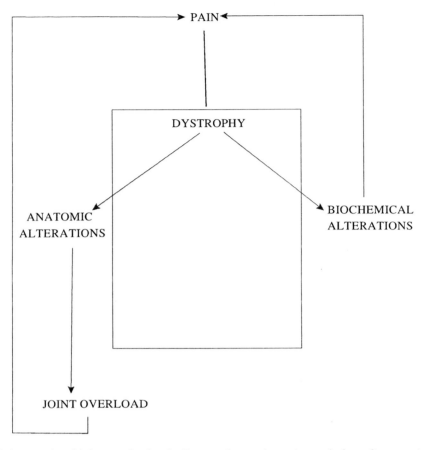

Figure 1. Vicious cycle of joint overload pain. It may also apply to the evolution of osteoarthritis (see text).

OSTEOARTHRITIS

In practically all types of joint pain, the peripheral and central nervous system are involved. Hence, they are also involved in the evolution of osteoarthritis. The first observable change is the thickening of cortical bone under the articular cartilage, which induces an intra-osseous venous stasis and changes in the blood flow of that area. This leads to two consequences. First, nutrients for the articular cartilage and its nourishment are impaired, and therefore the articular cartilage moves into a fibrillated state. Second, cancellous bone is compressed by the intra-osseous venous hypertension, which causes early pain. The cartilage does not induce pain because it is not innervated.

This "intra-osseous engorgement pain syndrome" is characterised by a dull, aching or throbbing pain felt diffusely around the joint that usually worsens toward the end of the day, is aggravated by activity, and persists at rest. Arnoldi et al.[2] studied a group of patients with pain in the knee or hip. The joints of these patients were examined by means of bilateral intra-osseous phlebography, intra-osseous pressure measurements, and 99mTC polyphosphate scintigraphy. These studies showed a direct correlation between pain intensity and the degree of intra-osseous hypertension.

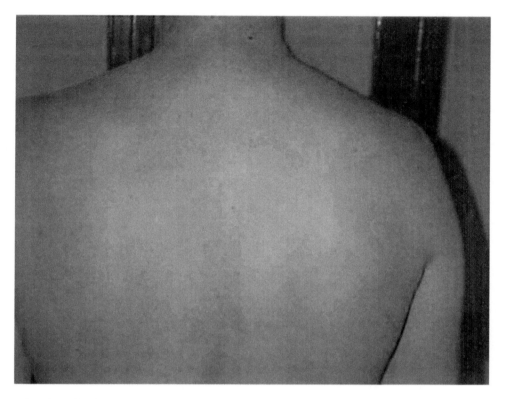

Figure 2. Muscular hypotrophy of the right rotator cuff in a patient in which a scapulo- humeral periarthritis started 24 hours before.

A rule of immediate clinical evidence is that pain induces dystrophies. These dystrophies are probably caused by reflexes starting from the painful area, and ending, probably through sympathetic efferents, in well-defined zones for each pain localization. For instance, an acute periarthritis of the shoulder induces hypotrophy of the rotator cuff muscles. A similar phenomenon (left rotator cuff hypotrophy) was observed by the authors in many patients a few hours after an acute myocardial infection [3].

The terms "dystrophy" or "hypotrophy" are used here with a meaning that is different from the one common in the field of neurology. Our definition includes indeed also tenderness or spontaneous pain of the involved muscles. For example, in the knee, dystrophy after the onset of pain involves many muscles surrounding the joint and mainly the quadriceps muscle. It follows that the axis of the knees changes either in various or in valgus; therefore, the forces acting on those joints become pathologically altered, thus increasing pain. A similar mechanism acts for the hallux valgus in painful flat feet.

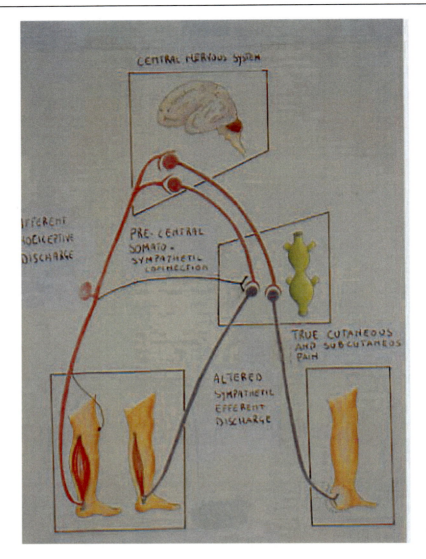

Figure 3. Reflex pain and muscular dystrophy induced by somato-sympathetic vicious cycles.

Pain therapy in these cases not only provides a symptomatic remedy but is also to be considered as a treatment that can block the worsening of the disease. There is evidence that the sympathetic nervous system is reflexively involved in the pathogenesis of these vicious cycles.

More recent research demonstrates neurogenic acceleration in osteoarthritis. Other factors that contribute to pain in osteoarthritis are: synovitis (which is much less important than in inflammatory arthritides), periarticular myalgic spots or trigger points, bursitis, tendonitis and enthesopaty around the affected joint.

INFLAMMATORY ARTHRITIDES

Most studies on joint inflammation focus primarily on tissue factors and much less on the active role of the nervous system. The hypothesis that the nervous system may play an important role in the pathogenesis of rheumatoid arthritis derives from clinical observations. For example, in hemiplegic patients who later develop rheumatoid arthritis, the joints of the paretic side are completely spared, while, as a rule, the disease develops symmetrically.

The symmetrical distribution of joint involvement, its ordinate centripetal evolution, and the fact that the distal interphalangeal joints are usually spared are also clues of nervous system involvement in the pathogenesis of the disease.

The non-involvement of distal interphalangeal joints in rheumatoid arthritis is probably due to the fact that proprioceptive innervation of these joints is less developed than that of the proximal ones. In two patients we have observed a typical rheumatoid arthritis starting from distal interphalangeal joints. The patients who, by the nature of their work, had mechanically overstressed distal joints. Therefore, these joints developed a range of movement greater than that of other persons.

Studies on animals demonstrate that during experimental arthritis in the rat also proprioceptors can activate silent synapses with second order nociceptors located in the dorsal horns. The findings have a clinical counterpart. An inflamed joint indeed is often painless when it is relaxed, but even very little movements induce an unbearable pain.

Nowadays it is well established that inflammation, swelling, hyperalgesia and pain within a joint are caused by a complex interaction of substances produced and released by many cells, nerve terminals included.

This type of activation is not typical of the joints but may involve many other tissues. The contribution of nerve terminals is referred to as "neurogenic inflammation"[5]. Normal joints have both afferent (sensory) and efferent (motor and sympathetic) innervations. Fast-conducting large, myelinated A fibers innervating the joint capsule arise from specialised encapsulated structures located at their peripheral ends. They are important for proprioception and detection of joint movements. Slow conducting unmyelinated fibers and finely myelinated axons are named "free nerve endings". These afferent fibers provide the overwhelming majority of joint afferent innervation. They transmit diffuse, burning or aching pain sensations, regulate synovial microvascular function, and release neuropeptides into the surrounding tissues.

Recent developments in immunochemical techniques have provided fresh insight into joint innervation. Substantially improved resolution and characterisation of individual fibers have been made possible by using antiserum against specific neuronal markers combined with sensitive staining methods. The use of these techniques has revealed vastly increased small diameter nerve fibers in the joints, compared with previous studies using standard histology methods.

Small diameter nerve fibers were found in all sections of normal joint tissues, scattered throughout the fibrous capsule, ligaments, tendon and synovium. Many of the small-diameter nerves found in normal synovium were immunonoreactive for neuropeptides. These included fibers containing immunoreactive substance P (SP), calcitonin-gene-related peptide (CGRP) and vasointestinal peptide, which are considered to be markers of sensory fibers, as well as nerves containing immunoreactive neuropeptide Y (NPY), found in most peripheral noradrenergic neurones. Many SP and CGRP immunoreactive nerves were found in perivascular areas and on the synovial surface. It was also shown that, in acute and chronic phases of inflammation, the density of CGRP was enhanced in peripheral nervous terminals and in dorsal root ganglion nervons. Further, recently it has been shown that serum levels of SP in patients with rheumatoid arthritis are significantly higher than in healthy control individuals [6]. It is not yet clear whether the SP high serum levels derive from the synovial fluid or express a systemic involvement of the disease. When pooled together, these data indicate that changes in neuropeptide content and in the proportion of nerves producing neuropeptides are associated with inflammation. Thus, it is plausible that sensory neuropeptides may contribute to arthritis both for the abundant nerve supply and for the possible upregulation in the joints of sensory neurones containing these proinflammatory substances.

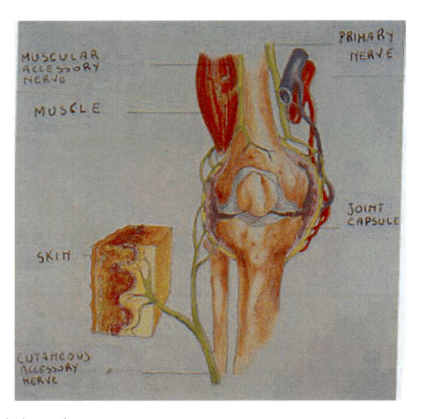

Figure 4. Joint innervation.

Dissection studies have shown that every joint has a dual nerve supply. This supply includes primary nerves that penetrate the capsule as independent branches of adjacent peripheral nerves and accessory nerves sending a branch to the joint, and another either to the muscle (articulo-muscular nerves) or to the skin and subcutaneous tissues (articulo-cutaneous nerves).

The definition of joint position and the detection of joint motion are monitored separately by a combination of multiple inputs from different receptors of various somatic structures. Nerve endings in muscles and skin as well as in the joint capsule mediate sensation of joint position and movement. Patients who have undergone capsulotomy along with total knee or hip replacement or surgical removal of interphalangeal joints of the hand still retain good awareness of joint position. Indeed, joint replacement may partially reverse the impairment of joint position sensation that results from articular inflammation. It has been suggested that impaired proprioception may contribute to the propensity for arthritis to develop in hypermobile subjects. In the non-inflamed joints, most sensory fibers do not respond to movement within the normal range. In the acutely inflamed joints, however, these nerve fibers become sensitised by mediators, such as bradykinin and prostaglandins, so that normal movements induce pain.

Pain on joint movements within the normal range is a characteristic symptom of patients with chronically inflamed joints caused, for example, by rheumatoid arthritis. In the course of acute inflammation, e.g., infections and attacks of gouty arthritis, joints become painful even at rest.

One aspect of pain perception is that the sensitivity of the inflamed tissues changes. For instance, patients with esophagitis or gastritis feel liquids when they drink, and this sensation is often unpleasant, even if the liquids are slightly warm or cold. These sensations are not perceived if the mucosa is not inflamed.

"Silent nociceptors" which spontaneously fire or start firing after slight movement or normally nonpainful stimuli (peripheral sensitisation), may explain one of the most important mechanisms of pain from inflamed joints. Afferent nerve fibers from the joint also play an important role in the reflex inhibition of muscle contraction. During the development of inflammation induced in laboratory animals by kaolin and carrageenan, these proprioceptive units increase their responses to joint movements and inhibit spindle discharge. This reflex muscle inhibition may explain complex symptoms described by patients with painful knees and hands ranging from the abrupt "giving away" and "dropping" (pseudocramp: "Very often things fall from my hands!") to the rapid quadriceps wasting observed in patients with acutely swollen knees. Descending inputs from the central nervous system and sympathetic abnormal discharge may contribute to these symptoms.

PHYSIOLOGY AND PATHOPHYSIOLOGY OF JOINT SYMPATHETIC INNERVATION

Sympathetic nerve fibers surround blood vessels, particularly in the deeper regions of the normal synovium. The autonomic innervation of the joint is involved in different functions, such as direct modulation of sensory receptors, vasomotor changes, quick and slow changes of micro vessel permeability and of tissue imbibiton, release of active metabolites, control over some enzymatic reactions, and modulation of immune cells. These functions can shift in time and intermingle. Sympathetic nerves contain and release both classic neurotransmitters (norepinephrine) and neuropeptides (NPY). In the arthritic joint, the NPY-ergic perivascular fibers even enter the vessel wall [7].

Clinical data on the role of sympathetic efferents in maintaining joint pain and inflammation seem controversial. In chronic joint pain and inflammation, such as that caused by rheumatoid arthritis, sympathetic blockade exerts a beneficial but unfortunately transient effect on pain and swelling. Reversible sympathetic block in the course of an acute attack of arthritis, such as podagra induce instead worsening of pain and inflammation (personal observation). It may thus be supposed that in the two pathologic conditions (chronic and acute arthritis), the sympathetic nerves exert an opposite function. With respect to the role of sympathetic efferent for maintaining and worsening chronic pain, the reader is referred to the wide variety of literature that deals with these topics, for example, reflex sympathetic dystrophies, algodystrophies and sympathetically maintained or dependent pain.

To summarise, in the course of chronic arthritis, sympathetic neurotransmitters facilitate transmission of nociceptive information by sensory fibers and enhance synovial inflammation. Unfortunately, surgical denervation of the sympathetic nerves is not a good treatment because several days after the sympathectomy, a denervation hypersensitivity to circulating catecolamines develops and induces worsening of the symptoms [8]. It has been recently demonstrated that vagal activity may also influence neurogenic inflammation and pain. In the presence of subdiaphragmatic (or celiac branch) vagotomy, sympathetically dependent pain and inflammation were increased by four orders of magnitude compared with results in vagus-intact animals (9).

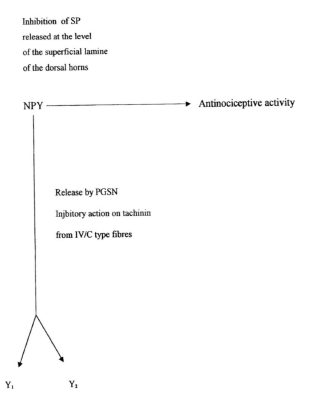

Figure 5. The central and peripheral actions of neuropeptide Y (NPY) are depicted. SP = Substance P, PGSN = Post-ganglionic sympathetic nerves. Y_1 and Y_2 = Peripheral receptors of NPY.

In order to clarify the effects of the sympathetic nerves in the course of an acute attack of arthritis, it is necessary to explain the mechanisms of the accompanying symptoms on the skin and subcutaneous tissues surrounding the inflamed joint (which have already been described by the Roman physician Celsius). One may wonder why inflammation inside the joint manifests itself with signs on the skin and subcutaneous tissues that contribute to the acute pain. To understand this phenomenon, let us examine some studies on experimental inflammation induced on the skin.

Many algogenic substances (e.g., histamine, cantharidine, and SP), when injected into the derma, induce a reaction that was first described by Lewis [4]. The reaction is caused by a substance released by tissues that Lewis called "substance H". Subsequently it was found that this substance was histamine. When it is intradermally injected, as other algogenic substances, it induces the following three phenomena, known as the "Lewis triple reaction":

(a) An area of redness that spreads a few millimeters around the injected area and that reaches its maximum 1 minute after the injection and then becomes bluish. This reaction is caused by a local vasodilator effect; (b) A cutaneous erythematous area of a brighter red (secondary hyperalgesia), that spreads over 1cm beyond the area of initial red discoloration and develops more slowly. This reaction is probably caused by activation of axon reflexes; (c) A blister appears 1 to 2 minutes after the injection and replaces the initial red discoloration. This reaction is caused by an increased capillary permeability.

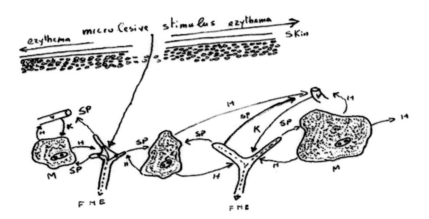

Figure 6. Mechanism of erithema spreading from the site of the microlesion; this stimulus induces excitation of the free nociceptive endings (FNE). The signal does not only transit to the central nervous system but also proceeds antidromically along the terminal branches of the nerve (axon reflexes) which release substance P (SP) and other polypeptides involved in pain and inflammation. SP in turn induces liberation of histamine (H) from the surrounding mastocytes (M). SP and H act on microvessels (V) which increase their permeability, and consequently other inflammatory and pain mediators such as kinins (K) pass from the blood to the surrounding tissues. Both H and K excite neighbour FNE and the phenomenon so spreads.

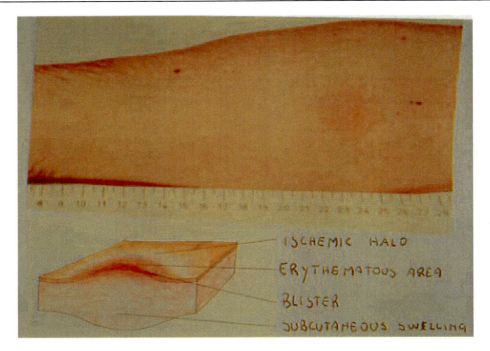

Figure 7. Phenomena observed 1min. after intradermal injection of histamine (870pM). The blister, the erythematous area and the surrounding ischemic (pale) halo are evident. The subject feels a recurrent burning pain. Down: a schematic drawing.

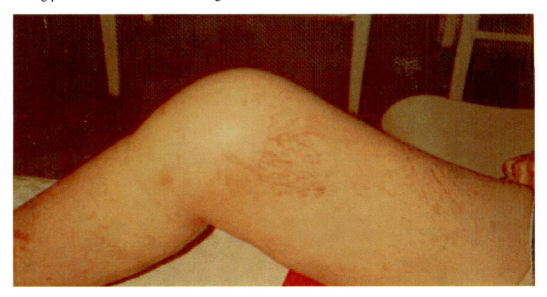

Figure 8. Teleangectasias suddenly stop around an ischemic and swollen areaof the medial aspect of a painful knee.

Erythema is the most interesting phenomenon of this triple reaction. This phenomenon is probably caused by the nociceptive and damaging stimuli which induce release of neuropeptides by C fibber free endings, that in turn, determine a complex activation of many tissue substances involved in inflammation. In line with an oversimplified model, liberation of SP by free endings induces release of histamine by neighbour mastocytes, which in turn excites other nerve endings, and so forth. This accounts for the spreading of erythema.

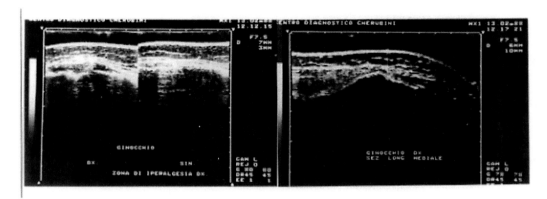

Figure 9. Echographic images of the medial surfaces of the knee of a patient with acute arthitis and pain of the right knee. Left echography. The thickness of subcutaneous tissues of the right knee (right) are higher than in the left knee (left). Right echography. Detailed examination of the painful knee. The thickness of subcutaneous layers increases exactly under the hyperalgesic skin. From the authors personal archives.

However, if this mechanism is true - and many experimental data support it - why does the erythema stop? One possible explanation derives from studies in which an ischemic halo of regular shape was observed developing around the erythematous area. This white halo, although visible on first viewing, was much more evident in thermographic studies. The temperature of the ischemic skin was 4° to 5°C lower than the erythematous area and 2° to 3°C lower than before the experiment [10]. This white halo, which stops the spreading of the erythema, is probably produced via a reflex arc with a sympathetic efferent branch. In fact, if the reaction is induced in an upper limb of which the stellate ganglion was previously blocked by local anaesthetics, the white halo does not appear, and the erythematous reaction is absolutely enormous. The white halo has also been observed surrounding the inflamed skin in the course of a spontaneous attack of acute arthritis (personal observations). This is the probable reason for worsening of pain and inflammation if an acute attack of gouty arthritis is treated by a reversible sympathetic block. Another clinical demonstration of this reflex is the observation that teleangectasias stop all around the hyperalgesic area of a painful knee.

Another observed phenomenon is the increased thickness of subcutaneous tissues under the erythematous area. This phenomenon was demonstrated by means of echografic studies of an acutely inflamed and swollen knee [11].

For further understanding of the described phenomena and of their relation to joint pain, the concept of erythralgia on the skin, first described by Lewis [12], comes into play. Erythralgia is a phenomenon characterised by redness, increase of cutaneous temperature, subcutaneous swelling and allodynia or hyperalgesia. The concept of erythralgia may be extended from the skin to mucosal and synovial tissues. Arthroscopic studies of acutely inflamed joints and gastroscopies of the inflamed mucosa in the course of an acute gastritis have confirmed these findings.

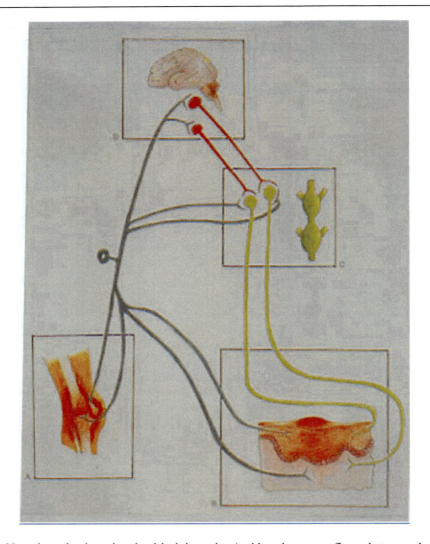

Figure 10. Neural mechanisms involved in joint pain. Antidromic axon reflexes between the inflamed joints (A) and the superficial tissues (B) release at this level painful and proinflammatory substances which induce red discoloration, pain and swelling. Joint afferents give also precentral (C) and central (D) synapses to sympathetic efferents to the skin and subcutaneous tissues (B).

Another rule of pain is that erythralgia induces reflexes. For instance, synovial erythralgia induces the described secondary hyperalgesia in the skin of an inflamed joint, probably through axon reflexes running on the articulocutaneous nerves, which release inflammatory polypeptides in the skin and subcutaneous tissues. The anaesthetic block of these nerves inhibits the superficial signs of an acute arthritis and the quality of pain changes from stubbing and burning to a pain that is deeper and better tolerated. The reversible block of the sympathetic ganglia induces instead worsening of pain and the appearance of other symptoms, and the erythralgic area spreads.

Another phenomenon is referred pain from the joint, with the same characteristics of referred pain from inflamed viscera. This referred pain is always located on well defined superficial and muscular areas. These areas should be known for local therapies. This is probably a sympathetically maintained pain and should be considered one of the causes of joint pain. It can therefore be concluded that sympathetic nerves act in two ways. On the one hand, they are involved in protection of the inflamed joint and on the other hand, they maintain and probably worsen pain through vicious cycles involving some of the mechanisms responsible for pain. The physiologic reason for this apparent paradox may be that, when sympathetic nerves over discharge, they release large amounts of NPY, which has analgesic and anti-inflammatory properties [13, 14].

The Scenario of an Inflamed Joint

Evidence is accumulating that implicates neuropeptides, SP in particular, in early pathogenetic mechanisms of rheumatoid arthritis and other chronic arthritides. Kinins, prostaglandins and leukotrienes lower the activation threshold of peripheral unmyelinated afferent fibers (sensitisation). These fibers release inflammatory mediators when neurons are activated, thus contributing to inflammation. SP, the best studied of these substances, can stimulate the release of other mediators, such as leukotrienes, which in turn stimulate lymphocyte and synovial proliferation and induce release of interleukin-1, tumour necrosis factor (TNF-), and interleukin-6 from monocytes. Also these substances can sensitise or even excite nociceptors. They are key factors for the pathologic alterations observed in rheumatoid arthritis.

It is clear, then, that separation between neurogenic and tissue inflammation is artificial and should be used only for teaching purposes. Inflammation indeed involves all tissues, nerves included, and the initial event (often unknown) may start acting on nerves, tissues or both. The cascade of events is characterised by interactions that result in a progressive worsening of the disease. The distinction between neuropeptides and cytokines is to be abandoned because neuropeptides should be considered as cytokines, produced and released mainly by nerve terminals, having, as other cytokines, paracrine and autocrine activity.

A further complication is introduced by the fact that some opioids can modulate the immune system. Metenkefalin, for instance, enhances ß- cell antibody production, inhibits oxygen radicals production from macrophages, and is a chemotactic factor. As with SP, immunoreactive metenkefalin is present in synovial fluid, and it is produced by local nerves, monocytes, lymphocytes, and chondrocytes.

Opioid receptors of nerve endings are upregulated during inflammation. This may account for the observation that the peripheral antinociceptive effect of exogenous opioids is enhanced in inflammation [15]. These observations may also explain a finding from our clinic, confirmed by others: the injection of 10 mg of morphine into an inflamed joint results in pain relief, and inflammation decreases. Morphine injection is in many cases more powerful than standard injection of steroids, regardless of whether they are combined with local anaesthetics.

Central Nervous System and Traditional Hormones

Pain sensation is up-regulated or down-regulated in the central nervous system (CNS), from the spinal cord to the brain, by central sensitisation or "gating" of nociceptive inputs.

Thus, although the normal joint may respond predictably to painful stimuli, there is often a poor correlation between apparent joint disease and perceived pain in chronic arthritis.

It has been observed that following stroke or peripheral nerve injuries, the development of rheumatoid arthritis is either prevented or ameliorated in the affected limb. This observation was the first recognition of the involvement of the nervous system in the pathogenesis of the disease. A lot of subsequent work has established intimate and intricate associations among the central nervous system, the endocrine system, and immuno-inflammatory mechanisms. The predominant interaction is with the hypothalamic-pituitary-adrenal axis, which mediates the secretion of corticotropin releasing hormone, which then in turn stimulates the pituitary gland to release corticotropin.

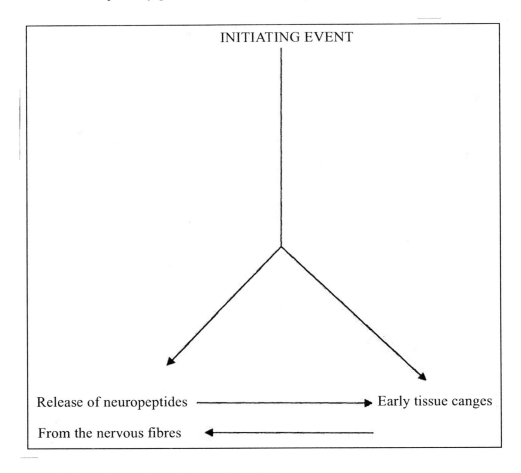

Figure 11. Early pathogenetic mechanisms of arthritides.

A subsequent stimulation of the adrenal cortex leads to glucocorticoid release, with its known potent anti-inflammatory effect. Many factors can interact within the CNS to modify this pathway. Of particular relevance is the observation that the hypothalamic–pituitary adrenal axis is defective in rheumatoid arthritis, and the cortisol responses to inflammation are abnormally low. This hypothalamic irregularity in rheumatoid arthritis involves other substances, including the excessive production of prolactin, a pro-inflammatory neuropeptide.

Thyroid stimulating hormone decreases in articular rheumatism, but increases in the presence of systemic manifestations of rheumatoid arthritis. The role of these and other findings in the pathogenesis and maintenance of the disease is still to be clarified [16].

Even less clear is the role of central SP. The increased serum, cerebrospinal, dorsal horn SP in arthritis inhibits the immune system, according to some authors, but increases nociceptive joint pain according to others. Also controversial are the findings regarding central neuropeptides and spinal opioidergic systems associated with chronic inflammatory pain in the rat. Inhibition of serotonin metabolism and enhancement of dopaminergic systems in the hypothalamus and sensory-motor cortex were observed in arthritic rats, but it was also shown that central serotonin exerts a proinflammatory role.

Central neurones (including the spinal cord, preoptic area, hypothalamus and hippocampus among others) of arthritic rats express C-FOS only after repeated noxious stimulation of the inflamed joints. Similar results could be obtained with other models of pain as well. These findings demonstrate that central neurons may become "memory cells" in neuropathic pain and arthritis. A single hypothesis that correlates the peripheral and central nervous system is impossible to conceive because too much information is lacking concerning the relationship between these two components.

Rheumatoid Arthritis

When rheumatoid arthritis involves only somatic structures, it is characterised by joint inflammation, bony erosions, and destruction of other periarticular structures (e.g. tendons and ligaments) which results, in late stages of the disease, in severely crippled joints. Inflammatory flares along the course of the disease follow two patterns: 1) a monocyclic flare that lasts from a few days to months (if it is not adequately treated) and is followed by a definitive remission, and 2) a polycyclic series of flares followed by remissions. The frequency and duration of flares and the duration of the apparently inactive periods vary from one individual to another. A third pattern is characterised by unremitting inflammation that tends to worsen. Symptomatic therapies in this case work less well than in the other two patterns.

It should be emphasised that joint inflammation and destruction often occur uncoupled, and it is not uncommon to see a patient with severely crippled joints who had few, if any, inflammatory flares with very little pain whose only symptom is morning stiffness. Although it is easy to control pain and inflammation in the first two patterns described above, it is very difficult to stop bony erosions. A reliable sign that the disease will develop into erosions and other joint damages is the high level of C-reactive protein, which does not decrease, even if the patient is treated with very strong and combined immunosuppressors. New therapies for rheumatoid arthritis should focus not only on reduction and control of external signs of joint inflammation, but should also include attempts to reduce or stop joint destruction.

It has recently been shown that TNF and interleukin-1 are master cytokines in the process of human rheumatoid arthritis. Studies in experimental models revealed that TNF is indeed a pivotal cytokine in joint swelling and that interleukine-1 is the dominant collagen-destructive cytokine. The production of interleukin-1 may occur independently of TNF [17].

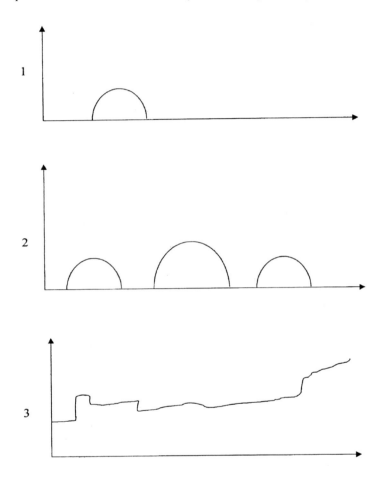

Figure 12. Inflammatory flares along the course of rheumatoid arthritis. 1) Monocyclic. 2) Polycyclic. 3) Unremitting.

Another debated aspect of rheumatoid arthritis is whether the clinical course of seropositive and seronegative forms of the disease is similar or whether these two forms should be considered different pathologic entities. The word "seropositive" indicates that the disease is accompanied by high titres of IgM rheumatoid factor detected with the classical methods: latex test and Waaler-Rose. According to our experience, seronegative and seropositive are two aspects of the disease that do not influence its course and prognosis. More sophisticated laboratory methods have shwn in many cases high titles of IgG and IgA rheumatoid factors in seronegative patients. Another relevant observation is that during the course of the disease, patients may change from seronegative to seropositive.

Seronegative Spondiloarthropaties

Seronegative spondyloarthropaties consttute a very large area of rheumatology that includes reactive arthritides (Reiter's disease), ankylosing spondylitis, psoriatic arthritis, and other similar conditions. The histocompatibility antigen B27 is a risk factor for development of spondylitis. Spondylitis is in fact much more frequent in B27 positive than in B27 negative individuals. These diseases primarly involve the enthesis, i.e, the zone where the tendon attaches to the bone.

Ankylosing spondylitis should be suspected in a young male with morning stiffness and pain in the back, mainly involving the lower lumbar spine and the sacrum, which do not ameliorate with standard anti-inflammatory analgesic drugs. The diagnosis of ankylosing spondylitis is not difficult after a good clinical assessment along with the appropriate laboratory and imaging techniques.

The focus here is not the inflamed enthesis, which acts as a trigger point with characteristics similar to those observed in myofascial trigger points (e.g, local pain or tenderness and radiation of pain). The only difference is in the location and the radiation patterns. It should be noted, however, that both myofascial and enthesic trigger points are located in areas of transition from one tissue to another (muscle belly and tendon for myofascial trigger points, tendon and bone for the enthesic ones). It is possible that stretching forces in these areas are less damped than in other somatic structures, therefore possibly generating pain.

Regarding the 10:1 ratio of ankylosing spondylitis in male patients when B27 is equally expressed in both genders, we have observed that B27 positive female patients often develop a lumbsacral pain with the same characteristics as those observed in male patients and also develop a sacroileitis. The only difference is that in male patients the disease develops along the spine and toward rhizomelic joints, whereas in female patients it does not. The reason for this is unknown.

Gout

Crystal arthropaties are a group of rheumatic diseases characterised by deposition of different types of crystals in different organs. Among the involved crystals we mention for instance uric acid (gout), calcium pyrophosphate dehydrate (condrocalcinosis) and calcium oxalate. The most frequent of these diseases is gout. Hyperuricemia and gout are not synonyms. Gout indeed is characterised by clinical symptoms and not all the hyperuricemic individuals have those.

It is impossible to describe a natural clinical history for gout since different types of gout may develop independently. These clinical syndromes include gouty arthritis, tophaceus gout, uric acid nephrolithiasis and gouty nephropathy. In its narrower and perhaps more commonly used definition, gout refers to arthritis caused by uric acid crystals.

Acute gout is characterised by the rapidity of onset and build-up of pain, with associated swelling and redness of the affected joint. In over half of the initial attacks, this occurs in the first metatarsophalangeal joint, and in time, this joint is affected in some 90% of patients with gout. This may be due to the fact that this joint is the cooler of the body and this may facilitate crystal formation within the joint. The attacks occur during the night probably because uric acid enters into the joint during the day in water solution. Water comes out the joint during the night when the patient is lying without uric acid so that the synovial uric acid concentration increases and crystallization is promoted.

Nowadays the acute gouty attacks are well controlled by drugs as colchicine and indomethacine and prevented by xantine-oxidase inhibitors (allopurinol) or by uricuric agents (probenecid, sulfinpyrazone and others).

The Universe or Arthralgies

Joints are structures with the highest sensitivity to pain. Arthralgias may be present in every disease (mainly if accompanied by fever). They disappear a few days after recovery. Of particular interest is the group of patients often called "weather predictors". These patients begin to feel pain 1 to 2 days before it starts raining. The reason for this phenomenon is not clear. Research on this phenomenon includes a study in which such patients were put in a chamber where the barometric pressure could be changed. The patients started to feel pain when the barometric pressure of the chamber was lowered. It was concluded that these patients feel the lowering of barometric pressure that precedes rain. Nevertheless, the biologic influences of barometric pressure on the body remain unknown [18].

Arthralgias, however, cannot be underestimated, as they are in many cases a symptom of serious inflammatory connective diseases or the heralds of such diseases.

A young female patient with diffuse arthralgias and long-lasting morning stiffness may develop lupus erythematosus; very intense arthralgias and long lasting morning stiffness mainly of the little joints of the hands and wrists may accompany Sjögren's syndrome.

Lastly, breast implantation, augmentation mammoplasty with silicone, gel implants and some cosmetics may induce very severe arthralgias that continue until the cause is removed. Some cases of scleroderma are also described.

Therapy

The drugs used for joint pain fall generally into two classes: symptomatic and disease modifying. This dualism, however, raises more questions than it answers. For example, every person affected by rheumatoid arthritis from the past century has probably taken aspirin or aspirin-like drugs. Who can say if the evolution of the disease was different before these drugs were available? In India, where these drugs are much less common, one of the authors observed the devastating level of arthritides compared with that in Western countries.

Pharmaceutical companies continue to search for new anti-inflammatory and analgesic medications that are also relatively free of side effects. The ideal drug has not yet be found and physicians must distinguish reality from fashion. "Pro-drugs", for example, named because only the first metabolite after the hepatic pass was active, entered the market a few years ago and are now almost totally forgotten.

Currently, the COX1-COX2 (cyclooxigenase 1 and 2) hypothesis is gaining recognition. COX1 and COX2 are two isoforms of COX. COX1 is called "constitutive" because it is always present to produce prostaglandin exerting physiologic functions, such as protection of the gastric mucosa. COX2 is called "inducible" because it works only after inflammatory stimuli. A drug with the capacity to block COX2 and not COX1 would, according to this hypothesis, be the best treatment for pain and inflammation. Some drugs recently available in the market inhibit much more COX2 than COX1 and research on more selective drugs, such as rofecoxib [19] and elecoxib [20] is on the way. It is important to note that these are pure laboratory results and that side effects, such as bleeding from the stomach and gastric ulcer are still a possibility and no endoscopy studies in treated patients were published [21]. Moreover, these drugs may induce asthma in individuals who are predisposed to it. This side effect was also observed for aspirin at the beginning of this century. Lastly, it should be remembered that an adverse effect of treatment with aspirin-like drugs is acute renal failure, particularly in a subset of patients who are in a state of effective volume depletion. This risk may increase if these drugs are associated with cyclosporin, a disease-modifying drug that is potentially nephrotoxic.

Corticosteroids are considered midway between symptomatic and disease-modifying drugs. They are the treatment of choice in polymyalgia rheumatica and giant cell artheritis but must be used with caution in rheumatoid arthritis, and only when they are absolutely necessary to control inflammation. The daily dosage must be tapered when pain and inflammation are under reasonable control. An alternate-day regimen for tapering is suggested. Chronic administration of these drugs leads to side effects that are worse than the disease itself. They cannot be stopped in cortisone-addicted patients because the atrophic suppressed adrenal cortex is unable to synthesise physiologic cortisol once again, and interruption of the therapy may be life threatening.

Intraarticular effusions should be aspirated and steroids combined or not with local anaesthetics should be injected inside the joint at a variable dosage according to the intensity of inflammation. This treatment can be repeated two to three times. If swelling recurs, the treatment of choice is synoviectomy. This may be obtained with surgical procedures or injecting into the joint radionuclides. The latter is the methods currently used in our clinic [22].

Physical therapies that do not produce heat may also be helpful. Rehabilitation is of paramount importance.

Disease modifying drugs for the treatment of osteoarthritis, the so-called "condroprotectors" should be treated as if they arose from a book of folk medicine.

Self-administration of over-the-counter (OTC) medications for pain is a pressing problem. It has been reported that 58.7% to 95.9% of the participants, in a study on adolescents, take OTC medications for pain in every area, including head, ear, throat, muscle, joint and back pains [23]. Information about these medications was obtained from a variety of sources, primarily parents. Self-administration was widespread; 58.3% to 75.9% of adolescents reported taking an over the counter (OTC) medication for pain without first checking with an adult in the previous three months. Females tended to self-administer medication more than males in this age group. Higher levels of pain frequency and intensity were related to higher levels of self-administration for all pains except those of the muscles, joints or back. Adolescents reported that they began to self-administer medications between the ages of 11 and 12. The OTC medication used was often inappropriate.

CONCLUSIONS

The focus of this chapter was on joint pain, but it should be remembered that many joint diseases are accompanied by diffuse muscular pain and tenderness. Because fibromyalgia syndrome has gained great acceptance and awareness in both the medical and the lay community., the possibility of overdiagnosis exists. Careful diagnosis of this disease is recommended, as misdiagnosis could have tremendous consequences on the patient's health.

Muscle Pain

The diseases in which muscular pain is the main or a relevant accompanying symptom are so many that only a few can be described.

Diseases with Diffuse and Painful Muscular Involvement

Early and disseminated chronic Lyme disease: The erythema migraine is often accompanied by fatigue, fever and chills, myalgia, arthralgia, headache and paraesthesias. Myalgia, headache and paraesthesiaa may reflect early neurological dissemination. About 60% of untreated individuals develop arthritis from weeks to years after the onset of illness. Frank arthritis may be preceded by months or even years of intermittent migratory myalgias, arthralgias and periarticular pain. A fibromyalgia alone was observed in 20% of patients.

HIV: HIV infected patients may develop a myopathy as a result of polymyositis like inflammatory muscle disease, ridovudine therapy or opportunistic infections (e.g. toxoplasmosis). Most patients with HIV associated polymyositis present with an insidious onset of proximal muscle weakness and hypotropy, as well as muscle pain and tenderness (often diffuse, mimicking fibromyalgia). In approximately 50% of patients with myopathy, it is the initial manifestation of HIV infection, while in the remainder myopathy develops after the occurrence of opportunistic infections. Most patients with either inflammatory myopathy associated with HIV-1 or ridovuline induced myopathy have elevation of muscle enzymes and EMG abnormalities. Indeed, in one study, 16% of all HIV-infected individuals taking rivoduline for more than 6 months developed abnormally elevated muscle enzymes, though only a few became symptomatic.

Sarcoidosis: The aetiology of sarcoidosis is unknown. A variety of infective and non-infective agents have been implicated, but there is no proof that any one agent is responsible. Sarcoid myopathy is usually asymptomatic. In acute sarcoidosis with erythema nodosum asymptomatic granulomatous myopathy is common and random muscle biopsy may contribute to establishing the diagnosis. Sarcoid myopathy may also be symptomatic in acute disease and presents with fever, severe muscle pain and tenderness involving proximal girdle muscles.

Reactive arthritides: The prototype of these arthritides is the rheumatic fever, which has now disappeared in the Western countries. This disease unfortunately left a heredity in the minds of physicians who interpreted muscular pain in fibromyalgia (previously called fibrositis) as secondary to an infective disease working somewhere. Tonsils, appendix and other organs were cut and extracted in these poor patients since they were considered to be the foci of the disease. After those interventions fibromyalgia did not improve. Fortunately these beliefs are slowly changing.

Reactive arthritides are secondary to many infective agents, such as yersinia, mycoplasma, borrelia, neisseria (gonorrhoeae, etc.), clamidia (trachomatis, etc.), campylobacter, streptococci, shigella, etc. These agents are located in the bowels, in the genitourinary tract, throat or elsewhere. These infections may trigger mono-oligoarthropaties, sacroileitis or enthesipathies. For treatment antirheumatic drugs have to be combined with antibiotics.

Vasculitides: Vasculitides are a universe of diseases. Many of them are accompanied by myalgias. As examples we mention only microscopic polyangiitis and Takayasu's arteritis.

Arthralgias and/or diffuse myalgias are present in about 50% of patients affected with microscopic polyangiitis. Such symptoms are often a non-specific initial clinical presentation of this disease.

Myalgia is found infrequently but can be severe in Takayasu's arteritis.

Endocrinopathies: In this context we will mention only hypothyroidism. The myopathy of hypothyroidism may have a wide spectrum of muscle complaints, including proximal muscle pain, stiffness and hypertrophy (Hoffmann's syndrome). Muscular weakness may or may not be accompanied by myalgias. Muscle biopsy findings are usually normal, although occasional fiber destruction and mucinous infiltrates have been reported in some patients. The peculiar nature of this myopaty could suggest either polymyalgia rheumatica (when stiff, painful muscles predominate) or polymyositis (when the creatinkinase level is elevated).

Genetic diseases: Familial Mediterranean fever could serve as an example. Muscle pain occurs in about 20% of patients with familial Mediterranean fever. Usually the pain is not severe, appears in the lower extremities after exertion, lasts from a few hours to 1 to 2 days and subsides with rest or non-steroidal anti-inflammatory drugs. In 12% of patients with familial Mediterranean fever a syndrome of protracted febrile myalgia develops. It is characterized by severe, debilitating myalgia accompanied by fever, abdominal pain, a high erythrocyte sedimentation rate, and leucocytosis. In patients who are treated with non-steroidal anti-inflammatory drugs the attacks last 6 to 8 weeks but they subside promptly after a high dose of prednisone.

Since colchicine, that is used in the therapy of this disease, is known to induce neuropathy and myopathy in rare cases, it is important to differentiate colchicine induced myopathy from an attack of protracted febrile myalgia.

Disorders of fat metabolism: Patients with disorders of fatty acid metabolism often report episodes of muscle pain. Exercise, particularly in the fasting state, may sometimes be the precipitating factor. It is unlikely that metabolic depletion is the immediate cause of pain in these patients. Probably exercise mobilizes free fatty acids from body fat depots and muscle triglycerides. Yet, because fatty transport into the mythochondria is defective in these patients, the free fatty acids (mostly stearic and palmitic) accumulate within the muscle fibers and due to their detergent effect, damage the muscle fiber membranes.

Osteoporosis: In more than 50% of women with postmenopausal osteoporosis fibromyalgia is observed. This fibromyalgia may develop, because a number of local factors, such as prostaglandins (mainly PGE2), insuline-like growth factor, interleukins 1, 6 and 11, TNFα, transforming growth factor β, which are very high in osteoporosis, play an important role stimulating, on one hand, osteoclasts proliferation and sensitising or exciting muscular nociceptors, on the other.

Drugs: There are many drugs which may induce myalgia as a side effect. We mention here only drugs used in the treatment of rheumatic diseases: chloroquine and hydroxychloroquine, gold salts, D-penicilline and colchicines. In this context we will describe only myopathy induced by corticosteroids as these drugs are the most widely used for the treatment of rheumatic diseases. The development of myalgias and muscle weakness tend to parallel the development of other adverse effects of corticosteroids, particularly osteoporosis.

Steroid induced myopathy is not strictly dose dependent, but it is less common with doses of prednisone less than 30mg per day and is an uncommon effect of alternate day treatment.

Myopathy may develop after only short exposure and may have an insidious or abrupt onset. It is usually most severe in the pelvic girdle, with lesser involvement of shoulder girdle and distal muscles. Myalgias in the setting of high-dose corticosteroids treatment suggest the clinical diagnosis.

Diagnosis is very difficult in the setting of systemic lupus erythematosus or polymyositis, where an inflammatory myopathy may obscure the diagnosis. Elevated urine creatine in the presence of normal serum concentrations of muscle enzymes such as creatine kinase and aldolase is probably the best distinguishing feature, although this test has been questioned. Muscle biopsies show selective atrophy of type II fibers; glycogen-synthetase, β-hydroxyl-CoA, and citric acid synthetase are lower in patients with corticosteroid induced myopathy compared to normal muscles. The myopathic alterations are potentially reversible by decreasing corticosteroid dosage and increasing exercise.

In conclusion the two forms of myopathy induced by corticosteroids are:

a)   a generalised muscle atrophy after short term treatment with large doses;
b)   proximal limb muscle weakness after extended treatment with moderate doses.

Diffuse Connective Tissue Disease with Chronic Myalgia

In these diseases muscular pain may be an important but not the main symptom.

Lupus erythematosus systemicus: Myalgia, very often similar to fibromyalgia, muscle weakness and tenderness have been reported in up to 60% of patients with lupus, although a true myositis is confined to about 5% of these patients. Treatment with corticosteroids and chlorochine may cause a myopathy, but in the main the myalgia experienced by patients is independent. Histologically a vacual myopathy has been described in lupus. This is identified by the presence of plump swollen sarcolemmal nuclei with other prominent vacuolated nuclei, centrally located within the muscle fiber. Immunoglobulin deposition is often seen in the muscles of these patients, but this is irrespective of whether they have clinically overt muscle disease and seems to relate better to minor fibers damage as a secondary event, rather than to a primary inflammatory myopathy.

Unless an overlap syndrome is present, creatine kinase levels rarely exceed 1000 I.U. Other causes of elevated muscle enzymes such as hypothyroidism, drugs, vigorous exercise or intramuscolar injections should be excluded. Electromyography and muscle biopsy findings range from normal to those seen in classical polymyositis. Low to moderate dose steroids (e.g., about 20 mg. of prednisone a day) suffice for treatment of lupus myositis.

Mixed connective tissue disease: Myalgias are common and about 2/3 of patients develop an inflammatory myopathy that is similar to polymyositis. Very often myositis may occur acutely in a patient who has other mild features and prompts the diagnosis of mixed connective tissue disease. The prognosis seems more favourable than in polymyositis/dermatomyositis with less corticosteroid treatment needed. No demonstrable weakness, EMG abnormalities, or muscle enzyme elevations are present. It is often unclear whether the symptom represents a low-grade myositis or an associated fibromyalgia syndrome.

In children inflammatory infiltration of skeletal muscle has been reported at autopsy, without clinical or laboratory evidence of muscle disease.

Sjögren's syndrome: Arthralgias and/or myalgias with morning stiffness are experienced (continuously or episodically) by 70% of patients with primary Sjögren's syndrome. It is always important to rule out hypothyroidism (which is relatively common in this population) and to look for disordered sleep patterns, especially when the patient rises from bed in the morning with significant fatigue. Such sleep disorders may be due to polydipsia/polyuria or nocturnal myoclonus. The component of fatigue due to active autoimmune disease is difficult to assess.

Scleroderma: In most instances weakness and atrophy of skeletal muscle result from disuse secondary to joint contractures or chronic disease. Approximately 20% of patients have a primary myopathy. Typically this is a subtle process with weakness detected only by the examining physician.

Serum muscle enzyme elevation and muscle biopsy showing focal replacement of myofibrils with collagenous connective tissue and perimysial-epimysial fibrosis without inflammatory changes have been described. A minority of patients exhibit more pronounced proximal muscle weakness and electrophysiologic, biochemical and pathological evidence of polymyositis. These persons have been variously classified as having scleroderma with myositis or scleroderma in overlap with polymyositis.

Active polymyositis due to scleroderma or attributable to an overlap syndrome should be treated with moderate doses of corticosteroids (prednisone: 20-30mg per day). Methotrexate, penicillamine, azathioprine or another immune-suppressive agent can be added in the event that the response is incomplete.

In contrast, bland myopathy with minimal or no elevation of serum creatine kinase and little or no progression of pain and weakness should be treated with low dose non-steroidal anti-inflammatory agents.

Non-specific musculo-skeletal complaints such as arthralgias and myalgias are one of the earliest symptoms of scleroderma. Pain on motion of the ankle, wrists, knee or elbow may be accompanied by a coarse friction rub caused by inflammation and fibrosis of the tendon sheat or adjacent tissues.

Polymyositis, dermatomyositis, inclusion body myositis: In these diseases muscular pain is rare and muscle weakness predominates. This may be due to the fact that histologically these diseases are characterised not only by muscular inflammation, but also by a severe muscular hypotrophy with damage of muscular nerve fibers.

Diseases in Which Chronic Muscular Pain is the Main Symptom

The more frequent diseases of this group are: fibromyalgia, myofascial syndromes and polymyalgia rheumatica.

Primary fibromyalgia with or without chronic fatigue: Fibromyalgia, previously called fibrositis, is a disease that has recently been extensively studied so that triennial "Myopain" meetings are organised. Yet the aetiology and pathogenesis of this disease are still obscure.

Fibromyalgic muscles do not apparently differ from healthy muscles. As noted above, muscle inflammation, as that seen in polymyositis, is accompanied by muscle weakness more than pain. Therefore, peripheral and central hypotheses still need confirmation.

The age of onset is about 40-50 years, but the disease can be seen also in younger patients.

The disease prevails in females (females/males: 8/1) and epidemiological studies on prevalence range from less than 1% in Denmark to 11% in Norway. This great difference may be due to the fact that the diagnostic criteria vary in different countries.

We observed a constitutional predisposition to develop this disease (fibrositic diathesis) that is hypergia-dysergia and laxity of somatic structures. The predisposed women often have painful and exceeding fat, tenderness everywhere, teleangectasias, haemorrhoids, phlebectasias, restless legs, epistaxis in their history, etc. If dermographia (secondary hyperalgesia) is induced on their skin, rubbing the stunt portion of the needle that is inside the reflex hammer results in an abnormally red demographia, large and even pomphoid. If a wasp or a mosquito pinks their skin, a wide area of pomphoid, itchy redness develops all around. All the muscles of the body are tender, in their full length. Similar findings are observed in subcutaneous tissues and when fat rolling them. A highly evident reactive hyperaemia is observed on the skin after these manoeuvres. In other words, these patients have what can be called "tender bodies".

The cardinal symptom of fibromyalgia is diffuse chronic pain. The pain often begins in one location, particularly the neck and shoulders, but then becomes more generalised. Usually patients state that "it hurts all over" and they have difficulty locating the site of pain arising from articular or non-articular tissues. Patients describe the muscle pain often as burning, radiating or gnawing and the intensity of the pain as modest or severe but varying greatly. Most patients also report profound fatigue. This is often notable when arising from sleep but is also marked in the mid-afternoon. Seemingly minor activity also intensifies their symptoms. Patients are stiff in the morning and feel unrefreshed, even if they have slept 8-10 hours. They usually recognise that they sleep "lightly", waking frequently during early morning and having difficulty getting back to sleep, often affected by restless legs (dysfunctional sleep).

Headaches, either "tension type" or typical migraine, and symptoms suggestive of irritable bowel syndrome (called in the fifthies by the Italian Florentine school "chronic dysreactive abdomen") are present in more than 50% of patients. True Raynaud's phenomenon or a Raynaud's-like excess sensitivity to cold have also been commonly reported. In many patients, multiple other seemingly unrelated somatic symptoms, such as dizziness, difficulty to concentrate, dry eyes and dry mouth, palpitations, and sensitivity to foods, medications, and allergenes are common and may give rise to the suspicion of a somatoform disorder [24].

We have studied fibromyalgia by administering a questionnaire (devised by the authors, validated also in English) to 250 consecutive patients suffering from "chronic fibromyalgia" (Unpublished study). Factor analysis yielded the following six independent factors – the first four strong and the last two weaker ones: 1) Cognitive: catastrophising, "external control" beliefs; 2) Emotional: alexythymia; 3) Behavioral: a lot of useless unfocused activities, restlessness; 4) Relational: need for support; 5) Lack of reactivity; 6) Lack of autonomy.

These factors indicate dysfunctional psychological characteristics. It is impossible to determine if the factors are primary or are due to the chronic suffering of the patients. Be it as it may, it seems likely that they could be modified with psychotherapeutic means, such as cognitive-behavioral therapy.

A committee of the American College of Rheumatology proposed the following criteria for the diagnosis of fibromyalgia [25]: 1) History of widespread pain; 2) Pain in 11 of 18 tender point sites (predetermined by the committee) on digital palpation.

There are some difficulties with these criteria. For instance, tender points are found also in myofascial pain (myalgic spots). Further, pain often radiates, and if it does, it radiates not infrequently a little around the myalgic spot. Moreover, it seems problematic to speak about tender points in patients who complain of tenderness all over.

Table 1: Main differential characteristics between fibromyalgia and myofascial pain

	FIBROMYALGIA	MYOFASCIAL PAIN
Spontaneous pain	Diffuse	Locali
Induced pain	Muscles and subcutaneous tissues	Muscles (trigger points or myalgic spots)
Females/males ratio	8/1	0.6
Sleep	Often dysfunctional	Rare insomnia and directly caused by pain
Irritable colon	yes	Not
Restless legs syndrome	Frequent	Present only if myofascial pain involves anterior tibial muscles
Fibrositic diathesis (see text)	Yes	Not
Dermographia	Hyper reaction	Normal
Therapy	Systemic	Often local
Therapy results	Often poor	Often good

A large number of pharmacological and non-pharmacological interventions have been proposed for treating fibromyalgia. One issue about which most authors agree is that the steroidal and non-steroidal anti-inflammatory drugs do not work. The most efficacious drugs seem to be tricyclic antidepressants administered at doses lower than those used for treating depression (e.g., amitriptyline 10+25mg per day). The patients sleep better, do not wake up in the early morning, and thus are better able to face the day. Recent trials are under way with gabapentin. Table 1 presents the main differences between fibromyalgia and myofascial pain.

More recently another syndrome was defined - the chronic fatigue syndrome, in which chronic fatigue predominates. It may or may not follow a 7-10 days continuous fever of unknown etiology. Due to the fatigue, the work capacity and performance of the patients are reduced by at least 50%. Since the great majority of fibromyalgic patients suffer also from chronic fatigue, the overlap between these two diseases is very wide. Consequently it is an open issue whether they are two separate diseases or two manifestations of the same disease.

Myofascial pain: Myofascial pain affects muscles in localised areas. Almost all muscles may be involved. Trigger points and myalgic spots are typical findings. Trigger points, when they are stimulated by digital palpation or spontaneously, radiate pain to distant locations or induce pain in well defined areas which are not connected with the trigger itself (target areas). Radiation patterns and target areas do not follow a somatomeric distribution. Somato-somatic and somato-sympathetic reflexes may be involved. In contrast, myalgic spots are tender, muscular zones with no radiation of pain.

Since almost all muscles may be involved, a great number of syndromes have been described (for a complete description see for example reference 28). In the present context only a few select diseases due to myofascial pain will be described.

Pain From Temporomandibular Disfunctions

Many temporo-mandibular dysfunctions are of muscular origin. The masseter muscle is mainly involved, but other masticator muscles, such as the temporal muscle, the internal and external pterygoid muscles and the digastric muscles may contribute to the dysfunction. Pain increases while chewing. Odontoiatric techniques to reduce a forward hyperlussation of the temporal condyle together with other interventions may be of some help.

Tension Type Headache

This type of pain is very frequent. It is often secondary to tenderness of some muscles of the neck, which assume the character of the trigger points, and of some muscles of the skull. Pain radiates over the occipit and even to frontal areas of the skull involving the whole skull bilaterally as a helmet. Pain is often accompanied by subjective vertigoes and/or loss of equilibrium that may be present even without pain. It is commonly believed that this symptom is due to ischaemia along the distribution of the vertebro-basilar arteries following cervical osteoarthritis. This is unlikely since vertebral arteries are well protected inside the spine and an eco-color-doppler does not show alterations. Another more likely reason may have to do with the role the neck fulfills in regard to equilibrium, being a structure interposed between two mobile platforms – the head and the trunk. Thus, vertigoes and loss of equilibrium are probably due to the fact that proprioceptive information from the neck exerts an important role for the equilibrium function. Indeed, experience shows that if we block with local anaesthetics trigger points of the neck, pain as well as the other symptoms disappear within few seconds.

Two sets of observations demonstrate the validity of the suggested interpretation. One concerns astronauts, who now do not glide any more in space as they used to years ago, but stand in the upright position as they were trained to adjust their proprioception by exercising neck movements. Another example is a cat that falls from a window on the back, but lands standing. During the fall it rotates first the neck and then the body. If hypertonic saline (a strong algogenic stimulus) is injected in the cat's neck, thus interfering with this function, the cat falls striking the back.

Scapulo-humeral periarthritis and cervico-brachialgias. Trigger points and myalgic spots of a scapulo-humeral periarthritis are many but only a few dominate. These are the points or spots that are to be blocked if reversible block with local anaesthetics is the chosen treatment.

Diagnosis has to be very accurate as shoulder pain may be an early sign of Pancoast's disease and cancer of the superior sulcus [26]. In many of these cases pain is accompanied by a Bernard-Horner's syndrome of the same side. Pain on a shoulder, mainly the left, can be referred by myocardial ischaemia or infarction [27]. This pain may evolve into a shoulder-hand syndrome that is very difficult to treat [28]

Rotator cuff dystrophy (hypotrophia plus tenderness) is an early consequence as it may be seen also a few hours after the onset of pain.

There are many and varied causes of cervicobrachialgia. One frequent and not well known cause is secondary to myofascial pain from the scalenus anterior muscle. When this muscle is painful and contracted it narrows the thoracic outlet. To reach with a needle the scalenus anterior is not difficult as it is found back to the clavicular branch of the sterno-cleido-mastoid muscle near and beneath the clavicle. Pain radiates along the upper limb and the Adson's manoevre results positive. If this muscle is blocked with local anaesthetics, Adson's manoeuvre becomes negative and cervicobrachial pain disappears (unpublished observations). Many nocturnal algo paraesthesic syndromes are secondary to myofascial pain.

Back pain: Back pain secondary to myofascial involvement of spinal and paraspinal muscles, tendons and ligaments may constitute a diagnostic problem. The reason is that pain at a dorsal level, for example, can radiate anteriorly to the abdominal wall or chest just as diseases of the abdominal wall or chest may radiate back (e.g., myocardial infarction, acute pancreatitis). Another example is myofascial low back pain which may simulate a true sciatica and the Lasegue's sign is positive because of the contracture of the gluteus major muscle. Medical tests may not suffice in these and similar cases so that clinical observation searching for the areas of superficial and deep hyperalgesia are mandatory.

Tennis and golf players elbow: Some tennis and golf players feel pain on the back of the hand when they grip the racket. This area is a target of trigger points located in the elbow. Notably, one of the main causes of trigger points is repetitive microtraumas of the kind that are often observed in sport medicine.

Pubalgia (groin pain): Groin is a frequently observed symptom in soccer and football players, due to repetitive and sudden stretching of the proximal attachment of the abductor muscles of the thigh. In many cases the patients have to stop playing if they are not properly and very early treated at the level of the trigger points, for example, with local anaesthetics.

Coxofemural Periarthritis

This pain and accompanying symptoms may be confused with pain following osteoarthritis of the hip. Some objective signs can distinguish these two conditions: movements of the hip are completely blocked, in osteoarthritis for anatomical reasons, in periarthritis for pain. In periarthritis the block is elastic so that an attempt to increase the passive movement (for instance, by intrarotation and hyperabduction) causes the joint to move a little more but pain increases. The two key points to be blocked are: (a) lateral (midway between the great trochanter and the superior-anterior spine of the pelvic

bone); and (b) anterior (corresponding to the proximal insertion of abductor muscles and near to the femoral artery, vein and plexus).

Restless legs: This syndrome was first described in 1945 by Eckbom who divided it into "asthenia crurum paraesthesica" and "asthenia crurum dolorosa" [29]. Some patients, mainly women, feel a boring sensation that is unrest of the legs defined by them as restlessness. Parasthesias, such as tingling or "pins and pricks" are often accompanying symptoms. These symptoms occur mainly when the patients lie in bed or are forced to maintain the legs flexed (sitting at the theatre etc.). They are often undervalued by the physician and by the family and interpreted as being of neurotic origin. Therefore these patients seldom speak about these symptoms even with a physician. Luganesi interpreted restless legs as a sleep disturbance [30]. Instead, we observed in most of these patients tenderness of the upper and lower third of the tibialis anterior muscle. These areas of tenderness may induce a deranged proprioceptive input that increases when these muscles are slightly stretched in the lying position. To our mind, this is the main cause of the symptom. It is rarely observed at the level of the upper limbs because they have a wider cortical representation and are therefore less automatic.

Heel Pain

This pain is mostly observed in people exercising different kinds of sport activities which stretch the triceps surae muscle. Heel pain may be a target of a trigger point located at the junction of the triceps belly with the Achilles tendon.

Pain on the dorsal aspect of the foot: Also this kind of pain is often seen in sport medicine. The trigger point is located on the distal third of the tibialis anterior muscle. Blocks with local anaesthetics and resting of the painful muscle may help a lot by disrupting a vicious cycle. The newly reached steady state can be maintained for a long time unless promoting factors (i.e. arteriopathies of the lower limbs) re-create this vicious cycle [31]. In this case, whenever possible, the causative factor should be removed.

Local corticosteroids may be combined with local anaesthetics when inflammation is a contributing factor to the pain. When pain is in an acute phase, it is better to avoid infiltrative manoeuvres and to wait for a spontaneous reduction of the pain, helping the patient with analgesics, warm packs, etc.

There are three major contraindications of trigger points injections: (a) Severe acute muscular pain mainly due to muscle injury or trauma; (b) Allergies to local anaesthetics; and

(c) Coagulation disorders or those treated with anticoagulants. If the contraindications are considered, injecting trigger points with proper dosages of local anaesthetics is harmless.

Drugs can be used as a single agent or in combination with trigger point injections. Drugs that may be prescribed include flunarizine in tension type headache and restless legs syndrome, magnesium, ademetonium, slight myorelaxants and tricyclic antidepressants.

Polymyalgia rheumatica and giant cell arthritis: These diseases are often discussed together although it is doubtful that they are two different expressions of the same disease. Most patients with classic polymyalgia rheumatica do not develop clinical or biopsy-proven giant cell arteritis, even if followed for many years. This was true also before corticosteroids were available. Conversely, there are patients with giant cell artheritis, but without polymyalgia rheumatica and muscular pain.

A classic symptom of polymyalgia rheumatica is the primary involvement of the shoulder girdle muscles. In contrast, muscular pain, from its onset, mostly involves not only the shoulder girdle, but also muscles of the neck, lower back, hips, thighs, etc. mimicking in many cases fibromyalgia. These so called "pain of the elderlies" are actually a true polymyalgia rheumatica, which has to be properly treated with corticosteroids. The differential diagnosis between polymyalgia rheumatica and fibromyalgia is easy with an accurate clinical examination and proper blood exams (e.g. erythrocyte sedimentation rate and C reactive protein).

CONCLUSION

If soft-tissue rheumatism is suspected, measuring creatine-kinase may be required to exclude myositis, which however is usually obvious from a clinical point of view. It is necessary to exclude other causes of myalgia, such as anxiety, depression, fibromyalgia, thyroid diseases, Parkinson's disease, widespread malignancies (e.g. multiple myeloma), and toxic (e.g. alcoholic) and metabolic (e.g. diabetes) myopathies. Creatin kinase is the most reliable enzyme test in polymyositis and dermatomyositis, with plasma activity level correlating with disease activity.

Muscle weakness and pain is a common symptom also of rheumatic diseases in which the main or only involvement is at the joint level. Symptoms that are more characteristic of soft tissue involvement are probably secondary and due to somato-sympathetic reflexes between the inflamed joint and those tissues.

REFERENCES

[1]   Zoppi M. and Beneforti E.: Joint pain. *Current Review of Pain.* 3 (1999) 121-129.
[2]   Arnoldi C.C., Djurhuus J.C. and Heertordt J.: Intraosseous plebography, intraosseous pressure measurements and 99m TC polyphosphate scintigraphy, in patients with various painful conditions in the hip and knee. Acta Orthop. *Scand.* 51 (1980) 19-28.

[3]   Zoppi M., Morelli A. and Zamponi A.: Mechanisms of pain in rheumatic diseases. In: M. Hyodo, T. Oyama and M. Swerdlow (Eds.). Pain Clinic 4ht, VSP, *Utrecht*; 1992, pp. 81-83.

[4]   Geppetti G. and Holzer P.: *Neurogenic inflammation.* CRC Press, Boca Raton, 1996.

[5]   Zoppi M., Cesaretti S. and Anichini M.: Substance P in the serum of patients with rheumatoid arthritis. *Rev. Rhum. Engl. Ed.* 64 (1997) 19-22.

[6]   Schwab W., Bilgicyldirim A. and Funl R.H.: Microtopography of the autonomic nerves in the rat knee: a fluorescence microscopic study. *Anat. Rec.* 247 (1997) 109-118.

[7]   Maresca M., Nuzzaci G. and Zoppi M.: Muscular pain in chronic occlusive arterial diseases of the limbs. *Adv. Pain Res.Ther.,* 7(1984) 521-538.

[8]   Green P.C., Miao F.S. and Strausbough R.: Endocrine and vagal controls of sympathetically dependent neurogenic inflammation. Ann. N.Y. *Acad. Sci.,* 840 (1998) 282-288.

[9]   Zoppi M., Liotto R. and Zamponi A.: Rheumatic pain. In: P. Raj, S. Erdine and D. Niv (Eds*.). Management of Pain: a World Perspective.* Monduzzi, Bologna, 1995, pp.227-231 .

[10]   Galletti R., Obletter G., Giamberardino M.A.: Pain in osteoarthritis of the knee. In: M. Zoppi (Ed.). *The Pain Clinic,* Raven Press, New York, 1990, pp.183-190.

[11]   Lewis T.: *Pain.* Macmillan, London, 1942.

[12]   Larsson S., Ekblom A., and Henzikson K.: Immunoreactive tachynins, calcitonin gene-related peptide and neuropeptide Y in human synovial fluid from inflamed knee joints. *Neurosci. Lett.* 100 (1995) 326-329.

[13]   Salo P.: The role of joint innervation in the pathogenesis of arthritis. *Can.J. Surg.,* 42 (1999) 91-100.

[14]   Stein C.: Interaction of immune- competent cells and nociceptors. Prog. Pain. *Res.Manage.* 2 (1994) 285-303.

[15]   Baerwald C.C. and Panayi G.S.: Neurohormonal mechanisms in rheumatoid arthritis. Scand. *J. Rheumatol.* 26 (1997) 1-3.

[16]   Van den Berg W.B.: Joint inflammation and cartilage destruction may occur uncoupled. Springer Semin. *Immunopathol.* 20 (1998) 149-164.

[17]   Quick D.C.: Joint pain and weather: a critical review of the literature. *Minn. Med.,* 80 (1997) 25-29.

[18]   Scott L.J. and Lamb H.M.: Rofecoxib. *Drugs.* 58 (1999) 499-505.

[19]   Geis G.S.: Update on clinical developments with celecoxib, a new specific COX-2 inhibitor: what can we expect? *Scand. J. Rheumatol.* 109 (1999) 31-37

[20]   McKenna F.: COX-2: Separating with from reality. *Scand. J. Rheumatol.* 109 (1999) 19-29.

[21]   Zoppi M. and Beneforti E.: Mechanism and treatment of joint pain. *Manage. Pain World Perpect.* 3 (1998) 153-158.

[22]   Chambers C.T., Reid G.J. and McGrath P.J.: Self administration of over-the-counter medication for pain among adolescents. *Arch. Pediatr. Adolesc. Med.,* 151 (1997) 449-455.

[23]   Goldenberg L.: Fibromyalgia and related syndromes. In: J.H. Klipper and P.A. Dieppe (Eds.). *Rheumatology.* Mosby, London, 1998, pp 4-15-1-12.

[24] Wolfe F. et al.: The American College of Rheumatology 1990 criteria for the classification of fibromyalgia. Report of the Multicenter Criteria *Committee.Arthritis Rheum.*, 33 (1990) 160-172.

[25] Marino C., Zoppi M., Morelli U., Buoncristiano U. and Pagni E.: Pain in early cancer of the lungs. *Pain*, 27 (1986) 57-62.

[26] Procacci P., Zoppi M. and Maresca M.: Heart, vascular and haemopathic pain. In: P.D. Wall and R. Melzack (Eds.) *Textbook of Pain* (4th ed.) Churchill Livingstone, Edinburgh, 1999, pp. 621-639.

[27] Zoppi M.: The shoulder-hand syndrome, a paraneoplastic disease. *Internal Medicine*, 5 (1997) 119-121.

[28] Eckbom K.A.: Restless legs. Acta Med. *Scand. Suppl.* 158 (1945) 1-123.

[29] Lugaresi E., Caccagna G., Mantovani M. and Lebrun R.: Some periodic phenomena arising during drowsiness and sleep in man. *Electroenceph. Clin. Neurophysiol.* 32 (1972) 701-705.

[30] Maresca M., Nuzzaci G. and Zoppi M.: Muscular pain in chronic occlusive arterial diseases of the limbs. *Advances in Pain. Research and Therapy* 7 (1984) 521-527.

[31] Sydenham, T: London: G. Kettilby, 1683 (Reprinted as On Go Works of Thomas Sydenham,MD, 3rd ed., vol. 2. Birmingham, AL: Classics of Medicine Library; 1979; pp. 124-5).

In: The Handbook of Chronic Pain
Editors: S. Kreitler, D. Beltrutti, et al., pp. 533-550

ISBN 978-1-60021-044-0
© 2007 Nova Science Publishers, Inc.

Chapter 28

Pain and Suffering in Cancer

Shulamith Kreitler, and Ofer Merimsky

PREVALENCE OF CANCER PAIN

Cancer is a ubiquitous disease: an estimated 6.35 million new cases are diagnosed worldwide annually, and the number of surviving cancer patients increases steadily due to improved detection and treatment (Bonica and Ekstrom, 1990). Pain is among the most common symptoms associated with cancer. About 70% of cancer patients suffer from severe pain at some time in the course of their disease; 25% have pain when they are first diagnosed, 30-60% during active therapy, 75% if their disease is advanced, and 25% when they die (Bonica, 1990; Twycross and Lack, 1983). The incidence of cancer pain is so high that it has justifiably been identified as a world-wide health problem of the highest priority (WHO, 1986).

Pain seems to be related to stage of disease: persistent severe disease-related pain occurs in 5-10% of patients with nonmetastatic disease (Daut and Cleeland, 1982) but the rates increase to 20-40% in patients with metastatic disease (Cleeland, 1984).

Pain varies with type of cancer. The lowest rates are reported for patients with leukemia (5%) or lymphoma (20%), higher rates (50-75%) for patients with lung, gastrointestinal or genitourinary tumors, and the highest rates (85%) for patients with cervix or primary bone tumors (Foley, 1975). It is generally estimated that about 20% of the pain is cancer-induced, about 75% is treatment-dependent, and about 5% is unrelated to the cancer or treatment (e.g., cervical or lumbar osteoarthritis, thoracic and abdominal aneurysms, and diabetic neuropathy).

PAIN SYNDROMES IN CANCER

The major mechanisms involved in causing cancer pain are invasion of pain-sensitive sites or organs by tumor mass, obstruction of vascular and lymphatic channels, compression or infiltration of nerves, necrosis, distention of a hollow viscus, tissue inflammation and edema. An important distinction usually drawn in regard to cancer pain is between primary nociceptive pain (caused by stimulation of pain receptors) and neuropathic pain (painful sensations caused by injury to peripheral or central nervous system structures) (Patt and Burton, 1999).

Cancer pain syndromes are often defined in terms of distinct etiologies and pathophysiologies. They are associated with particular pain characteristics and have important implications in regard to prognosis and treatment (Cherny and Portnoy, 1999). The two major types are acute and chronic pain syndromes. The acute pain syndromes are mostly related to diagnostic or therapeutic procedures and include the following: 1. Pain due to diagnostic interventions (e.g., bone marrow biopsy, lumbar puncture, myelography); 2. Postoperative pain; 3. Pain due to analgesic procedures (e.g., epidural injection, strontium-induced pain); 4. Pain due to therapeutic interventions (e.g., pleurodesis, nephrostomy insertion, intercostal catheter, porth-a-cath insertion); 5. Pain due to chemotherapy infusion techniques (e.g., intravenous infusion pain, hepathic artery infusion pain, intraperitoneal chemotherapy abdominal pain); 6. Pain due to chemotherapy toxicity (e.g., pain along the vein in association with dacarbazine infusion, extravasation of drugs, mucositis, taxol-induced, corticosteroid-induced, diffuse bone pain, pain due to acute tumor reaction to chemotherapy as seen in soft tissue sarcoma); 7. Pain due to radiotherapy (e.g., burns, subacute myelopathy, early-onset brachial plexopathy); 8. Pain due to immunotherapy (e.g., interferon-induced); 9. Pain due to hormonal therapy (e.g., flare phenomena in breast or prostate cancer); 10. Pain due to a variety of other causes, mainly infection (e.g., herpetic neuralgia), vascular events (e.g., superior vena cava obstruction) or supportive care (Granulocyte Colony Stimulating Factor causes low back pain, ondansetrone causes headache).

The chronic pain syndromes are mostly tumor-related and include the following: 1. Headache and facial pain (e.g., due to intracerebral tumor, leptomeningeal metastases, cranial neuralgias); 2. Somatic pain (e.g., multifocal or generalized bone pain, pelvis and hip pain, muscle pain); 3. Visceral pain (e.g., chronic intestinal obstruction, hepatic distension syndrome, adrenal pain syndrome); and 4. Neuropathic pain (e.g., cervical or brachial plexopathy, paraneoplastic peripheral neuropathy, nerve tumors).

However, some chronic pain syndromes are associated with cancer treatments, due mainly to: 1. Radiation (e.g., plexopathies, burning perineum syndrome, soft tissue fibrosis); 2. Surgery (e.g., phantom pain syndromes, postradical neck dissection pain); 3. Chemotherapy (e.g., chronic peripheral neuropathy, plexopathy due to intra-arterial infusion); and 4. Hormonal therapy (e.g., gynecomastia in prostate cancer).

EFFECTS OF CANCER PAIN

Following Cecily Saunders (1967), the pain of cancer patients is often referred to as "total pain" because of its all-encompassing nature and multi-dimensional effects, especially if it is not totally relieved by analgesics (Hanks, 1991). Pain has physical, emotional, cognitive and behavioral effects. It interferes with the ability to eat, to sleep, to think, to function physically, or to interact with others (Cleeland et al., 1996; Ferrel, 1995; Feuz and Rapin, 1994). Further, it is correlated with fatigue (Burrows et al., 1998), intensifies psychological distress and mood disturbance, enhances the sense of vulnerability and loss of control and increases thinking about catastrophic outcomes (Ferrel, 1995). Hence, pain may seriously reduce the patient's quality of life (Padilla et al., 1990).

The effects of cancer pain may be detected in many domains of the patient's life, primarily the physical, emotional, cognitive, interpersonal and behavioral. By reducing the sense of physical strength and limiting the number, nature and duration of motor or motor-dependent activities, the pain may appreciably lower physical well-being. In the cognitive domain it affects adversely functions, such as attention, memory, concentration, learning, interest and curiosity, decision making and problem solving, all of which are involved in a broad array of activities. In the emotional sphere, there are two major trends of effects. On the one hand, pain may promote negative emotions, mainly anxiety, fear, depression, and anger, which may be manifested in different degrees (e.g., the range for anger runs from slight irritability to explosive attacks of rage). On the other hand, pain may depress positive emotions, mainly affection, joy, pleasure and hope. In the interpersonal domain, major adverse effects of the pain were detected in regard to keeping up social relations, communicating with others, and being interested in others. Social interactions may become gradually focused on getting and maintaining social support and other needed help from others. In the general behavioral field, pain may reduce or practically eliminate motivation for a great number of activities, with a resultant narrowing down of the behavioral range. The effects of pain in the different domains may interact and enhance one another. Thus, limiting the range of physical activities may increase frustration, which could be promote manifestations of anger or depression, which in turn may cause problems in the interpersonal field, and so on (Rummans et al., 1998; Ward et al., 1998).

However, the effects of pain are not necessarily all negative. The need to reduce activities may bring about focusing on a particularly creative or satisfying activity that the individual has long desired to do or a newly discovered one; it may deepen relations with beloved ones; it may enhance joy and love; it may lead to the promotion or discovery of spiritual needs and of new meanings of life and existence. This does not mean in any way that efforts to control pain are to be limited, but that in case these efforts are not completely successful at least some patients may still find ways to maintain a certain tolerable or even good level of quality of life.

PAIN AND SUFFERING

Pain in cancer often interacts with the other more general sources of suffering in cancer. The most common identified factors of distress are physical symptoms in addition to pain (e.g., fatigue, drowsiness, nausea, cough, inability to sleep), distress related to health-care services (e.g., problems of communication, expenses, unavailability, inefficiency), problems with the family (e.g., conflicts, lack of empathy, inability to help beloved ones), and mainly psychological and existential concerns. Changes in life-style, activities, body image, professional and role functioning, social relations, cognitive performance and emotional state impair the patient's sense of identity, independence, control over oneself and one's life and feeling of personal integrity. Fear of death, of the void, of the unknown and even of pain and suffering may combine with regret about past mistakes, with despair because of unfulfilled aspirations and sometimes with religious concerns too. Thus, the total situation includes components of distress which constitute a breeding ground for existential suffering (Fishman, 1992; Strang, 1997). Under these circumstances the physical and spiritual or psychological pain tend to coalesce, so that they become symbolically integrated with each other in a way that affects both the patient's experience of the situation and the results of treatment. Some patients may not always be aware whether their pain is physical or psychological. When their physical pain has been controlled to some extent, their suffering may still persist. Other patients may stick to the physical pain in order to avoid the psychological pain. The salient connotations of suffering in the case of cancer pain are one reason why cancer pain has often been regarded as different from other types of pain (Turk and Fernandez, 1990). However it may be, the potential integration of pain with suffering highlights the importance of targeting the alleviation of suffering as an integral aspect of the treatment of pain in cancer (Cherny, 2000).

PAIN AND PSYCHIATRIC SYMPTOMS

Pain affects the frequency of psychiatric symptoms in cancer patients. Patients with pain had more psychiatric symptoms than those without pain, especially adjustment disorder with depressed or anxious mood (69%) and major depression (15%). In addition, pain may bring about distortions in psychological and personality factors, while relief of pain is often attended by decrease or even disappearance of psychiatric disorders (Cleeland and Tearman 1986). On the other hand, some of the often used analgesics may also be responsible for psychiatric disorders. ,F for example, high doses of dexamethasone that are sometimes used in epidural spinal cord compression may cause major depression, or sometimes steroid psychosis,; opioids (e.g., morphine sulfate, oxycodone) that are used in advanced disease may cause confusional states (Breitbart and Payne, 2000).

PAIN AND SUICIDE

Although the rate of suicide in cancer patients is on the whole low, this population of patients is at increased risk (Breitbart, 1987).aUncontrolled pain has often been mentioned as a major risk factor for suicide by cancer patients (Massie, Gagnon and Holland, 1994). However, the evidence shows that when pain is uncontrolled, cancer patients indeed tend to have increased suicidal ideation, probably because unrelieved pain impairs their sense of control and increases their fear of further suffering. But thoughts about suicide do not necessarily represent an intent to actually commit suicide. Suicide risk increases due to factors other than the pain itself, such as mood disturbance, delirium, loss of hope and of control (Breitbart and Payne, 2000).

PAIN AND EUTHANASIA

In the heated discussions on the legal, ethical and public aspects of euthanasia and physician-assisted suicide, pain is often cited as a major motivation, justification or opposing argument for euthanasia. It is assumed (by health professionals and the public) that patients request hastened death because they are in pain or want to avoid pain (Foley, 1995). Further, the supporters of euthanasia emphasize that every individual should be given the option of avoiding pain and suffering through hastened death (Kaplan and Bratman, 1999-2000). In contrast, the opponents of euthanasia claim that before proceeding with euthanasia other simpler and available procedures for attaining pain relief are to be offered and applied (Cherny, 1996; Valverius, Nilstun and Nilsson, 2000). Empirical studies show that the relation of pain to desire for death is anything but simple and straightforward. Indeed, some studies indicate that pain increases desire for assisted suicide, so that the stronger the pain, the more intense the desire (Chochinov, Wilson, Enns et al., 1995; Rosenfeld, Galieta, Breitbart et al., 1998). Yet, the majority of studies show that pain is mostly not a first-order reason for the patient's interest in assisted suicide. Patients mention pain as a reason less often than, but appears after other reasons, such as fear of becoming a burden on one's family or of losing dignity and lack of social support (Back, Wallace, Starks and Pearlman, 1996). Further, pain does not figure alone as the reason for interest in assisted suicide, but as part of a series of physical factors (e.g., physical symptoms, disease status) (Massie, Gagnon and Holland, 1994). In general, the desire for hastened death is more a function of psychological and psychiatric factors, such as depression than of pain and physical problems (Cherny, 1996).

However, the desire for hastened death is an issue that deserves consideration apart from the operational implication of aiding the patient to die. The desire is unstable (Chochinov, Tataryn, Clinch and Dudgeon, 1999), it increases when the patient is lonely and depressed (Rosenfeld, 2000), it decreases after getting social support and exposure to empathic listening (Hornik, 1998; Severson, 1997) and it does not seem to be a function of current pain (Emanuel, Fairclough, Daniels and Clarridge, 1996; Sullivan, Rapp, Fitzgibbon and Chapman, 1997). It is also possible that considering the option of euthanasia expresses the patient's need to gain a modicum of control in a situation marked by extreme helplessness.

These observations suggest that the desire for hastened death may be a cry for help, when basic psychological and physical needs are unmet. Taking care of these needs may well result in a significant decrease in the patient's interest in assisted suicide.

EFFECTS OF PSYCHOLOGICAL FACTORS ON PAIN

Psychological factors were found to affect the degree of pain. Patients with higher levels of anxiety and depression tend to report pain more often than patients low in anxiety and depression (Bond and Pearson, 1969; McKegney, Bailey and Yates, 1981; Spiegel and Bloom, 1983). Further, patients who observe in their daily activities marked impairment are apt to report increased pain intensity (Payne, 1995). Patients diagnosed as having psychological impairment have more pain in the late stages of cancer (McKegney et al., 1981; Bond et al., 1969). If patients have maladaptive coping strategies, lower levels of self-efficacy and distress due to the disease or treatment, they are liable to have higher pain intensity in later stages of the disease (Syrjala and Chapko, 1995). The meaning assigned to the pain is an important factor in accounting for pain intensity and for the effects of pain on quality of life. Women with metastatic breast cancer report more intense pain if they interpret it as a sign of the spread of their disease than if they believe it is due to another causeanother cause (Spiegel and Bloom, 1983). Similarly, if the patients believe that a new pain is related to their disease it interferes more with their pleasure and daily life than if they assume it is due to another cause unrelated (Daut and Cleeland, 1982).

UNDERTREATMENT OF PAIN IN CANCER

Despite the availability of medical and psychological treatment options, cancer pain seems still to be undertreated (Portenoy 1999) world-wide (e.g., Zenz, Zenz, Tryba et al., 1995). In order to reduce the magnitude of the problem, it is important to analyze some of its causes. Barriers to proper pain control in cancer may be found in patients, in doctors, in institutional organization and in interactions between these factors.

Patients tend to underreport their pain, mainly because cancer patients often consider pain as denoting spread of disease and deterioration in their health state. Likewise, prescription of morphine, which often follows complaints about pain, may indicate to the patient that the doctor may soon be unable to help him or her any more and that death is nearing. Some patients may be reluctant to take analgesics because they are afraid of becoming addicted or tolerant to the pain medications, and are worried about side effects of the drugs. Moreover, cancer patients often feel helpless and on the lookout for measures they could undertake in order to promote their state of health, especially since empowerment seems to be the politically correct thing to do. Overcoming pain appears to be something patients can do for themselves, without depending on anyone. Finally, patients may underreport pain because they may feel that doctors are not that keen to get the information. Hence, they fear that reporting pain may be considered as indicating that one is not not being a "good" patient, and may distract the physicians from the main task of treating the underlying disease.

Some physicians tend to undertreat pain when the patient is over 70 years old, a woman, or has good functional status, or when they do not quite accept the patient's estimate of the pain as highly severe or do not ascribe it to the cancer (Cleeland, Gonin, Hatfield et al., 1994). These factors gain in importance in view of the two following findings. First, the discrepancy between patients' and clinicians' estimates of pain increases when pain severity is high (Grossman, Sheidler, Sweden et al., 1991). Second, when pain persists or does not respond sufficiently to analgesics, it is often ascribed to psychological factors rather than to medical ones (Foley, 1985; Twycross and Lack, 1983). Further attitudes of doctors contributing to undertreatment of pain are considering pain control as difficult, often unsuccessful and indicative of failure of medical attempts to cure the patient. Moreover, they may not always be adequately informed about new pharmacologic or surgical options for treating pain and how to integrate psychotropic drugs and psychological measures in the comprehensive treatment of pain (Sampson, 1994). Physicians may be concerned about minimizing addiction and substance abuse as well as minimizing side effects of the drugs, such as possible respiratory depression in advanced patients (Vainio, 1989). However, studies showed that increased need for analgesics results mostly from disease progression or increased tolerance, which is distinct from addiction. If addiction occurs then it is mostly in individuals with drug abuse prior to the onset of cancer. Further, in terminal patients with respiratory failure, administering subcutaneous morphine actually improved dyspnea (Bruera, MacMillan, Pither et al., 1990).

Improving patient education, physicians' attitudes, and doctor-patient communication are often mentioned as prerequisites for raising pain treatment in cancer to the optimal level (Von Roenn et al., 1993).

BASIC PRINCIPLES OF THE PHARMACOLOGIC TREATMENT OF PAIN IN CANCER PATIENTS

WHO Analgesic Ladder. Drug therapy is the cornerstone of the treatment of cancer pain. Pharmacologic therapy follows basically the World Health Organization guidelines which define a three-step ladder for analgesic pain management (Ventafridda, Caraceni and Gamba, 1990). Three main principles inspire this approach. First, the goal is freedom from pain. Second, the selection of analgesics is to proceed in line with the severity of pain. Third, pain management is to be tailored to the needs of the patient, selecting on each step of the ladder the drug which best fits the individual's characteristics. Accordingly, on each level the simplest dosage schedules and least invasive pain control modalities are used first. If pain persists, substitution of drugs within the same category is attempted or dose and potency of the drug are increased before proceeding to the next step. The dosage is scheduled on a regular basis in order to maintain continuously the level of drug that helps prevent recurrence of pain. On each level, drugs of the preceding level may be added, as well as adjuvant drugs.

Step 1: Mild to moderate pain: For pain at this intensity level nonopioid analgesics (NSAIDs e.g., cox-2 inhibitors, naproxene, aspirin, ibuprofen) and paracetamol, dypirone, propoxyphene and acetaminophen (it resembles NSAIDs in analgesic potency but lacks peripheral anti-inflammatory activity) are recommended. The major underlying mechanism consists in bringing about a reduction of prostaglandins in the tissues. Their main characteristics are that they have a ceiling effect for analgesia, do not produce tolerance or dependence, are administered through oral tablets, capsules or liquid, have antipyretic effects and their major side effects include gastrointestinal reactions (from mild discomfort to gastric ulceration), hepatic dysfunction, renal failure and bleeding.

Step 2: Mild to moderate pain (which has not been or could not be controlled by NSAIDs): The recommendation focuses on so-called weak opioids (e.g., oxycodone, hydrocodone, codeine) or opioid-like agents (tramadol) which may be combined with NSAIDs. Tramadol is a pain reliever which affects chemicals and receptors in the body that are associated with pain. Tramadol is used to relieve moderate to moderately severe pain. It differs from other opioids by combining a weak opioid and a monoaminergic mode of action. It is effective in different types of moderate-to-severe pain, including neuropathic pain. Moreover, as the mode of action of tramadol does not overlap with that of NSAIDs, it is a useful agent to be combined with these drugs. Tramadol induces fewer opioid adverse reactions for a given level of analgesia compared with traditional opioids. Common adverse reactions of tramadol such as nausea and dizziness, which usually occur only at the beginning of therapy and attenuate over time, can be further minimized by up-titrating the drug over several days.

Step 3: Moderate to severe pain: For pain at this intensity level opioids, usually of the "strong" type are recommended.

Opioids analgesics: Types. Opioids are classified, on the basis of their affinity to opioid receptors, into three classes: (a) full morphine-like agonists, whose effectiveness with increasing doses is not limited by a "ceiling", and they do not antagonize the effect of other full agonists ingested simultaneously (e.g., morphine, methadone, levorphanol, fentanyl); (b) partial agonists, which are less effective at the opioid receptor and are subject to a "ceiling" effect (e.g., buprenorphine), and (c) mixed agonist-antagonists, which are neutral or block at one type of opioid receptor while activating another opioid receptor (e.g., pentazocine, butorphanol, nalbuphine). Their analgesic effectiveness is limited by a dose-dependent "ceiling" effect. They can reverse opioid effects and precipitate withdrawal symptoms in patients who are opioid dependent or tolerant).

Opioids: Tolerance, dependence and addiction: The three mentioned phenomena are relevant in regard to opioids and are often confused with one another. Tolerance indicates a markedly diminished analgesic effect with continued use of a drug or the need for greatly increased amounts of the drug in order to maintain a given or desired effect of analgesia over time. Physical dependence is characterized by the onset of withdrawal symptoms if the opioid is suddenly stopped or an opioid antagonist is administered. Addiction (or psychological dependence) denotes a compulsive behavior of drug abuse, manifested in a craving for the drug, in undertaking extraordinary efforts to get and use it for goals other than pain relief, and in failure to cut down or control its use despite awareness that its continued use causes physical or psychological problems. Tolerance and physical dependence often occur together but are not necessarily accompanied by addiction. The former two are rather frequent in cancer patients, whereas addiction is rare and almost never occurs in patients without a previous history of drug abuse (Kanner and Foley, 1981).

Opioids: Half-life, onset and duration of analgesia. The opioids vary in their plasma half life, and analgesic onset and duration. Opioid analgesics with long half-lives (15-30 hours, e.g. methadone, levorphanol) require about 5 days to attain a steady state, but tend to accumulate with early initial dosing, so that they bring about delayed toxicity effects. Morphine and oxycodone have a much shorter half-life (2-3 hours). Further, Oopioids vary greatly in the duration of analgesia they provide. For example, immediate-release preparations of morphine or oxycodone often provide only 3 hours of analgesia so that they need to be administered on a round-the-clock basis, in contrast to levorphanol or methadone which may provide up to 6 hours of relief, or longer-lasting sustained release oral preparations (of morphine, e.g., Oramorph SR sustained release or of oxycontin) which provide relief for 8-12 hours, or transdermal fentanyl patches which may act for 48 to 72 hours. However, the longer-lasting preparations may have a delayed analgesic onset (e.g., fentanyl patch 12-18 hours) and may need to be complemented by other drugs for acute or breakthrough pain. Facts of this kind may significantly affect the patients' quality of life. In selecting drugs for pain-control, it is advisable to take into account psychological effects in addition to medical and pain-dependent considerations. Thus, longer-lasting drugs may be more adequate for patients who want to be freed from thoughts about pain control, whereas drugs that need to be administered round-the-clock may be more adequate for patients whose well-being depends on being constantly "in control".

Opioid: Routes of administration. There are various routes of administering opioid analgesics that vary also in their quality of life effects. Oral administration is usually preferred because of its convenience and low cost. The rectal route is safe and inexpensive, suitable for patients who have nausea or vomiting, but inappropriate for those with diarrhea, rectal lesions, mucositis, trombocytopenia or neutropenia. The transdermal route is appropriate for stable pain when no rapid dose titration is necessary. Intravenous administration provides the most rapid onset of analgesia but it is of shorter duration than with other routes. Hence, when continuous pain-control is required, continuous intravenous access or subcutaneous infusion may be used. Patient-controlled analgesia (PCA) helps the patient maintain control by matching drug delivery to analgesic needs, orally or by a portable pump. Intraspinal drug administration is an invasive route with several disadvantages (e.g., mechanical problems, infection potential) but provides profound analgesia without motor, sensory or sympathetic blockade in cases of intractable pain especially in the lower body part.

Opioids: Side effects: Side effects are a major disadvantage of opioids. Common side-effects include constipation, nausea and vomiting, respiratory depression or a subacute overdose manifested as slowly progressive somnolence and respiratory depression, as well as dry mouth, urinary retention, pruritus, myoclonus and sleep disturbances. Also psychological side-effects are frequent, mainly sedation, mental clouding, and delirium, often accompanied by attentional deficits, disorientation, and perceptual disturbances, such as illusions and visual hallucinations. Some of the side effects become weaker or disappear with continued use of the drug, and some can be controlled by the use of adjuvant agents and other drugs.

Adjuvant drugs. The need to supplement the opioid treatment of pain by other drugs may arise because of unpleasant or dangerous side-effects and increased tolerance, or because the pain is only semi-responsive to opioids (e.g., bone metastasis, nerve compression), not responsive to opioids (e.g., muscle spasm), or can be treated more specifically (e.g., functional gastrointestinal pains). Thus, in the treatment of cancer pain adjuvant drugs are often used, during all stages of the analgesic ladder, in order to enhance the analgesic effect of opioids, treat concurrent symptoms that may exacerbate pain, or provide independent analgesia for particular kinds of pain. The major kinds of adjuvant drugs are (Breitbart adand Payne, 2000):

a) *Corticosteroids:* They may contribute to controlling pain directly or indirectly, by affecting neuropathic pain or pain resulting from inflammatory processes, or elevated intracranial pressure and epidural spinal cord compression; by reducing cerebral and spinal cord edema; by improving appetite and combating nausea; and by elevating mood. The major side effects are psychiatric, gastrointestinal and immunosuppressive.

b) *Anticonvulsants:* They are used mainly for neuropathic pain characterized by continuous or lancinating dystenias.

c) *Oral local anesthetics:* They are used mainly for neuropathic pain with dystenias, especially when antidepressants are not well tolerated or anticonvulsants are ineffective.

d) *Neuroleptics:* They are used mainly for treating chronic pain syndromes, especially in cases suffering from dose-limiting side effects of other drugs.

e) *Bisphosphonates:* They are used mainly for preventing pathologic fractures and for treating bone pain.

f) *Antidepressants:* They were found to have an analgesic effect in different types of pain, chronic neuropathic and nonneuropathic pain syndromes, probably through both their serotonergic and noradrenergic properties, as well as their antihistaminic and direct neuronal effects. They are used as adjuvant analgesics most often for potentiating the analgesic effects of opioids, and thus enabling even a reduction in their use. The tricyclic antidepressants (e.g., amitriptyline) are the most widely studied and used antidepressants for analgesia, but the use of heterocyclic and noncyclic antidepressants as well as of fluoxetine is increasing. The effect is often biphasic with peaks after a few days or hours and after 2-4 weeks.

g) *Psychostimulants:* One main use of psychostimulants (e.g., dextroamphetamine, modafinil) is as potent adjuvant analgesics alone but mainly in combination with opioids. A second important effect they have is to diminish sedation side-effects of narcotic analgesics, thereby improving, for example, cognitive functioning of patients getting continuous infusion of opioids. In addition, they stimulate appetite, decrease fatigue and elevate the patient's overall sense of well-being. Modafinil has been used in patients with non-malignant pain syndromes, and is reported to improve opioid-induced sedation. There have been reports on the use of modafinil for the treatment of fatigue in various neurological syndromes (Webster, 2003). Its role in cancer patients treated by narcotics needs to be elucidated.

h) *Chemotherapy:* cChemotherapeutic agents are widely and commonly used in patients with metastatic cancer in order to palliate cancer-related symptoms. Cancer- related pain might result from the primary tumor (eg: e.g., lung cancer involving the pleura and chest wall) or from organ involvement by metastases (e.g., bone and liver metastases from lung cancer). The decision of which chemotherapy should be used for this purpose in a particular patient is based primarily on the chemosensitivity of the tumor and on the tolerability of the patient to possible side effects. Chemotherapy may be combined with radiation therapy, with analgesic therapy or with any modality used for pain control.

NON-PHARMACOLOGIC TREATMENT OF PAIN IN CANCER PATIENTS

Non-pharmacologic therapies include a variety of more and less invasive approaches, which may be used, each in line with its potentials and risks, for different reasons, such as psychological resistance of the patient to opioids, patients' desire to apply all available means or specific therapies, failure to attain adequate pain control by means of drugs, and inability to stabilize a satisfactory balance between analgesia and side effects of opioids. The more aggressive or destructive procedures (see d. and e. below), such as coeliac plexus blocks or percutaneous cordotomy, have been promoted by some clinicians because despite their destructiveness, their effect is localized, in contrast to opioids which affect the whole body and the whole person with much more adverse impact on quality of life (Lipton, 1989). The major non-pharmacologic approaches are the following:

(a) *Radiation therapy*: Local or hemi-body radiation may enhance the effectiveness of analgesic drugs and other noninvasive therapies by affecting directly the cause of pain (viz. by reducing tumor bulk), while minimizing adverse effects on normal cells and repair of damaged tissue.

An example for palliative radiation therapy is spinal cord compression unamenable by surgery or chemotherapy (Kovner, 1999,; Merimsky, 2004a)

(b) *Surgery*: Curative excision or palliative debulking of a tumor may reduce pain directly or relieve symptoms of compression or obstruction. It is especially true in cases of spinal cord compression, in which laminectomy, vertebrectomy, tumor debulking, and spine stabilization are used for pain alleviation together with relief of cord compression and restoration of neurological functions. A second example of palliative surgery is major amputations such as forequarter amputation or hemipelvectomy applied in cases of soft tissue and bone sarcomas that are uncontrolled by any other treatment modality. (Merimsky, 1997,; Merimsky, 2001,; Merimsky, 2004b) . Less extensive surgery, viz. surgical internal fixation of fractures and impending fractures of long bones with lytic lesions is applied in cases with metastatic renal cell carcinoma (Kollender, 2000,; Bickels, 2002).

(c) *Local anesthetic*: Intractable localized or regional pain may be handled by the relatively brief application of an intra-axial infusion with opioids and/or local anesthetics. Pain relief is temporary but sympathetic sensation and function are preserved while supraspinal side-effects are prevented.

(d) *Sympathetic blocks*: Nerve blocks of a permanent nature are attained by using neurolytic agents in regard to leading neural pathways or ganglions, for example, ganglion impar, superior hypogastric, or celiac plexus block. A study with pancreatic cancer patients showed that celiac plexus block prevented a marked decrease in the patients' quality of life by providing a long-lasting analgesic effect, as well as reducing morphine consumption and its side-effects (Kawamata, Ishitani and Ishikawa, 1996).

(e) *Nerve blocks by surgical means*: Surgical neurolysis is possible at every level of the neuraxis (e.g., face-unilateral, chest wall, upper or lower abdomen), and is mostly attended by neurologic complications. The most frequent procedure is cordotomy that consists in blocking the spino-thalamic pathway for pain relief on the opposite body side.

(f) *Physical interventions*: Physical therapies are used primarily for the generalized weakness and pains associated with cancer diagnosis and therapy. They include the following techniques: 1. cutaneous stimulation, for example, by applying heat (e.g., hot pack, heating pad, diathermy), cold (e.g., flexible ice pack), massage, pressure or vibration to the aching body area (counterindicated on irradiated skin); 2. Exercise, useful for subacute and chronic pain due to its beneficial effects on weak muscles, stiff joints, impaired coordination and balance (counterindicated when bone fractures are likely); 3. Repositioning, designed to prevent or alleviate pain in the immobilized patient; 4. Immobilizing, by means of adjustable elastic or thermoplastic braces, designed to reduce breakthrough pain induced by movement of the spine or a limb or to stabilize fractures and otherwise compromised limbs or joints; 5. Counterstimulation, by means of transcutaneous electrical nerve stimulation (TENS), applied to large myelinated peripheral nerve fibers in order to inhibit pain transmission, or by means of acupuncture.

PSYCHOLOGICALLY-BASED TREATMENTS OF PAIN IN CANCER PATIENTS

There is an important role for psychological treatments of pain in regard to cancer pain, both because of their potential effect on the physical pain and because of the psychological effects and connotations of suffering that accompany cancer pain.

The psychological treatments of pain in general apply also in the case of this population of patients, but they need to be selected and adapted for the special needs and characteristics of cancer patients. First, because the pain is often of at least moderate intensity and continuous, it is recommended that the treatments do not require a too long period of preparation before they have a real effect on pain alleviation. Second, in view of the reduction in the sense of control of many patients, it is desirable to select treatments that enable the patients to feel that they have some kind of control over the pain and themselves. Third, because of the tendency of pain in cancer to affect a variety of domains, the selected treatments should address different components of pain and of its impact.

Psychological treatments of pain may be grouped into four groupskinds: sensory, affective, cognitive or behavioral (see chapter 19, this book). In view of the above considerations, the most highly recommended treatments for cancer pain are the following: (a) Treatments focused on the sensory component: guided imagery, suggestion and autosuggestion, relaxation and meditation, distraction and displacement, music therapy and hypnosis; (b) Treatments focused on the affective component: Supportive therapies, meaning-based control of negative emotions, a modified version of dynamic psychotherapy, and art therapy; (c) Treatments focused on the cognitive component: educational-didactive information based therapy, cognitive-attitudes based therapy, and cognitive coping; and (d) Treatments focused on the behavioral component: family therapy and cognitive-orientation therapy. The less recommended treatments are biofeedback, (because of limitations in generalizing the technique beyond the training period, (Fotopoulos, Graham and Cook, 1979), dynamic psychotherapy, (because of the length of time before it takes effect;), and conditioning, environmental and behavioral therapies, (because of the length of preparatory training they require, and their reduced reliance on the patient's active control).

In this context we will review briefly the major components of the recommended techniques (see chapters 19 and 21 for more extensive descriptions). The major elements in the sensory-focused therapies are the active use of fantasy and of distraction in order to control pain. Thus, the patient may be taught and encouraged to construct fantasy images transforming the nature, intensity, location, duration and context of the sensation of pain, relying mainly on suggestion or imagery in a relaxed state or deeper hypnotic state (Fishman, 1990; Levitan, 1992). Relaxation techniques aim at reducing physiological and psychological arousal by images, by muscular acts or positions or by meditative means. They help to alleviate pain intensity directly or by serving as context for further imagery-based techniques. Conjointedly, distraction by means of fantasy, cognitions or actions may be practiced (e.g., by focusing on some pleasant image, a thought, a problem, or engaging in doing something, such as counting, or praying). A technique like music therapy which focuses on listening to music may be used primarily as an aid to constructing pain-controlling images or for distraction or both.

The major elements in the affective-focused therapies are cathartic relief and reduction of negative emotions, mainly anxiety, fear, depression, despair, frustration, anger and distress accompanying the cancer pain. The supportive, psychotherapeutic and art therapies all provide frameworks for relief through expressing one's distress and sharing it, as well as getting encouragement from others. Learning specific means for overcoming negative emotions is served in particular by the meaning-based technique, psychotherapy and art therapy. The meaning-based therapy consists in learning to process inputs in terms of processes enabling anxiety control (e.g., action) and unlearning to process them in terms of processes enhancing anxiety (e.g., metaphors, emotional connotations). Psychotherapy and art therapy, when adequately structured, enable the patient to get insight into psychological tendencies, partly nonunconscious, that enhance pain and suffering (e.g., considering the pain as punishment for one's "sins") and acquire approaches that enable controlling pain (e.g., focusing on fulfilling one's long-standing wishes).

The cognitive-focused therapies provide the patient with an array of cognitions that may help in pain control. These include informations about the cause and functioning of pain and medical means for controlling it (e.g., drugs),; attitudes and beliefs in regard to pain that enable reducing its harmful effects (e.g., 'enhanced pain does not necessarily indicate disease progression;' or ' it is possible to function and enjoy life despite the pain'),; a variety of cognitive coping means that promote pain control (e.g., self-statements emphasizing pain as a challenge); and the avoidance of coping mechanisms that maintain or increase pain (e.g., catastrophizing, over-dramatizing the pain, self-pity).

The behavior-focused therapies target reducing or preventing the development of behaviors that maintain the pain and broaden its impact. The most useful means in this context are control by means of family therapy, and by increasing cognitive support for cognitions that combat pain (viz. cognitive-orientation therapy).

In sum, best effects of psychological therapies are attained by enabling each patient to use a variety of means. The advantages of this approach are first, each patient will be able to find out which means are best suited to his or her tendencies and goals; second, the chances are increased that the different components of pain – sensory, affective, cognitive and behavioral – will be addressed; and third, the broad range of alternative therapies will insure that when one or another loses its effectiveness temporarily or indefinitely other techniques may be applied for pain control.

GENERAL CONCLUSIONS

Cancer pain is one of the more complex and negative facets of malignancy. Its prevalence, intensity, duration and connotations are complicating factors that have led many to doubt whether its management can be handled by the same means as other kinds of pain. In contrast to these views, the approach that has come to dominate the field in recent years is based on the assumption that the principles of general pain management apply in this case too with certain adjustments and adaptations.

First, pain should be identified and recognized as an important and basic aspect of the disease. Awareness of this fact on the part of health professionals and of patients would facilitate communication about pain, consulting about treatments, and readiness of physicians to treat pain as well as readiness of patients to cooperate in pain treatments even if these treatments are merely "palliative" rather than curative.

Second, an attempt is to be made to consider cancer pain in a matter-of-fact manner, dissociated as much as possible from connotations of suffering and death that tend to be evoked in the case of malignancies. Weeding out the extra baggage of significations that serve to enhance the patient's load of distress may promote circumscribing the problem and rendering it more manageable and treatable.

Third, psychological approaches to the treatment of pain are to be considered as an integral component of the treatment of cancer pain on all levels rather than one among several available approaches designed to be applied when one or another of the applied treatments has failed or has not functioned up to the expected level. Hence, psychological pain treatments do not constitute one level in the WHO ladder but are to be considered as part of each step on the ladder, possibly as a support railing for climbing up or down the ladder. The message beyond the metaphor is that psychological pain treatments should accompany all other pain treatments in cancer pain, enhancing their effect and thus in the very least slowing down progression up the ladder.

REFERENCES

Back, A. L., Wallace, J. I., Starks, H. E. and Pearlman, R. A. (1996). Physician-assisted suicide and euthanasia in Washington State. Patient requests and physician responses. *JAMA, 275,* 919-925.

Bickels, L., and Merimsky, O. (2002). Bone metastases of renal cell carcinoma: the role of surgery. *Israel Medical Association Journal,* 4, 376-378.

Bond, M. R., and Pearson, I. B. (1969). Psychological aspects of pain women with advanced cancer of the cervix. *Journal of Psychosomatic Research,* 13, 13-19.

Bonica, J. J. (1987). Cancer pain. In J. J. Bonica (Ed.), *The management of pain,* Vol. 1 (2nd ed.) (pp. 400-460). Philadelphia: Lea and Febiger.

Bonica, J. J., and Ekstrom, J. L. (1990). Systemic opioids for the management of cancer pain: An updated review. *Advanced Pain Research and Therapy, 14,* 425-446.

Breitbart, W. (1987). Suicide in cancer patients. *Oncology, 1,* 49-53

Breitbart, W., Passik, S. D., and Rosenfeld, B. D. (1999) Cancer, mind and spirit. In P. D. Wall and R. Melzack (Eds.), *Textbook of pain* (4th ed.) (pp. 1065-1112). Edinburgh: Churchill Livingstone.

Breitbart, W., and Payne, D. (2000). Psychiatric aspects of pain management in patients with advanced cancer and AIDS. In H. Chochinov and W. Breitbart Eds.*), Handbook of psychiatry in palliative medicine* (pp. 131-159). New York: Oxford University Press. Bruera, E., MacMillan, K., Pither, J., and MacDonald, R. M. (1990). Effects of morphine on the dyspnea of terminal cancer patients. *Journal of Pain and Symptom Management,* 5,341-344.

Burrows, M., Dibble, S. L., and Miaskowski, C. (1998). Differences in outcomes among patients experiencing different types of cancer-related pain. *Oncological Nursing Forum, 25,* 735-741.

Cherny, N. I. (1996). The problem of inadequately relieved suffering. *Journal of Social Issues, 52,* 13-30.

Cherny, N. I. (2000). The treatment of suffering in patients with advanced cancer. In H. Chochinov and W. Breitbart Eds.), *Handbook of psychiatry in palliative medicine* (pp. 375-396). New York: Oxford University Press.

Cherny, N. I., and Portenoy, R. K. (1999). Cancer pain: Principles of assessment and syndromes. In P. D. Wall and R. Melzack (Eds.), *Textbook of pain* (4th ed.) (pp. 1017-1064).Edinburgh: Churchill Livingstone.

Chochinov, H. M., Wilson, K. G., Enns, M., Mowchun, N., Lander, S., Levitt, M. and Clinch, J. J. (1995). Desire for death in the terminally ill. *American Journal of Psychiatry, 152,* 1185-1191.

Chochinov, H. M., Tataryn, D., Clinch, J. J., and Dudgeon, D.(1999). Will to live in the terminally ill. *Lancet, 354 (9181),* 816-819.

Cleeland, C. S. (1984). The impact of pain on the patient with cancer. *Cancer, 58,* 2635-2641.

Cleeland, C. S., Gonin, R., Hatfield, A. K., et al. (1994). Pain and its treatment in outpatients with metastatic cancer: the Eastern Cooperative Oncology group's outpatient study. *New England Journal of Medicine, 330,* 592-596.

Cleeland, C. S., and Tearman, B. H. (1986). Behavioral control of cancer pain. In D. Holzman and D. Turk (Eds.), *Pain management* (pp. 193-212). New York: Pergamon.

Cleeland, C. S., Nakamura, Y., Howland, E. W., Morgan, N. R., Edwards, K. R., and Bakonja, M. (1996). Effects of oral morphine on cold pessor tolerance time and neuropsychological performance. *Neuropsychopharmacology, 15,* 252-262.

Daut, R. L., and Cleeland, C. S. (1982). The prevalence and severity of pain in cancer. *Cancer, 50,* 1913-1918.

Emanuel, E. J., Fairclough, C. L., Daniels, E. R. and Clarridge, B. R. (1996). Euthanasia and physician-assisted suicide: attitudes and experiences of oncology patients, oncologists and the public. *Lancet, 347, 1805*-1810.

Ferrel, B. R. (1995). The impact of pain on quality of life: A decade of research. *Nursing Clinics of North America, 30,* 609-624.

Feuz, A., and Rapin, C. H. (1994). An observational study of the role of pain control and food adaptation of elderly patients with terminal cancer. *Journal of the American Dietetic Association, 94,* 767-770.

Fishman, B. (1990). The treatment of suffering in patients with cancer pain. In K. Foley, J. Bonica and V.Ventafridda (Eds.), *Advances in Pain Research and Therapy*, Vol. 16 (pp.301-316). New York: Raven Press.

Fishman, B. (1992). The cognitive behavioral persspective on pain management in terminal illness. *Hospice Journal, 8,* 73-88.

Foley, K. M. (1975). Pain syndromes in patients with cancer. In J. J. Bonica, V. Ventafriddi, R. B. Fink, L. E. Jones, and Loeser, J. D. (Eds.), *Advances in pain research and therapy*, Vol. 2 (pp. 59-75). New York: Raven Press.

Foley, K. M. (1995). Pain, physician-assisted suicide and euthanasia. *Pain Forum, 4,* 163-178.

Fotopoulos, S. S., Graham, C., and Cook, M. R. (1979). Psychophysiologic control of cancer pain. In J. J. Bonica and V. Ventafridda (Eds.) *Advances in Pain Research and Therapy*, Vol. 2 (pp. 231-244). New York: Raven Press.

Grossman, S. A., Sheidler, V. R., Sweden, K., Mucenski, J., and Piantadosi, S. (1991). Correlations of patient and caregiver ratings of cancer pain. *Journal of Pain and Symptom Management, 6,* 53-57.

Hanks, G. W. (1991). Opioid responsive and opioid non-responsive pain in cancer. *British Medical Bulletin, 47,* 718-731.

Hornik, M. (1998). Physician-assisted suicide and euthanasia's impact on the frail elderly: A social worker's response. *Journal of Long Term Home Health Care, 17,* 34-41.

Kanner, R. M., and Foley, K. M. (1981). Patterns of narcotic use in a cancer pain clinic. *Annals of the New York Academy of Science, 362,* 161-172.

Kaplan, K. J., and Bratman, E. (1999-2000). Palliative care, assisted suicide and euthanasia: Nationwide questionnaire to Swedish physicians. *Omega: Journal of Death and Dying, 40,* 27-41.

Kawamata, M., Ishitani, K., and Ishikawa, K. et al., (1996). Comparison between celiac plexus block and morphine treatment on quality of life on patients with pancreatic cancer pain. *Pain, 64,* 597-602.

Kollender, Y., Bickels, J., Price, W. M., Kellar, K. L., Chen, J., Merimsky, O., Meller, I., and Malawer, M. M. (2000). Metastatic renal cell carcinoma of bone: indications and technique of surgical intervention. *Journal of Urology, 164*, 1505-1508.

Kovner, F., Spigel, S., Rider, I., Otremsky, I., Ron, I., Shohat, E., Rabey, J. M., Avram, J.,Merimsky, O., Wigler, N., Chaitchik, S., and Inbar, M. (1999). Radiation therapy of metastatic spinal cord compression. Multidisciplinary team diagnosis and treatment. *Journal of Neurooncology, 42,* 85-92.

Levitan, A. (1992). The use of hypnosis with cancer patients. *Psychiatry in Medicine, 10,* 119-131.

Lipton, S. (1989). Pain relief in active patients with cancer: The early use of nerve blocks improves the quality of life. *British Medical Journal, 298*, 37-38.

Massie, M., Gagnon, P., and Holland, J. (1994). Depression and suicide in patients with cancer. *Journal of Pain Symptom Management, 9*, 352-331.

McKegney, F. P., Bailey, C. R., and Yates, J. W. (1981). Prediction and management of pain in patients with advanced cancer. *General Hospital Psychiatry, 3*, 95-101.

Merimsky, O., Kollender, Y., Inbar, M., Chaitchik, S., and Meller, I. (1997). Palliative major amputation and quality of life in cancer patients. *Acta Oncologica, 36,* 151-157.

Merimsky, O., Kollender, Y., Inbar, M., Lev-Chelouche, D., Gutman, M., Issakov, J., Mazeh,D., Shabat, S., Bickels, J., and Meller, I. (2001). Is forequarter amputation justified for palliation of intractable cancer symptoms? *Oncology, 60*, 55-59.

Merimsky, O., Kollender, Y., Bokstein, F., Issakov, J., Flusser, G., Inbar, M. J., Meller, I., and Bickels, J. (2004a). Radiotherapy for spinal cord compression in patients with soft-tissue sarcoma. *International Journal of Radiation Oncology, Biology, Physics, 58*, 1468-1473.

Merimsky, O., Kollender, Y., Inbar, M., Meller, I., and Bickels, J. (2004b). Palliative treatment for advanced or metastatic osteosarcoma. *Israel Medical Association Journal, 6*, 34-38.

Padilla, G., Ferrell, B., Grant, M., and Rhiner, M. (1990). Defining the content domain of quality of life for cancer patients with pain. *Cancer Nursing, 13,* 108-115.

Patt, R. B., and Burton, A. W. (1999). Pain associated with advanced malignancy, including adjuvant analgesic drugs in cancer pain mangement. In G. M. Aronoff (Ed.), *Evaluation and treatment of chronic pain* (3rd ed.) (pp. 337-376). Baltimore, MD: Williams and Wilkins.

Payne, D. (1995). *Cognition in cancer pain.* Unpublished Dissertation.

Portenoy, R. K., Payne, D., and Jacobsen, P. (1999). Breakthrough pain: Characteristics and impact in patients with cancer pain. *Pain, 81,* 129-134.

Rosenfeld, B. (2000). Assisted suicide, depression, and the right to die. *Psychology, Public Policy, and Law, 6,* 467-488.

Rosenfeld, B., Galieta, M., Breitbart, W., and Krivo, S. (1998). Interest in physician-assisted suicide among terminally ill AIDS patients: measuring and understanding desire for death. Paper presented at Biennial Conference of the American Psychology-Law Society, Redondo Beach, Calif.

Rummans, T. A., Frost, M., Suman, V. J., Taylor, M., Novotny, P., Gendron, T.,Johnson, R., Hartmann, L., Dose, A.-M., and Evans, R. W. (1998). Quality of life and pain in patients with recurrent breast and gynecologic cancer. *Psychosomatics, 39*, 437-445

Saunders, C. M. (1967). *The management of terminal illness.* London: Hospital Medicine Publications.

Sampson, C. C. (1994). Management of cancer pain: Guideline overview. *Journal of the National Medical Association, 86*, 571-573, 634.

Severson, K. T. (1997). Dying cancer patients: Choices at the end of life. *Journal of Pain and Symptom Manangement, 14*, 94-98.

Spiegel, D., and Bloom, J. R. (1983). Pain in metastatic breast cancer. Cancer, 52, 341-345.

Strang, P. (1997). Existential consequences of unrelieved cancer pain. *Palliative Medicine, 11*, 299-305.

Sullivan, M., Rapp, S., Fitzgibbon, D. and Chapman, C. R. (1997). Pain and the choice to hasten death in patients with painful metastatic cancer. *Journal of Palliative Care, 13*, 18-28.

Syrjala, K., and Chapko, M. (1995). Evidence for a biopsychosocial model of cancer treatment-related pain. *Pain, 61*, 69-79.

Turk, D. C., and Fernandez, E. (1990). On the putative uniqueness of cancer pain: Do psychological principles apply? *Behavior Research and Therapy, 28*, 1-13.

Twycross, R. G., and Lack, S. A. (1983). *Symptom control in far advanced cancer: Pain relief.* London: Pitman Books.

Vainio, A. (1989). Practicing physicians' experiences of treating patients with cancer pain. *Acta Oncologica, 28*, 177-182.

Valverius, E., Nilstun, T. and Nilsson, B. (2000). Gender, pain and doctor involvement: High school student attitudes toward doctor-assisted suicide. *Palliative Medicine, 14*, 141-148

Ventafridda, V., Caraceni, A., and Gamba, A. (1990). Field testing of the WHO Guidelines for Cancer Pain Relief: Summary report of demonstration projects. In K. M. Foley, J. J. Bonica and V. Ventafridda (Eds.), *Proceedings of the 2nd International Congress on Pain, Vol. 16* (pp. 155-165). New York: Raven Press.

Von Roenn, J. H., Cleeland, C. S., Gonin, R., Hatfield, A. K., and Pandya, K. J. (1993). Physician attitudes and practice in cancer pain management. A survey from the Eastern Cooperative Oncology Group. *Annals of Internal Medicine, 119*, 121-126.

Ward, S. E., Carlson, D. K., Hughes, S. H., Kwekkeboom, K. L., and Donovan, H. S. (1998). The impact on quality of life of patient-related barriers to pain management. *Research in Nursing and Health, 21*, 405-413.

Webster, L., Andrews, M., and Stoddard, G. (2003). Modafinil treatment of opioid-induced sedation. *Pain Medicine, 4*, 135-40. World Health Organization (1986). *Cancer pain relief.* Geneva: Author.

Zenz, M., Zenz, T., Tryba, M., and Strumpf, M. (1995). Severe undertreatment of cancer pain: A 3-year survey of the German situation. *Journal of Pain and Symptom Management, 10*, 187-191.

Part IX:
Organization of a Pain Service

In: The Handbook of Chronic Pain
Editors: S. Kreitler, D. Beltrutti, et al., pp. 553-560

ISBN 978-1-60021-044-0
© 2007 Nova Science Publishers, Inc.

Chapter 29

Pain Treatment Facilities: Terminology and Characteristics

Diego Beltrutti, Francesco Marino, Aldo Lamberto,
Mauro Nicoscia, and Alfredo Fogliardi

ETYMOLOGY AND DEFINITION OF TERMS

Originating from the Greek word for pain, *algos*, clinics for pain diagnosis and treatment have come to be called centers of "algology". However, this term may cause confusion, since the branch of biology that studies algae is also known as algology, and it is only recently that Webster's dictionary has incorporated a definition of algology that refers to the study of pain. Some specialists in Europe have suggested that the term "antalgology" be used to define the science of evaluating and treating persistent pain, and "antalgic centers" be used to define those places where this medical discipline is practiced. In order to avoid confusion the most popular general terms to define an institution that deals with pain are "pain treatment facility" or "pain clinic."

The more specific term "pain clinic" is currently used to define a center where ambulatory patients with chronic pain are examined and treated. In such centers, specialists (usually anesthesiologists) examine patients and provide consultation in order to determine appropriate use of antalgic therapies. A "modality-oriented clinic" is a facility that generally provides a specific type of therapy, such as transcutaneous electrical nerve stimulation (TENS), acupuncture, or biofeedback, in the absence of comprehensive assessment and management programs.

Major healthcare facilities or other clinics that have anesthesiologists competent in pain medicine are generally referred to as "centers for diagnosis and pain therapy". The term "center for antalgic therapy" suggests a unique and exclusive interest in outpatient pain therapy, especially if it includes the term "ambulatory." In contrast, the term "center for diagnosis and pain therapy" is used when the institution or clinic provides both diagnosis and treatment, generally for both inpatients and outpatients.

Nowadays, many centers add the term "palliative care" to emphasize that, in addition to the dealing with chronic pain conditions, there is also a specialized unit that focuses on care for patients in terminal conditions, such as cancer.

Within the international medical community, the term "pain clinic" may have different connotations. For some, it may connote the place where you relegate patients when other options have been exhausted, such as cancer patients suffering tremendous pain and for whom the classical treatments do not provide relief. However, for others, the pain clinic is a place where patients who have pain in spite of negative diagnostic tests can have recourse to further evaluation, care and understanding. Often, the staff of a pain clinic may not get the recognition that they deserve because of their ability to keep their patience and maintain optimism with patients whom their colleagues may have classified as "psychiatric cases".

Some centers have very strict admission policies, whereby admission is exclusively dependent on recommendation by a family doctor or on consultation by a specialist, accompanied by a formal application on with a physician's letterhead. In other centers patients are accepted also on the basis of self-referral and may be examined at their own request.

Nearly all centers provide accessibility to hospitalized patients as well as outpatients.

GROWTH OF PAIN MANAGEMENT CENTERS

In 1953, J. J. Bonica published a text on pain that soon became the international "bible" for those anesthesiologists with an interest in the diagnosis and treatment of pain [1]. Establishment of the first recognized pain center dates back to 1961, when Bonica opened a pain clinic at the University of Washington at Seattle. The following years in the United States have witnessed a spectacular growth of centers for the evaluation and therapy of pain. As an indication of the growth one only has to consider that there were only 17 pain clinics operating in the U.S. in 1976, which increased to 285 by 1979 and to more than 1,000 by 1986 [2]. These centers varied in size, number of the staff, and available budget [3], and while some were only used for in-patients, others only treated outpatients. Some centers consisted of a single specialist, usually an anesthesiologist (mono-disciplinary center), but other centers were able to provide a comprehensive program of collaborative research, diagnosis, and treatment (multidisciplinary centers).

In Europe, ambulatory antalgic therapy was initiated at the hospital level in the 1970's. However, this approach in the university setting goes back to the middle 1960's when anesthesiologists who visited Bonica's pain clinic learned about this new medical branch and took it back with them to their institutions.

Pain treatment centers went through a period of disorderly growth until it became clear that it was imperative to establish some structure and guidelines. The first step took place with the 1972 charter of the International Association for the Study of Pain (IASP). Under the guidance of J.J. Bonica, an association of worldwide dimensions was created where specialists from different countries and different branches (ranging from basic science to research and clinical practice) would be able to discuss and develop new strategies and solutions for fighting pain [4].

According to Bonica's proposal, there are only three basic requirements for instituting a well-functioning pain center [5]:

a) A passion for "pain medicine" among those establishing and working in the center.
b) Practical and clinical experience in the field and the desire to keep informed of new developments, approaches, and therapies for diagnosing and treating pain.
c) The ability to function as part of a group.

Europe certainly did not lag behind. The first IASP world congress took place in Florence in 1975, and the following year saw the founding of national chapters of IASP with the purpose of promoting the study and diffusion of pain therapy in various countries worldwide. However, for many years in Europe, the field of antalgic therapy was supported by the initiative of pioneers who often had to work individually, sustained mainly by their will and commitment [6-7-8].

In the absence of precise standards, the terms categorizing pain centers often did not show the real potential of the center. The facilities ranged from monodisciplinary centers, in which there was only a single physician in charge of pain therapy, to centers in which anesthesiologists, neurosurgeons, rehabilitators, psychiatrists, and psychologists worked in collaboration with nurses and other medical professionals (multidisciplinary centers). In monodisciplinary centers, a single type of therapy was generally practiced that was dependent on the capability and specialty of the physician running the center. The therapy was performed by anesthesiologists in their spare time, and although it was generally limited to nerve blocks, it could also have included TENS, acupuncture and other basic therapies.

In the North American setting, the terminology for these centers includes "pain clinic", "pain unit", and "pain center." These terms may refer to different types of clinical facilities that vary in the number of physicians committed to the program, the therapies used, the kind of pain treated, the internal organization, and inclusion of research and teaching in addition to diagnosis and treatment.

The terms interdisciplinary and multidisciplinary have not been used synonymously. A multidisciplinary center is a facility where patients are examined by a series of different specialists who suggest successive therapeutic regimens. In contrast, an interdisciplinary center does not provide a series of temporal therapies as in a multidisciplinary model, but offers an integrated approach to pain management where therapies interact and complement one another.

At present it is generally assumed that the best therapeutic results are obtained not by a series of therapies, but rather by an integrated protocol designed in collaboration with different specialists.

A "pain center" is always an interdisciplinary facility where a patient can be examined by specialists who work in collaboration and who exchange information with the purpose to obtaining the best therapeutic result.

APPROACHES TO TREATMENT

Pain centers can be characterized in terms of their basic approach to pain management which can be physiopathologic, psychiatric/psychological, or rehabilitative.

Centers using a physiopathologic approach rely on interventions that modify a physiopathologic process without delving into the complexity of the phenomenon of chronic pain. Hence, this approach focuses on control of peripheral nociceptive disorders and uses primarily nerve blocks for the treatment of acute pain, post-surgical pain, and some types of chronic pain.

Centers that focus on the psychiatric/psychological approach evaluate the pain as a physical manifestation related to a state of conflict or emotional stress. The pain patients are often treated with psychopharmacologic agents and/or psychotherapy. This approach is fairly specific, and by itself is not adequate for treating chronic pain [9-10].

Currently, the most widely accepted approach to treating chronic pain is rehabilitation. It is an integrative approach that takes into account medical-physiologic, physical, social, occupational, and economic factors.

Notably, the rehabilitative approach treats not only the patient in isolation but incorporates in the treatment also the family environment. The goals of rehabilitative therapy are to improve the functioning of the patients, reduce drug dependence, limit medical resource utilization, and return the patients to their "role" in their family, occupation, and society.

The year 1987 was important for the rehabilitative approach to antalgic therapy because during that year the Commission on Accreditation of Rehabilitation Facilities (CARF), established in 1966, devoted to accreditation of pain control facilities [11]. CARF currently evaluates and accredits rehabilitative facilities for both inpatients and outpatients in the U.S., Canada, Sweden, and France, and is expanding its role in Europe. However, no such accreditation program is available in Italy and therefore there are currently no precise regulations or criteria for inpatient or outpatient rehabilitative pain centers.

Since CARF guidelines are only applied to rehabilitative facilities, there is still some reluctance in the U.S. on behalf of family doctors to send the patients to a pain clinic because the level of professionalism and experience in an unaccredited pain clinic may not be known.

GUIDELINES OF IASP

The following guidelines [12] have been recommended by the IASP for pain clinic nomenclature:

a)   A modality-oriented clinic is one which "offers a specific type of treatment and does not provide comprehensive assessment or management." Examples include facilities that focus on use of TENS (transcutaneous electrical nerve stimulation), acupuncture, biofeedback, or nerve blocks. These kinds of centers do not offer a global, interdisciplinary approach that integrates techniques in the management of chronic pain, and do not provide diagnostic facilities.

b) A pain clinic is "facility focusing upon the diagnosis and management of patients with chronic pain." This kind of center can be specific for certain problems such as migraine, or for certain anatomic areas such as low back pain. The guidelines of IASP state that this term should not be used for those centers operated by a solo practitioner. Therefore, a pain clinic represents a facility in which, although there are different physicians and paramedical staff, they still do not offer a full interdisciplinary approach to diagnosis and treatment.

c) A multidisciplinary pain clinic is "a facility staffed by physicians of different specialties and other non-physician health care providers who specialize in the diagnosis and management of patients with chronic pain." Diagnostic and treatment facilities are available to both inpatients and outpatients. The main difference between a multidisciplinary pain clinic and a multidisciplinary pain center is that the former does not have provisions for teaching and research activities.

d) A multidisciplinary pain center is an organization that provides "health care professionals and basic scientists which includes research, teaching and patient care related to acute and chronic pain." The clinical programs must be supervised by a clinically trained director specializing in antalgic therapy with the cooperation of physicians, psychologists, nurses, physiotherapists, occupational therapists, social workers, and occupational consultants. These centers have intervention programs available for inpatients and outpatients. The patients are provided with integrated programs of evaluation, often performed in a single day, and personalized management programs tailored for specific needs. In the U.S. it is currently emphasized that the director of such a center be a physician specializing in pain medicine who is part of national or international associations for the study of pain and who actively attends meetings for this study and educational programs [13].

Not all pain cases represent complex clinical conditions requiring all of the diagnostic and therapeutic techniques available in a pain center. However, when a difficult and complex case does present itself, it is necessary that all the advanced integrative and multidisciplinary approaches be available as suggested by the IASP guidelines.

QUALITY CONTROL

With the increasing importance of pain management and the growth of pain clinics and centers comes the recognized need to establish and promote standards of care. Since pain medicine is a relatively young science, there is still little guidance by regulatory agencies on maintaining quality and performance standards in these centers. While some facilities are managed by experienced physicians and health care workers, others are run by personnel with little training in anesthesiology or pain management. Consequently, there is a wide range in quality of care. Similarly, differences exist in the types of clinics, with some providing very specific services for a limited range of pain pathologies (e.g. non-malignant pain), and others establishing multidisciplinary approaches to pain management that incorporate research and teaching in their programs.

In addition to pain centers that are part of universities or hospitals, private pain centers have also been established. However, many of these are not only unconnected with a hospital or teaching center, but may not even be based on sound medical principles. Often, these so-called "healing centers and institutes" are advertised in newspapers, on radio, and on television as self-proclaimed "experts" able to intervene in different pathologies. More and more frequently, medical associations have been warning the public and regulatory authorities that behind officious-sounding "well-being" or "wellness" institutes" are charlatans such as "prano-therapists" "massagists" or "estheticians" who call themselves healers and try to take advantage of people who may be desperately seeking pain relief, especially if not managed by more traditional therapies. As a result, many people including some within the medical profession, may understandably be suspicious of pain centers, and may not give credibility even to those legitimate institutes that provide a different approach to what may be commonly practiced.

CLINICAL GOALS OF A PAIN CENTER

Although the goals of some pain centers may depend upon the types of management programs they utilize and the types of pain that they treat, some goals are common to all centers:

- Providing medical and psychosocial evaluation of the patient prior to starting any treatment.
- Providing an interdisciplinary perspective from specialists of different medical branches who work together during diagnosis, therapy, and follow-up. These specialists do not send the patients through an endless round of consultations and tests, but rather the specialists meet and discuss each case and reach a consensus regarding therapeutic conduct.
- Personalizing the treatment based on the characteristics of the individual patient and problem.
- Obtaining good antalgic effect with minimum analgesic dosage.
- Helping the patient to improve their daily function and emotional state.
- Offering the possibility of a return to work and daily life.
- Offering the families a responsibility in home management of the patient.
- Providing services to both inpatients and outpatients.
- Including behavioral therapy (operant, respondent and classic conditioning) as part of a comprehensive program that can help modify the patient's behavior.
- Instituting a follow-up program in order to maintain and evaluate the results.
- Offering pharmacological or psychological intervention program to help control the anxiety and depression that accompanies pain.

Conclusions

Despite the recent growth of facilities dedicated to the management of pain, the successful future of pain centers depends on a series of factors. The most important one is the expansion of our present knowledge in the field of pain management and prevention, especially with regard to chronic pain syndromes. Family doctors need to be better trained to recognize chronic pain syndromes at an early stage and understand that the onset of these syndromes may result from inadequate or delayed pain management. Studies on patients treated in chronic pain programs show that they can attain significant improvement in their functional status and psychological state, as well as a reduction of disability and in the consumption of analgesic drugs [14].

It can be expected that the next few years will continue to witness growth in the number of ambulatory pain centers. It is especially important that in addition to an increase in number, there is an increase in quality. This quality can be expressed not only by providing global and interdisciplinary treatment, but also by presenting data demonstrating both short- and long-term outcomes [15-16].

Adequate and effective treatment of pain can result in reductions in post-operative recovery time, improvement in post-surgical results, reductions in the development of chronic pain, and improved patient function and quality of life. Therefore, a comprehensive and efficient approach to antalgic therapy for both acute and chronic pain, such as that provided by qualified pain centers, not only provides better patient outcomes, but also lowers the economic burden by reducing overall health resource utilization and increasing productivity [17].

References

[1]   Bonica JJ. The Management of Pain. Lea and Febiger, 1953.

[2]   Dickerson CC. Pain centers: a survey and analysis of past, present and future functioning. In: CD Tollison (Ed). Handbook of Chronic Pain Management. Williams Wilkins, Baltimore, 664-78.1989.

[3]   Bonica JJ. Organization and function of pain clinics. In: JJ Bonica (Ed.) Advances in Neurology, vol. 4. Raven Press, New York, 433-43. 1976.

[4]   Brena SF. Pain control facilities: roots, organization and function. In: SF Brena, SL Chapman (Eds) Chronic Pain, New York, Spectrum Pubblications, 11-20. 1983.

[5]   Bonica JJ, Benedetti C, Murphy TM. Function of pain clinics and pain centres. In: M. Swerdlow (Ed.) Relief of Intractable Pain. Elsevier, Amsterdam. 65-84. 1983.

[6]   Lipton. S. Currents views on the management of a pain relief centre. In: M Swerdlow. The Therapy of Pain. MTP Press Lancaster, 57-78. 1986.

[7]   Mushin WW, Swerdlow M, Lipton S. The pain centre, *Practitioner* 218, 439-443.1977.

[8]   Swerdlow M. The value of clinics for the relief of chronic pain. *Journal of Medical Ethics* 4, 117-126.1978.

[9]   Vasudevan SV, Linch NT. Pain centers organizationa and outcome. Rehabilitation Medicine-Adding Life to Years (special issue). *West J Med.* 154, 532-35.1991.

[10]   Tyrer SP. Psychology, Psychiatry and Chronic pain. Butterworth-Heinemann, Oxford, 1992.

[11]   Commission on Accreditation of Rehabilitation Facilities: standards manual for organization serving people with disabilities. Tucson, AZ.:author.

[12]   Pain Treatment Centers at a Crossroads. (Eds) MJM Cohen and JN Campbell. IASP Press. Progress in Pain Research and Management, Vol. 7, 1996.

[13]   Karjalainen K, Malmivaara A, van Tulder M, et al. Multidisciplinary biopsychosocial rehabilitation for subacute low back pain among working age adults. *Cochrane Database Syst Rev.* 2003; (2): CD002193.

[14]   Stieg RL. The cost effectivness of pain treatment: Who cares? *Clin J Pain.*6, 301-304.1990.

[15]   Wilder-Smith OH, Mohrle JJ, Dolin PJ, Martin NC. The management of chronic pain in Switzerland: a comparative survey of Swiss medical specialists treating chronic pain. Eur *J Pain.* 2001;5:285-98

[16]   Wulf H. Epidural analgesia in postoperative pain therapy. A review. *Anaesthesist.* 1998 47:501-10.

[17]   Thunberg KA, Hallberg LR. The need for organizational development in pain clinics: a case study. *Disabil Rehabil.* 2002 ;24:755-62

In: The Handbook of Chronic Pain
Editors: S. Kreitler, D. Beltrutti, et al., pp. 561-566

ISBN 978-1-60021-044-0
© 2007 Nova Science Publishers, Inc.

Chapter 30

Burnout and Other Problems of the Health Professional Treating Pain

S. Kreitler, D. Beltrutti, D. Niv and A. Lamberto

JOB BURNOUT: ITS NATURE AND MANIFESTATIONS

Job burnout is a common psychological syndrome that develops in response to chronic interpersonal stressors on the job. Its three major components are: (a) overwhelming exhaustion, (b) feelings of cynicism and detachment from the job, and (c) a sense of ineffectiveness and lack of accomplishment. Exhaustion refers to the individual's feelings of being overextended and depleted of one's emotional and physical resources. Cynicism refers to the negative, critical, excessively detached and impersonal response to various aspects of the job. Reduced efficacy refers to feelings of incompetence and a lack of achievement and productivity at work. The syndrome develops in stages, with exhaustion preceding the emergence of cynicism, until finally lowered efficacy and depressed self-esteem set in (Maslach and Goldberg, 1998). Although the onset is slow and may be covered up in the beginning, it cannot be overlooked when it gets to the point that one cares increasingly less about oneself, one's co-workers and the recipients of one's services. Yet, at least the exhaustion and the cynicism are as much a result of burnout as they are means of stopping the erosion by halting one's involvement in the work. When one stops giving of oneself and caring about what goes on on the job, the burnout process may be expected to grind to a halt. Finally, although an individual who suffers of burnout seems to be an inefficient and detached worker, it is to be noted that it is a problem promoted precisely by the opposite tendencies, that is, excessive devotion to work, and striving for the highest standards of excellence (Freudenberger, 1975).

In sum, burnout seems to be a frequent phenomenon, injurious both to the organization in which one works, because of the lowered efficiency on the job, and to the individual worker, because of the effects on mental and physical health it may have (Cooper and Payne, 1988).

BURNOUT IN THE HEALTH PROFESSIONS

The vulnerability of health professionals to burnout is by now a well-known phenomenon (Farber, 1983). It has been documented very often in regard to doctors and nurses in the different domains and in different countries (Chao-ping et al., 2003; Graham et al., 2002; Grassi and Magnani, 2000; LeBlanc et al., 2001; McManus et al., 2002; Peltzer et al., 2003). Some of the more obvious contributing factors are the following: pressures exerted by the suffering of the patients and their needs, the necessity to give and care for the patients, the responsibility involved in the work, the financial demands of the health services, the growing costs of medication and medical instrumentation, the desire and difficulties of matching what is needed with what is possible in patient treatment, the stress of trying to keep updated in view of the constantly increasing loads of potentially relevant information, keeping one's status both both in the communities of practitioners and of academics, not to mention the additional factors of professional competition, the risks of being sued and the long working hours.

There is however one factor in the health professions that seems to be particularly important in promoting burnout: the emotional involvement in the caretaking setup. Surprisingly, earlier research did not find much evidence to support this expectation. Rather, it showed that client-related stressors, such as treating chronically ill or terminal patients, correlated less with burnout than common job-related stressors, such as workload or time pressure. However, the conclusions changed when more recent studies focused explicitly on the role of emotions in the job, such as emotional requirements to display emotions, to react to emotions or to be empathetic. The contribution of such factors to burnout over and beyond job-related stressor became evident.

PAIN THERAPISTS AND BURNOUT

As workers providing human services and as health professionals it is obvious that individuals who deal with treating pain patients would be at special risk to suffer of burnout. But it seems to us that burnout is not the only risk or danger threatening pain therapists. It is our objective to highlight specific difficulties inherent in treating pain patients. Discussing these difficulties may render pain therapists less vulnerable to burnout and moreoverbeyond that, perhaps help them able to turn the difficulties into means for improving their professional achievements as well as their own well-being.

SPECIAL DIFFICULTIES OF BEING A PAIN THERAPIST

Empathy and Compassion

A major difficulty which constitutes a serious overload factor is empathy. Empathy is the ability to imagine oneself in the position of another person, feeling that person's feelings, be they positive or negative. It consists not merely in reacting to the other's feelings but actually experiencing those feelings as if they were evoked in oneself. This ability was shown to play an important role in the domain of esthetic experiences, ethical moral responses, and above all in therapeutic endeavors of caring for others – in the capacity of a doctor, a psychologist, a nurse or a social worker. In the specific field of pain therapy, it is evident that empathy is evoked and re-evoked continuously as an integral component of the therapeutic process. This in itself would count as risk factor for emotional exhaustion.

Over and beyond empathy as such, a more specific problem has recently been identified, which is of particular relevance for pain therapists. It has been called "compassion fatigue" and is particularly prevalent in professionals who work with suffering people (Huggard, 2003). It differs from burnout and should not be confused with it. It is described as a state of tension and preoccupation with the suffering clients, persistent excessive arousal, overreacting to suffering of the other, and a tendency to re-experience the suffering to which one has been exposed. Notably, some of the manifestations of compassion fatigue resemble critical incident stress or secondary post-traumatic stress, for example, avoidance of reminders of the stimuli of suffering. Compassion fatigue emerges as a likely outcome of caring too much or too often for the other human being in pain.

Compassion fatigue may be evoked in any one of the health professions, but it is to be expected particularly in the context of pain therapy because of the specific affinity of pain with suffering. Pain is not just one more symptom in a very long array of physical and psychophysical symptoms that patients present. It is perhaps more than other symptoms representative of suffering. As such it is more likely to evoke empathy, caring, and compassion in the health professionals in attendance.

A most recent study sheds light on the origins of compassion fatigue, at least in pain therapists (Singer et al., 2004). The study was designed to examine whether any parts of the physiological process involved in reacting to a painful stimulus occur also in another person who is not experiencing any painful stimulus but merely empathizing with someone who is. The first stage consisted in delivering a painful electric shock to the hands of 16 women and tracing the reactions in their brain by functional magnetic resonance imaging (fMRI). The results showed that there was activationthe brains were activated in several areas, including both sensory and emotional regions. in their brainsin the brains of the women . In the next stage they delivered an electric shock to the hands of each woman's partner. The women were allowed to see the administration of the shock but not the faces of their partners, so as to prevent reactions to the sight of their suffering friend. The fMRI showed that the women's brains were activated in exactly the same emotional areas as when their own hand was being hurt. Hence, when we watch someone in pain, we react emotionally exactly as if the pain occurred to us, in our own bodies. The important implication is that empathy for pain is not merely an "as if" reaction but an actual pain experience, with all the actual affective trimmings that accompany it. Further, the brain activation and the evoked emotion were stronger in those with a stronger emotional bond. It is likely, that this enhancing factor exists most often in the case of pain therapists taking care of a patient, especially one with whom they are familiar.

Anger, Frustration and Other Emotions

Pain therapists face further fairly unique challenges in their work. Emotions other than empathy may often be involved in the treatment of a pain patient. Treating chronic pain entails being in contact with the patient for a fairly long period of time. This makes for a closer bond between the therapist and the patient. The formal objective of the relationship, accepted by both parties, is to overcome the pain. This however is not always possible. Indeed, it is mostly impossible, at least not right away, that is, not as fast as both parties would like it to happen. The result may be frustration as well as anger on the part of both therapist and patient. It is likely that these emotions will be evoked in the first phases of the treatment, if the patient's expectations of combating the pain completely are not met. Many patients are even frustrated by the realization that analgesics mostly just reduce the pain but do not make it disappear completely. Yet, these emotions are even more likely in late phases of the treatment, when both parties realize that the pain behaves as if it iswere here to stay and that its removal would not be as easy as desired.

On top of this potentially stressful framework, pain therapist and chronic pain patient may get into the throes of what has been called "the pain game". This "game" consists in the patient's assuming a challenging attitude toward the pain therapist: "Here I am suffering of my pain for over X years, and I have been treated by a Z number of pain experts, some of them really big shots in the field. Now, let's see, doctor, how you are getting on top of my pain problem, I can hardly wait and see who is going to come out of this battle with an upper hand – you or my pain!?" This or a similar structuring of the situation is not making things emotionally easier for either party.

Patient-Related Difficulties

The difficulties called here "patient-related" have to do partly with medical aspects and partly with psychological features of the chronic pain patient. Pain may be medically a difficult problem to resolve, regardless of whether the organic damage is or is not identified. In many cases there is additional co-morbidity which may complicate the situation both directly and indirectly insofar as it limits the range of medication or other treatments that may be applied. In chronic pain patients the situation is often further complicated by psychological factors, such as depression, and personality disorders of the patient that even if they have preceded the pain problem they are liable to be exacerbated by it. This renders prolonged contact with the patient even more difficult. In addition to these psychological problems, there are often social, economic and legal-forensic issues concerning the pain patient that pain therapists need to take notice of, handle, and react to.

Circumstantial Difficulties

Only two of the diverse "circumstantial" problems will be noted here. The first has to do with team work. In pain therapy more than (and probably, sooner than) in any other medical domain the necessity of team work between different professions has been recognized and implemented. This includes not only the physician and nurse, as in many other medical domains, but also the psychologist, the art therapist, the social worker and other professionals who may contribute to the patient's well-being. Interdisciplinary cooperation is undoubtedly a blessing, but it takes a lot to make it work properly so that all involved professionals feel that they can contribute their best and not pay an undue price in stress.

Another circumstantial problem may have to do with the overall status of pain therapy within the context of medicine proper. Pain has only fairly recently been recognized as a disease in itself rather than an accompaniment of other medical disorders. Accordingly, pain therapy has only belatedly been recognized as a medical discipline in its own right. Yet, on the fringes there persists a certain unclarity concerning the status of pain therapy as a curative or palliative field, especially since in the domain of pain, palliation is considered as an integral component of the therapeutic procedure. Unclarities of this type are important insofar as palliation is unfortunately still all too often accorded a lower status than the curative disciplines.

What Can Be Done to Cure or Palliate the Described Ailments?

The therapeutic means for the difficulties of pain treatment are to be applied on the individual level and on the organizational one. The means at the disposal of the individual are too well known to deserve a detailed presentation. They include relaxation, vacation, variation at work, recognizing one's limits, setting realistic goals, taking care of oneself, learning proper communication skills, and so on. Research has shown that organizational changes are often more useful than individual means for combating burnout (Maslach et al., 2001). Be it as it may, it is unlikely that the health services would be changed mainly in order to help pain therapists.

There may however be some clues embedded within the pain therapy situation itself that may be helpful. The first is the team of health professionals engaged in pain therapy. This team itself may serve as the tool for helping pain therapists themselves to cope with the complexities of the situation by acting as co-therapists for each other. The other is the recognition of pain therapists that they may be the pioneers of the new medicine both in regard to the team work between the different health professionals and in regard to incorporating palliation into the very fabric of curative medicine. The paradigm being laboriously forged in the pain clinics of nowadays may well be the common structure that will characterize the medicine of tomorrow.

REFERENCES

Chao-ping, L., Kan, S., and Zheng-xue, L. (2003). An investigation of job burnout of doctor and nurse. *Chinese Journal of Clinical Psychology, 11,* 170-172.

Cooper, C. L., and Payne, R. (Eds.) (1988). Causes, coping and consequences of stress at work. Chichester, UK: Wiley.

Farber, B. A. (Ed.) (1983). Stress and burnout in the human service professions. New York: Pergamon Press.

Freudenberger, H.J. (1975). The staff burnout syndrome in alternative institutions. *Psychotherapy: Theory, Research, Practice, 12,* 72-83.

Graham, J., Potts, H. W. W., and Ramirez, A. J. (2002). Stress and burnout in doctors. *Lancet, 360,* 1975-1976.

Grassi, L., *Psychosomatics, 69*and Magnani, K. (2000). Psychiatric morbidity and burnout in the medical profession: An Italian studyof geneal practioners and hospital physicians. *Psychotherapy and Psychosomatics, 69,* 329-334.

Huggard, P. (2003). Compassion fatigue: How much can I give? *Medical Education, 37,* 163-164.

Le Blanc, P. M., Bakker, A. B., Peeters, M. C. W., van Heesch, N. C. A., and Schaufeli, W. B. (2001). Emotional job demands and burnout among oncology care provides. *Anxiety, Stress and Coping, 14,* 243-263.

Maslach, C. (1982). *Burnout: The cost of caring.* Englewood Cliffs, NJ: Prentice-Hall.

Maslach, C., and Goldberg, J. (1998). Prevention of burnout: new perspectives. *Applied and Preventive Prey. Psychology, 7,* 63-74.

Maslach, C., Schaufeli, W.B., and Leiter, M.P. (2001) Job burnout. *Annual Review of Psychology, 52,* 397-422.

McManus, I. C., Winder, B. C., and Gordon, D. (2002). The causal links between stress adn and burnout in a longitudinal study of UK doctors. *Lancet, 359,* 2089-2090.

Peltzer, K., Mashego, T.-A., and Mabeba, M.(2003). Occupational stress adn and burnout among South African medical practitioners. *Stress and Health, 19,* 275-280.

Singer, T. et al. (2004). Empathy for pain involves the affective but not sensory components of pain. *Science, 303,* 1157-1162.

Zapf, D., Seifert, C., Schmutte, B., and Mertini, H. (2001). Emotion work and job stressors and their effects on burnout. *Psychology and Health, 16,* 527-546.

Index

B

D

E

H

I

J

K

L

M

manipulation, 209, 256, 413, 415
mapping, 350
market, 518, 519
marriage, 103, 107
masking, 452, 474
mass, 230, 255, 383, 390, 534
masseter, 419, 442, 526
mast cells, 35, 186
mastectomy, 239
mastery, 364
mastoid, 283, 527
matrix, 311
meals, 146, 380, 425, 454
meanings, 97, 108, 116, 163, 175, 307, 317, 535
measurement, 58, 97, 127, 151, 164, 331, 419, 442,
    448, 468
measures, 13, 14, 18, 79, 81, 85, 86, 89, 104, 118,
    122, 148, 165, 170, 172, 173, 174, 179, 210, 223,
    262, 325, 326, 327, 334, 337, 342, 344, 347, 352,
    368, 387, 410, 412, 430, 433, 501, 538, 539
meat, 426
media, 309, 311
median, 49, 70, 168, 222, 256, 261, 270, 278, 279,
    287, 470, 472
mediastinum, 284
mediation, 20, 132, 203, 487
medication, 66, 67, 74, 80, 85, 86, 87, 88, 91, 92,
    109, 110, 151, 170, 172, 173, 190, 192, 193, 196,
    198, 241, 266, 299, 311, 323, 324, 325, 326, 327,
    328, 329, 332, 339, 345, 368, 369, 371, 372, 401,
    424, 455, 462, 519, 530, 562, 564
Mediterranean, 521
medulla, 12, 19, 192, 200, 386
medulla oblongata, 386
MEG, 14, 15, 350
melanoma, 280, 396
melatonin, 415, 455
melting, 409
melts, 302
membership, 141
membranes, 187, 189, 445
memory, 10, 14, 15, 65, 317, 456, 515, 535
men, 58, 116, 117, 121, 126, 174, 177, 472, 485,
    489, 490, 495
menarche, 139
menopause, 447
menstruation, 403, 424
mental disorder, 19, 49, 55, 162, 459
mental health, 79, 98, 120, 168, 435, 497
mental illness, 177

mental processes, 327
mental state, 380
mesons, 275
messages, 61, 62, 63, 303, 306, 380
messenger RNA, 62
messengers, 7, 139
metabolic acidosis, 392
metabolic pathways, 439
metabolism, 439, 515, 521
metabolites, 389, 409, 507
metal salts, 384
metaphor, 546
metastasis, 278, 281, 385, 389, 394, 416, 542
metastatic cancer, 82, 158, 231, 247, 277, 282, 542,
    547, 550
metastatic disease, 80, 278, 282, 283, 533
metastatic lung cancer, 284
methodology, 270, 344
methylprednisolone, 193
Mg^{2+}, 9
Miami, 97
mice, 22, 27, 28, 29, 30, 35, 37, 38, 39, 186, 202,
    203, 205, 430
microcirculation, 258, 259, 270
microscopy, 258
microspheres, 198
midbrain, 12, 13
migraine headache, 58, 159, 194, 321, 343, 348, 350,
    351, 352, 402, 460, 461, 462, 464
migraines, 435, 442
migrainous neuralgia, 243, 453
migration, 267
milligrams, 428
Millon Clinical Multiaxial Inventory, 129, 177
minority, 118, 231, 523
misconceptions, 367
misunderstanding, 111
mixing, 317
mobility, 69, 78, 79, 80, 81, 160, 167, 258, 362, 363,
    387
mode, 302, 305, 306, 308, 310, 312, 313, 314, 442,
    540
modeling, 102, 313, 349
models, 102, 106, 108, 109, 111, 186, 187, 190, 191,
    192, 194, 202, 204, 264, 311, 361, 364, 368, 373,
    376, 403, 459, 476, 486, 487, 515, 516
moderators, 355
modern society, 405
moisture, 393
molecules, 10, 33, 38, 204, 383

N

O

P

Q

R

T

U

V